PAIN MANAGEMENT – CURRENT ISSUES AND OPINIONS

Edited by **Gabor B. Racz** and **Carl E. Noe**

Pain Management – Current Issues and Opinions
Edited by Gabor B. Racz and Carl E. Noe

Published by InTech
Janeza Trdine 9, 51000 Rijeka, Croatia

Publishing Process Manager Ivana Zec

Technical Editor Teodora Smiljanic

Cover Designer InTech Design Team

Additional hard copies can be obtained from orders@intechopen.com

Pain Management – Current Issues and Opinions,
Edited by Gabor B. Racz and Carl E. Noe
p. cm.
ISBN 978-953-307-813-7

For EU product safety concerns:
IN TECH d.o.o., Prolaz Marije Krucifikse Kozulić 3, 51000 Rijeka, Croatia,
info@intechopen.com or visit our website at intechopen.com.

Meet the editors

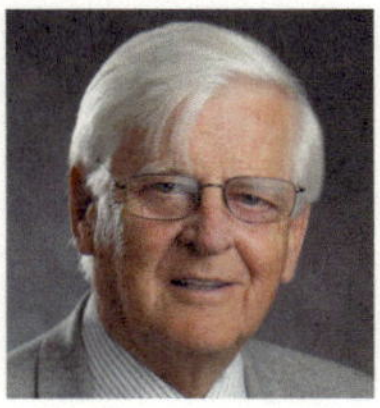

Professor Dr Gabor B. Racz is a Grover Murray professor and Chairman Emeritus of the Department of Anesthesiology at Texas Tech University Health Science Center in Lubbock Texas, USA. He is a founder of the International Pain Institute at Texas Tech, the World Institute of Pain, and the Texas Pain Society. He is an international leader in the field of pain.

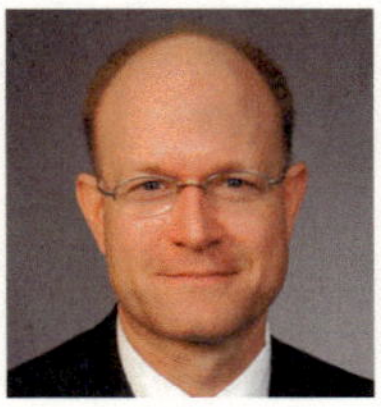

Professor Dr Carl E. Noe trained under Dr Racz, and he is a professor of Anesthesiology and Pain Management at the University of Texas Southwestern Medical Center in Dallas, Texas. He is the Medical Director of the Eugene McDermott Center for Pain Management, Division Director, Medical Director of the Parkland Memorial Hospital Pain Clinic, and Director of the Pain Fellowship Program.

Contents

Preface

Recently, the Institute of Medicine in the United States assembled a panel to look at the issue of pain and its treatment. The comprehensive report has outlined that there is a great deal of suffering, and an excessive amount of money is being spent on many ineffective treatments for treating pain, and the associated costs with the disability that is the consequence of poorly-treated pain is even more staggering.

Despite this, significant gains have indeed been achieved over the past 20 years in the treatment of pain by interventional pain and other pain specialists. The evidence is accumulating, and the etiologies of painful conditions are also better understood.

Policy makers need to include input from physicians recognized in interventional pain training and experience, as well as other practicing physicians, in order to avoid excluding data from studies regarding one camp of pain practitioners which may be unknown to another camp of practitioners. Interventional pain management should not be isolated from interdisciplinary and pharmacological pain management camps, and the field should evolve to a point where patients are evaluated and treated using the best of all worlds.

The reader must always be careful and maintain personal selectiveness for incorporating those areas that are indeed in the best interest of the patient that suffers from pain. The material contained within this book has been assembled more for quality rather than completeness. One may wish to have other and different areas covered, but there is only so much that can be accomplished in a limited amount of time and space. There is a significant amount covered in the various parts on opioids which must be looked at, as treatment of pain in many parts of the world is heavily opioid dependent.

It is interesting to note that in the United States over the last couple of years, the mortality rate from prescribed opioids has exceeded that for motor vehicle-induced mortality. When opioids are used, the nature of the medication is such that it is subject to diversion and abuse. Disciplining patients should not be the responsibility of the physician, but verifying the use interestingly helps to maintain the appropriate use. For example, urine tests two to six times per year, qualitative and quantitative is followed by a one-third reduction in the inappropriate use of the medication. Physicians need to look at whatever is in the best interest of the patient, and clearly the unintended overuse is not.

Dr Noe and myself go back for many years in the arena of interventional pain evaluation, research, teaching, and treatment.The clear recognition is that we could not have fulfilled the rolls that one has to fulfill without the complete devotion to our partners, Laura, Dr Noe's devoted wife, and Enid, my beautiful wife of 50 years this year. After a very brief discussion between my friend, Dr Carl Noe, and myself, we felt that the most appropriate way for us to express our gratitude is by dedicating this book to them.

We hope that the readers will find information that will make them think and improve their outlook on a fair and balanced vision of pain and its treatment, regardless of which branch of medicine they practice.

The purpose of this project is to bring the best minds together from around the world quickly and on an ongoing basis to make a world with less pain, hence the title *Painless*. The electronic format will leverage technology to allow for rapid additions of new material and updates of this initial presentation. We look forward to this global conversation with you.

Gabor B. Racz, MD, FIPP, ABIPP
Grover E. Murray Professor
Professor and Chairman Emeritus
Texas Tech University Health Sciences Center
USA

Part 1

Pain Science

1

Intrathecal Studies on Animal Pain Models

Jen-Kun Cheng
Mackay Memorial Hospital/Mackay Medical College
Taiwan

1. Introduction

Spinal and epidural anesthesia have been widely used in clinical settings for the management of peri-operative, neuropathic and cancer pain (Dureja et al., 2010; Hong, 2010; Mercadante, 1999). They provide another route for the analgesic administration in addition to oral or systemic absorption. Since the pain pathway initiate with primary and secondary neurons located in dorsal root ganglion and spinal cord, respectively, the ***intrathecal*** (spinal) route may provide an effective alternative for less drug dosage and fewer side effects, compared with systemic administration.

In recent decades, many animal pain models have been developed to explore the possible mechanisms involved in the pathogenesis of clinically relevant pain statuses, such as postoperative (Brennan et al., 1996), neuropathic (Kim & Chung, 1992), inflammatory (Wheeler-Aceto et al., 1990) and cancer pain (Clohisy & Mantyh, 2003). These studies not only help to extent our understanding on pain mechanisms but also provide novel promising agents or targets for the management of different pain situations (Mogil et al., 2010). In this chapter, we present various animal pain models, emphasizing on *intrathecal* studies, and potential therapeutic molecular targets and analgesics found in latest years. In addition, the related neurotoxicity studies and morphine-induced tolerance will be mentioned.

2. Intrathecal animal pain studies

The first mentioned *intrathecal* study using rat animal model was reported by Yaksh, beginning with the study of *intrathecal* morphine (Yaksh et al., 1977). For *intrathecal* drug administration, a polyethylene catheter is inserted *intrathecally* in rats during inhalation anesthesia (LoPachin et al., 1981). The catheter is passed caudally from the cisterna magnum to the level of lumbar enlargement. Since the development of *intrathecal* catheterization, lots of studies explored the pharmacology and pain pathways using *intrathecal* space as a route of drug administration, either in basic researches or clinical studies. The *intrathecal* studies on various pain models provide a lot of promising analgesics for the management of different pain statuses.

2.1 Postoperative pain model

The postoperative or incisional pain model was proposed by Brennan in 1996 (Brennan et al., 1996). A 1-cm longitudinal incision is made through skin, fascia and muscle of the plantar aspect of the hindpaw in anesthetized rats. The lesion produced reliable and quantifiable mechanical allodynia and thermal hyperalgesia around the wound and spontaneous nociceptive behaviors for about one week, which mimics the clinical course of postoperative pain. Selective denervations of the rat hindpaw prior to foot incision reveal both the sural and tibial nerves are responsible for the nociception transmission from the incision. This model helps to better understand mechanisms of sensitization caused by surgery and provide promising therapeutics for postoperative pain management (Kang & Brennan, 2009).

2.2 Inflammatory formalin pain model

The formalin test involves subcutaneous injection of 5% formaldehyde (50 μl) at the plantar surface of the rat hindpaw, using a 27-gauge needle. After injection, the rat displays characteristic nociceptive behaviors, flinching, shaking, biting and licking of the injected paw. Two phases of nociceptive behaviors are observed after formalin injection as described previously (Abbott et al., 1995). Phase 1 is initiated within seconds after injection and it lasts for about 5–10min. After several minutes quiescent, a second phase of flinching occurs and peaks at 25–35 min after injection.

The formalin-induced nociceptive response in rats is believed to be an inflammatory pain and involves central sensitization in the spinal cord (Abbott et al., 1995). The hindpaw injection of formalin induces tissue injury leading to acute (phase 1) and facilitated (phase 2) states of pain. The phase 2 response is believed to be a persistent input-induced nociceptive behavior mediated through central sensitization (Coderre & Melzack, 1992). LTP of C-fiber-evoked field potentials in the spinal superficial dorsal horn has been reported in the formalin-injected rats (Sandkuhler & Liu, 1998). *Intrathecal* injection of T-type Ca^{2+} channel blockers (mibefradil and Ni^{2+}) has been reported to attenuate formalin-induced pain behaviours, either phase 1 or 2, indicating the important role of T-type Ca^{2+} channel in the spinal central sensitization (Cheng et al., 2007). Other chemical irritants, such as complete Freund's adjuvant (CFA), carrageenan or capsaicin, could also be used to be injected subcutaneously into the plantar surface of rat hindpaw to induce pain behaviors (Duarte et al., 2011; Thorpe et al., 2011; Yu et al., 2011).

2.3 Nerve injury-induced neuropathic pain model

Nerve injuries due to trauma, chemotherapy, diabetic mellitus or tumor invasion may induce neuropathic pain, which is usually refractory to conventional analgesic agents, including opioids and non-steroid anti-inflammatory agents. For the past decades, several animal models have been developed to mimic the clinical conditions and explore the possible mechanisms underlying neuropathic pain. Among these neuropathic pain models, nerve injury-induced neuropathic pain (NINP) models, such as spinal nerve ligation, spared nerve injury and chronic constriction injury, are most often studied (Ji & Strichartz, 2004).

Several targets have been proposed to be involved in the pathogenesis of NINP, such as NMDA receptors (Szekely et al., 2002) and ion channels (Rogers et al., 2006). Recently, new molecules have been emerging as promising targets for the treatment of NINP, such as purinergic receptors (Donnelly-Roberts et al., 2008), cannabinoid receptors (Lynch & Campbell, 2011), transient receptor potential V1 (TRPV1) receptor (Facer et al., 2007), chemokine receptors (White et al., 2007), acid-sensing ion channel (Mazzuca et al., 2007; Poirot et al., 2006), annexin 2 light chain p11 (Foulkes et al., 2006) and matrix metalloproteinase (Kawasaki et al., 2008a).

The L5/6 spinal nerve ligation neuropathic pain model was reported by Kim and Chung in 1992 (Kim & Chung, 1992). This model involves a tight ligation of L5 and L6 spinal nerves of animals under anesthesia. The nociceptive behavioral assessments also consist of von Frey hair test (Chaplan et al., 1994) and radiant heat test (Hargreaves et al., 1988) for the quantification of mechanical allodynia and thermal hyperalgesia, respectively, on the affected hindpaw. Compared with postoperative pain model and formalin inflammatory pain model, this model induced chronic nociceptive behaviors lasting for several weeks. This chronic pain model helps to reveal the possible mechanisms involved in the development and maintenance of nerve injury-induced pain, either the neuronal components or glial components.

Spared nerve injury pain model was developed by Decosterd and Woolf in 2000 (Decosterd & Woolf, 2000). An adaptation of spared nerve injury surgery was later developed in the mouse (Bourquin et al., 2006). This model involves a lesion of two of the three terminal branches of the sciatic nerve (tibial and common peroneal nerves) leaving the remaining sural nerve intact. The spared nerve injury model differs from the L5/6 spinal ligation pain model in that the co-mingling of distal intact axons with degenerating axons is restricted, and it permits behavioral testing of the non-injured skin territories adjacent to the denervated areas. The mechanical (von Frey and pinprick) sensitivity and thermal (hot and cold) responsiveness is increased in the ipsilateral sural territory.

2.4 Cancer pain model

Cancer pain significantly affects the diagnosis, quality of life and survival of patients with cancer. Tumor growth may produce inflammation in tumor bearing tissues, which will release inflammatory mediators to stimulate nociceptors. Tumor growth may also compress the peripheral nerves in tumor bearing tissues, inducing nerve injury. Therefore, cancer pain is likely to share mechanisms of inflammatory pain and neuropathic pain, although this pain may have distinct mechanisms (Ghilardi et al., 2010). Whether inflammation or nerve injury dominates during tumor growth may depend on the interactions between tumor cells and surrounding tissues (Cain et al., 2001).

In recent years, several laboratories have developed cancer pain models by inoculation of tumor cells into a hindpaw of mouse (Constantin et al., 2008). Animals inoculated with melanoma cells into the plantar of the hindpaw show marked pain hypersensitivity and peripheral nerve degeneration (Gao et al., 2009a). We have used this melanoma cancer pain model to test the anti-tumor growth and analgesic effects of JNK inhibitor (Gao et al., 2009a). Other cancer pain models include breast, prostate and bone cancer pain models (Bloom et al., 2011; Ghilardi et al., 2010; Jimenez-Andrade et al., 2010). These cancer pain models may possess different pathophysiologies for pain induction. For example, intramedullary injection of breast cancer cells could induce periosteal sprouting of CGRP(+) sensory fibers and pain, both of which could be blocked by anti-nerve growth factor (NGF) (Bloom et al., 2011). Inhibitor of NGF receptor TrkA has been shown to attenuate bone cancer pain and tumor-induced sprouting of sensory nerve fibers (Ghilardi et al., 2010). Similarly, NGF also plays an important role in the induction of prostate cancer-induced sensory fiber sprouting and bone pain (Jimenez-Andrade et al., 2010).

3. Potential therapeutic molecular targets for pain management

Voltage-gated ion channels and glial cells have all been found to be promising therapeutic targets for pain management. Voltage-gated ion channels are a class of transmembrane ion channels that are activated by changes in membrane potential; these types of ion channels are especially critical in excitable cells, including neuronal, cardiac and skeletal cells (Szu-Yu Ho & Rasband, 2011), or even cancer cell migration (Cuddapah & Sontheimer, 2011). Since voltage-gated ion channels are important for neuronal excitability, conduction and transmission, they have long been the targets of interest in the field of pain research.

3.1 Voltage-gated Na^+ channels

Voltage-gated Na^+ channels are essential for the initiation of action potentials which are crucial for nerve conduction. Their activation and inactivation are strongly gated by the membrane potential of neuronal cells, but their properties can also be modulated by G-proteins or protein kinases (Kakimura et al., 2010). Voltage-gated Na^+ channels are constituted by the pore-forming α−subunit and auxiliary β-subunits. Up to now, nine α−subunits (Nav1.1-1.9) and four β-subunits (β1-4) have been identified (Catterall et al., 2005). The Na^+ channels can be either sensitive (Nav1.1, Nav1.2, Nav1.3, Nav1.6) or resistant (Nav1.4, Nav1.5, Nav1.7, Nav1.8, Nav1.9) to tetrodotoxin (TTX), a toxin found in the liver of puffer fish. Neuronal cells contain most of the Na^+ channel subtypes but Nav1.4 and Nav1.5, respectively, are mainly in skeletal and cardiac muscles (Jarecki et al., 2010). Nav1.1, Nav1.3, Nav1.6, Nav1.7, Nav1.8 and Nav1.9 have been found in adult dorsal root ganglion (DRG) sensory neurons and these isoforms can be important for the firing properties of sensory neurons (Hunanyan et al., 2011). After spared nerve injury in rats, altered neuronal electrogenesis in DRG neurons, such as accelerated re-priming of TTX-sensitive Na^+ currents, was observed and may be due to a complex regulation of voltage-gated Na^+ channels (Berta et al., 2008; Wang et al., 2011).

Several lines of evidence indicate that Nav1.7, and Nav1.8 are involved in pain regulation, especially NINP (Lampert et al., 2010). Nav1.7 and Nav1.8 channels have been shown to accumulate in neuroma endings in humans with neuropathic pain (Kretschmer et al., 2002). This accumulation may be due to a loss of myelin inhibition or target determined transfer of Na^+ channels (Aurilio et al., 2008). Loss of Nav1.7 function may lead to complete insensitivity to pain in humans (Cox et al., 2010). Compounds possessing Nav1.7 blocking effects have been reported to reverse nerve injury-induced mechanical allodynia (Tyagarajan et al., 2010). Nav1.8 is increased in sciatic nerve after nerve injury and *intrathecal* antisense oligoneucleotide directed against Nav1.8 is effective in neuropathic pain models (Joshi et al., 2006). A μΩ-conotoxin MrVIB was found to be a preferential Nav1.8 blocker and could reverse partial sciatic nerve ligation-induced mechanical allodynia and thermal hyperalgesia, when given *intrathecally* (Ekberg et al., 2006). Intraperitoneal administration of A-803467, a selective Nav1.8 blocker, has been reported to attenuate nerve injury-induced mechanical allodynia (Jarvis et al., 2007). Nonetheless, Nassar et al. found that mice lacking Nav1.7 and Nav1.8 still develop neuropathic pain after spinal nerve ligation (Nassar et al., 2005). Recent studies also revealed a role of Nav1.3 (Mo et al., 2011) and Nav1.9 (Leo et al., 2010) in the development of neuropathic pain. For normal nerve conduction, Nav1.1 family is involved (Catterall et al., 2010). Therefore, the selective Nav1.3, Nav1.7, Nav1.8 and Nav1.9 channel blockers will have clinical potential in the treatment of neuropathic pain since they do not affect normal neuronal conduction.

Besides the pore-forming α-subunit, β2 subunit was reported to be up-regulated in injured and non-injured sensory neurons after peripheral nerve injuries (Pertin et al., 2005) and the development of spared nerve injury-induced mechanical allodynia is attenuated in β2-null mice (Lopez-Santiago et al., 2006), suggesting the important role of β2 subunit in NINP. The involvement of Na^+ channel β2 subunit in neuropathic and inflammatory pain has been extensively reviewed (Brackenbury & Isom, 2008).

In addition to changes in protein expression, phosphorylation-induce change of conductance or gating property of Na^+ channels may also lead to enhanced neuronal excitability and NINP (Aurilio et al., 2008). The activation of presynaptic delta-opioid receptor by enkephalin has been reported to prevent the increase in neuronal $Na_V1.7$ in DRG through inhibition of PKC and p38 (Chattopadhyay et al., 2008). Tumor necrosis factor-α (TNF-α), a pro-inflammatory cytokine involved in NINP formation (Schafers et al., 2003), was found to enhance TTX-resistant Na^+ currents in isolated DRG neurons *via* a TNF receptor 1- and p38-dependent mechanism (Jin & Gereau, 2006). The Na^+ currents of isolated sensory neurons can be enhanced by protein kinase A and protein kinase C (Gold et al., 1998; Mo et al., 2011), both of which are involved in NINP (Gao et al., 2005; Song et al., 2006). Phosphorylation of TTX-S and TTX-R sodium channels involving both serine/threonine and tyrosine sites has been reported to contribute to painful diabetic neuropathy (Hong et al., 2004). Further studies are required to reveal the exact role of Na^+ channel phosphorylation in the pathogenesis of NINP.

3.2 Voltage-gated Ca^{2+} channels

Voltage-gated Ca^{2+} channels are involved in neuron excitability, neurotransmitter release, synaptic transmission and gene expression (Dolmetsch et al., 2001). Ca^{2+} channels are constituted by the pore-forming α-subunit and auxiliary subunits, β- and α2δ□subunits. They are classified into Cav1, Cav2 and Cav3 families based on their structure homology, but are categorized as L- (Cav1.1, Cav1.2 and Cav1.3), P/Q- (Cav2.1), N- (Cav2.2), R- (Cav2.3), and T- (Cav3.1, Cav3.2 and Cav3.3) type based on their sensitivity to specific blockers, activation/inactivation characteristics and current conductance (Catterall et al., 2002). Various Ca^{2+} channel blockers have been tested in the postoperative, inflammatory and neuropathic pain models (Cheng et al., 2007). The potential use of Ca^{2+} channel blockers for neuropathic pain treatment and roles of Ca^{2+} channels in ascending pain pathway have been well reviewed (Yaksh, 2006; Zamponi et al., 2009).

3.2.1 N-type Ca^{2+} channels

N-type Ca^{2+} channels are distributed in the dorsal root ganglia and spinal dorsal horn. It is generally believed that N-type Ca^{2+} channels are involved in the neurotransmitter release of spinal dorsal horn (Smith et al., 2002). Substance P, one of the neurotransmitter of primary sensory neurons, has been found to be mostly co-localized with N-type Ca^{2+} channels in the spinal dorsal horn (Westenbroek et al., 1998).

Several lines of evidence indicate that N-type Ca^{2+} channels play an important role in NINP. Mice lacking N-type Ca^{2+} channels exhibit reduced signs of neuropathic pain after spinal nerve ligation (Saegusa et al., 2001). *Intrathecal* small interference RNA knockdown of N-type Ca^{2+} channels reversed sciatic nerve constriction-induced tactile allodynia and thermal hyperalgesia (Altier et al., 2007).

New non-peptide compounds with N-type Ca^{2+} channel blocking property have been recently developed in pharmaceutical companies for the treatment of neuropathic pain (Knutsen et al., 2007). A highly reversible ω-conotoxin FVIA, a potent N-type Ca2+ channel blocker with fewer side effects, was found to possess analgesic effect in the formalin test and neuropathic pain models (Lee et al., 2010). Recent findings suggest that diminished Ca^{2+}

influx through N-type Ca^{2+} channels may contribute to sensory neuron dysfunction and pain after nerve injury (McCallum et al., 2011).

3.2.2 T-type Ca^{2+} channels

T-type Ca^{2+} channels are low-voltage activated Ca^{2+} channels. It can serve as an initiator to trigger the opening of high-voltage activated ion channels. In spinal dorsal horn, it may be involved in spontaneous neurotransmitter release and long term potentiation (LTP) (Ikeda et al., 2003). LTP, a form of synaptic plasticity, in the spinal dorsal horn is believed to contribute to the central sensitization of pain transmission (Ji et al., 2003), a wiring phenomenon usually observed in neuropathic pain (Romanelli & Esposito, 2004).
Among three subtypes of T-type Ca^{2+} channels, $Ca_V3.1$, $Ca_V3.2$ and $Ca_V3.3$, $Ca_V3.2$ mRNAs are mostly abundant in the spinal dorsal horn and are limited to the superficial layers (Talley et al., 1999). *Intrathecal* injection of the antisense oligonucleotide targeted to the α1-subunit of $Ca_V3.2$, but not $Ca_V3.3$ or $Ca_V3.1$, produced analgesic effect in both acute and neuropathic pain states (Bourinet et al., 2005), suggesting that $Ca_V3.2$ is much more involved in spinal nociceptive pathway than $Ca_V3.1$ and $Ca_V3.3$.
Subtype-specific blockers of T-type Ca^{2+} channels are not commercially available. However, mibefradil, a non-selective T-type Ca^{2+} channel blocker, when given systemically or intraplantarly, can reverse mechanical allodynia and thermal hyperalgesia induced by L5/6 spinal nerve ligation (Dogrul et al., 2003). Our recent work on *intrathecal* T-type Ca^{2+} channel blockers (mibefradil or Ni^{2+}) revealed their effectiveness in the second phase of formalin test (Cheng et al., 2007). In these years, small molecules with potent blocking effect on T-type Ca^{2+} channels, such as KYS05090, have been developed (Doddareddy et al., 2007; Seo et al., 2007). Recent studies revealed spinal T-type Ca^{2+} (Cav3.2 and Cav3.3 but not Cav3.1) channels may play an important role in the pathogenesis of chronic compression of DRG-induced neuropathic pain (Wen et al., 2010). In addition, Cav3.2-dependent activation of extracellular signal-regulated kinase in the anterior nucleus of paraventricular thalamus was found to contribute to the development of acid-induced chronic mechanical hyperalgesia (Chen et al., 2010).

3.2.3 P/Q- and R-type Ca^{2+} channels

Compared with N-type Ca^{2+} channel, it seems P/Q type is much less important in NINP. Only one study using transgenic mice revealed its involvement in chronic constriction injury-induced mechanical allodynia (Luvisetto et al., 2006). The hypoalgesic behaviors of P/Q-type Ca^{2+} channel mutant mouse suggest P/Q-type Ca^{2+} channel has a pro-nociceptive role (Fukumoto et al., 2009). As for R-type Ca^{2+} channel, its blocker SNX-482 could inhibit C-fiber and Aδ-fiber-mediated neuronal responses after L5/6 spinal nerve ligation, when administered ***intrathecally*** (Matthews et al., 2007). Moreover, the responses to innocuous mechanical and thermal stimuli were more sensitive to SNX-482 in nerve-ligated rats than control animals (Matthews et al., 2007). These findings suggest spinal R-type Ca^{2+} channel could be a potential therapeutic target for NINP. Blocking the R-type Ca^{2+} channel has been reported to enhance morphine analgesia and reduce morphine-induced tolerance (Yokoyama et al., 2004).

3.2.4 α2δ subunit of Ca^{2+} channels

α2δ subunit is one of the modulatory subunits of Ca^{2+} channels, which could modulate the membrane targeting and conductance of α1 subunit of Ca^{2+} channel (Felix, 1999). Four isoforms ($\alpha2\delta$-1~4) were identified (Qin et al., 2002). The $\alpha2\delta$-1 subunit is up-regulated in dorsal root ganglion and dorsal spinal cord after peripheral nerve injury (Li et al., 2004). *Intrathecal* injection of $\alpha2\delta$-1 antisense oligonucleotide could block this up-regulation in spinal dorsal horn and diminish injury-induced tactile allodynia (Li et al., 2004). Over expression of $\alpha2\delta$-1 in spinal dorsal horn neurons could enhance Ca^{2+} currents, exaggerate dorsal horn neuronal responses to external stimuli and increase the nociceptive responses in neuropathic pain models (Li et al., 2006).

$\alpha2\delta$ subunit is the specific binding site in the central nervous system of gabapentin and its analogue pregabalin (Klugbauer et al., 2003), both of which have been shown to be effective in preclinical and clinical studies of neuropathic pain (Cheng & Chiou, 2006). Gabapentin was first designed as a chemical analogue of γ-aminobutyric acid, an inhibitory neurotransmitter, to treat spasticity and was later found to have anticonvulsant and antinociceptive activities in various seizure and pain models. A point mutation of the arginine 217 of $\alpha2\delta$-1 subunit, which is critical for gabapentin binding (Wang et al., 1999), was found to cause a loss of gabapentin-induced analgesia (Field et al., 2006). Recently, chronic *intrathecal* infusion of gabapentin was found to prevent nerve ligation-induced mechanical allodynia and thermal hyperalgesia without causing obvious neuropathological changes in spinal cord and cauda equine (Chu et al., 2011).

Gabapentin has been found to attenuate morphine-induced tolerance (Lin et al., 2005) and this finding may encourage the combined use of gabapentin with morphine in the treatment of neuropathic pain. It is interesting to note that $\alpha2\delta$-1 subunit was identified to be a receptor involved in excitatory synapse formation and gabapentin may act by blocking new synapse formation (Eroglu et al., 2009).

3.3 Voltage-gated K^+ channels

The opening of K^+ channel may lead to cell repolarization and make the neuron less excitable and down-regulation of K^+ channel in nociceptive neurons may decrease pain threshold. There are 12 different families of voltage-gated K^+ channels (Kv1 to Kv12) and all Kv channels are tetramers of α subunits (Ocana et al., 2004). A-type K^+ channel (A-channels) is a group of Kv channels that are activated transiently and inactivated rapidly. Five A-channels Kv1.4, Kv3.4, Kv4.1, Kv4.2, and Kv4.3 were found in mammals (Chien et al., 2007; Mienville et al., 1999; Serodio et al., 1996). Except for Kv3.4 with high-voltage activation, the other four are activated at low voltages (Coetzee et al., 1999). Kv1.4 proteins in the somata of DRG neurons are greatly reduced in the L5/6 spinal nerve ligation pain model (Rasband et al., 2001). The expression of Kv1.4 is also reduced in the small-/medium sized (Aδ-/C-) trigeminal ganglion neurons after temporomandibular joint inflammation (Takeda et al., 2008). Gene expressions of Kv1.2, Kv1.4, and Kv4.2 are down-regulated in the DRG following sciatic nerve transection (Park et al., 2003). Recent study also revealed the Kv1.2 expression is decreased in DRG neurons from rats with irritable bowel syndrome, a visceral pain model (Luo et al., 2011). The expression of Kv3.4 and Kv4.3 in DRG neurons were found to be also decreased after spinal nerve ligation and ***intrathecal*** injections of antisense oligodeoxynucleotides against Kv3.4 or Kv4.3 in naïve rats could induce mechanical hypersensitivity (Chien et al., 2007). New compounds with A-type K^+ channel opening activity, such as KW-7158 (Sculptoreanu et al., 2004), may prove to be effective for the treatment of NINP.

The Kv7 channel (also known as KCNQ) opener retigabine has been reported to be effective in sciatic chronic constrict injury (Blackburn-Munro & Jensen, 2003) and L5 spinal nerve ligation (Dost et al., 2004) pain models. It is important to note that the antiallodynic effect of retigabine could be inhibited by linopirdine, a selective KCNQ channel blocker, indicating the involvement of KCNQ channel opening in the effect of retigabine (Dost et al., 2004). When directly applied to the spinal cord, retigabine inhibited the Aδ and C fiber-mediated response of dorsal horn neurons to noxious stimuli (Passmore et al., 2003). Recently, the selective cyclooxygenase-2 (COX-2) inhibitor celecoxib was found to enhance Kv7.2-7.4, Kv7.2/7.3 and Kv7.3/7.5 currents expressed in HEK 293 cells, providing a novel mechanism for its antinociceptive effect (Du et al., 2011b). Based on these reports, further efforts may be needed to develop subtype-specific K^+ channel openers and to test their effects in NINP models.

Just as voltage-gated Na^+ channels, K^+ channels could also be modulated by phosphorylation (Sergeant et al., 2005). The Kv4.2 current of spinal dorsal horn neurons could be inhibited by extracellular signal-regulated kinase (ERK)-induced phosphorylation (Hu et al., 2003). Genetic elimination of Kv4.2 increases excitability of dorsal horn neurons and sensitivity to tactile and thermal stimuli (Hu et al., 2006). This modulation of Kv4.2 by ERK may underlie the induction of central sensitization, a cellular mechanism of NINP (Ji et al., 2003). The role of Kv channels in different trigeminal neuropathic and inflammatory pain models was recently reviewed (Takeda et al., 2011).

3.4 Other K^+ channels

In addition to Kv channels, there are other K^+ channels that are important for pain modulation, such as G-protein coupled inwardly rectifying (GIRK or Kir3), ATP-sensitive (K_{ATP} or Kir6), Ca^{2+}-activated (KCa) and two-pore (K_{2P}) K^+ channels (Gutman et al., 2003). Activation of K_{ATP} channels was recently found to antagonize nociceptive behavior and hyper-excitability of DRG neurons from rats (Du et al., 2011a). Following partial sciatic nerve ligation, elevated tyrosine phosphorylation (pY12) of Kir3.1 was observed in the spinal superficial dorsal horn of wild type, but not Kir3.1 knock-out, mice (Ippolito et al., 2005). This phosphorylation may suppress channel conductance and accelerate channel deactivation (Ippolito et al., 2002), leading to enhanced neuronal excitability and could possibly contribute to the genesis of NINP. It is interesting to note that induced expression of Kir2.1 in chronically compressed DRG neurons can effectively suppress the neuronal excitability and, if induced at the beginning of the chronic compression, prevent the development of compression-induced hyperalgesia (Ma et al., 2010).

The TREK-1 channel is a member of mechano-gated K_{2P} family, one of the targets of inhalation anesthetics (Patel et al., 1999). TREK-1 is highly expressed in small sensory neurons and extensively co-localized with TRPV1 (Alloui et al., 2006). Mice with a disrupted TREK-1 gene are more sensitive to painful heat and low threshold mechanical stimuli and display an increased thermal and mechanical hyperalgesia in conditions of inflammation (Alloui et al., 2006). On the other hand, the TREK-1 null mice showed decreased sensitivity to acetone (less cold allodynia) after sciatic nerve ligation (Alloui et al., 2006). The chemotherapy drug oxaliplatin, which induces cold hypersensitivity, could lower the expression of TREK-1 (Descoeur et al., 2011). Future studies are needed to elucidate the role of TREK-1 channels in NINP. Similar as TREK-1, TREK-2 is also a member of the K_{2P} family. TREK-2 provide the major background K^+ conductance in cell body of small to medium-sized DRG neurons (Mathie, 2007), which are the major component of nociceptors. Based on these findings, it is also intriguing to investigate the role of TREK-2 in NINP (Huang & Yu, 2008).

Changes in the expression and function of voltage-gated ion channels in the pain pathway may contribute to the development and maintenance of NINP. Manipulations aiming at voltage-gated ion channels may provide novel strategies for the treatment of NINP. In addition to ion channel modulators, recent studies also reveal the promising roles of glial inhibitors, such as minocycline, and morphine in the management of NINP.

3.5 Microglia and astrocyte activation in nerve injury-induced neuropathic pain

During the last decade, the neuroimmune system, such as spinal glial cells, has been found to be critical for the development and maintenance of nerve injury-induced neuropathic pain (Watkins et al., 2007). Nerve injury not only induces morphological changes of microglia but also biochemical changes to induce pain. Nerve injury results in a up-regulation of P2X4 receptor (Tsuda et al., 2003) and CX3CR1 receptor in spinal cord microglia (Verge et al., 2004; Zhuang et al., 2007). *Intrathecal* blockade of P2X4 and CX3CR1 signaling attenuates NINP (Tsuda et al., 2003; Zhuang et al., 2007). The chemokine receptor CCR2 and the Toll-like recepotor-4 (TLR4) are also important for the formation of neuropathic pain *via* microglial activation (Abbadie et al., 2003; Tanga et al., 2005). Phosphorylation of p38 in microglia via activation of P2X4 receptor could increase the synthesis and release of the neurotrophin BDNF and pro-inflammatory cytokines (IL-1β, IL-6, and TNF-α), all of which could enhance nociceptive transmission in the spinal cord (Coull et al., 2005; Ji & Suter, 2007; Kawasaki et al., 2008b; Wang et al., 2010)

Our study using continuous *intrathecal* infusion of minocycline, a microglia inhibitor, revealed its effectiveness in attenuating the development of nerve injury-induced pain and no obvious spinal neurotoxicity was observed after the infusion (Lin et al., 2007). Other glial modulators, such as AV-411 (Ledeboer et al., 2006) and pentoxifylline (Mika et al., 2007), also possessed analgesic effect in NINP models. In addition to glial activation, compliment activation was recently found to participate in spinal nerve ligation-induced pain (Levin et al., 2008). Similar with gabapentin, minocycline could also attenuate morphine-induced tolerance (Cui et al., 2008) and this made itself a promising drug to be co-administered with morphine in the treatment of neuropathic pain. It is worthwhile to note that the attenuation effect of minocycline on morphine-induced tolerance is associated with inhibition of p38 activation in spinal microglia caused by chronic morphine (Cui et al., 2008).

In contrast to microglia, which is important for the development phase of NINP (Ji & Suter, 2007), astrocytes activation was critical for the maintenance phase of NINP (Zhuang et al., 2006). JNK-induced MCP-1 production and JAK-STAT3 pathway in spinal cord astrocytes was found to contribute to the maintenance of NINP (Gao et al., 2009b; Tsuda et al., 2011). The role of astrocyte activation and kinases involved in glial activation after nerve injury have been well reviewed (Gao & Ji, 2010; Ji et al., 2009).

4. Morphine in nerve injury-induced neuropathic pain

Morphine is the main drug used in pain clinics, especially in cancer pain. Recent animal studies also revealed the effectiveness of morphine in NINP models (Mika et al., 2007; Zhang et al., 2005). However, acute and chronic use of morphine can induce hyperalgesia and analgesia tolerance (Mao et al., 1994), which often lead to increased drug consumption and unwanted side-effects.

4.1 Glial non-opioid/p38 pathway in morphine-induced analgesia and tolerance

Using the tail flick test, Tseng's group has shown that morphine could induce anti-analgesia, which could be prevented by *levo-*, *dextro*naloxone **(a non-opioid ligand)** and p38 inhibitor *via* a glial non-opioid mechanism (Wu et al., 2006a; Wu et al., 2006b; Wu et al., 2005). From the works of Tseng's group, it could be summarized that 1) both *dextro-* and *levo-*morphine and lipopolysaccharide (LPS), a toll-like receptor (TLR)-4 agonist, could induce anti-analgesia, which could be prevented by *dextro-*, *levo-*naloxone and p38 inhibitor; 2) the anti-analgesia-inducing potency is: *dextro-*morphine > *levo-*morphine, and the reversal potency is: *levo-*naloxone > *dextro-*naloxone, which may imply the different binding affinities of *dextro/levo-* morphine and naloxone to the putative non-opioid receptor or TLR-4 (Hutchinson et al., 2007).

Inspired by the studies of Hong's group showing naloxone could attenuate LPS-induced microglial activation and neuronal damage (Liu et al., 2000), Watkin's group further tested the possible involvement of the putative nonopioid/TLR-4 pathway in NINP. They found *dextro-*naloxone, *levo-*naltrexone, and LPS-antagonist possess analgesic effects in chronic constriction neuropathic pain model (Hutchinson et al., 2007). Taken together with the role of glial p38 activation in NINP (Jin et al., 2003) and morphine-induced tolerance (Cui et al., 2006), it is possible that the putative glia non-opioid/TLR-4 pathway is important for the development of NINP and morphine-induced tolerance (Cui et al., 2006).

4.2 Intrathecal studies on morphine tolerance

Morphine has long been used *intrathecally* in the management of cancer and non-cancer chronic pain (Plummer et al., 1991; Roberts et al., 2001). However, the long-term use of morphine is associated with severe side-effects and tolerance (Osenbach & Harvey, 2001). Recently, many studies have revealed that *intrathecal* morphine could induce glial activation and neuro-inflammation in the spinal cord (Muscoli et al., 2010; Zhang et al., 2011). Several therapeutic targets have been found, including cytokine receptors, kappa-opioid receptors, N-methyl-D-aspartate receptors, and Toll-like receptors (Hameed et al., 2010; Lewis et al., 2010). Recently, tumor necrosis factor (TNF)-α antagonist etanercept was found to reverse morphine-induced tolerance and block morphine-induced neuroinflammation in the microglia (Shen et al., 2011). *Intrathecal* gabapentin and minocycline could also enhance the antinociceptive effects of morphine and attenuate morphine-induced tolerance (Habibi-Asl et al., 2009; Hutchinson et al., 2008; Lin et al., 2005). These promising agents may be co-administered with *intrathecal* morphine to improve the pain management for cancer patients (Christo & Mazloomdoost, 2008; Mercadante et al., 2004).

5. Intrathecal neurotoxicity studies

For a drug to be tested *intrathecally* in clinical trials, it is imperative to examine its neurotoxic effects first in animals (Bennett et al., 2000; Smith et al., 2008). For instance, *intrathecal* lidocaine has been found to induce neuropathological changes in the spinal cord and cauda equina (Kirihara et al., 2003). Other analgesics, such as adenosine, sufentanil, alfentanil and morphine have all been tested *intrathecally* in animal studies to examine their potential neurotoxicity (Chiari et al., 1999; Sabbe et al., 1994; Westin et al., 2010). Recently, chronic *intrathecal* infusion of minocycline or gabapentin has been reported to cause no grossly neurotoxicity in animal studies (Chu et al., 2011; Lin et al., 2007), supporting the *intrathecal* use of these agents for pain management.

6. Conclusion

Intrathecal space has been a route for spinal anesthesia and analgesics. This space also provides us a way to explore the possible mechanisms involved in pain transmission. Since pain is a major world-wide issue in clinical settings, more and more *intrathecal* animal studies have been undertaken to explore the possible mechanisms involved in the formation of different pain statuses and help to develop promising analgesics to alleviate the suffering of pain patients. These efforts will eventually help to provide better pain managements in clinical settings.

7. Acknowledgment

This chapter was supported by a John J. Bonica Trainee Fellowship from the International Association for the Study of Pain (IASP), a grant of NSC 98-2314-B-195-002-MY3 from National Science Council, Taipei, Taiwan and grants MMH 10015 and 10044 from Mackay Memorial Hospital, Taipei, Taiwan to J.K.C.

8. References

Abbadie, C., Lindia, J.A., Cumiskey, A.M., Peterson, L.B., Mudgett, J.S., Bayne, E.K., DeMartino, J.A., MacIntyre, D.E. & Forrest, M.J. (2003). Impaired neuropathic pain responses in mice lacking the chemokine receptor CCR2. *Proc Natl Acad Sci U S A*, Vol.100, No.13, pp. 7947-7952.

Abbott, F.V., Franklin, K.B. & Westbrook, R.F. (1995). The formalin test: scoring properties of the first and second phases of the pain response in rats. *Pain*, Vol.60, No.1, pp. 91-102.

Alloui, A., Zimmermann, K., Mamet, J., Duprat, F., Noel, J., Chemin, J., Guy, N., Blondeau, N., Voilley, N., Rubat-Coudert, C., Borsotto, M., Romey, G., Heurteaux, C., Reeh, P., Eschalier, A. & Lazdunski, M. (2006). TREK-1, a K^+ channel involved in polymodal pain perception. *EMBO J*, Vol.25, No.11, pp. 2368-2376.

Altier, C., Dale, C.S., Kisilevsky, A.E., Chapman, K., Castiglioni, A.J., Matthews, E.A., Evans, R.M., Dickenson, A.H., Lipscombe, D., Vergnolle, N. & Zamponi, G.W. (2007). Differential role of N-type calcium channel splice isoforms in pain. *J Neurosci*, Vol.27, No.24, pp. 6363-6373.

Aurilio, C., Pota, V., Pace, M.C., Passavanti, M.B. & Barbarisi, M. (2008). Ionic channels and neuropathic pain: physiopathology and applications. *J Cell Physiol*, Vol.215, No.1, pp. 8-14.

Bennett, G., Deer, T., Du Pen, S., Rauck, R., Yaksh, T. & Hassenbusch, S.J. (2000). Future directions in the management of pain by intraspinal drug delivery. *J Pain Symptom Manage*, Vol.20, No.2, pp. S44-50.

Berta, T., Poirot, O., Pertin, M., Ji, R.R., Kellenberger, S. & Decosterd, I. (2008). Transcriptional and functional profiles of voltage-gated Na(+) channels in injured and non-injured DRG neurons in the SNI model of neuropathic pain. *Mol Cell Neurosci*, Vol.37, No.2, pp. 196-208.

Blackburn-Munro, G. & Jensen, B.S. (2003). The anticonvulsant retigabine attenuates nociceptive behaviours in rat models of persistent and neuropathic pain. *Eur J Pharmacol*, Vol.460, No.2-3, pp. 109-116.

Bloom, A.P., Jimenez-Andrade, J.M., Taylor, R.N., Castaneda-Corral, G., Kaczmarska, M.J., Freeman, K.T., Coughlin, K.A., Ghilardi, J.R., Kuskowski, M.A. & Mantyh, P.W. (2011). Breast Cancer-Induced Bone Remodeling, Skeletal Pain and Sprouting of Sensory Nerve Fibers. *J Pain*, pp.

Bourinet, E., Alloui, A., Monteil, A., Barrere, C., Couette, B., Poirot, O., Pages, A., McRory, J., Snutch, T.P., Eschalier, A. & Nargeot, J. (2005). Silencing of the $Ca_v3.2$ T-type calcium channel gene in sensory neurons demonstrates its major role in nociception. *EMBO J*, Vol.24, No.2, pp. 315-324.

Bourquin, A.F., Suveges, M., Pertin, M., Gilliard, N., Sardy, S., Davison, A.C., Spahn, D.R. & Decosterd, I. (2006). Assessment and analysis of mechanical allodynia-like behavior induced by spared nerve injury (SNI) in the mouse. *Pain*, Vol.122, No.1-2, pp. 14 e11-14.

Brackenbury, W.J. & Isom, L.L. (2008). Voltage-gated Na^+ channels: potential for beta subunits as therapeutic targets. *Expert Opin Ther Targets*, Vol.12, No.9, pp. 1191-1203.

Brennan, T.J., Vandermeulen, E.P. & Gebhart, G.F. (1996). Characterization of a rat model of incisional pain. *Pain*, Vol.64, No.3, pp. 493-501.

Cain, D.M., Wacnik, P.W., Turner, M., Wendelschafer-Crabb, G., Kennedy, W.R., Wilcox, G.L. & Simone, D.A. (2001). Functional interactions between tumor and peripheral nerve: changes in excitability and morphology of primary afferent fibers in a murine model of cancer pain. *J Neurosci*, Vol.21, No.23, pp. 9367-9376.

Catterall, W.A., Goldin, A.L. & Waxman, S.G. (2005). International Union of Pharmacology. XLVII. Nomenclature and structure-function relationships of voltage-gated sodium channels. *Pharmacol Rev*, Vol.57, No.4, pp. 397-409.

Catterall, W.A., Kalume, F. & Oakley, J.C. (2010). $Na_V1.1$ channels and epilepsy. *J Physiol*, Vol.588, No.Pt 11, pp. 1849-1859.

Catterall, W.A., Striessnig, J., Snutch, T.P. & Perez-Reyes, E. (2002). Voltage-gated calcium channels. *The IUPHAR compendium of voltage-gated ion channels*, pp. 32-56.

Chaplan, S.R., Bach, F.W., Pogrel, J.W., Chung, J.M. & Yaksh, T.L. (1994). Quantitative assessment of tactile allodynia in the rat paw. *J Neurosci Methods*, Vol.53, No.1, pp. 55-63.

Chattopadhyay, M., Mata, M. & Fink, D.J. (2008). Continuous delta-opioid receptor activation reduces neuronal voltage-gated sodium channel (NaV1.7) levels through activation of protein kinase C in painful diabetic neuropathy. *J Neurosci*, Vol.28, No.26, pp. 6652-6658.

Chen, W.K., Liu, I.Y., Chang, Y.T., Chen, Y.C., Chen, C.C., Yen, C.T. & Shin, H.S. (2010). Ca(v)3.2 T-type Ca^{2+} channel-dependent activation of ERK in paraventricular thalamus modulates acid-induced chronic muscle pain. *J Neurosci*, Vol.30, No.31, pp. 10360-10368.

Cheng, J.K. & Chiou, L.C. (2006). Mechanisms of the antinociceptive action of gabapentin. *J Pharmacol Sci*, Vol.100, No.5, pp. 471-486.

Cheng, J.K., Lin, C.S., Chen, C.C., Yang, J.R. & Chiou, L.C. (2007). Effects of intrathecal injection of T-type calcium channel blockers in the rat formalin test. *Behav Pharmacol*, Vol.18, No.1, pp. 1-8.

Chiari, A., Yaksh, T.L., Myers, R.R., Provencher, J., Moore, L., Lee, C.S. & Eisenach, J.C. (1999). Preclinical toxicity screening of intrathecal adenosine in rats and dogs. *Anesthesiology*, Vol.91, No.3, pp. 824-832.

Chien, L.Y., Cheng, J.K., Chu, D., Cheng, C.F. & Tsaur, M.L. (2007). Reduced expression of A-type potassium channels in primary sensory neurons induces mechanical hypersensitivity. *J Neurosci*, Vol.27, No.37, pp. 9855-9865.

Christo, P.J. & Mazloomdoost, D. (2008). Interventional pain treatments for cancer pain. *Ann N Y Acad Sci*, Vol.1138, pp. 299-328.

Chu, L.C., Tsaur, M.L., Lin, C.S., Hung, Y.C., Wang, T.Y., Chen, C.C. & Cheng, J.K. (2011). Chronic intrathecal infusion of gabapentin prevents nerve ligation-induced pain in rats. *Br J Anaesth*, Vol.106, No.5, pp. 699-705.

Clohisy, D.R. & Mantyh, P.W. (2003). Bone cancer pain. *Cancer*, Vol.97, No.3 Suppl, pp. 866-873.

Coderre, T.J. & Melzack, R. (1992). The contribution of excitatory amino acids to central sensitization and persistent nociception after formalin-induced tissue injury. *J Neurosci*, Vol.12, No.9, pp. 3665-3670.

Coetzee, W.A., Amarillo, Y., Chiu, J., Chow, A., Lau, D., McCormack, T., Moreno, H., Nadal, M.S., Ozaita, A., Pountney, D., Saganich, M., Vega-Saenz de Miera, E. & Rudy, B. (1999). Molecular diversity of K+ channels. *Ann N Y Acad Sci*, Vol.868, pp. 233-285.

Constantin, C.E., Mair, N., Sailer, C.A., Andratsch, M., Xu, Z.Z., Blumer, M.J., Scherbakov, N., Davis, J.B., Bluethmann, H., Ji, R.R. & Kress, M. (2008). Endogenous tumor necrosis factor alpha (TNFalpha) requires TNF receptor type 2 to generate heat hyperalgesia in a mouse cancer model. *J Neurosci*, Vol.28, No.19, pp. 5072-5081.

Coull, J.A., Beggs, S., Boudreau, D., Boivin, D., Tsuda, M., Inoue, K., Gravel, C., Salter, M.W. & De Koninck, Y. (2005). BDNF from microglia causes the shift in neuronal anion gradient underlying neuropathic pain. *Nature*, Vol.438, No.7070, pp. 1017-1021.

Cox, J.J., Sheynin, J., Shorer, Z., Reimann, F., Nicholas, A.K., Zubovic, L., Baralle, M., Wraige, E., Manor, E., Levy, J., Woods, C.G. & Parvari, R. (2010). Congenital insensitivity to pain: novel SCN9A missense and in-frame deletion mutations. *Hum Mutat*, Vol.31, No.9, pp. E1670-1686.

Cuddapah, V.A. & Sontheimer, H. (2011). Ion Channels and the Control of Cancer Cell Migration. *Am J Physiol Cell Physiol*, pp.

Cui, Y., Chen, Y., Zhi, J.L., Guo, R.X., Feng, J.Q. & Chen, P.X. (2006). Activation of p38 mitogen-activated protein kinase in spinal microglia mediates morphine antinociceptive tolerance. *Brain Res*, Vol.1069, No.1, pp. 235-243.

Cui, Y., Liao, X.X., Liu, W., Guo, R.X., Wu, Z.Z., Zhao, C.M., Chen, P.X. & Feng, J.Q. (2008). A novel role of minocycline: attenuating morphine antinociceptive tolerance by inhibition of p38 MAPK in the activated spinal microglia. *Brain Behav Immun*, Vol.22, No.1, pp. 114-123.

Decosterd, I. & Woolf, C.J. (2000). Spared nerve injury: an animal model of persistent peripheral neuropathic pain. *Pain*, Vol.87, No.2, pp. 149-158.

Descoeur, J., Pereira, V., Pizzoccaro, A., Francois, A., Ling, B., Maffre, V., Couette, B., Busserolles, J., Courteix, C., Noel, J., Lazdunski, M., Eschalier, A., Authier, N. & Bourinet, E. (2011). Oxaliplatin-induced cold hypersensitivity is due to remodelling of ion channel expression in nociceptors. *EMBO Mol Med*, Vol.3, No.5, pp. 266-278.

Doddareddy, M.R., Choo, H., Cho, Y.S., Rhim, H., Koh, H.Y., Lee, J.H., Jeong, S.W. & Pae, A.N. (2007). 3D pharmacophore based virtual screening of T-type calcium channel blockers. *Bioorg Med Chem*, Vol.15, No.2, pp. 1091-1105.

Dogrul, A., Gardell, L.R., Ossipov, M.H., Tulunay, F.C., Lai, J. & Porreca, F. (2003). Reversal of experimental neuropathic pain by T-type calcium channel blockers. *Pain*, Vol.105, No.1-2, pp. 159-168.

Dolmetsch, R.E., Pajvani, U., Fife, K., Spotts, J.M. & Greenberg, M.E. (2001). Signaling to the nucleus by an L-type calcium channel-calmodulin complex through the MAP kinase pathway. *Science*, Vol.294, No.5541, pp. 333-339.

Donnelly-Roberts, D., McGaraughty, S., Shieh, C.C., Honore, P. & Jarvis, M.F. (2008). Painful purinergic receptors. *J Pharmacol Exp Ther*, Vol.324, No.2, pp. 409-415.

Dost, R., Rostock, A. & Rundfeldt, C. (2004). The anti-hyperalgesic activity of retigabine is mediated by KCNQ potassium channel activation. *Naunyn Schmiedebergs Arch Pharmacol*, Vol.369, No.4, pp. 382-390.

Du, X., Wang, C. & Zhang, H. (2011a). Activation of ATP-sensitive potassium channels antagonize nociceptive behavior and hyperexcitability of DRG neurons from rats. *Mol Pain*, Vol.7, No.1, pp. 35.

Du, X., Zhang, X., Qi, J., An, H., Li, J., Wan, Y., Fu, Y., Gao, H., Gao, Z., Zhan, Y. & Zhang, H. (2011b). Characteristics and molecular basis of celecoxib modulation on Kv7 potassium channels. *Br J Pharmacol*, pp.

Duarte, D.B., Duan, J.H., Nicol, G.D., Vasko, M.R. & Hingtgen, C.M. (2011). Reduced expression of SynGAP, a neuronal GTPase activating protein, enhances capsaicin-induced peripheral sensitization. *J Neurophysiol*, pp.

Dureja, G.P., Usmani, H., Khan, M., Tahseen, M. & Jamal, A. (2010). Efficacy of intrathecal midazolam with or without epidural methylprednisolone for management of post-herpetic neuralgia involving lumbosacral dermatomes. *Pain Physician*, Vol.13, No.3, pp. 213-221.

Ekberg, J., Jayamanne, A., Vaughan, C.W., Aslan, S., Thomas, L., Mould, J., Drinkwater, R., Baker, M.D., Abrahamsen, B., Wood, J.N., Adams, D.J., Christie, M.J. & Lewis, R.J. (2006). muO-conotoxin MrVIB selectively blocks Nav1.8 sensory neuron specific sodium channels and chronic pain behavior without motor deficits. *Proc Natl Acad Sci U S A*, Vol.103, No.45, pp. 17030-17035.

Eroglu, C., Allen, N.J., Susman, M.W., O'Rourke, N.A., Park, C.Y., Ozkan, E., Chakraborty, C., Mulinyawe, S.B., Annis, D.S., Huberman, A.D., Green, E.M., Lawler, J., Dolmetsch, R., Garcia, K.C., Smith, S.J., Luo, Z.D., Rosenthal, A., Mosher, D.F. & Barres, B.A. (2009). Gabapentin receptor alpha2delta-1 is a neuronal thrombospondin receptor responsible for excitatory CNS synaptogenesis. *Cell*, Vol.139, No.2, pp. 380-392.

Facer, P., Casula, M.A., Smith, G.D., Benham, C.D., Chessell, I.P., Bountra, C., Sinisi, M., Birch, R. & Anand, P. (2007). Differential expression of the capsaicin receptor TRPV1 and related novel receptors TRPV3, TRPV4 and TRPM8 in normal human tissues and changes in traumatic and diabetic neuropathy. *BMC Neurol*, Vol.7, pp. 11.

Felix, R. (1999). Voltage-dependent Ca^{2+} channel $\alpha_2\delta$ auxiliary subunit: structure, function and regulation. *Receptors Channels*, Vol.6, No.5, pp. 351-362.

Field, M.J., Cox, P.J., Stott, E., Melrose, H., Offord, J., Su, T.Z., Bramwell, S., Corradini, L., England, S., Winks, J., Kinloch, R.A., Hendrich, J., Dolphin, A.C., Webb, T. & Williams, D. (2006). Identification of the alpha2-delta-1 subunit of voltage-dependent calcium channels as a molecular target for pain mediating the analgesic actions of pregabalin. *Proc Natl Acad Sci U S A*, Vol.103, No.46, pp. 17537-17542.

Foulkes, T., Nassar, M.A., Lane, T., Matthews, E.A., Baker, M.D., Gerke, V., Okuse, K., Dickenson, A.H. & Wood, J.N. (2006). Deletion of annexin 2 light chain p11 in nociceptors causes deficits in somatosensory coding and pain behavior. *J Neurosci*, Vol.26, No.41, pp. 10499-10507.

Fukumoto, N., Obama, Y., Kitamura, N., Niimi, K., Takahashi, E., Itakura, C. & Shibuya, I. (2009). Hypoalgesic behaviors of P/Q-type voltage-gated Ca^{2+} channel mutant mouse, rolling mouse Nagoya. *Neuroscience*, Vol.160, No.1, pp. 165-173.

Gao, X., Kim, H.K., Chung, J.M. & Chung, K. (2005). Enhancement of NMDA receptor phosphorylation of the spinal dorsal horn and nucleus gracilis neurons in neuropathic rats. *Pain*, Vol.116, No.1-2, pp. 62-72.

Gao, Y.J., Cheng, J.K., Zeng, Q., Xu, Z.Z., Decosterd, I., Xu, X. & Ji, R.R. (2009a). Selective inhibition of JNK with a peptide inhibitor attenuates pain hypersensitivity and tumor growth in a mouse skin cancer pain model. *Exp Neurol*, Vol.219, No.1, pp. 146-155.

Gao, Y.J. & Ji, R.R. (2010). Targeting astrocyte signaling for chronic pain. *Neurotherapeutics*, Vol.7, No.4, pp. 482-493.

Gao, Y.J., Zhang, L., Samad, O.A., Suter, M.R., Yasuhiko, K., Xu, Z.Z., Park, J.Y., Lind, A.L., Ma, Q. & Ji, R.R. (2009b). JNK-induced MCP-1 production in spinal cord astrocytes contributes to central sensitization and neuropathic pain. *J Neurosci*, Vol.29, No.13, pp. 4096-4108.

Ghilardi, J.R., Freeman, K.T., Jimenez-Andrade, J.M., Mantyh, W.G., Bloom, A.P., Kuskowski, M.A. & Mantyh, P.W. (2010). Administration of a tropomyosin receptor kinase inhibitor attenuates sarcoma-induced nerve sprouting, neuroma formation and bone cancer pain. *Mol Pain*, Vol.6, pp. 87.

Gold, M.S., Levine, J.D. & Correa, A.M. (1998). Modulation of TTX-R INa by PKC and PKA and their role in PGE2-induced sensitization of rat sensory neurons in vitro. *J Neurosci*, Vol.18, No.24, pp. 10345-10355.

Gutman, G.A., Chandy, K.G., Adelman, J.P., Aiyar, J., Bayliss, D.A., Clapham, D.E., Covarriubias, M., Desir, G.V., Furuichi, K., Ganetzky, B., Garcia, M.L., Grissmer, S., Jan, L.Y., Karschin, A., Kim, D., Kuperschmidt, S., Kurachi, Y., Lazdunski, M., Lesage, F., Lester, H.A., McKinnon, D., Nichols, C.G., O'Kelly, I., Robbins, J., Robertson, G.A., Rudy, B., Sanguinetti, M., Seino, S., Stuehmer, W., Tamkun, M.M., Vandenberg, C.A., Wei, A., Wulff, H. & Wymore, R.S. (2003). International Union of Pharmacology. XLI. Compendium of voltage-gated ion channels: potassium channels. *Pharmacol Rev*, Vol.55, No.4, pp. 583-586.

Habibi-Asl, B., Hassanzadeh, K. & Charkhpour, M. (2009). Central administration of minocycline and riluzole prevents morphine-induced tolerance in rats. *Anesth Analg*, Vol.109, No.3, pp. 936-942.

Hameed, H., Hameed, M. & Christo, P.J. (2010). The effect of morphine on glial cells as a potential therapeutic target for pharmacological development of analgesic drugs. *Curr Pain Headache Rep*, Vol.14, No.2, pp. 96-104.

Hargreaves, K., Dubner, R., Brown, F., Flores, C. & Joris, J. (1988). A new and sensitive method for measuring thermal nociception in cutaneous hyperalgesia. *Pain*, Vol.32, No.1, pp. 77-88.

Hong, R.W. (2010). Less is more: the recent history of neuraxial labor analgesia. *Am J Ther*, Vol.17, No.5, pp. 492-497.

Hong, S., Morrow, T.J., Paulson, P.E., Isom, L.L. & Wiley, J.W. (2004). Early painful diabetic neuropathy is associated with differential changes in tetrodotoxin-sensitive and -resistant sodium channels in dorsal root ganglion neurons in the rat. *J Biol Chem*, Vol.279, No.28, pp. 29341-29350.

Hu, H.J., Carrasquillo, Y., Karim, F., Jung, W.E., Nerbonne, J.M., Schwarz, T.L. & Gereau, R.W.t. (2006). The kv4.2 potassium channel subunit is required for pain plasticity. *Neuron*, Vol.50, No.1, pp. 89-100.

Hu, H.J., Glauner, K.S. & Gereau, R.W.t. (2003). ERK integrates PKA and PKC signaling in superficial dorsal horn neurons. I. Modulation of A-type K^+ currents. *J Neurophysiol*, Vol.90, No.3, pp. 1671-1679.

Huang, D. & Yu, B. (2008). Recent advance and possible future in TREK-2: a two-pore potassium channel may involved in the process of NPP, brain ischemia and memory impairment. *Med Hypotheses*, Vol.70, No.3, pp. 618-624.

Hunanyan, A.S., Alessi, V., Patel, S., Pearse, D.D., Matthews, G. & Arvanian, V.L. (2011). Alterations of action potentials and the localization of Nav1.6 sodium channels in spared axons after hemisection injury of the spinal cord in adult rats. *J Neurophysiol*, Vol.105, No.3, pp. 1033-1044.

Hutchinson, M.R., Bland, S.T., Johnson, K.W., Rice, K.C., Maier, S.F. & Watkins, L.R. (2007). Opioid-induced glial activation: mechanisms of activation and implications for opioid analgesia, dependence, and reward. *ScientificWorldJournal*, Vol.7, pp. 98-111.

Hutchinson, M.R., Northcutt, A.L., Chao, L.W., Kearney, J.J., Zhang, Y., Berkelhammer, D.L., Loram, L.C., Rozeske, R.R., Bland, S.T., Maier, S.F., Gleeson, T.T. & Watkins, L.R. (2008). Minocycline suppresses morphine-induced respiratory depression, suppresses morphine-induced reward, and enhances systemic morphine-induced analgesia. *Brain Behav Immun*, Vol.22, No.8, pp. 1248-1256.

Ikeda, H., Heinke, B., Ruscheweyh, R. & Sandkuhler, J. (2003). Synaptic plasticity in spinal lamina I projection neurons that mediate hyperalgesia. *Science*, Vol.299, No.5610, pp. 1237-1240.

Ippolito, D.L., Temkin, P.A., Rogalski, S.L. & Chavkin, C. (2002). N-terminal tyrosine residues within the potassium channel Kir3 modulate GTPase activity of Galphai. *J Biol Chem*, Vol.277, No.36, pp. 32692-32696.

Ippolito, D.L., Xu, M., Bruchas, M.R., Wickman, K. & Chavkin, C. (2005). Tyrosine phosphorylation of K(ir)3.1 in spinal cord is induced by acute inflammation, chronic neuropathic pain, and behavioral stress. *J Biol Chem*, Vol.280, No.50, pp. 41683-41693.

Jarecki, B.W., Piekarz, A.D., Jackson, J.O., 2nd & Cummins, T.R. (2010). Human voltage-gated sodium channel mutations that cause inherited neuronal and muscle channelopathies increase resurgent sodium currents. *J Clin Invest*, Vol.120, No.1, pp. 369-378.

Jarvis, M.F., Honore, P., Shieh, C.C., Chapman, M., Joshi, S., Zhang, X.F., Kort, M., Carroll, W., Marron, B., Atkinson, R., Thomas, J., Liu, D., Krambis, M., Liu, Y.,

McGaraughty, S., Chu, K., Roeloffs, R., Zhong, C., Mikusa, J.P., Hernandez, G., Gauvin, D., Wade, C., Zhu, C., Pai, M., Scanio, M., Shi, L., Drizin, I., Gregg, R., Matulenko, M., Hakeem, A., Gross, M., Johnson, M., Marsh, K., Wagoner, P.K., Sullivan, J.P., Faltynek, C.R. & Krafte, D.S. (2007). A-803467, a potent and selective Nav1.8 sodium channel blocker, attenuates neuropathic and inflammatory pain in the rat. *Proc Natl Acad Sci U S A*, Vol.104, No.20, pp. 8520-8525.

Ji, R.R., Gereau, R.W.t., Malcangio, M. & Strichartz, G.R. (2009). MAP kinase and pain. *Brain Res Rev*, Vol.60, No.1, pp. 135-148.

Ji, R.R., Kohno, T., Moore, K.A. & Woolf, C.J. (2003). Central sensitization and LTP: do pain and memory share similar mechanisms? *Trends Neurosci*, Vol.26, No.12, pp. 696-705.

Ji, R.R. & Strichartz, G. (2004). Cell signaling and the genesis of neuropathic pain. *Sci STKE*, Vol.252 pp. reE14.

Ji, R.R. & Suter, M.R. (2007). p38 MAPK, microglial signaling, and neuropathic pain. *Mol Pain*, Vol.3, pp. 33.

Jimenez-Andrade, J.M., Bloom, A.P., Stake, J.I., Mantyh, W.G., Taylor, R.N., Freeman, K.T., Ghilardi, J.R., Kuskowski, M.A. & Mantyh, P.W. (2010). Pathological sprouting of adult nociceptors in chronic prostate cancer-induced bone pain. *J Neurosci*, Vol.30, No.44, pp. 14649-14656.

Jin, S.X., Zhuang, Z.Y., Woolf, C.J. & Ji, R.R. (2003). p38 mitogen-activated protein kinase is activated after a spinal nerve ligation in spinal cord microglia and dorsal root ganglion neurons and contributes to the generation of neuropathic pain. *J Neurosci*, Vol.23, No.10, pp. 4017-4022.

Jin, X. & Gereau, R.W.t. (2006). Acute p38-mediated modulation of tetrodotoxin-resistant sodium channels in mouse sensory neurons by tumor necrosis factor-alpha. *J Neurosci*, Vol.26, No.1, pp. 246-255.

Joshi, S.K., Mikusa, J.P., Hernandez, G., Baker, S., Shieh, C.C., Neelands, T., Zhang, X.F., Niforatos, W., Kage, K., Han, P., Krafte, D., Faltynek, C., Sullivan, J.P., Jarvis, M.F. & Honore, P. (2006). Involvement of the TTX-resistant sodium channel Nav 1.8 in inflammatory and neuropathic, but not post-operative, pain states. *Pain*, Vol.123, No.1-2, pp. 75-82.

Kakimura, J., Zheng, T., Uryu, N. & Ogata, N. (2010). Regulation of the spontaneous augmentation of Na(V)1.9 in mouse dorsal root ganglion neurons: effect of PKA and PKC pathways. *Mar Drugs*, Vol.8, No.3, pp. 728-740.

Kang, S. & Brennan, T.J. (2009). Chemosensitivity and mechanosensitivity of nociceptors from incised rat hindpaw skin. *Anesthesiology*, Vol.111, No.1, pp. 155-164.

Kawasaki, Y., Xu, Z.Z., Wang, X., Park, J.Y., Zhuang, Z.Y., Tan, P.H., Gao, Y.J., Roy, K., Corfas, G., Lo, E.H. & Ji, R.R. (2008a). Distinct roles of matrix metalloproteases in the early- and late-phase development of neuropathic pain. *Nat Med*, Vol.14, No.3, pp. 331-336.

Kawasaki, Y., Zhang, L., Cheng, J.K. & Ji, R.R. (2008b). Cytokine mechanisms of central sensitization: distinct and overlapping role of interleukin-1beta, interleukin-6, and tumor necrosis factor-alpha in regulating synaptic and neuronal activity in the superficial spinal cord. *J Neurosci*, Vol.28, No.20, pp. 5189-5194.

Kim, S.H. & Chung, J.M. (1992). An experimental model for peripheral neuropathy produced by segmental spinal nerve ligation in the rat. *Pain*, Vol.50, No.3, pp. 355-363.

Kirihara, Y., Saito, Y., Sakura, S., Hashimoto, K., Kishimoto, T. & Yasui, Y. (2003). Comparative neurotoxicity of intrathecal and epidural lidocaine in rats. *Anesthesiology*, Vol.99, No.4, pp. 961-968.

Klugbauer, N., Marais, E. & Hofmann, F. (2003). Calcium channel alpha2delta subunits: differential expression, function, and drug binding. *J Bioenerg Biomembr*, Vol.35, No.6, pp. 639-647.

Knutsen, L.J., Hobbs, C.J., Earnshaw, C.G., Fiumana, A., Gilbert, J., Mellor, S.L., Radford, F., Smith, N.J., Birch, P.J., Russell Burley, J., Ward, S.D. & James, I.F. (2007). Synthesis and SAR of novel 2-arylthiazolidinones as selective analgesic N-type calcium channel blockers. *Bioorg Med Chem Lett*, Vol.17, No.3, pp. 662-667.

Kretschmer, T., Happel, L.T., England, J.D., Nguyen, D.H., Tiel, R.L., Beuerman, R.W. & Kline, D.G. (2002). Accumulation of PN1 and PN3 sodium channels in painful human neuroma-evidence from immunocytochemistry. *Acta Neurochir (Wien)*, Vol.144, No.8, pp. 803-810; discussion 810.

Lampert, A., O'Reilly, A.O., Reeh, P. & Leffler, A. (2010). Sodium channelopathies and pain. *Pflugers Arch*, Vol.460, No.2, pp. 249-263.

Ledeboer, A., Liu, T., Shumilla, J.A., Mahoney, J.H., Vijay, S., Gross, M.I., Vargas, J.A., Sultzbaugh, L., Claypool, M.D., Sanftner, L.M., Watkins, L.R. & Johnson, K.W. (2006). The glial modulatory drug AV411 attenuates mechanical allodynia in rat models of neuropathic pain. *Neuron Glia Biol*, Vol.2, No.4, pp. 279-291.

Lee, S., Kim, Y., Back, S.K., Choi, H.W., Lee, J.Y., Jung, H.H., Ryu, J.H., Suh, H.W., Na, H.S., Kim, H.J., Rhim, H. & Kim, J.I. (2010). Analgesic effect of highly reversible omega-conotoxin FVIA on N type Ca^{2+} channels. *Mol Pain*, Vol.6, pp. 97.

Leo, S., D'Hooge, R. & Meert, T. (2010). Exploring the role of nociceptor-specific sodium channels in pain transmission using Nav1.8 and Nav1.9 knockout mice. *Behav Brain Res*, Vol.208, No.1, pp. 149-157.

Levin, M.E., Jin, J.G., Ji, R.R., Tong, J., Pomonis, J.D., Lavery, D.J., Miller, S.W. & Chiang, L.W. (2008). Complement activation in the peripheral nervous system following the spinal nerve ligation model of neuropathic pain. *Pain*, Vol.137, No.1, pp. 182-201.

Lewis, S.S., Hutchinson, M.R., Rezvani, N., Loram, L.C., Zhang, Y., Maier, S.F., Rice, K.C. & Watkins, L.R. (2010). Evidence that intrathecal morphine-3-glucuronide may cause pain enhancement via toll-like receptor 4/MD-2 and interleukin-1beta. *Neuroscience*, Vol.165, No.2, pp. 569-583.

Li, C.Y., Song, Y.H., Higuera, E.S. & Luo, Z.D. (2004). Spinal dorsal horn calcium channel $\alpha_2\delta$-1 subunit upregulation contributes to peripheral nerve injury-induced tactile allodynia. *J Neurosci*, Vol.24, No.39, pp. 8494-8499.

Li, C.Y., Zhang, X.L., Matthews, E.A., Li, K.W., Kurwa, A., Boroujerdi, A., Gross, J., Gold, M.S., Dickenson, A.H., Feng, G. & Luo, Z.D. (2006). Calcium channel alpha2delta1 subunit mediates spinal hyperexcitability in pain modulation. *Pain*, Vol.125, No.1-2, pp. 20-34.

Lin, C.S., Tsaur, M.L., Chen, C.C., Wang, T.Y., Lin, C.F., Lai, Y.L., Hsu, T.C., Pan, Y.Y., Yang, C.H. & Cheng, J.K. (2007). Chronic intrathecal infusion of minocycline prevents the development of spinal-nerve ligation-induced pain in rats. *Reg Anesth Pain Med*, Vol.32, No.3, pp. 209-216.

Lin, J.A., Lee, M.S., Wu, C.T., Yeh, C.C., Lin, S.L., Wen, Z.H. & Wong, C.S. (2005). Attenuation of morphine tolerance by intrathecal gabapentin is associated with suppression of morphine-evoked excitatory amino acid release in the rat spinal cord. *Brain Res*, Vol.1054, No.2 pp. 167-173.

Liu, B., Du, L. & Hong, J.S. (2000). Naloxone protects rat dopaminergic neurons against inflammatory damage through inhibition of microglia activation and superoxide generation. *J Pharmacol Exp Ther*, Vol.293, No.2, pp. 607-617.

LoPachin, R.M., Rudy, T.A. & Yaksh, T.L. (1981). An improved method for chronic catheterization of the rat spinal subarachnoid space. *Physiol Behav*, Vol.27, No.3, pp. 559-561.

Lopez-Santiago, L.F., Pertin, M., Morisod, X., Chen, C., Hong, S., Wiley, J., Decosterd, I. & Isom, L.L. (2006). Sodium channel beta2 subunits regulate tetrodotoxin-sensitive sodium channels in small dorsal root ganglion neurons and modulate the response to pain. *J Neurosci*, Vol.26, No.30, pp. 7984-7994.

Luo, J.L., Qin, H.Y., Wong, C.K., Tsang, S.Y., Huang, Y. & Bian, Z.X. (2011). Enhanced Excitability and Down-Regulated Voltage-Gated Potassium Channels in Colonic DRG Neurons from Neonatal Maternal Separation Rats. *J Pain*, Vol.12, No.5, pp. 600-609.

Luvisetto, S., Marinelli, S., Panasiti, M.S., D'Amato, F.R., Fletcher, C.F., Pavone, F. & Pietrobon, D. (2006). Pain sensitivity in mice lacking the Ca(v)2.1alpha1 subunit of P/Q-type Ca^{2+} channels. *Neuroscience*, Vol.142, No.3, pp. 823-832.

Lynch, M.E. & Campbell, F. (2011). Cannabinoids for Treatment of Chronic Non-Cancer Pain; a Systematic Review of Randomized Trials. *Br J Clin Pharmacol*, pp.

Ma, C., Rosenzweig, J., Zhang, P., Johns, D.C. & LaMotte, R.H. (2010). Expression of inwardly rectifying potassium channels by an inducible adenoviral vector reduced the neuronal hyperexcitability and hyperalgesia produced by chronic compression of the spinal ganglion. *Mol Pain*, Vol.6, pp. 65.

Mao, J., Price, D.D. & Mayer, D.J. (1994). Thermal hyperalgesia in association with the development of morphine tolerance in rats: roles of excitatory amino acid receptors and protein kinase C. *J Neurosci*, Vol.14, No.4, pp. 2301-2312.

Mathie, A. (2007). Neuronal two-pore-domain potassium channels and their regulation by G protein-coupled receptors. *J Physiol*, Vol.578, No.Pt 2, pp. 377-385.

Matthews, E.A., Bee, L.A., Stephens, G.J. & Dickenson, A.H. (2007). The Cav2.3 calcium channel antagonist SNX-482 reduces dorsal horn neuronal responses in a rat model of chronic neuropathic pain. *Eur J Neurosci*, Vol.25, No.12, pp. 3561-3569.

Mazzuca, M., Heurteaux, C., Alloui, A., Diochot, S., Baron, A., Voilley, N., Blondeau, N., Escoubas, P., Gelot, A., Cupo, A., Zimmer, A., Zimmer, A.M., Eschalier, A. & Lazdunski, M. (2007). A tarantula peptide against pain via ASIC1a channels and opioid mechanisms. *Nat Neurosci*, Vol.10, No.8, pp. 943-945.

McCallum, J.B., Wu, H.E., Tang, Q., Kwok, W.M. & Hogan, Q.H. (2011). Subtype-specific reduction of voltage-gated calcium current in medium-sized dorsal root ganglion neurons after painful peripheral nerve injury. *Neuroscience*, Vol.179, pp. 244-255.

Mercadante, S. (1999). Neuraxial techniques for cancer pain: an opinion about unresolved therapeutic dilemmas. *Reg Anesth Pain Med*, Vol.24, No.1, pp. 74-83.

Mercadante, S., Villari, P. & Ferrera, P. (2004). Dialogues on complex analgesic strategies for difficult pain syndromes. *Support Care Cancer*, Vol.12, No.8, pp. 599-603.

Mienville, J.M., Maric, I., Maric, D. & Clay, J.R. (1999). Loss of IA expression and increased excitability in postnatal rat Cajal-Retzius cells. *J Neurophysiol*, Vol.82, No.3, pp. 1303-1310.

Mika, J., Osikowicz, M., Makuch, W. & Przewlocka, B. (2007). Minocycline and pentoxifylline attenuate allodynia and hyperalgesia and potentiate the effects of morphine in rat and mouse models of neuropathic pain. *Eur J Pharmacol*, Vol.560, No.2-3, pp. 142-149.

Mo, G., Grant, R., O'Donnell, D., Ragsdale, D.S., Cao, C.Q. & Seguela, P. (2011). Neuropathic Nav1.3-mediated sensitization to P2X activation is regulated by protein kinase C. *Mol Pain*, Vol.7, pp. 14.

Mogil, J.S., Davis, K.D. & Derbyshire, S.W. (2010). The necessity of animal models in pain research. *Pain*, Vol.151, No.1, pp. 12-17.

Muscoli, C., Doyle, T., Dagostino, C., Bryant, L., Chen, Z., Watkins, L.R., Ryerse, J., Bieberich, E., Neumman, W. & Salvemini, D. (2010). Counter-regulation of opioid analgesia by glial-derived bioactive sphingolipids. *J Neurosci*, Vol.30, No.46, pp. 15400-15408.

Nassar, M.A., Levato, A., Stirling, L.C. & Wood, J.N. (2005). Neuropathic pain develops normally in mice lacking both Na(v)1.7 and Na(v)1.8. *Mol Pain*, Vol.1, pp. 24.

Ocana, M., Cendan, C.M., Cobos, E.J., Entrena, J.M. & Baeyens, J.M. (2004). Potassium channels and pain: present realities and future opportunities. *Eur J Pharmacol*, Vol.500, No.1-3, pp. 203-219.

Osenbach, R.K. & Harvey, S. (2001). Neuraxial infusion in patients with chronic intractable cancer and noncancer pain. *Curr Pain Headache Rep*, Vol.5, No.3, pp. 241-249.

Park, S.Y., Choi, J.Y., Kim, R.U., Lee, Y.S., Cho, H.J. & Kim, D.S. (2003). Downregulation of voltage-gated potassium channel alpha gene expression by axotomy and neurotrophins in rat dorsal root ganglia. *Mol Cells*, Vol.16, No.2, pp. 256-259.

Passmore, G.M., Selyanko, A.A., Mistry, M., Al-Qatari, M., Marsh, S.J., Matthews, E.A., Dickenson, A.H., Brown, T.A., Burbidge, S.A., Main, M. & Brown, D.A. (2003). KCNQ/M currents in sensory neurons: significance for pain therapy. *J Neurosci*, Vol.23, No.18, pp. 7227-7236.

Patel, A.J., Honore, E., Lesage, F., Fink, M., Romey, G. & Lazdunski, M. (1999). Inhalational anesthetics activate two-pore-domain background K^+ channels. *Nat Neurosci*, Vol.2, No.5, pp. 422-426.

Pertin, M., Ji, R.R., Berta, T., Powell, A.J., Karchewski, L., Tate, S.N., Isom, L.L., Woolf, C.J., Gilliard, N., Spahn, D.R. & Decosterd, I. (2005). Upregulation of the voltage-gated sodium channel beta2 subunit in neuropathic pain models: characterization of expression in injured and non-injured primary sensory neurons. *J Neurosci*, Vol.25, No.47, pp. 10970-10980.

Plummer, J.L., Cherry, D.A., Cousins, M.J., Gourlay, G.K., Onley, M.M. & Evans, K.H. (1991). Long-term spinal administration of morphine in cancer and non-cancer pain: a retrospective study. *Pain*, Vol.44, No.3, pp. 215-220.

Poirot, O., Berta, T., Decosterd, I. & Kellenberger, S. (2006). Distinct ASIC currents are expressed in rat putative nociceptors and are modulated by nerve injury. *J Physiol*, Vol.576, No.Pt 1, pp. 215-234.

Qin, N., Yagel, S., Momplaisir, M.L., Codd, E.E. & D'Andrea, M.R. (2002). Molecular cloning and characterization of the human voltage-gated calcium channel $\alpha_2\delta$-4 subunit. *Mol Pharmacol*, Vol.62, No.3, pp. 485-496.

Rasband, M.N., Park, E.W., Vanderah, T.W., Lai, J., Porreca, F. & Trimmer, J.S. (2001). Distinct potassium channels on pain-sensing neurons. *Proc Natl Acad Sci U S A*, Vol.98, No.23, pp. 13373-13378.

Roberts, L.J., Finch, P.M., Goucke, C.R. & Price, L.M. (2001). Outcome of intrathecal opioids in chronic non-cancer pain. *Eur J Pain*, Vol.5, No.4, pp. 353-361.

Rogers, M., Tang, L., Madge, D.J. & Stevens, E.B. (2006). The role of sodium channels in neuropathic pain. *Semin Cell Dev Biol*, Vol.17, No.5, pp. 571-581.

Romanelli, P. & Esposito, V. (2004). The functional anatomy of neuropathic pain. *Neurosurg Clin N Am*, Vol.15, No.3, pp. 257-268.

Sabbe, M.B., Grafe, M.R., Mjanger, E., Tiseo, P.J., Hill, H.F. & Yaksh, T.L. (1994). Spinal delivery of sufentanil, alfentanil, and morphine in dogs. Physiologic and toxicologic investigations. *Anesthesiology*, Vol.81, No.4, pp. 899-920.

Saegusa, H., Kurihara, T., Zong, S., Kazuno, A., Matsuda, Y., Nonaka, T., Han, W., Toriyama, H. & Tanabe, T. (2001). Suppression of inflammatory and neuropathic pain symptoms in mice lacking the N-type Ca^{2+} channel. *EMBO J*, Vol.20, No.10, pp. 2349-2356.

Sandkuhler, J. & Liu, X. (1998). Induction of long-term potentiation at spinal synapses by noxious stimulation or nerve injury. *Eur J Neurosci*, Vol.10, No.7, pp. 2476-2480.

Schafers, M., Svensson, C.I., Sommer, C. & Sorkin, L.S. (2003). Tumor necrosis factor-alpha induces mechanical allodynia after spinal nerve ligation by activation of p38 MAPK in primary sensory neurons. *J Neurosci*, Vol.23, No.7, pp. 2517-2521.

Sculptoreanu, A., Yoshimura, N. & de Groat, W.C. (2004). KW-7158 [(2S)-(+)-3,3,3-trifluoro-2-hydroxy-2-methyl-N-(5,5,10-trioxo-4,10-dihydro thieno[3,2-c][1]benzothiepin-9-yl)propanamide] enhances A-type K^+ currents in neurons of the dorsal root ganglion of the adult rat. *J Pharmacol Exp Ther*, Vol.310, No.1, pp. 159-168.

Seo, H.N., Choi, J.Y., Choe, Y.J., Kim, Y., Rhim, H., Lee, S.H., Kim, J., Joo, D.J. & Lee, J.Y. (2007). Discovery of potent T-type calcium channel blocker. *Bioorg Med Chem Lett*, Vol.17, No.21, pp. 5740-5743.

Sergeant, G.P., Ohya, S., Reihill, J.A., Perrino, B.A., Amberg, G.C., Imaizumi, Y., Horowitz, B., Sanders, K.M. & Koh, S.D. (2005). Regulation of Kv4.3 currents by Ca^{2+}/calmodulin-dependent protein kinase II. *Am J Physiol Cell Physiol*, Vol.288, No.2, pp. C304-313.

Serodio, P., Vega-Saenz de Miera, E. & Rudy, B. (1996). Cloning of a novel component of A-type K^+ channels operating at subthreshold potentials with unique expression in heart and brain. *J Neurophysiol*, Vol.75, No.5, pp. 2174-2179.

Shen, C.H., Tsai, R.Y., Shih, M.S., Lin, S.L., Tai, Y.H., Chien, C.C. & Wong, C.S. (2011). Etanercept restores the antinociceptive effect of morphine and suppresses spinal neuroinflammation in morphine-tolerant rats. *Anesth Analg*, Vol.112, No.2, pp. 454-459.

Smith, H.S., Deer, T.R., Staats, P.S., Singh, V., Sehgal, N. & Cordner, H. (2008). Intrathecal drug delivery. *Pain Physician*, Vol.11, No.2 Suppl, pp. S89-S104.

Smith, M.T., Cabot, P.J., Ross, F.B., Robertson, A.D. & Lewis, R.J. (2002). The novel N-type calcium channel blocker, AM336, produces potent dose-dependent antinociception after intrathecal dosing in rats and inhibits substance P release in rat spinal cord slices. *Pain*, Vol.96, No.1-2, pp. 119-127.

Song, X.J., Wang, Z.B., Gan, Q. & Walters, E.T. (2006). cAMP and cGMP contribute to sensory neuron hyperexcitability and hyperalgesia in rats with dorsal root ganglia compression. *J Neurophysiol*, Vol.95, No.1, pp. 479-492.

Szekely, J.I., Torok, K. & Mate, G. (2002). The role of ionotropic glutamate receptors in nociception with special regard to the AMPA binding sites. *Curr Pharm Des*, Vol.8, No.10, pp. 887-912.

Szu-Yu Ho, T. & Rasband, M.N. (2011). Maintenance of neuronal polarity. *Dev Neurobiol*, Vol.71, No.6, pp. 474-482.

Takeda, M., Tanimoto, T., Nasu, M. & Matsumoto, S. (2008). Temporomandibular joint inflammation decreases the voltage-gated K^+ channel subtype 1.4-immunoreactivity of trigeminal ganglion neurons in rats. *Eur J Pain*, Vol.12, No.2, pp. 189-195.

Takeda, M., Tsuboi, Y., Kitagawa, J., Nakagawa, K., Iwata, K. & Matsumoto, S. (2011). Potassium channels as a potential therapeutic target for trigeminal neuropathic and inflammatory pain. *Mol Pain*, Vol.7, pp. 5.

Talley, E.M., Cribbs, L.L., Lee, J.H., Daud, A., Perez-Reyes, E. & Bayliss, D.A. (1999). Differential distribution of three members of a gene family encoding low voltage-activated (T-type) calcium channels. *J Neurosci*, Vol.19, No.6, pp. 1895-1911.

Tanga, F.Y., Nutile-McMenemy, N. & DeLeo, J.A. (2005). The CNS role of Toll-like receptor 4 in innate neuroimmunity and painful neuropathy. *Proc Natl Acad Sci U S A*, Vol.102, No.16, pp. 5856-5861.

Thorpe, L.B., Goldie, M. & Dolan, S. (2011). Central and Local Administration of Gingko Biloba Extract EGb 761(R) Inhibits Thermal Hyperalgesia and Inflammation in the Rat Carrageenan Model. *Anesth Analg*, Vol.112, No.5, pp. 1226-1231.

Tsuda, M., Kohro, Y., Yano, T., Tsujikawa, T., Kitano, J., Tozaki-Saitoh, H., Koyanagi, S., Ohdo, S., Ji, R.R., Salter, M.W. & Inoue, K. (2011). JAK-STAT3 pathway regulates spinal astrocyte proliferation and neuropathic pain maintenance in rats. *Brain*, Vol.134, No.Pt 4, pp. 1127-1139.

Tsuda, M., Shigemoto-Mogami, Y., Koizumi, S., Mizokoshi, A., Kohsaka, S., Salter, M.W. & Inoue, K. (2003). P2X4 receptors induced in spinal microglia gate tactile allodynia after nerve injury. *Nature*, Vol.424, No.6950, pp. 778-783.

Tyagarajan, S., Chakravarty, P.K., Zhou, B., Taylor, B., Eid, R., Fisher, M.H., Parsons, W.H., Wyvratt, M.J., Lyons, K.A., Klatt, T., Li, X., Kumar, S., Williams, B., Felix, J., Priest, B.T., Brochu, R.M., Warren, V., Smith, M., Garcia, M., Kaczorowski, G.J., Martin, W.J., Abbadie, C., McGowan, E., Jochnowitz, N., Weber, A. & Duffy, J.L. (2010). Discovery of a novel class of biphenyl pyrazole sodium channel blockers for treatment of neuropathic pain. *Bioorg Med Chem Lett*, Vol.20, No.24, pp. 7479-7482.

Verge, G.M., Milligan, E.D., Maier, S.F., Watkins, L.R., Naeve, G.S. & Foster, A.C. (2004). Fractalkine (CX3CL1) and fractalkine receptor (CX3CR1) distribution in spinal cord and dorsal root ganglia under basal and neuropathic pain conditions. *Eur J Neurosci*, Vol.20, No.5, pp. 1150-1160.

Wang, M., Offord, J., Oxender, D.L. & Su, T.Z. (1999). Structural requirement of the calcium-channel subunit $\alpha_2\delta$ for gabapentin binding. *Biochem J*, Vol.342 (Pt 2), pp. 313-320.

Wang, W., Gu, J., Li, Y.Q. & Tao, Y.X. (2011). Are voltage-gated sodium channels on the dorsal root ganglion involved in the development of neuropathic pain? *Mol Pain*, Vol.7, pp. 16.

Wang, Z., Ma, W., Chabot, J.G. & Quirion, R. (2010). Calcitonin gene-related peptide as a regulator of neuronal CaMKII-CREB, microglial p38-NFkappaB and astroglial ERK-Stat1/3 cascades mediating the development of tolerance to morphine-induced analgesia. *Pain*, Vol.151, No.1, pp. 194-205.

Watkins, L.R., Hutchinson, M.R., Ledeboer, A., Wieseler-Frank, J., Milligan, E.D. & Maier, S.F. (2007). Norman Cousins Lecture. Glia as the "bad guys": implications for improving clinical pain control and the clinical utility of opioids. *Brain Behav Immun*, Vol.21, No.2, pp. 131-146.

Wen, X.J., Xu, S.Y., Chen, Z.X., Yang, C.X., Liang, H. & Li, H. (2010). The roles of T-type calcium channel in the development of neuropathic pain following chronic compression of rat dorsal root ganglia. *Pharmacology*, Vol.85, No.5, pp. 295-300.

Westenbroek, R.E., Hoskins, L. & Catterall, W.A. (1998). Localization of Ca^{2+} channel subtypes on rat spinal motor neurons, interneurons, and nerve terminals. *J Neurosci*, Vol.18, No.16, pp. 6319-6330.

Westin, B.D., Walker, S.M., Deumens, R., Grafe, M. & Yaksh, T.L. (2010). Validation of a preclinical spinal safety model: effects of intrathecal morphine in the neonatal rat. *Anesthesiology*, Vol.113, No.1, pp. 183-199.

Wheeler-Aceto, H., Porreca, F. & Cowan, A. (1990). The rat paw formalin test: comparison of noxious agents. *Pain*, Vol.40, No.2, pp. 229-238.

White, F.A., Jung, H. & Miller, R.J. (2007). Chemokines and the pathophysiology of neuropathic pain. *Proc Natl Acad Sci U S A*, Vol.104, No.51, pp. 20151-20158.

Wu, H.E., Sun, H.S., Cheng, C.W., Terashvili, M. & Tseng, L.F. (2006a). dextro-Naloxone or levo-naloxone reverses the attenuation of morphine antinociception induced by lipopolysaccharide in the mouse spinal cord via a non-opioid mechanism. *Eur J Neurosci*, Vol.24, No.9, pp. 2575-2580.

Wu, H.E., Sun, H.S., Cheng, C.W. & Tseng, L.F. (2006b). p38 mitogen-activated protein kinase inhibitor SB203580 reverses the antianalgesia induced by dextro-morphine or morphine in the mouse spinal cord. *Eur J Pharmacol*, Vol.550, No.1-3, pp. 91-94.

Wu, H.E., Thompson, J., Sun, H.S., Terashvili, M. & Tseng, L.F. (2005). Antianalgesia: stereoselective action of dextro-morphine over levo-morphine on glia in the mouse spinal cord. *J Pharmacol Exp Ther*, Vol.314, No.3, pp. 1101-1108.

Yaksh, T.L. (2006). Calcium channels as therapeutic targets in neuropathic pain. *J Pain*, Vol.7, No.1 Suppl 1, pp. S13-30.

Yaksh, T.L., Kohl, R.L. & Rudy, T.A. (1977). Induction of tolerance and withdrawal in rats receiving morphine in the spinal subarachnoid space. *Eur J Pharmacol*, Vol.42, No.3, pp. 275-284.

Yokoyama, K., Kurihara, T., Saegusa, H., Zong, S., Makita, K. & Tanabe, T. (2004). Blocking the R-type (Cav2.3) Ca^{2+} channel enhanced morphine analgesia and reduced morphine tolerance. *Eur J Neurosci*, Vol.20, No.12, pp. 3516-3519.

Yu, Y.Q., Zhao, F., Guan, S.M. & Chen, J. (2011). Antisense-Mediated Knockdown of Na(V)1.8, but Not Na(V)1.9, Generates Inhibitory Effects on Complete Freund's Adjuvant-Induced Inflammatory Pain in Rat. *PLoS One*, Vol.6, No.5, pp. e19865.

Zamponi, G.W., Lewis, R.J., Todorovic, S.M., Arneric, S.P. & Snutch, T.P. (2009). Role of voltage-gated calcium channels in ascending pain pathways. *Brain Res Rev*, Vol.60, No.1, pp. 84-89.

Zhang, Y., Conklin, D.R., Li, X. & Eisenach, J.C. (2005). Intrathecal morphine reduces allodynia after peripheral nerve injury in rats via activation of a spinal A1 adenosine receptor. *Anesthesiology*, Vol.102, No.2, pp. 416-420.

Zhang, Y., Li, H., Li, Y., Sun, X., Zhu, M., Hanley, G., Lesage, G. & Yin, D. (2011). Essential role of toll-like receptor 2 in morphine-induced microglia activation in mice. *Neurosci Lett*, Vol.489, No.1, pp. 43-47.

Zhuang, Z.Y., Kawasaki, Y., Tan, P.H., Wen, Y.R., Huang, J. & Ji, R.R. (2007). Role of the CX3CR1/p38 MAPK pathway in spinal microglia for the development of neuropathic pain following nerve injury-induced cleavage of fractalkine. *Brain Behav Immun*, Vol.21, No.5, pp. 642-651.

Zhuang, Z.Y., Wen, Y.R., Zhang, D.R., Borsello, T., Bonny, C., Strichartz, G.R., Decosterd, I. & Ji, R.R. (2006). A peptide c-Jun N-terminal kinase (JNK) inhibitor blocks mechanical allodynia after spinal nerve ligation: respective roles of JNK activation in primary sensory neurons and spinal astrocytes for neuropathic pain development and maintenance. *J Neurosci*, Vol.26, No.13, pp. 3551-3560.

2

Polymer Based Therapies for the Treatment of Chronic Pain

Pradeep K. Dhal, Diego A. Gianolio and Robert J. Miller*
Drug and Biomaterial R&D
Genzyme Corporation – A Sanofi Company, Waltham, MA, USA

1. Introduction

Since chronic pain manifests functional limitation, it is the leading cause of longer term disability [1, 2]. In the US alone, an estimated 75 million people suffer from chronic pain [3]. In addition to chronic pain, proper management of postoperative acute pain impacts the clinical outcome of patients undergoing surgery [4]. Opioid family of analgesics and non-steroidal anti-inflammatory drugs (NSAIDs) are the main stays of current pharmacological agents available for the management of chronic pain [5, 6]. However, current therapies for pain management show modest efficacy and are associated with significant side effects. The major adverse effects of oral NSAIDs are gastrointestinal bleeding, gastric ulcer, renal failure and cardiovascular risks (in particular with selective COX-2 inhibitors) [7, 8]. The side effects of opioid family therapies include constipation, nausea, cognitive impairment and most importantly addiction [9, 10]. Thus, development of safer and effective treatment of chronic pain is an important goal of current pharmaceutical research.

In recent years numerous efforts have been made to develop long-acting opioid analgesics and NSAIDs to modulate their pharmacokinetic profiles. Some of these include sustained release formulations and topical gels [11, 12]. Biological agents such as antibody against nerve growth factor (NGF) have also been evaluated as therapies for chronic pain. The anti-NGF antibody acts by sequestering NGF and thus inhibits its interaction with the NGF-receptor on the sensory neurons [13].

Polymeric approach offers an attractive route to develop novel therapeutic agents for effective management of chronic pain. Interesting physical and chemical characteristics of synthetic and natural polymers enable them as promising materials for biomedical applications such as therapeutic agents, drug delivery carriers, and medical devices [14, 15]. A number of polymer derived therapies have been commercialized in the marketplace [16, 17]. The present article reviews the current state of research and development efforts to discover and develop biomedical polymer as therapeutic agents for the treatment of chronic pain. While use of polymer-derived agents for the treatment of different kinds of pains will be highlighted, the primary focus of the present article pertains to management of pain arising from osteoarthritis. Furthermore, role of polymers as intrinsically pain relieving agents either alone or as chemical conjugates of low molecular weight pain modulating agents are described in this article. The research and development efforts to develop control release formulations of low molecular weight pain therapies are outside the scope of this article. There are in fact a number of interesting articles that describe this aspect of pain management therapies [18, 19].

2. Osteoarthritis pain

Osteoarthritis (OA) is one of the most prevalent musculo-skeletal degenerative diseases [20]. Although OA affects joints of the knee, hip, hand, and spine, knee is the most affected joint [21]. As a result of pain and reduced mobility, OA leads to significant loss of quality of life. Since OA is generally considered to be a result of mechanical "wear and tear" of joints, it typically affects people over the age of 60. However, its onset can be expedited at younger age due to other factors including obesity, genetic factors, and joint injury [22, 23]. Approximately 10% of the world's adult population over the age of 60 has been affected by OA [24]. Therefore, the economic burden of this disease, which includes healthcare costs and loss of productivity, is significant. These expenditures are likely to escalate with aging population. At present approximately 27 million people in the US suffer from OA and it has been estimated that by the year 2030 25% of the US adult population (a third of which of working age) will be affected by OA [25].

Although OA manifests a broad clinical syndrome, its primary cause has been attributed to the progressive breakdown of articular cartilage and chondrocytes within the synovial joints. This degeneration leads to narrowing of the joint space, suchondral sclerosis, and synovial inflammation. Breakdown of the cartilage results in alternation in joint mechanics, which further exacerbates the disease [26, 27]. In OA, concentrations of a number of mediators of inflammation such as cytokines, chemokines, and proteolytic enzymes like matrix metalloproteinases (MMPs) as well as free radicals are elevated in the synovial fluid that catalyze further degradation of cartilage [28, 29]. This process results in a self-sustaining degenerative circle that hinders the natural process of cartilage repair.

In spite of years of intensive research in tissue engineering, there has been no breakthrough to regenerate physiologically viable articular cartilage [30]. Also, no therapeutic agent has been developed that demonstrates structure modifying efficacy in OA patients [31]. The current therapies for OA are largely symptomatic in alleviating the chronic pain. These agents largely include anti-inflammatory agents, NSAIDs, and opioid family of analgesics. The relative efficacies of these therapies to relieve OA associated chronic pain have been modest at best [32, 33]. As mentioned earlier, long term use of these pharmacological agents results in major side effects (see above). In order to minimize systemic side effects associated with oral NSAIDs, topical agents containing the active agents have been developed. These delivery systems are expected to deliver the drugs in high concentrations locally and would reduce systemic side effects [34]. However, efficacy of these topical therapies is modest. In recent years, other novel therapeutic approaches for the management of OA pain has been pursued that include antibodies targeting NGF and antagonist of **T**ransient **R**eceptor **P**otential **V**anilloid (TRPV) family of ion channels [35, 36]. One of the attractive therapeutic options for treating OA associated pain are polymer based viscosupplements. The following section describes the state of viscosupplement based treatments for OA pain.

3. Hyaluronic acid derived viscosupplements

3.1 Hyaluronic acid and its biology

Hyaluronic acid or hyaluronan (HA) is a polysaccharide that belongs to the glycosaminoglycan class of biological macromolecules. This highly viscous anionic biopolymer is composed of β-1, 3-D-glucuronic acid and β-1, 4-N-acetyl-D-glucosamine arranged in an alternate fashion along the polymer backbone (Fig. 1). HA is ubiquitous in nature and is produced by every tissue of higher organisms and some bacteria. The biopolymer is found in the extracellular matrices (particularly in soft connective tissues), synovial fluid, and cartilage. HA is endogenously synthesized by chondrocytes and synoviocytes [37-39]. After being released into the synovial space, HA accumulates on the surfaces of cartilage and ligament. Endogenously synthesized HA is generally of very high molecular weight (in the range of 3 -5 million Dalton) and its fully hydrated form assumes a globular shape [40]. Unique viscoelastic properties of HA enables it to maintain rheological homeostasis of the synovial fluid in the joints and plays a critical role in providing lubrication, elasticity, and shock absorption to joint tissues. Furthermore, by providing a coat on the surface of articular cartilage, HA protects the cartilage and blocks the loss of proteoglycan from the cartilage matrix into the synovial space [41]. In healthy joint of human knee, the normal concentration of HA in the synovial fluid is in the range of 2.5 - 4.0 mg/mL. However, under pathological conditions such as osteoarthritis, the concentration of HA is significantly reduced (estimated to be ~ 1 - 2 mg/mL) [42]. Furthermore, the biopolymer undergoes degradation under diseased conditions with substantial reduction in molecular weight. A combination of lowering in concentration and molecular weights leads to lowering in viscosity and elasticity of synovial fluid and consequently adverse impact on joint function. Thus, catabolic degradation of HA directly correlates with the onset OA.

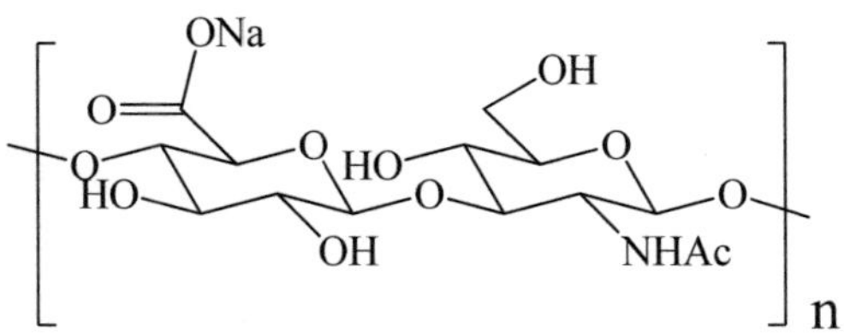

Fig. 1. Chemical structure of hyaluronic acid.

3.2 HA derivatives for the treatment of osteoarthritis

In addition to acting as a lubricant for the joint, HA has been reported to impart anti-inflammatory, anabolic, and chondroprotective effects [43, 44]. Since OA onset is attributed to degradation of high molecular weight HA and its concentration in the synovial fluid, increase in HA concentration either by increasing the rate of the proteoglycan biosynthesis or by incorporating HA exogenously to the joint space would improve joint function and relieve OA associated chronic pain. Therefore, the effect of intraarticular administration of exogenous HA to restore rheological properties of the synovial fluid have been extensively studied [45].

In order to maintain desired viscoelastic property of synovial fluid, the exogenous HA needs to have high molecular weight. It has been observed that the frequency and the amount of exogenous HA injected can be lowered by increasing the molecular weight of HA based exogenous viscosupplement. Towards that end, a variety of synthetic approaches have been undertaken to engineer high molecular weight HA derivatives [46]. In general, the desired rheological properties of HA based viscosupplements are achieved by crosslinking of naturally occurring linear HA to produce higher molecular weight compounds.

Functional group richness of HA has rendered it to be an important precursor material for the design and synthesis of numerous biomaterials with tuned physicochemical and biological properties that have found broad applications in biomedicine and biosurgery [47, 48]. HA offers three kinds of functional groups that can be used for chemical modification: carboxylic acid, primary and secondary hydroxyl, and N-acetyl (after removal of acetyl group to generate primary amine). While carboxyl groups can be modified to introduce amide and ester bonds, the hydroxyl groups can be subjected to reaction with various electrophiles such as epoxides, alkyl halides, alkyl tosylates, vinyl sulfones, etc. However, since HA is unstable at low pH, the chemical reactions employed for its modification must be selected very carefully so that they are mild and compatible to HA. This is necessary to avoid undesired degradation of HA to lower molecular weight. Furthermore, the byproducts of these reactions must be benign for both short- and long-term uses. Over the years, a great deal of research efforts have been put forth to synthesize chemically modified HA [49].

In order to synthesize HA derived viscosupplements, linear HA has been subjected to crosslinking reactions with a number of bifunctional reagents such as diepoxides, divinyl sulfone, epichlorohydrin etc [50, 51]. Some representative examples of crosslinking chemistries that were carried out to prepare HA based hydrogels are shown in Figure 2.

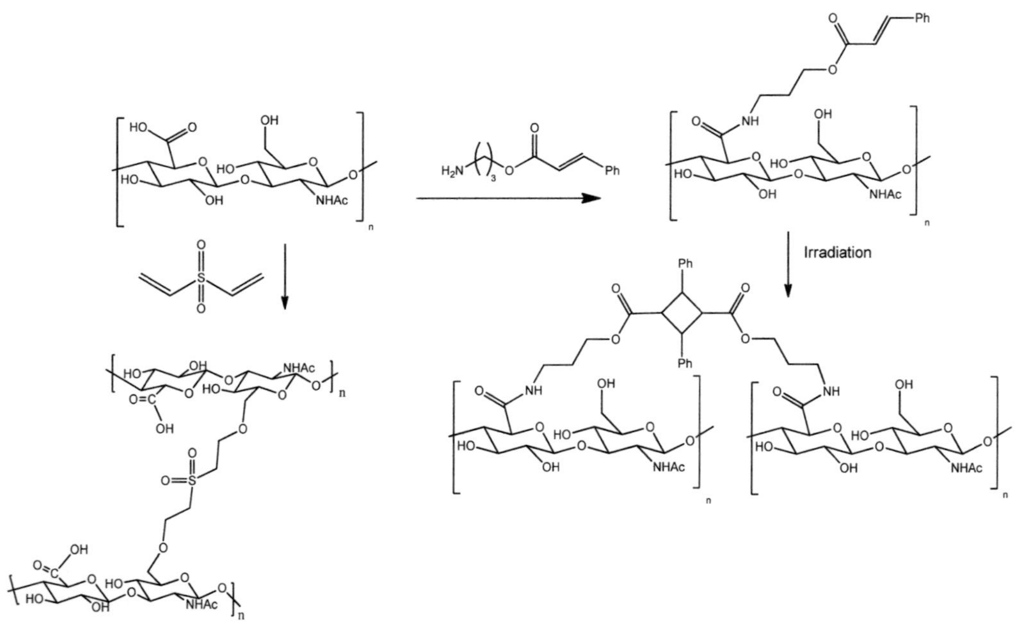

Fig. 2. Representative examples of crosslinking chemistries used to prepare HA hydrogels.

Several factors need to be taken into consideration while optimizing HA derived viscosupplementation products. For example, the rheological properties need to be tuned so that they match with those of native synovial fluid. The hydrogels must be free from any reagents that could trigger an inflammatory response associated with an exogenous material. The molecular weight of the hydrogel is critical to obtain desired clinical benefits since HA is prone to degradation and this process is accelerated in a diseased joint. A variety of HA derived crosslinked viscosupplements have been approved for human use.

The precursor HA for these preparations are obtained either from avian sources or by biofermentation in bacteria. Table 1 summarizes some important features of representative HA based viscosupplements that are marketed for intraarticular injection in the knee to relieve OA pain [52]. Particularly, these products differ by their molecular weights, which influence their rheological properties and hence residence time in the joint.

Brand name	Generic name	HA source	Modification type	Molecular weight (kDa)
Artz®/Supartz®	Sodium hyaluronate	Avian	N/A	600 - 1,200
Euflexxa®	Sodium hyaluronate	Biofermentation	N/A	2,400 - 3,600
Hyalgan®	Sodium hyaluronate	Avian	N/A	500 - 730
Intragel®	Sodium hyaluronate	Biofermentation	N/A	800 - 1, 200
Orthovisc®	High mol. Wt. hyaluronan	Biofermentation	Chemical Modification	1,100 - 2,900
Synvisc®	Hylan G-F 20	Avian	Cross-linked	6,000

Table 1. Representative examples of clinically approved hyaluronic acid (HA) based viscosupplementation products (reference 45).

One of the most effective viscosupplement that has been approved for clinical use is Synvisc® (Hylan G-F 20) and its single injection formulation, Synvisc-One® [53]. The main components of Synvisc® are HA lightly crosslinked with formaldehyde (Hylan A) and divinyl sulfone crosslinked hylan A (Hylan B). Synvisc® contains 90% (v/v) of Hylan A and 10% (v/v) of hylan B and its chemical structure is shown in Figure 3. Synvisc® has been approved for the treatment of pain associated with mild to moderate OA. In subsequent clinical studies it has been observed that intraarticular injection of Synvisc® resulted in significant pain relief in the carpometacapal joint, temporomandibular joint and the hip [54]. These findings suggest that pain relief from the intraarticular injections of HA-derived viscosupplements is not limited to knee. Since, OA of the hip is the second most common form of arthritis after OA of the knee, additional clinical investigation of the role of viscosupplements in relieving chronic pain arising from hip arthritis is warranted.

The biological mechanisms underlying the pharmacological action of HA derived viscosupplements to relieve OA pain are not completely understood. It was initially thought that since there is a reduced level of HA in OA joints, intraarticular injection of exogenous HA restores the rheological properties of synovial fluid to the level present in healthy joints. However, while the half-life of exogenous HA in the synovial fluid is only few days, its clinical effect in reducing OA pain has been found to be maintained for several months [55]. This indicates that mechanism of action of HA derived viscosupplements is of multifactorial nature and is a combination of physical and biological effects. A number of *in vitro* studies have been carried out to investigate the biological activities of HA [56]. The results of these studies suggest that HA exhibits chondroprotective and anti-inflammatory effects in the synoviocytes by preventing invasion of inflammatory cells to the joint space. Biological activity of HA has also been attributed to down regulation of the gene expression of various inflammatory cytokines and catabolic enzymes like aggrecanase. Furthermore, being a natural ligand of the cell surface receptor CD44, HA has been thought to impart its effect by modulating CD44-mediated metabolism. In another *in vitro* study, when synovial fibroblasts were cultured with high molecular weight HA, newly synthesized HA molecules were found. These biological effects of exogenous HA may result in overall cartilage protection [57, 58]. Thus, well controlled clinical studies would shed further light on the chondro-protection properties of exogenous HA like Synvisc and lead to the discovery of novel therapies with disease modifying properties.

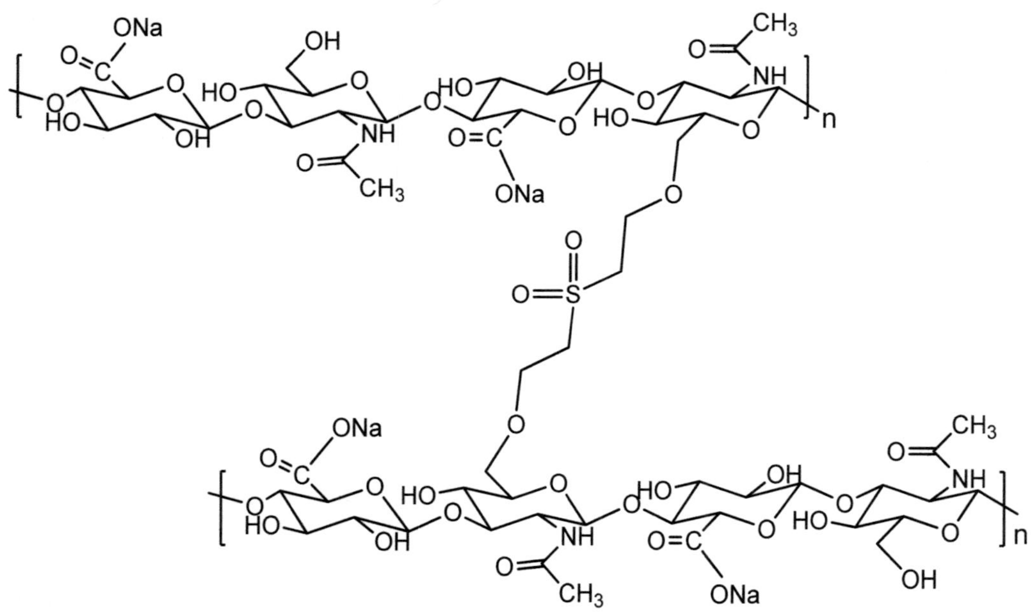

Fig. 3. Structure of Hylan B component of Synvisc®.

3.3 HA-steroid combinations for the treatment of chronic pain

One of the shortcomings of HA derived viscosupplements is their slower onset of action to reduce OA pain relative to low molecular weight drugs such as NSAIDs and steroids. Therefore, the viscosupplements are generally administered weekly over a course of three to five weeks. As described earlier, unlike traditional pain killers, pain relief from viscosupplements lasts much longer (up to several months). Although intraarticular injection of corticosteroids achieves maximum benefit within few days of injection, repeated injection of these catabolic agents can have adverse effect [59]. In order to achieve fast and longer lasting pain relief while minimizing the side effects of steroids, combination therapy of HA and corticosteroids have been envisioned. Non-covalently bound admixtures of HA gel with steroids, where the steroid is dispersed within the HA hydrogel matrix have been investigated as combination therapy to treat OA pain. This approach allows sustained local delivery of the steroid at OA site and would overcome the side effects associated with steroid overdose. Figure 4 shows the structures of representative corticosteroids that have used to prepare HA derived drug-viscosupplement composites.

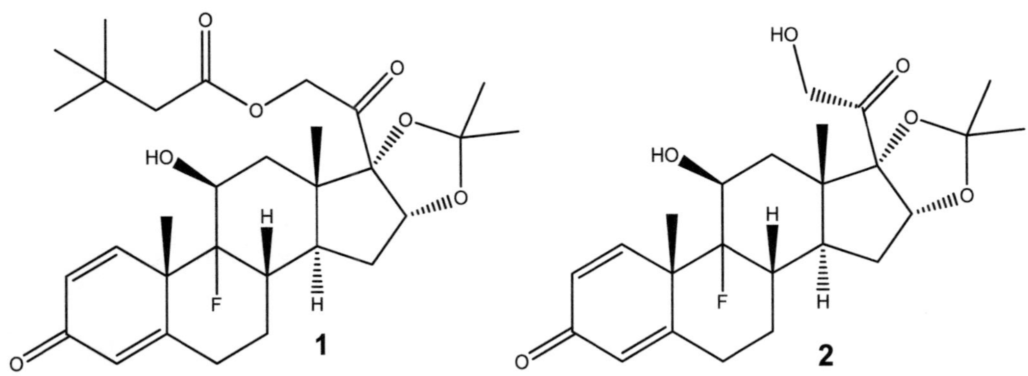

Fig. 4. Corticosteroids used to prepare HA-steroid composite hydrogel viscosupplements.

Preparation stable formulation of crosslinked HA hydrogel, Synvisc® with triamcinolone hexaacetonide (TAH) (Figure 4, **1**) was investigated by dispersing Tween-80 stabilized TAH colloidal suspension within a swollen gel of Syvisc® [60]. By optimizing the ratio of Synvisc® to TAH in the formulation mixture, a stable composite was obtained. The rheological properties of Synvisc® were not adversely affected by the presence of the hydrophobic corticosteroid and the composition was found to be stable in an accelerated shelf life test.

Another steroid-viscosupplement composite was prepared by crosslinking linear HA in the presence of triamcinolone acetonide (Figure 4, **2**). In this study, divinyl sulfone was allowed to react partially with HA to generate a linear HA structure with pendant vinyl sulfone group. To a solution of this vinyl sulfone functionalized HA was added a suspension of **2** and resulting reaction mixture was treated with α,ω-dithio polyethylene glycol (PEG) as the crosslinking agent. A crosslinked HA gel with relatively homogeneously distributed steroid particles within the gel matrix was obtained. The synthetic strategy adopted for the preparation of this dual-acting viscosupplement is shown in Figure 5 [61]. In a preliminary clinical study, this steroid-HA composite (Hydros-TA) showed faster pain relief compared to the corresponding native viscosupplement alone. Long term clinical study involving larger patient population needs to be carried out to demonstrate the clinical efficacy of such steroid-viscosupplement composites to treat OA associated chronic pain.

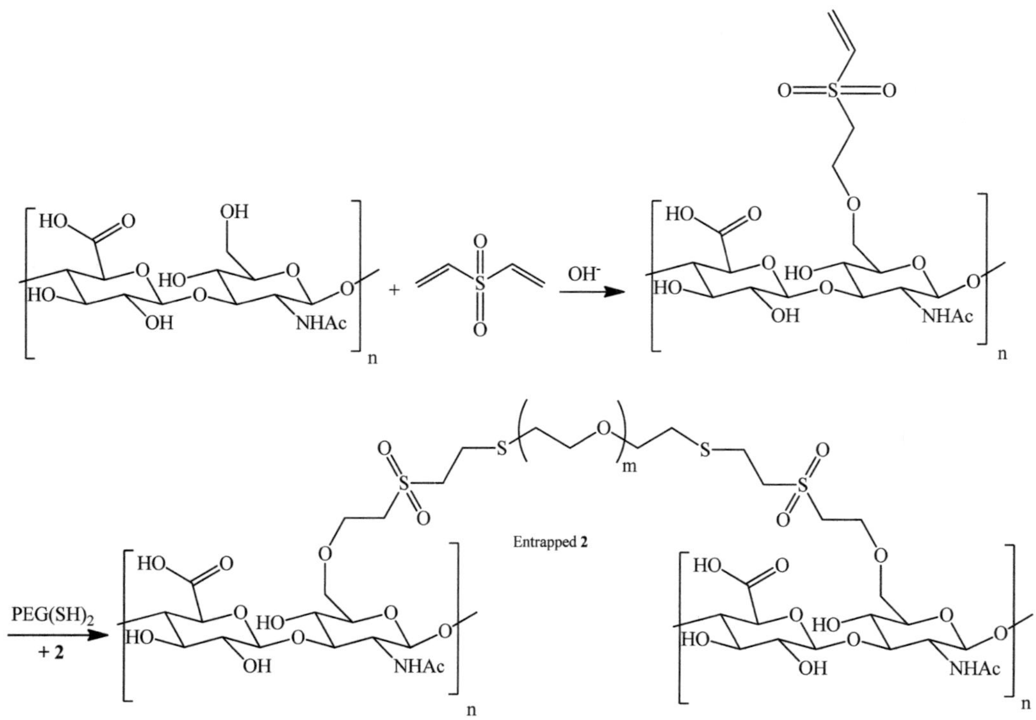

Fig. 5. Crosslinking of HA in the presence of a dispersion of triamcinolone acetonide to prepare viscosupplment-steroid composite hydrogel

3.4 Covalent conjugates of HA and low molecular pain killers

Intrinsic biocompatibility and its versatility for chemical modification make HA an attractive biomaterial to synthesize conjugated drug delivery systems. Chemical modification of HA has allowed the preparation of an array HA-drug conjugates and HA-protein conjugates as sustained-release carriers for drugs and biotherapeutics [62, 63]. Covalent conjugates of HA containing hydrogels with pain relieving agents have been explored as dual acting agents to treat chronic pain. This approach would offer a number of potential clinical benefits, that include: i) retaining viscosupplementation property of soluble HA, ii) minimizing the systemic exposure of NSAIDs and opioid family pain killers by localizing administration to the target site, iii) modulating the duration of action of these pain killers by incorporating appropriate conjugation chemistry to control the rate of cleavage of the drug from the HA gel, and iv) minimizing the frequency of administration of viscosupplement and the pain killer in the clinic. These features of the HA-drug conjugates could lead to better patient compliance and improved quality of life.

A series of HA derived functional hydrogels conjugated with local analgesics (e.g. bupivacaine) and opioid drugs (e.g. morphine) were synthesized in our laboratories as long acting treatments for chronic pain [64, 65]. Divinyl sulfone crosslinked HA hydrogel (Hylan B) was used as the polymer matrix for the synthesis of these drug conjugates. Appropriate linker arms were designed to tether these pain relieving agents to the HA matrix. Bupivacaine was conjugated to HA through a hydrolysable imide bond (Figure 6A). On the other hand, opioid drugs such as morphine, naloxone analogs were conjugated via a hydrolysable ester bonds (Figure 6B). A number of conjugates were synthesized by varying the nature of the linker arm, spacer length, and the amount of the drug loading. A systematic evaluation of the release kinetics of the drugs from the HA gel was carried out under *in vitro* conditions to identify an optimum composition. The optimum drug-HA conjugate from each class was evaluated *in vivo* for its biological activity. These drug-conjugated HA hydrogels exhibited therapeutic benefits by prolonging pain relief and were more effective than the individual agents and their admixtures. These preclinical research findings suggest that development of HA based viscosupplements conjugated with traditional pain relieving agents might lead to a promising new generation of long acting therapies for the treatment of OA associated chronic pain.

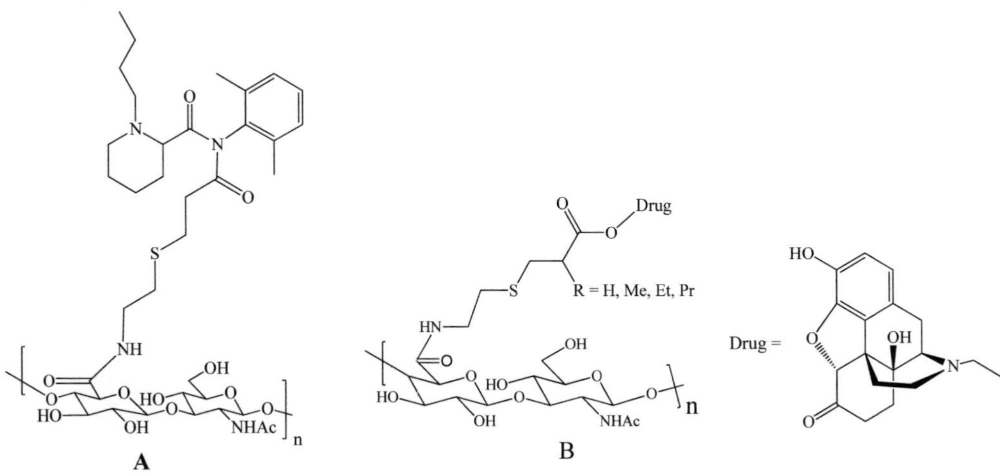

Fig. 6. HA conjugated local analgesics (A) and opioids.

In related work, conjugates of HA with methotrexate (MTX) were synthesized to achieve viscosupplementation and anti-inflammatory effect concurrently intraarticularly [66]. Increased levels of TNF-α have been found in the synovium of OA affected joints that can be mitigated by oral administration of MTX [67]. However, systemic administration of MTX is associated with certain side effects such as pneumonitis and myelosuppression [68]. Therefore, by localizing MTX to target joint by delivering it as a polymer conjugate, the systemic side effect could be minimized. After a careful structure-activity study by screening various linker arms and enzyme target groups, an optimized HA conjugate of MTX was identified (Figure 7). A peptiditic linker was chosen as target for cathepsin enzymes, which are over-expressed in OA joints. The polyethyleneglycol (PEG) linker was chosen to enable the peptide target to be accessible to the cathepsin enzyme in the joint environment. *In vitro* and *in vivo* studies revealed that the HA-MTX conjugate is capable of reducing joint pain and swelling of the knee. On the other hand, admixture of HA and MTX showed marginal efficacy.

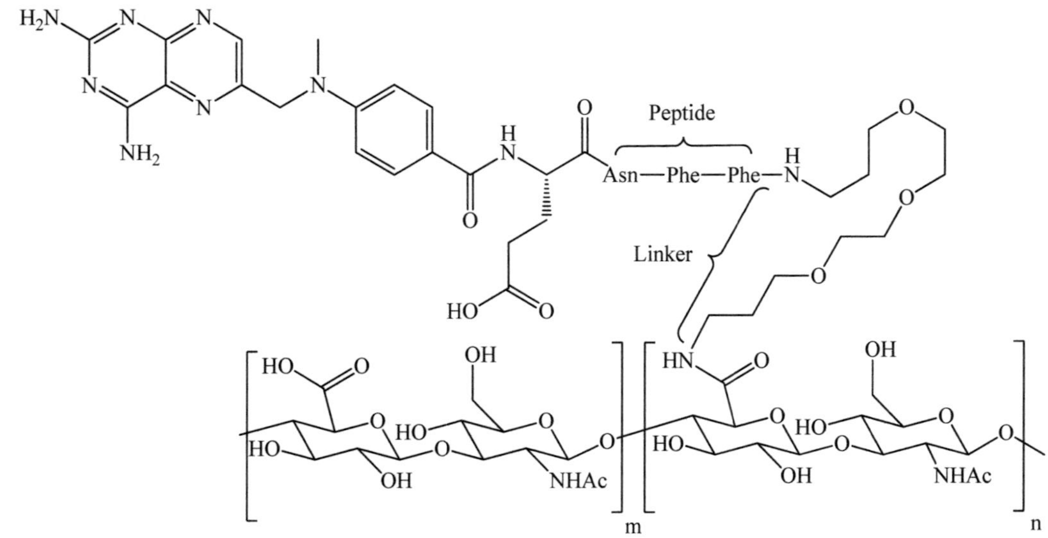

Fig. 7. HA conjugate of methotrexate as an intraarticular combination therapy for the treatment of OA pain.

4. Polymer-opioid conjugates and polymeric opioid derivatives

Besides being a first-line analgesic therapy for acute pain, opioids have been found to be useful in treating chronic pain. However, the adverse effects associated with their long term use limit the therapeutic benefits of opioid analgesics, thus leading to discontinuation of the therapy. Constipation (opioid-induced bowel dysfunction (OBD)) is one of the significant side effects associated with opioid therapies. OBD affects up to 80% of the patients undergoing opioid therapy. While other side effects associated with chronic use of opioids resolve with time, constipation continues to persist [69].

Efforts have been made to utilize polymeric approach to design and develop new generation of opioid analogs as pain killers. These polymeric compounds enable the patients to overcome OBD without losing the benefits of opioid therapy by limiting drugs' systemic absorption. Pegylation chemistry was utilized to synthesize these macromolecular opioids. The technology of pegylation has been successfully utilized to improve pharmacokinetic properties of a number of (bio)pharmaceutical agents [70]. Two representative polymer conjugated opioid derivatives are shown in Figure 8. These compounds consist of naloxol analogs linked to PEG chains through hydrolytically stable ether linkage [71, 72]. In preclinical studies, these pegylated opioid derivatives were found to maintain their centrally mediated analgesia, while antagonizing peripherally mediated constipation. One of the key conjugates, NKTR-118 (Figure 8A, n = 7) has proceeded to advanced clinical trial. In the phase II clinical trial, patients receiving NKTR-118 exhibited significant increase in bowel movement compared to patients receiving native naloxol, without compromising the analgesic property of the opioid [73]. NKTR-118 is currently undergoing phase III clinical trial.

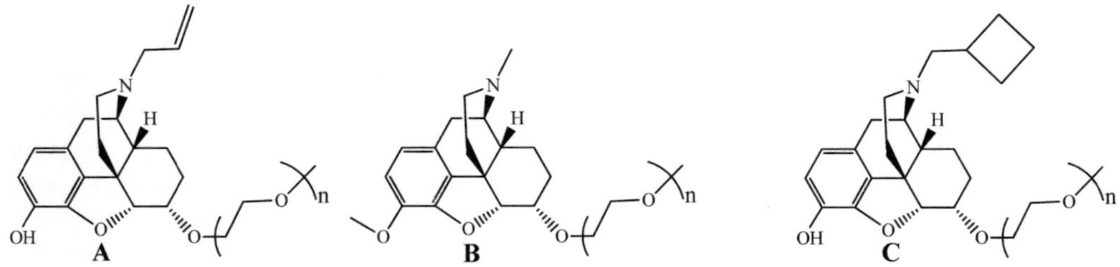

Fig. 8. Polymer modified naloxol derivatives to prevent opioid induced constipation.

Another interesting approach to develop polymeric pain relievers has been reported that utilizes a polymerization chemistry to synthesize poly(anhydride-esters), where the bioactive drug becomes part of the polymer backbone [74]. The general structure of this class of polymeric pain relievers is shown in Figure 9. Following this strategy, they were able to incorporate significant amounts (~ 62%) of the deliverable drug to the polymer chain. Hydrolytic degradation of these poly(anhydride-ester) polymers under physiological pH conditions releases the drug in a controlled manner. As a result, the side effects associated with the native drug (if released immediately) can be minimized. Some of the polymeric pain relievers reported are poly(anhydride-esters) containing the anti-inflammatory agent, salicylic acid and the opioid drug, morphine (Figure 10). Although syntheses of polymeric pain relievers based on these poly(anhydride-ester) scaffolds have been studied extensively, there is limited information about the biological activities of these polymers as treatments for chronic pain [75, 76]. Nevertheless, these polymeric opioids and anti-inflammatory agents offer a new perspective to develop novel treatments for chronic pain.

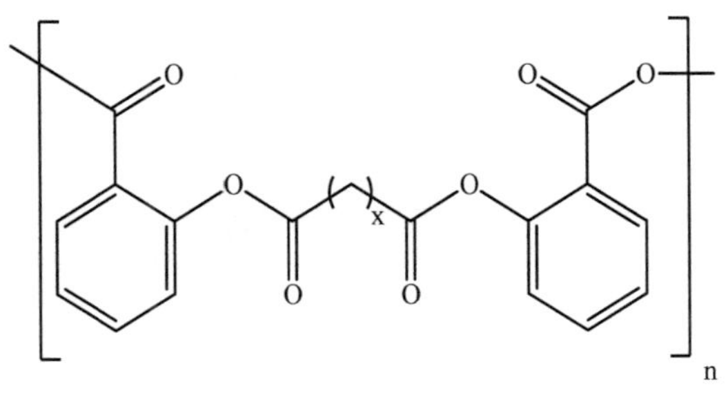

Fig. 9. Structure of salicylic acid-based poly(anhydride-esters) as polymeric anti-inflammatory agents.

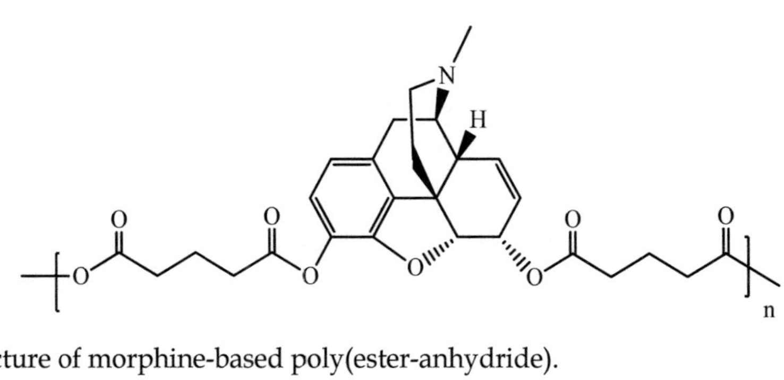

Fig. 10. Structure of morphine-based poly(ester-anhydride).

5. Conclusion

Because of its clinical relevance, development of novel pharmacologic agents for effective management of chronic pain continues to be an important goal of pharmaceutical research. Although numerous therapeutic agents with different modes of action have been developed to treat chronic pain, no single agent exhibits the most desired profile. For example, while opioids and NSAIDs remain the main stay of therapeutic options, concerns over their associated side effects have begun to limit their use. Polymeric approach offers a variety of options to develop a new generation of pain relievers, which include intrinsically bioactive polymers to different delivery systems for traditional pain killers. HA derived viscosupplements offer an attracting option to treat chronic pain due to excellent biocompatibility and various biological functions of HA. The ability to trigger various biological functions makes HA based viscosupplements as promising agents to not only relieve symptomatic effects of chronic OA pain, but also to bring about potentially disease modifying effects. Therapies comprising of polymers in combination with traditional pain killers (either as conjugates or as stable non-covalent formulations) have been found to minimize the side effects of the latter. By targeting the disease via different mechanisms of actions, these combination agents could become superior therapeutic options to treat chronic pain. With increasing understanding of the pathobiology of chronic pain and intense research in biomedical polymers, it will be possible to develop novel polymer based therapies in the near future that are safe and could act as structure modifying treatments for chronic pain.

6. References

[1] Smith B. H & Torrance N. (2011). Management of Chronic Pain in Primary Care. *Cur. Opin. Suppor. Palliat. Care*, Vol. 5, No.2, pp. 137-142

[2] Teets, R.Y.; Dahmer, S. & Scott, E. (2010). Integrative Medicine Approach to Chronic Pain. *Primary Care*, vol.37, No.2, 407-421.

[3] National Center for Health Statistics (2006), *Health, United States, 2006 with Chartbook on Trends in the Health of Americans*. Hyattsville, MD: Dept. of Health and Human Services, Centers for Disease Control and Prevention.

[4] Vadivelu, N.; Mitra, S. & Narayan, D. (2010). Recent Advances in Postoperative Pain Management. *Yale J. Biol. Med.* Vol.83, No.1, pp.11-25

[5] Turk, D. C.; Wilson, H.D. & Cahana, A. (2011). Treatment of Chronic Non-cancer Pain. *Lancet*, Vol. 377, No.9784, pp. 2226-2235

[6] Chan, B. K. B.; Tam, L. K.; Wat, C. Y.; Chung, Y. F. ; Tsui, S. L. & Cheung, C. W. (2011). Opioids in Chronic Non-cancer Pain. *Expert. Opin. Pharmacother.* , Vol. 12, No.5, pp.705-720

[7] Scanzello, C. R.; Moskowitz, N. K. & Gibofsky, A. (2010). The Post-NSAID Era: What to Use Now for the Pharmacologic Treatment of Pain and Inflammation in Osteoarthritis. *Cur. Rheomatol. Rep.*, Vol. 10, No.1, pp49-56

[8] Roth, S. H. (2011). Nonsteroidal Anti-Inflammatory Drug Gastropathy: New Avenues for Safety. *Clin. Interven. Aging.*, Vol. 6, pp 125-131

[9] Crofford, L. J. (2010). Adverse Effects of Chronic Opioid Therapy for Chronic Musculoskeletal Pain. *Nat. Rev. Rheumatol.* Vol. 6, No. 4, pp. 191-197

[10] Merza, Z. (2010). Chronic Use of Opioids and Endocrine System. *Hormone Metabol. Res.*, Vol. 42, No. 9, pp. 621-626.

[11] Weiniger, C. F.; Golovanevski, M.; Sokolsky-Papkov, M. & Domb, A. J. (2010). Review of Prolonged Local Anesthetic Action. *Expert. Opin. Drug. Deliv.*, Vol. 7, No.6, pp.737-752.

[12] Haroutiunian, S.; Drennan,D. A.; Lipman, A. G. (2010). Topical NSAID Therapy for Musculoskeletal Pain. *Pain. Med.*, Vol. 11, No. 4, pp.535-549

[13] Cattaneo, A. (2010). Tanezumab, a Recombinant Humanized mAb Against Nerve Growth Factor for the Treatment of Acute and Chronic Pain. *Cur. Opin. Mol. Ther.*, Vol. 12, No.1, pp.94-106

[14] Nair, L.S.& Laurencin, C. T. (2006). Polymers as Biomaterial for Tissue Engineering and Controlled Drug Delivery, *Adv. Biochem. Eng. Biotechnol.*, Vol. 102, No. 1, pp47-90

[15] Dhal, P. K., Huval, C. C. Holmes-Farley, S. R. & Jozefiak, T. J. Polymers as Drugs. *Adv. Polym. Sci.*, Vol. 192, No.1, pp 9-58 (2006)

[16] Duncan, R. (2003). The Dawning Era of Polymer Therapeutics. *Nat. Rev. Drug. Discov.*, Vol. 2, No. pp. 347-360

[17] Dhal, P. K. Polomoscanik, S.C.; Avila, L. Z.; Holmes-Farley, S.R. & Miller, R. J. (2009). Functional Polymers as Therapeutic Agents: Concept to Marketplace. *Adv. Drug Deliv. Rev.*, Vol. 61, No.13, pp1121-1130

[18] Manjanna, K. M.; Shivakumar, B. & Kumar, T. M. P. (2010). Microencapsulation: An Acclaimed Novel Drug-Delivery System for NSAIDs in Arthritis. *Crit. Rev. Therap. Drug Carr. Sys.*, Vol. 27, No.6, pp. 509-545

[19] Rainsfold, K. D.; Kean, W. F. & Ehrlich, G. E. (2008). Review of the Pharmaceutical Properties and Clinical Effects of the Topical NSAID Formulation, Diclofenac Epolamine. *Cur. Med. Res. Opin.*, Vol. 24, No.10, pp. 2967-2992

[20] Felson, D. T. (2004). An Update on the Pathogenesis and Epidemiology of Osteoarthritis. *Radiol. Clin. N. Am.* , Vol. 42, No. 1, pp. 1-9

[21] Kean, W. F. & Buchanan, W. F. (2004). Osteoarthritis: Symptoms, Sign, and Source of Pain. *Inflamm. Pharmacol.*, Vol. 12, No. 1, pp. 3-31

[22] Sharma, L.; Kapoor, D. & Issa, S. (2006). Epidemiology of Osteoarthritis: An Update. *Cur. Opin. Rheumatol.*, Vol. 18, No. 2, pp. 147- 156

[23] Spector, T. D. & MacGregor, A. J. (2004). Risk Factors for Osteoarthritis: Genetics. *Osteoarthr. Cartil.*, Vol. 12, pp. S39-S44

[24] WHO Scientific Group (2003). The Burden of Musculoskeletal Condition at the Start of the New Millennium. *World Health Organ. Tech. Rep. Ser.*, Vol. 919, pp 1-218

[25] Centers for Disease Control and Prevention (2010). Arthritis-related Statistics, August 2010. Available from: http://www.cdc.gov/arthritis/data_statistics/ arthritis_related_stats.htm

[26] Wieland, H. A.; Michaelis, M.; Kirschbaum, B. J. & Rudolphi, K. A. (2010). Osteoarthritis: An Untreatable Disease. *Nat. Rev. Drug. Discov.*, Vol. 4, No. 4, pp. 331-345

[27] Felson, D. T. & Neogi, T. (2004). Osteoarthritis: Is It a Disease of Cartilage or Bone? *Arthrit Rheumatol.*, Vol. 50, pp 341-344

[28] Roach, H. I.; Aigner, T.; Soder, S.; Haag, J.; Welkerling, H. (2007). Pathobiology of Osteoarthritis: Pathomechanisms and Potential Therapeutic Targets. *Cur. Drug. Targets*, Vol.8, No. 2, pp. 271- 282

[29] Burrage, P.S.; Mix, K. S. & Brinckerhiff, C. E. (2006). Matrix Metalloproteinases : Role in Arthritis. *Front. Biosci.*, Vol. 11, No. 1, pp 529-543
[30] Becerra, J.; Andrades, J. A.; Guerado, E.; Zamora-Navas, P.; Lopez-Puertas, J. M. & Reddi, A. H. (2010). Articular Cartilage: Structure and Regeneration. *Tissue Eng. Part B.*, Vol. 16, No. 6, pp. 617- 627
[31] Altman, R. D. (2005). Structure-/Disease-modifying Agents for Osteoarthritis. *Semin. Rheumatol. Arthritis*, Vol. 34, No. 6 (suppl. 2), pp. 3 -5
[32] Kroenke, K.; Krebbs, E. E. & Bair, M. J. (2009). Pharmacotherapy of Chronic Pain: A Synthesis of Recommendation from Systematic *Reviews. Gen. Hosp. Psychiatry*, Vol. 31, 206 -219
[33] Manchikanti, L & Singh, A. (2008). Therapeutic Opioids: A Ten-year Perspective on the Complexities and Complications of the Escalating Use, Abuse, and Nonmedical Use of Opioids. *Pain Physician*, Vol.11, No.2, pp. S63-S88
[34] Schuelert, N.; Russell, F. A. & McDougall, J. J. (2011). *Ortho. Res. Rev.*, Vol. 3, No. 1, pp. 1-8
[35] Seidel, M. F.; Herguijuela, M.; Forkert, R. & Otten, U. (2010). Nerve Growth Factor in Rheumatic Diseases. Semi. *Arthritis. Rheumatol.*, Vol. 40, No.2, pp. 109- 126
[36] Wong, G. Y. & Gavva, N. R. (2009). Therapeutic Potential of Vanilloid Receptor TRPV1 Agonists and Antagonists as Analgesics: Recent Advances and Setbacks. *Brain Res. Rev.*, Vol. 60, No. 1, pp. 267- 277
[37] Laurent, T. C. & Fraser, J. R. (1992). Hyaluronan. *FASEB J.*, Vol. 6, No. &, pp. 2397- 2404
[38] Yamada, T. & Kawasaki, T. (2005). Microbial Synthesis of Hyaluronan and Chtin: New Approaches. *J. Biosci. Bioeng.*, Vol. 99, No. 6, pp. 521- 528
[39] Balazs, E. (1982). The Physical Properties of Synovial Fluid and the Specific Role of Hyaluronic Acid. In *Disorders of the Knee,* Helfert A. J. (Ed), J. B. Lippincott, Philadelphia, pp. 61-74
[40] Scott, J. E. & Heatley, F. (1999). Hyaluronan Forms Specific Stable Tertiary Structures in Aqueous Solution: A ^{13}C NMR Study. *Proc. Natl. Acad. Sci. USA*, Vol. 96, No. 9, pp. 4850-4855
[41] Shen, B.; Wei, A.; Bhargav, D., Kishen, T. & Diwan, A. D. (2010). Hyaluronan: Its Potential Application in Intervertebral Disc Regeneration. *Ortho. Res. Rev.*, Vol. 2, No. 1, pp. 17-26
[42] Watterson, J. R. & Esdaile, J. M. (2000). Viscosupplementation: Therapeutic Mechanisms and Clinical Potential in Osteoarthritis of the Knee. *J. Am. Acad. Orthop. Surg.*, Vol. 8, No. 5, pp. 277- 284
[43] Volpi, N.; Schiller, J. & Stern, R. (2009). Role, Metabolism, Chemical Modification, and Applications of Hyaluronan. *Cur. Med. Chem.*, Vol. 16, No. 14, pp. 1718- 1745
[44] Bastow, E. R., Byers, S. & Golub, S. B. (2008). Hyaluronan Synthesis and Degradation in Cartilage and Bone. *Cell Mol. Life Sci.*, Vol. 65, No. 3, pp. 395- 413
[45] Gigante, A. & Callegari, L. (2011). The Role of Intra-articular Hyaluronan in the Treatment of Osteoarthritis. *Rheumatol. Int.*, Vol. 31, pp 427 -444
[46] Burdick, J. A. & Prestwich, G. D. (2011). Hyaluronic Hydrogels for Biomedical Applications. *Adv. Mater.*, Vol. 23, No.12, pp. H41-H56
[47] Avila, L. Z.; Gianolio, D. A.; Konowicz, P. A.; Philbrook, M.; Santos, M. R. & Miller, R. J. (2008). Drug Delivery and Medical Applications of Chemically Modified

Hyaluronan. In *Carbohydrate Chemistry, Biology and Medical Applications*. Garg, H.G.; Cowman, M. K. & Hales, C. A. (Eds.), Elsevier, Amsterdam, pp. 333- 357
[48] Leonelli, F.; La Bella, A.; Migneco, L. M.& Bettelo, R. M. (2007). Design, Synthesis and Applications of Hyaluronic acid- Paclitaxel Bioconjugates. *Molecules*, Vol. 13, pp. 360 -378
[49] Schante, C. E.; Zuber, G.; Herlin, C. & Vandamme, T. F. (2011). Chemical Modification of Hyaluronic Acid for the Synthesis of Derivatives for a Broad Range of Biomedical Applications. *Carbohy. Polym.*, Vol. 85, No.3, pp.469- 489
[50] Balazs, E. A. (2009). Therapeutic Use of Hyaluronan. *Struct. Chem.*, Vol. Vol.20, No. 2, pp. 341-349
[51] Allison, D. D. & Grande-Allen, K. J. (2006). Hyaluronan: A Powerful Tissue Engineering Tool. *Tissue. Eng.*, Vol. 12, No. 8, pp. 2131- 2140
[52] Abate, M.; Pulcini, D.; Di Iorio, A.& Schiavone, C. (2010). Viscosupplementa-tion with Intra-articular Hyaluronic Acid for the Treatment of Osteoarthritis in the Elderly. *Cur. Pharm. Des.*, Vol. 16, No. 6, pp. 331- 340.
[53] Stitik, T. P.; Kazi, A. & Kim, J.-H. (2008). Synvisc in Knee Osteoarthritis. *Future Rheumatol.*, Vol. 3, No. 3, pp. 215- 222
[54] Migliore, A.; Giovannangeli, F.; Granta, M. & Lagana, B. (2010). Hylan G-F 20: Review of Its Safety and Efficacy in the Management of Joint Pain in Osteoarthritis. *Clin. Med. Insights: Arthr. Musculo. Disord.*, Vol. 3, No. 1, pp 55-68
[55] Bagga, H.; Burkhardt, D.; Sambrook, P. & March, L. (2006). Long-term Effects of Intrarticular Hyaluronan on Synovial Fluids in Osteoarthritis of the Knee. *J. Rheumatol.*, Vol. 33, No. 5, pp. 946- 950
[56] Moreland, L. W. (2002). Intra-articular Hyaluronan and Hylans for the Treatment of Osteoarthritis: Mechanisms of Action. *Arthr. Res. Ther.*, Vol. 5, No. 2, pp. 54 - 67
[57] Waddell, D. D. (2007). Viscosupplementation with Hyaluronan for Osteoarthritis of Knee: Clinical Efficacy and Economic Implications. *Drug & Aging*, Vol. 24, No. 8, pp. 629- 642
[58] Altman, R. D. (2010).Non-avian-derived Hyaluronan for the Treatment of Osteoarthritis of the Knee. *Exper. Rev. Clin. Immunol.*, Vol. 6, No.1, pp. 21- 27
[59] Gossec, L.; Dougados, M. (2006). Do Intra-articular Therapies Work and Who Will Benefit Most? *Best Pract. Res. Clin. Rheumatol.*, Vol. 20, No. 1, pp 131 - 144
[60] Chang, G.; Voschin, E.; Yu, L.-P. & Skrabut, E. (2011). Stable Hyaluronan/Steroid Formulation. *United States Patent Application*, No.2011/00559918 A1
[61] Gravett, D. M; Daniloff, G. Y. & He, P. (2010). Modified Hyaluronic Acid Compositions and Related Methods. *Unites States Patent*, No. 7,829, 118 B1
[62] Varghese, O.P.; Sun, W.; Hilborn, J. & Ossipov, D. A. (2009). In-situ Crosslinkable High Molecular Weight Hyaluronan-bisphosphonate Conjugates for Localized Delivery and Cell-specific Targeting: A Hydrogel Linked Prodrug Approach. *J. Am. Chem. Soc.*, Vol. 131, No. 25, pp. 8781 - 8783
[63] Sun, L. T.; Buchholz, K. S.; Lotze, M. T. & Washburn, N. R. (2010). Cytokine Binding by Polysaccharide-Antibody Conjugates. *Mol. Pharm.*, Vol. 7, No. 5, pp. 1769 - 1777
[64] Gianolio, D. A.; Philbrook, M.; Avila, L. Z.; MacGreggor, H.; Duan, S. X.; Bernasconi, R.; Slavsky, M.; Dethlefsen, S.; Jarrett, P. K. & Miller, R. J. (2005). Synthesis and Evaluation of Hydrolyzable Hyaluronan-Tethered Bupivacaine Delivery Systems. *Bioconj. Chem.*, Vol. 16, No. 6, pp. 1512 - 1518

[65] Gianolio, D. A.; Philbrook, M.; Avila, L. Z.; Young, L. E.; Plate, L.; Santos, M. R.; Bernasconi, R.; Liu H.; Ahn, S., Sun, W. Jarrett, P. K. & Miller, R. J. (2008). Hyaluronan-Conjugated Opioid Depots: Synthetic Strategies and Release Kinetics *In Vitro* and *In vivo*. *Bioconj. Chem.*, Vol. 19, No. 9, pp. 1767 - 1774

[66] Homma, A.; Sato, H.; Okamachi, A. et. al. (2009).Novel Hyaluronic Acid- Methotrexate Conjugates for Osteoarthritis Treatment. *Bioorg. Med. Chem.*, Vol. 17, No. pp. 4647 – 4656

[67] Bondeson, J. (2010). Activated Synovial Macrophages as Targets for Osteoarthritis Drug Therapy. *Cur. Drug. Tar.*, Vol. 11, No. 5, pp. 576 - 585

[68] Hamstra, D. A.; Page, M.; Maybuam, J. & Rehemtulla, A. (2000). Expression of Endogenously Activated Secreted or Cell Surface Carboxypeptidase A Sensitizes Tumor Cells to Methotrexate-α-Peptide Prodrugs. *Cancer Res.*, Vol. 60, No. 3, pp 657.

[69] Asai, T. & Power, I. (1999). Naloxone Inhibits Gastric Emptying in Rats. *Anesth. Analg.*, Vol. 88, No. 1, pp. 204 – 208

[70] Harris, J. M. & Chess, R.B. (2003). Effect of Pegylation on Pharmaceuticals. *Nat. Rev. Drug. Discov.*, Vol. 2, No.3, pp. 214 - 221

[71] Jude-Fishburn, C. S.; Riley, T. A.; Zacarias, A. N. & Gursahani, H. (2011). Pegylated Opioids with Low Potential for Abuse and Side Effects. *PCT Int. Appl.*, WO 2011088140 A1

[72] Diego, L.; Atayee, R.; Helmons, P.; Hsiao, G & von Gunten, C.F. (2011). Novel Opioid Antagonists for Opioid-Induced Bowel Dysfunction. *Exper. Opin. Investig. Drugs*, Vol. 20, No. 8, pp. 1047- 1056

[73] Hipkin, R. W. & Dolle, R. E. (2010). Opioid Receptor Antagonists for Gastrointestinal Dysfunction. *Ann. Rep. Med. Chem.* Vol. 45, No. 1, 143 – 155

[74] Schemltzer, R. C. ; Johnson, M; Griffin, J. & Uhrich, K. (2008). Comparison of Salicylate Based Poly(anhydride-esters) formed via Melt Condensation versus Solution Polymerization. *J. Biomat. Sci. Polym. Edn.*, Vol. 19, No. 10, pp. 1295- 1306

[75] Feng, W. Yu, L. & Uhrich, K. E. (2008). Opioid-Based Poly(anhydride-esters): New Approach to Preventing Drug Abuse. *Polym. Prepr.*, Vol. 49, No. 2, pp. 454 – 455

[76] Rosario-Melendez, Roselin; Delgado-Rivera, Roberto; Yu, Lei & Uhrich, K. E. (2011). Synthesis, Characterization, and *In Vitro* Studies of a Morphine-Based Poly(anhydride- ester). *Polym. Mater. Sci. Eng.*, Vol. 105, No. 2, pp 833 - 835

3

Molecular Aspects of Opioid Receptors and Opioid Receptor Painkillers

Austin B. Yongye and Karina Martínez-Mayorga
Torrey Pines Institute for Molecular Studies, Port Saint Lucie, FL, USA

1. Introduction

The unpleasant sensation of pain is experienced by all human beings at a given point in life. When pain gets severe and/or chronic it requires medical treatment. For over a thousand years, opioid agonists have been employed therapeutically to treat pain, with the first reports of such use involving the alkaloid morphine dated to the second century B.C.(Waldhoer, Bartlett et al. 2004) The term *opioid* refers to any substance with opium-like activity. Opium is extracted from the juice of the poppy plant *Papaver somniferum*. Opium contains in excess of 20 different alkaloids, and for centuries its crude form was used for pain management and for its psychological effects. In 1806 the German pharmacist Sertürner isolated a pure substance from opium, which he called morphine after the Greek god of dreams, Morpheus. Thereafter other alkaloids such as codeine (1832) and papaverine (1848) were isolated.(Reisine and Pasternak 1996) These discoveries paved the way for the use of pure alkaloids as opposed to crude opium in the medical profession. It became apparent that these alkaloids had a high potential for abuse and addiction. However, it was not until 1973 that the first descriptions of the pharmacological properties of morphine, along with other agonists and antagonists, at the level of the receptor were reported.(Pert, Pasternak et al. 1973)

Opioid receptors are of therapeutic relevance because they constitute the primary targets in the clinical treatment of both acute and chronic pain. They are members of the superfamily of seven helix transmembrane (TM) proteins known as G-protein coupled receptors (GPCRs); so-called because they are coupled in the cytoplasmic side to a group of G_i/G_o hetero-trimeric proteins called G-proteins: G_α, G_β and G_γ.(Eguchi M 2004) Currently four types of opioid receptors have been identified: μ (mu for morphine), κ (kappa for ketocyclazocine), δ (delta for deferens given that it was originally discovered in the vas deferens of mice)(Waldhoer, Bartlett et al. 2004) and orphan opioid receptor-like 1. They are in turn sub-divided into additional subtypes on the basis of their ligand binding and pharmacological profiles: μ_1-μ_2, κ_1-κ_3, and δ_1-δ_2.(Pasternak 1993; Blakeney, Reid et al. 2007) The μ, κ and δ main types are the most studied, each playing a different role in pain sedation: the μ-receptor generates the most profound analgesia, but is also associated with constipation, respiratory depression, euphoria, tolerance, dependence and addition;(Schmauss and Yaksh 1984; Cowan, Zhu et al. 1988) the δ-receptor is involved in pain relief from thermal sources,(Mansour, Khachaturian et al. 1988) but like the μ-receptor, it is also associated with respiratory depression and addiction;(Abdelhamid, Sultana et al.

1991; Maldonado, Negus et al. 1992) the κ-receptor mediates pain originating from chemical stimuli,(Leighton, Johnson et al. 1987; Wollemann, Benyhe et al. 1993) but it promotes dysphoria, diuresis and sedation.(von Voigtlander, Lahti et al. 1983; Lahti, Mickelson et al. 1985) There is also evidence that opioid receptors exist as homo- or hetero-oligomeric complexes and that their pharmacological responses may be cross-modulated.(Zhu, King et al. 1999; Rutherford, Wang et al. 2008) For instance, Waldhoer M et al. used 6′-GNTI to demonstrate the existence of a δ-κ hetero-dimer *in vivo*.(Waldhoer, Fong et al. 2005) Furthermore, δ-opioid antagonists suppress some of the side effects of μ-opioid agonists such as dependence and tolerance while retaining their analgesic properties.(Ananthan 2006) The realization of this potential for cross-modulation generated interests in developing so-called bivalent ligands of opioid receptors.(Dietis, Guerrini et al. 2009; Balboni, Salvadori et al. 2011) One therapeutic relevance of opioid receptors worth mentioning is that opioid receptors antagonists such as naloxone are utilized clinically in the treatment of morphine and heroin addiction and overdose.(Blakeney, Reid et al. 2007) In this chapter, we summarize structural aspects of opioid receptors and opioid receptor ligands, with special emphasis on the μ-opioid receptor. The importance of the combined use of experimental information and computational models is highlighted.

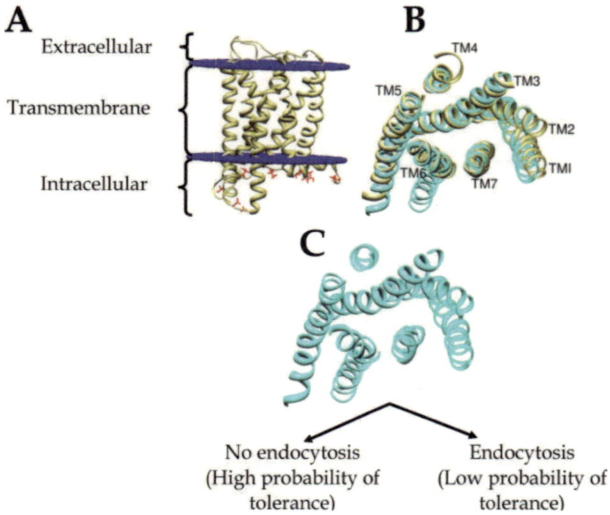

Fig. 1. (A) The three domains of the μ-opioid receptor. Intracellular serine, threonine and tyrosine residues are shown in red. (B) Extracellular perspective: the seven transmembrane helices are arranged sequentially in a counterclockwise direction. The modeled active and inactive structures are shown in cyan and tan, respectively. A substantial structural difference between the two states can be seen at TM6. (C) Hypothesized outcome of degree of ligand-induced receptor endocytosis. Homology models from Pogozheva, I. D., A. L. Lomize, et al. (1998), Fowler, C. B. et al. (2004).

2. Biochemical and biophysical characterization of the μ-opioid receptor

2.1 Structural studies of the μ-opioid receptor

The notion of preferential stabilization of distinct conformational states by agonists and non-agonists has been established experimentally and also demonstrated computationally (see Figure1). The experimental studies include: Li *et al.* (Li, Han et al. 2007) employing agonists and inverse-agonists of the muscarinic acetylcholine GPCR; Xu *et al.* (Xu, Sanz et al. 2008) identified inter-residue interaction differences between the active and inactive states for the μ-opioid receptor. From the computational side, molecular dynamics simulations studies suggest that μ-opioid receptor agonists and antagonists bind to the receptor with a set of interactions that are specific to each class.(Kolinski and Filipek 2008) In addition, MD simulations have been utilized to elucidate an increase in solvent exposure of the intracellular domains between helices 3 and 6, and different interactions between the arginine of the E/DRY motif for active and inactive GPCRs.(Fanelli and De Benedetti 2006)

2.2 Mechanism of activation of opioid receptors

To describe the mechanism of activation and action of opioid receptors it suffices to describe the cellular assembly of these receptors. Opioid receptors comprise three domains: an extracellular N-terminus, seven transmembrane α-helices and an intracellular C-terminus, Figure 1. The 7TM helices are arranged sequentially in a counter-clockwise manner when viewed from the extracellular side, and are linked by loops called EL1, EL2, EL3, IL1, IL2 and IL3. EL and IL denote extracellular loop and intracellular loop, respectively. Across the receptors the intracellular loops share the highest sequence homology (90%), followed by TM domains (70%), while the extracellular loops, the N- and C-termini show the greatest diversity.(Knapp, Malatynska et al. 1995) Coupling between the receptors and G-proteins occurs via the pertussis toxin sensitive G_α unit.

Activation and signaling from opioid receptors by different classes of ligands are regulated by a highly conserved mechanism.(Finn and Whistler 2001; Eguchi 2004) They are activated naturally by endogenous peptides, but also by exogenous opiates. Agonist-dependent opioid receptor activation induces conformational changes in the receptor, which promote exchange of G_α-bound GDP for unbound GTP, followed by dissociation of the G-proteins from the receptor. The G_α unit further dissociates from the $G_{\beta\gamma}$ units. Signal transduction occurs via GTP-bound G_α inhibiting adenylate cyclase, responsible for producing cyclic adenosine monophosphate (cAMP). Down-regulation of cAMP results in the reduction of voltage-dependent current and neurotransmitter release.(Eguchi 2004) Moreover, the threshold of voltage-dependent ion channels becomes more negative, decreasing inward flow of current responsible for spontaneous neuronal activity resulting in a drop in cellular excitability. cAMP reduction also leads to a decrease in neurotransmitter release by cAMP-dependent protein kinase. The G_β and G_γ subunits also play key roles in decreasing cell excitability by inhibiting voltage-gated Ca^{2+} channels, hyperpolarizing the membrane and up-regulating the conduction of potassium.(Eguchi 2004) These combined decreases in neurotransmitter release and excitability are manifested as analgesia. Finally, the inactive state is re-constituted when G_α-bound GTP is hydrolyzed to GDP, re-association with $G_{\beta\gamma}$ and recoupling with the receptor.

Numerous experimental approaches have been utilized to investigate GPCR structure and activation including: solution and solid-state NMR, fluorescence, IR and UV spectroscopy, spin-labeling, site-directed mutagenesis, substituted cysteine accessibility, disulphide cross-linking, engineering metal-binding sites, and identification of constitutively active mutants.(Gether 2000; Meng and Bourne 2001; Parnot, Miserey-Lenkei et al. 2002; Decaillot, Befort et al. 2003; Hubbell, Altenbach et al. 2003; Struts, Salgado et al. 2011) Experimentally and computationally, the importance of the lipid membrane should be recognized. It is well documented that membrane composition affects receptor function.(Botelho, Gibson et al. 2002; Botelho, Huber et al. 2006) From the computational side, molecular dynamics simulations showed that the modification of the original positioning of the lipids in the membrane influences the dynamics of the protein.(Lau, Grossfield et al. 2007) In addition, water flux though the transmembrane helices, has been proposed to affect rhodopsin activation. (Grossfield, Pitman et al. 2008) Lastly, the time scale involved in the activation of GPCRs is a challenging task. However, the combined use of computer power and experimental information allows for the generation of detailed structural information. For instance, 2000 ns molecular dynamics simulations and solid-state 2H-NMR data were combined to elucidate the protonation state of key residues directly involved in rhodopsin activation.(Martinez-Mayorga, Pitman et al. 2006) This exemplifies how computational models can provide detailed structural information not available otherwise.

Advances in crystallography and molecular engineering have provided the three-dimensional structures of a few GPCR's: rhodopsin,(Palczewski, Kumasaka et al. 2000; Ridge and Palczewski 2007; Choe, Kim et al. 2011) β-adrenergic receptor,(Kobilka and Schertler 2008) and adenosine receptor.(Jaakola, Griffith et al. 2008) In the absence of experimental structures of opioid receptors, the 2.6-Å resolution crystal structure of bovine rhodopsin(Palczewski, Kumasaka et al. 2000) has served as a template for generating homology models of these receptors,(Pogozheva, Lomize et al. 1998; Fowler, Pogozheva et al. 2004; Fowler, Pogozheva et al. 2004; Pogozheva, Przydzial et al. 2005) Like rhodopsin, opioid receptors belong to class A of the GPCR superfamily. The crystallographic structure of the active state of rhodopsin is now available (Choe, Kim et al. 2011) and can be contrasted with the large body of literature that suggests a common active conformation among the class-A GPCRs. (Karnik, Gogonea et al. 2003) In the activated state TM6 undergoes outward rigid-body translation toward TM5, but away from TM3 and TM7. As a result, a cavity opens up in the intracellular domain in contact with G-proteins. Similar movements have been also suggested for TM1-3 and TM7.(Lin and Sakmar 1996; Gether, Lin et al. 1997; Altenbach, Cai et al. 2001) A better understanding of these activation mechanisms at the molecular level could lead to new drugs geared towards the therapeutic regulation of their functions.

Decaillot FM et al. applied mutagenesis to study the mechanism of activation of the human δ-opioid receptor.(Decaillot, Befort et al. 2003) By analyzing 30 constitutively active mutants of this receptor, mutations hypothesized to produce distinct active conformations were grouped into four abutting areas of the receptor from the extracellular (group I) to the intracellular (group IV) domain. Details about the residues that form each group can be found in Decaillot FM. A sequential binding mechanism was proposed to activate the receptor.(Decaillot, Befort et al. 2003) Sequential binding in GPCRs is not uncommon. A similar mechanism has been postulated for the β2-adrenergic receptors.(Swaminath, Xiang et al. 2004) In the case of the δ-opioid receptor agonists bind to residues in group I comprising a hydrophobic region in EL3, weakening interactions with TM6 and TM7 in the extracellular domain thus initiating a signal. Next, the ligand enters the binding pocket disrupting interactions in groups II and III. Group II residues form a molecular switch that controls movements of TM3. Group III residues are closest to the binding site, consist of patches of hydrophilic and hydrophobic residues and form a network of interactions between residues derived from TM3, 6 and 7. The disruption of these interactions results in a receptor state that is susceptible to activation and helps propagate signals to the intracellular side. It was hypothesized that the amphiphilic nature of opiates and opioid ligands makes them complementary to residues in group III, i.e., the hydrophilic portion of the ligands disrupt the hydrogen-bonding network, while the hydrophobic portion compete with the hydrophobic residues. Finally, disrupting the interactions in group 4 residues results in the separation of TM6 and TM7 in the intracellular side and possibly destabilizing interactions with Gα and exposure to other secondary protein effectors.

Insights about the conformation of the activated state of the μ-opioid receptor are based on modeling experimental distance constraints derived from site-directed mutagenesis, inter-helix H-bonds, disulphide bonds, and engineered Zn^{2+} binding sites between the μ-opioid receptor and analogues of the receptor-bound conformation of a cyclic tetra-peptidomimetic, JOM6.(Fowler, Pogozheva et al. 2004) Structural data for the active state were also derived from disulphide bonds between TM5 and TM6 in the ACM3 muscarinic receptor,(Ward SD, JBC 2002) intrinsic allosteric Zn^{2+} binding sites in TM5 and TM6 of the β_2-adrenergic receptor,(Swaminath, Lee et al. 2003) engineered activating metal-coordination center akin to those between TM3 and TM7 in the β_2-adrenergic(Elling, Thirstrup et al. 1999) and tachykinin(Holst, Elling et al. 2000) receptors, between TM2 and TM3 of the MC4 melanocortin receptor. Finally one hydrogen bond constraint from the δ-opioid receptor(Decaillot, Befort et al. 2003) was introduced. A comparison between the modeled structures of the active and inactive states of the μ-opioid receptor is shown in Figure 1. A noticeable difference is seen in TM6 highlighting the rigid-body movement described for the δ-opioid receptor.

2.3 Internalization of opioid receptors and changes in downstream signaling

Signal transduction by the μ-opioid receptor is determined by properties of the ligand such as affinity, potency, efficacy, bio-availability and half-life, collectively defined as 'relative activity' or RA.(Martini and Whistler 2007) In addition, the length of time the receptor-ligand complex remains coupled to the G-protein, is controlled by receptor desensitization, endocytosis and to an extent the pharmacokinetic properties of the ligand. It has been noted that ligand activity and endocytosis do not have a linear relationship.(Martini and Whistler 2007) Hence, an interplay of relative activity versus endocytosis (RAVE) for each ligand determines the magnitude of the signal transduced. Thus each ligand-receptor complex has an associated RAVE value. As highlighted by Martini L et al.(Martini and Whistler 2007) endogenous peptides have good RA values at the μ-opioid receptor, and also induce significant desensitization and endocytosis. Based on this reasoning, the good balance between their RA and VE values explain why they do not induce tolerance. Another example is methadone. Methadone has comparable potency with encephalin and is also an equally good receptor internalizer.(Whistler, Chuang et al. 1999) Nonetheless, it has a longer half-life compared to other opioids, and consequently a larger RA value giving rise to a moderately higher RAVE value. The extension of the RAVE analysis to morphine is more complicated and invokes secondary protein effectors and region-selective differences in receptor endocytosis.(Martini and Whistler 2007) In general, agonists such as morphine with high RAVE values are more likely to induce tolerance. It has been demonstrated that the development of μ-opioid tolerance is inversely related to the ability of an agonist to promote receptor endocytosis or internalization.(Whistler, Chuang et al. 1999; Finn and Whistler 2001) This theory distinguishes two types of agonists based on their ability to stabilize different receptor conformational states, resulting in phosphorylation by different kinases. Depending on the type of kinase the receptor can be rapidly endocytosed, resensitized and recycled to the cell surface, preventing the development of tolerance.

The formation of an opioid ligand-receptor complex results in structural changes at the extracellular and transmembrane domains, which are propagated to the intracellular

domain followed by the dissociation of G-proteins; phosphorylation by G-protein coupled receptor kinases (GRK), protein kinase A (PKA) and C (PKC); and binding by other proteins such as β-arrestins.(Eguchi 2004) The phosphorylated receptor is endocytosed, whereby it is re-sensitized and recycled to the cell surface or it is marked for degradation. Unlike PKA and PKC, specific GRK-phosphorylation triggers the recruitment of β-arrestins, receptor internalization, resensitization and recycling to the cell surface. This dynamic recycling process has been suggested as crucial to circumvent development to drug tolerance. Tolerance-causing agonists impede receptor endocytosis and/or resensitization, while non-tolerance-inducing drugs promote rapid receptor desensitization-internalization-resensitization and recycling.(Martini and Whistler 2007)
The exact cause of development of tolerance is still a subject of debate. Nonetheless, it is generally accepted that chronic administration of opiates for analgesia gives rise to tolerance. The cellular mechanism of tolerance may involve downstream compensatory changes in neuronal circuits.(Eguchi 2004) The continual and sustained inhibition of adenylate cyclase activity triggers a positive feedback to compensate for the low intracellular levels of cAMP, resulting in the reversible superactivation of adenylate cyclase. This up-regulation of enzyme activity restores the cellular concentration of cAMP, resulting in cells being tolerant to the opiate and also dependent on it given that withdrawing the drug or introducing an antagonist gives rise to abnormally high levels of cAMP and also a restoration of the normal activity level of adenylate cyclase.(Sharma, Klee et al. 1975) The change is delayed but relatively stable and is known to be responsible for opiate tolerance and dependence.(Sharma, Klee et al. 1975) The combined inhibition and up-regulation of adenylyl cyclase provide a means of activating and deactivating neuronal circuits and may play a role in a memory process. It was later shown that the adenylate cyclase V and Gβγ played a role in this activation.(AvidorReiss, Nevo et al. 1996)

2.4 Point-mutation studies to identify key residue targets for phosphorylation

Mutation studies have been successful in identifying key cytosolic domains and residues of ligand-activated μ-opioid receptors, which are liable to phosphorylation, and potentially directly involved in agonist-dependent receptor internalization. (Celver, Lowe et al. 2001; El Kouhen, Burd et al. 2001; Celver, Xu et al. 2004) Truncation of the μ-opioid receptor at Ser363 produced a mutant that was not phosphorylated, and was endocytosed and recycled more slowly than the wild-type,(Qiu, Law et al. 2003) suggesting that phosphorylating residues in this segment may be important for internalization. Cleaving off the entire C-terminal resulted in increased agonist-independent internalization and recycling,(Waldhoer, Bartlett et al. 2004) indicating a greater exposure of some residues critical for the dynamic recycling machinery. Utilizing a single agonist, [D-Ala^2,MePhe^4,Gly^5-*ol*]enkephalin (DAMGO), the mutation of Thr180 to alanine in the second intracellular loop prevented receptor desensitization, while alanine scanning of serine or threonine in the third cytoplasmic loop did not inhibit receptor desensitization.(Celver, Lowe et al. 2001) In a DAMGO-induced receptor activation study, mutations of C-terminal serine/threonine residues identified three phosphorylation sites: Ser363, Thr370 and Ser375. The S375A mutant decreased the rate of receptor internalization, while the S363A and T370A double mutant accelerated the rate of internalization,(El Kouhen, Burd et al. 2001) which may suggest that the combined phosphorylation of Ser363 and Thr370 attenuates receptor internalization. Other studies employing etorphine and multiple mutations have also identified Ser356 and Ser363,(Burd, El-Kouhen et al. 1998) and Thr394 (using DAMGO)(Pak, Odowd et al. 1997; Wolf, Koch et al. 1999) as sites for phosphorylation that result in down-regulation of the μ-opioid receptor. Mutation of Ser356 and Ser363 simultaneously did not alter receptor phosphorylation, but the mutations prevented down-regulation of the receptor suggesting that the absence of down-regulation was not due to the removal of phosphorylation sites. Down-regulation may be occurring through a phosphorylation-independent mechanism or these two sites are not phosphorylated. This is contrary to later studies that demonstrated that Ser363 is phosphorylated.(El Kouhen, Burd et al. 2001) The T394A mutant is more rapidly internalized and resensitized relative to the wild-type μ-opioid receptor. These mutation studies show that multiple phosphorylation motifs may be needed for internalization and that not every phosphorylation site is phosphorylated.

3. Discovery and development of opioid receptor ligands

3.1 Endogenous opioid ligands

Extensive structural and pharmacological studies have been performed to understand the mechanisms of action of opioids as well as for the design of new and more efficient opioid-based painkillers. The opioid agonists propagate their analgesic effects by interacting with opioid receptors. They are both endogenously expressed peptides and exogenous opiates. The term opiate is reserved for foreign substances introduced into the body to target opioid receptors. The endogenous peptides enkephalins, dynorphins, β-endorphins and nociceptins are excised from their precursors pro-enkephalin, pro-dynorphin, pro-opiomelanocortin and pro-nociceptin/orphanin FQ, respectively. The majority of these peptides comprise a conserved N-terminal YGGF motif,(Gentilucci, Squassabia et al. 2007) except the uncharacteristically short peptides endomorphin-1 (YPWF-NH_2) and endomorphin-2 (YPFF-NH_2) that are considered analogues of the YGGF motif. A list of endogenous peptides, their precursors and receptor selectivity is presented in Table 1.

Peptide	Sequences	Precursor	Selectivity
Endomorphin-1	YPWF-NH_2	ND[a]	μ
Endomorphin-2	YPFF-NH_2		
β-endorphin	**YGGF**MTSEKSQTPLVTLFK NAIIKNAYKKGE	Pro-opiomelanocortin	μ=δ
[Leu[5]]enkephalin	**YGGF**L	Pro-enkephalin	δ
[Met[5]]enkephalin	**YGGF**M		
Metorphinamide	**YGGF**MRRV-NH_2		
Deltorphin A	YmFHLMD-NH_2	ND[a]	δ
Deltorphin I	YaFDVVG-NH_2		
Deltorphin II	YaFEVVG-NH_2		
Dynorphin A	**YGGF**LRRIRPKLKWDNQ	Pro-dynorphin	κ
Dynorphin A(1-8)	**YGGF**LRRI		
Dynorphin B	**YGGF**LRRQFKVVT		
α-neoendorphin	**YGGF**LRKYPK		
β-neoendorphin	**YGGF**LRKYP		
Nociceptin	FGGFTGARKSARKLANQ	Pro-nociceptin / Orphanin FQ	ORL-1[b]

[a] Not yet determined. The conserved YGGF sequence is shown in bold
[b] Orphan opioid receptor-like 1

Table 1. Endogenous opioid peptides, the precursor and receptor selectivity.

Endomorphin-1 and endomorphin-2 are highly potent, selective μ-opioid receptor endogenous peptides isolated from mammals, and elicit responses similar to that of morphine.(Zadina, Hackler et al. 1997; Horvath 2000) The endogenous peptides are advantageous in that they do not display any of the side effects of opiates (see below); however, they are not effective in clinical settings because of *in vivo* degradation by peptidases.(Witt, Gillespie et al. 2001) Notwithstanding their degradation, these peptides and their analogues have been utilized extensively as tools to probe receptor categorization and structure-activity relationships.(Hruby and Agnes 1999; Gentilucci, Squassabia et al. 2007) The exogenous opiates on the other hand are more effective in pain management, but present numerous undesirable side effects, some of which are highlighted below. As such, several efforts are being undertaken to identify beneficial analgesics with minimal to no side effects.

3.2 Potent opioid-based analgesics

Interests in identifying more effective analgesics have led to the reporting of a large number potent opioid peptide and non-peptide compounds that are generally classified as agonists or antagonists.(Pan 1998; Stevens, Jones et al. 2000; Eguchi 2004; Waldhoer, Bartlett et al. 2004; Gentilucci, Squassabia et al. 2007; Prisinzano and Rothman 2008; Volpe, Tobin et al. 2011) In spite of the multitude of known opioid compounds, only a relatively small number has been approved for clinical use. The majority of these prescribed analgesics are relatively selective for the μ-opioid receptor,(Volpe, Tobin et al. 2011) though at sufficiently higher doses interactions with the other opioid receptors will occur. While some of these compounds are selective for either the μ (morphine), κ (salvinorin A), or δ (naltrindole) opioid receptors, some are non-selective and display mixed agonist/antagonist responses, for example buprenorphine, pentazocine and butorphanol. Buprenorphine is a partial μ-agonist and partial κ-antagonist that is administered clinically for opioid detoxification and maintenance.(Blakeney, Reid et al. 2007)

Compound	Receptor	Function[a]	Compound	Receptor	Function[a]
Morphine*	M	A	Cyclazocine*	μ/κ	A/AN
Fentanyl*	"	"	Pentazocine*	"	"
Hydrocodone*	"	"	Nalbuphine*	"	"
Levorphanol*	"	"	SIOM	Δ	A
Meperidine*	"	"	SCN-80	"	"
Sufentanyl*	"	"	TAN-67	"	"
Methadone*	"	"	Ketocyclazocine	K	A
Oxycodone*	"	"	Ethyl Ketocyclazocine	"	"
Oxymorphone*	"	"	U-50,488	"	"
Codeine*	"	"	Salvinorin A	"	"
Naloxone*	"	AN	6′-GNTI[a]	"	"
Buprenorphine*	μ/κ	A/AN	5′-GNTI[a]	"	AN
Butorphanol*	"	"	Bremazocine	μ/δ/κ	A/AN

A = agonist; AN = antagonist
*Currently in clinical use. [a] GNTI: guanidino-naltrindole

Table 2. Opioid receptor ligands.

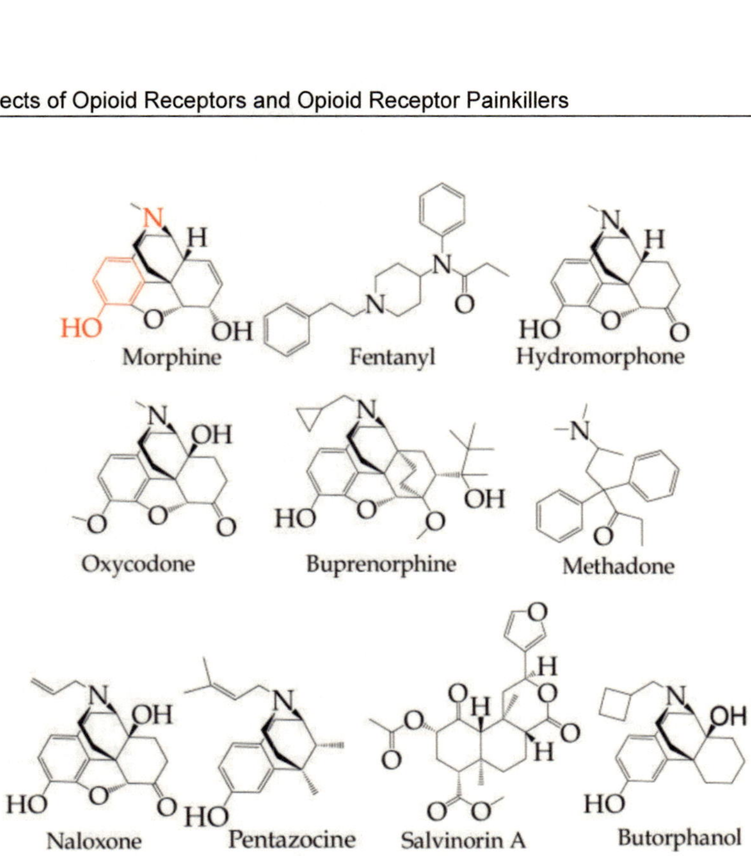

Fig. 2. The chemical structures of some exogenous opiates. The classical "message" tyramine moiety is colored in red in the structure of morphine.

The classification of some opioid compounds is given in Table 2. The chemical structures of selected compounds are shown in Figure 2. Several factors affect the potency of an analgesic, including route of administration, whether they act as full or partial agonists, ability to cross the blood-brain barrier (physico-chemical properties) and their effects on other major physiological systems.(Volpe, Tobin et al. 2011) Some potency comparisons with morphine worth mentioning include the following: fentanyl when administered intramuscularly is about 100 fold more potent; hydromorphone is 6-8 fold more potent;(Inturrisi 2002) and oral oxycodone is about 1.8 times more potent.(Curtis, Johnson et al. 1999) Though a partial agonist buprenorphine is reported to be 25-40 times more potent than morphine.(Blakeney, Reid et al. 2007)

3.3 Pharmacophoric features of opioid ligands

Numerous structure-activity relations (SAR) studies have been carried out on opioid receptor ligands to determine features that drive affinity or efficacy with the goal of generating more effective therapeutic compounds,(Eguchi 2004; Metcalf and Coop 2005; Prisinzano and Rothman 2008; Yongye, Appel et al. 2009, amongst others). SAR studies employing site-directed substitutions and constraints of endogenous peptides, as well as modifications of morphine have provided valuable insights about the pharmacophoric features, ligand selectivity and biological roles of opioid receptors.(Blakeney, Reid et al. 2007) For example it has been determined that a positively charged amine group, an aromatic moiety and a hydrophobic group result in tight binding of morphine. A salt-bridge is formed between the protonated amine and an aspartate residue in TM3, π-π stacking interactions between the aromatic group and residues in the binding pocket and hydrophobic-hydrophobic interactions. In endogenous peptides the N-terminal tyrosine contains a protonated amine and aromatic group, akin to the aromatic ring (A) and basic nitrogen (N) in morphine, Figure 3. This moiety termed tyramine is common to a majority of opioids, though there are some notable potent and selective opiates that lack this classical pharmacophore: Salvinorin A was the first highly potent, non-nitrogen opiate agonist selective towards the κ-opioid receptor;(Roth, Baner et al. 2002) one of its analogues, herkinorin became the first non-nitrogenous agonist selective towards the μ-opioid receptor.(Harding, Tidgewell et al. 2005) Furthermore, the phenylalanine side chain in endogenous peptides mimics the hydrophobic feature (B) of morphine (ring C). It should be pointed out that due to size differences between the peptides and morphine, the interactions between their respective hydrophobic features (B) and the receptor are different.

The observation of the occurrence of a common structural feature amongst opioid ligands gave rise to the "message-address" concept of ligand-receptor interactions, i.e., the same message (signal transduction) is delivered to different addresses (receptors). For the endogenous peptides the message comprises the conserved YGGF motif, with the exceptions cited in Table 1, while for the opiates the tyramine moiety represents the message. The other varied segments of the ligands make up the address and confer selectivity.

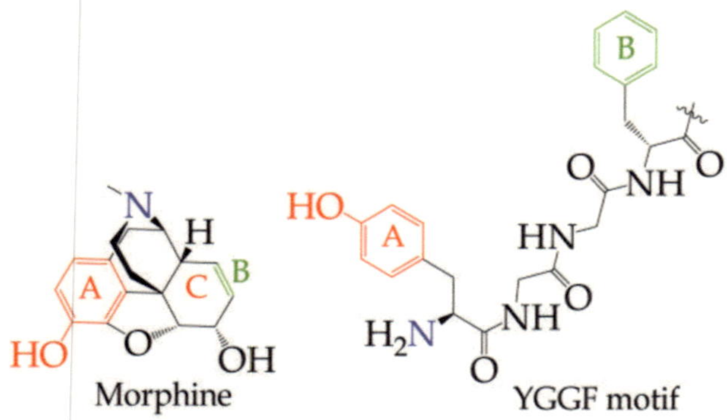

Fig. 3. Chemical structures of morphine and the truncated "message" motif of an endogenous peptide. The YGGF represents amino acids: Y, tyrosine; G, glycine and F, phenylalanine.

Generating pharmacophore models for opioid receptors have followed two traditional approaches: ligand-based or docking-based. Ligand-based methods involve identifying and superimposing common substructures of low energy conformers from which features that drive biological activity are determined. However, because of the inherent difficulties of superimposing structurally different scaffolds these efforts have typically revolved around congeneric series. See Shim J et al.(Shim, Coop et al. 2011) and references therein. In ligand-based virtual screenings via multi-conformer ensembles, the quality and coverage of the conformational ensemble are important. The production of the conformers can be computationally intensive, especially for compounds with a large number of rotatable bonds. Thus, reducing the size of multi-conformer databases and the number of query conformers, while simultaneously reproducing the bioactive conformer with good accuracy, is of crucial interest. A recent protocol that takes into account these aspects has been proposed.(Yongye, Bender et al. 2010) This protocol and other important aspects of conformational coverage in ligand-based virtual screening methods have been recently revised.(Musafia and Senderowitz 2010) On the other hand, docking-based approaches are most valuable when experimental structures of receptors are available. The absence of experimental opioid receptor structures means docking-based methods must rely on homology models. Moreover, for docking-based virtual screening, one has to contend with no induced fit and the possibility of different binding modes.

The identification of enkephalins and δ-opioid receptors fueled interests in developing ligands that target this receptor. The observation that co-administration of δ-opioid receptor antagonists with μ-opioid receptor agonists produced analgesia without the side effect of μ-only agonists further served as motivation to identify δ-selective opioids. Hence, considerable efforts have been devoted to studying the SAR of δ-opioid receptor ligands using both pharmacophore and quantitative structure-activity relationship modeling. See Bernard D et al.(Bernard, Coop et al. 2007) and references therein. Employing the *conformationally sampled pharmacophore* (CSP) approach Bernard D et al. were able to differentiate between δ-opioid receptor agonists and antagonists.(Bernard, Coop et al. 2003; Bernard, Coop et al. 2005) An advantage of the CSP method is the inclusion of high energy conformers in describing pharmacophores, the justification stemming from the fact that ligands may bind in higher energy conformers stabilized by intermolecular interactions with receptors. The CSP methodology was later applied to peptide and nonpeptide agonists to derive pharmacophore models of δ-opioid receptor ligands.(Bernard, Coop et al. 2007) Three pharmacophore points were considered: aromatic (A), basic nitrogen (N) and hydrophobic group (B).

Utilizing efficacy as the activity index, CSP was extended to five peptides and twenty nonpeptides comprising μ-opioid receptor ligands, to derive an aggregate pharmacophore. By analyzing a diverse group of agonists, partial agonists and antagonists the following conclusions were derived: interactions with the B or hydrophobic site of oripavines (etorphine, buprenorphine and diprenorphine) modulated the degree of agonism; agonists with bulky B groups adopt a pose in which interactions occur with both the basic amine and the B site; agonists with large N-substituents are oriented such that the substituents occupy the position of the traditional B site. The resultant pharmacophore is an aromatic group (A), a basic amine (N), a hydrophobic group (B) and N-substituents (S). The investigators claim that such an approach would facilitate efforts to develop compounds that possess both μ-agonistic and δ-antagonistic properties even though the cell lines only expressed the μ-opioid receptor.(Shim, Coop et al. 2011) Furthermore, depending on the structural class of the ligand, N-subsituents can enhance agonism or antagonism. For example, *N*-allyl and *N*-cyclopropylmethyl substituents in etorphines give rise to better agonists compared to morphine,(Gorin and Marshall 1977) while they induce antagonism in 4,5-epoxymorphinans.(Shim, Coop et al. 2011)

The currently known κ-opioid receptor agonists have been classified into eight structural classes(Yamaotsu and Hirono 2011): peptides (dynorphins), benzomorphans (pentazocine), morphinans (butorphanol), arylacetamines (U-69593), diazabicyclononanones (HZ2), bicyclic guanidines (TPI-614-1), benzodiazepines (±tifluadom) and neocleorodane diterpenes (salvinorin A). A comprehensive review of these classes and the history of the development of κ-opioid receptor ligand pharmacophores was published recently by Yamaotsu N et al.(Yamaotsu and Hirono 2011) Evidently, the structural diversity of these classes making it difficult to construct a consensus pharmacophore model. Previous SAR and pharmacophore analyses of κ-opioid receptor ligands are typically confined to structural analogues. Yamaotsu N et al. proposed a consensus pharmacophore encompassing all eight classes using seven compounds in both the training and test sets. Superposition was based on the physico-chemical properties of groups of atoms. The consensus pharmacophore comprised three hydrophobic groups, a hydrogen bond donor and three hydrogen bond acceptors. These pharmacophoric features were employed to describe four binding orientations of the different classes of ligands for the κ-opioid receptor. It remains to be determined how this consensus pharmacophore will perform in virtual screening: for example screening a database, requiring that a given number of features match, followed by biological evaluation of the top scoring compounds. Additionally, in the search of opioid receptor ligands, structure similarity(Martinez-Mayorga, Medina-Franco et al. 2008; Yongye, Appel et al. 2009) and chemoinformatic analyses(Medina-Franco, Martínez-Mayorga et al. 2009) have been employed to develop SAR and to characterize highly dense combinatorial libraries.

3.4 Identification of opioid receptor ligands

A large and growing body of literature has reported the identification of opioid receptor ligands. In particular, improvements in high-throughput chemical synthesis have made possible the rapid and efficient generation of molecules, giving rise to thousands or millions of compounds in combinatorial libraries. Advances in molecular biology have also enabled the evaluation of millions of individual compounds against a number of different biological targets via high-throughput screening (HTS). However, some high content assays, such as *in vivo* studies, are not amenable to the high-throughput miniaturization required to screen millions of individual compounds. In such cases, screening libraries using a mixture-based format(Houghten, Pinilla et al. 1999; Pinilla, Appel et al. 2003; Houghten, Dooley et al. 2006) (also known as positional scanning-synthetic combinatorial libraries or PS-SCL) enables the evaluation of thousands to millions of molecules in approximately a hundred to a few hundred samples. PS-SCL have been used to successfully identify active molecules for a variety of biological targets. (Houghten, Pinilla et al. 1999; Pinilla, Appel et al. 2003; Houghten, Pinilla et al. 2008) In the case of opioid receptors highly active peptides (Dooley, Chung et al. 1994; Houghten, Dooley et al. 2006) and peptidomimetics have been identified. (Houghten, Dooley et al. 2006) This technique has recently found new applications in the search of conotoxins (Armishaw, Singh et al.) and *in-vivo* screening (Reilley, Giulianotti et al.). A step forward in the development of peptides with therapeutic relevance corresponds to the formation of cyclic structures. Cyclic peptides are therapeutically attractive due to their high bioavailability, potential selectivity, and scaffold novelty. In addition, the presence of D-residues induces conformational preferences not followed by peptides consisting of only naturally abundant L-residues. Therefore, the development of synthetic schemes and comprehending how amino acids induce turns in peptides is significant in peptide design. For example, a successful method for the synthesis of cyclic peptides by the intramolecular aminolysis of peptide thioesters, has been recently reported,(Li, Yongye et al. 2009) and the corresponding explicit solvent molecular dynamics simulations were produced and analyzed.(Yongye, Li et al. 2009) The cyclic tetra-peptidomimetic, JOM6, (Fowler, Pogozheva et al. 2004) is an example of a conformationally constrained peptide that retains activity against the μ-opioid receptor. It is anticipated that research will continue in this direction.

The search of opioid receptor ligands using experimental screening of combinatorial libraries has been complemented using computational methods. *In silico* methods can be incorporated at different stages of the drug discovery process, from library design to lead optimization. (Brooijmans and Kuntz 2003) Computational methods are largely applied to corporate chemical collections (Bajorath 2002) as well as combinatorial chemical libraries. (Houghten, Pinilla et al. 2008) However, limited efforts have been reported so far to explicitly integrate information from mixture-based combinatorial libraries and computational techniques (López-Vallejo, Caulfield et al. 2011; Yongye, Pinilla et al. 2011). The structural analogy contained in combinatorial libraries in general and in mixture-based libraries in particular deserves particular considerations. Virtual screening may assist in downsizing large compound libraries and the selection of a smaller set of promising hits, whereas mixture-based screening may screen out some of the false positives of virtual screening. The integration of mixture-based combinatorial library screening data and virtual screening information has been undertaken. In the particular case of opioid receptors, the predicted activity obtained from the experimental mixture-based screening of a large library of bicyclic guanidines was combined with structural similarity methods. This approach allowed categorizing the molecules as actives, activity cliffs, diverse compounds and missed hits.(Yongye, Pinilla et al. 2011)

4. Conclusions

Ever since the discovery of opioid receptors as the principal mediators of analgesia and the identification of endogenous peptides as well as opiates that elicit analgesic responses, considerable efforts have been devoted to finding compounds that target these receptors with the aim of alleviating the sensation of pain. While the endogenous peptides do not display any side effects, their use in clinical settings is hampered because of *in vivo* degradation by protein-digesting enzymes. Opiates are more effective, but adverse side effects such as tolerance, dependence and addiction limit their prolonged usage; thus the continual search for more efficient analgesics. Several compounds have been reported as opioid receptor ligands, however, only a relatively few are currently prescribed in clinical settings with morphine being the prototypical μ-opioid agonist. A high proportion of opioid-based drugs is selective toward the μ-opioid receptor, and still retains untoward side effects prompting extensive studies about the molecular origins of these undesirable properties.

This review focuses on structural aspects of opioid receptors and opioid receptor ligands, with special emphasis on the μ-opioid receptor. The information presented here can be summarized as follows:

1. Considerable evidence now point to the existence of opioid receptors as homo- or hetero-oligomeric complexes and that their pharmacological responses may be cross-modulated. For example the co-administration of a μ-opioid agonist with a δ-opioid antagonist suppressed side effects such as dependence and tolerance while retaining μ-agonist induced analgesia. The realization of this potential for cross-modulation has generated interests in the development of bivalent ligands. The ligands may be individual compounds that possess mixed agonist/antagonist properties or a separate agonist and antagonist tethered through a linker. Future directions of research in analgesia will continue to point towards agonists with acceptable side effects, designing bivalent ligands, or ligands with mixed receptor specificities and functions.

2. While the exact mechanisms of development of tolerance are still under debate, the current models suggest a combination of ligand-induced conformational changes and receptor desensitization, as well as down-stream compensatory changes of secondary effectors.
3. Promising computational methods such as consensus pharmacophore models using different structural scaffold might serve a role in identifying ligands with mixed secondary functional profiles. Understanding the cross-talk between the different signaling pathways of the opioid receptors will also be significant.
4. Production and analysis of a large number of compounds with potential affinity to opioid receptors are possible. However, considerably more work will need to be done to understand and design compounds with high analgesic effect and lower side effects. To that end, a more detailed understanding of the signaling process upon opioid receptor activation is needed.

5. Acknowledgement

This work was supported by the State of Florida, Executive Officer of the Governor's Office of Tourism, Trade and Economic Development.

6. References

Abdelhamid, E. E., M. Sultana, *et al.* (1991). "Selective blockage of delta-opioid receptors prevents the development of morphine-tolerance and dependence in mice." Journal of Pharmacology and Experimental Therapeutics 258(1): 299-303.

Altenbach, C., K. W. Cai, *et al.* (2001). "Structure and function in rhodopsin: Mapping light-dependent changes in distance between residue 65 in helix TM1 and residues in the sequence 306-319 at the cytoplasmic end of helix TM7 and in helix H8." Biochemistry 40(51): 15483-15492.

Ananthan, S. (2006). "Opioid ligands with mixed m/d opioid receptor interactions: An emerging approach to novel analgesics." AAPS J. 8(1): E118-E125.

Armishaw, C. J., N. Singh, *et al.* (2010). "A synthetic combinatorial strategy for developing alpha-conotoxin analogs as potent alpha7 nicotinic acetylcholine receptor antagonists." J. Biol. Chem. 285: 1809-1821.

AvidorReiss, T., I. Nevo, *et al.* (1996). "Chronic opioid treatment induces adenylyl cyclase V superactivation - Involvement of G beta gamma." Journal of Biological Chemistry 271(35): 21309-21315.

Bajorath, J. (2002). "Integration of virtual and high-throughput screening." Nat. Rev. Drug Discov. 1(11): 882.

Balboni, G., S. Salvadori, *et al.* (2011). "Opioid bifunctional ligands from morphine and the opioid pharmacophore Dmt-Tic." European Journal of Medicinal Chemistry 46(2): 799-803.

Bernard, D., A. Coop, *et al.* (2003). "2D conformationally sampled pharmacophore: A ligand-based pharmacophore to differentiate delta opioid agonists from antagonists." Journal of the American Chemical Society 125(10): 3101-3107.

Bernard, D., A. Coop, *et al.* (2005). "Conformationally sampled pharmacophore for peptidic delta opioid ligands." Journal of Medicinal Chemistry 48(24): 7773-7780.

Bernard, D., A. Coop, *et al.* (2007). "Quantitative conformationally sampled pharmacophore for delta opioid ligands: Reevaluation of hydrophobic moieties essential for biological activity." Journal of Medicinal Chemistry 50(8): 1799-1809.

Blakeney, J. S., R. C. Reid, *et al.* (2007). "Nonpeptidic ligands for peptide-activated G protein-coupled receptors." Chemical Reviews 107(7): 2960-3041.

Botelho, A. V., N. J. Gibson, *et al.* (2002). "Conformational energetics of rhodopsin modulated by nonlamellar-forming lipids." Biochemistry 41(20): 6354-6368.

Botelho, A. V., T. Huber, *et al.* (2006). "Curvature and hydrophobic forces drive oligomerization and modulate activity of rhodopsin in membranes." Biophysical journal 91(12): 4464-4477.

Brooijmans, N. and I. D. Kuntz (2003). "Molecular recognition and docking algorithms." Annu Rev Biophys Biomol Struct. 32: 335-373.

Burd, A. L., R. El-Kouhen, *et al.* (1998). "Identification of serine 356 and serine 363 as the amino acids involved in etorphine-induced down-regulation of the mu-opioid receptor." Journal of Biological Chemistry 273(51): 34488-34495.

Celver, J., M. Xu, *et al.* (2004). "Distinct domains of the mu-opioid receptor control uncoupling and internalization." Molecular Pharmacology 65(3): 528-537.

Celver, J. P., J. Lowe, *et al.* (2001). "Threonine 180 is required for G-protein-coupled receptor kinase 3- and beta-arrestin 2-mediated desensitization of the mu-opioid receptor in Xenopus oocytes." Journal of Biological Chemistry 276(7): 4894-4900.

Choe, H. W., Y. J. Kim, *et al.* (2011). "Crystal structure of metarhodopsin II." Nature 471(7340): 651-U137.

Cowan, A., X. Z. Zhu, *et al.* (1988). "Direct dependence studies in rats with agents selective for different types of opioid receptor." Journal of Pharmacology and Experimental Therapeutics 246(3): 950-955.

Curtis, G. B., G. H. Johnson, *et al.* (1999). "Relative potency of controlled-release oxycodone and controlled-release morphine in a postoperative pain model." European Journal of Clinical Pharmacology 55(6): 425-429.

Decaillot, F. M., K. Befort, *et al.* (2003). "Opioid receptor random mutagenesis reveals a mechanism for G protein-coupled receptor activation." Nature Structural Biology 10(8): 629-636.

Dietis, N., R. Guerrini, *et al.* (2009). "Simultaneous targeting of multiple opioid receptors: a strategy to improve side-effect profile." British Journal of Anaesthesia 103(1): 38-49.

Dooley, C. T., N. N. Chung, *et al.* (1994). "An all D-amino-acid opioid peptide with central analgesic activity from a combinatorial library." Science 266(5193): 2019-2022.

Eguchi, M. (2004). "Recent advances in selective opioid receptor agonists and antagonists." Medicinal Research Reviews 24(2): 182-212.

El Kouhen, R., A. L. Burd, *et al.* (2001). "Phosphorylation of Ser363, Thr370 and Ser375 residues within the carboxyl tail differentially regulates μ-opioid receptor internalization." Journal of Biological Chemistry 276(16): 12774-12780.

Elling, C. E., K. Thirstrup, *et al.* (1999). "Conversion of agonist site to metal-ion chelator site in the beta(2)-adrenergic receptor." Proceedings of the National Academy of Sciences of the United States of America 96(22): 12322-12327.

Fanelli, F. and P. G. De Benedetti (2006). "Inactive and active states and supramolecular organization of GPCRs: insights from computational modeling." Journal of Computer-Aided Molecular Design 20(7-8): 449-461.

Finn, A. K. and J. L. Whistler (2001). "Endocytosis of the mu opioid receptor reduces tolerance and a cellular hallmark of opiate withdrawal." Neuron 32(5): 829-839.

Fowler, C. B., I. D. Pogozheva, *et al.* (2004). "Refinement of a homology model of the μ-opioid receptor using distance constraints from intrinsic and engineered zinc-binding sites." Biochemistry 43: 8700-8710.

Fowler, C. B., I. D. Pogozheva, *et al.* (2004). "Complex of an active μ-opioid receptor with a cyclic peptide agonist modeled from experimental constraints." Biochemistry 43: 15796-15810.

Gentilucci, L., F. Squassabia, *et al.* (2007). "Re-discussion of the importance of ionic interactions in stabilizing ligand-opioid receptor complex and in activating signal transduction." Current Drug Targets 8(1): 185-196.

Gether, U. (2000). "Uncovering molecular mechanisms involved in activation of G protein-coupled receptors." Endocrine Reviews 21(1): 90-113.

Gether, U., S. Lin, *et al.* (1997). "Agonists induce conformational changes in transmembrane domains III and VI of the beta(2) adrenoceptor." Embo Journal 16(22): 6737-6747.

Gorin, F. A. and G. R. Marshall (1977). "Proposal for biologically-active conformation of opiates and enkephalin." Proceedings of the National Academy of Sciences of the United States of America 74(11): 5179-5183.

Grossfield, A., M. C. Pitman, *et al.* (2008). "Internal Hydration Increases during Activation of the G-Protein-Coupled Receptor Rhodopsin." J. Mol. Biol. 381(2): 478-486.

Harding, W. W., K. Tidgewell, *et al.* (2005). "Neoclerodane diterpenes as a novel scaffold for mu opioid receptor ligands." Journal of Medicinal Chemistry 48(15): 4765-4771.

Holst, B., C. E. Elling, *et al.* (2000). "Partial agonism through a zinc-ion switch constructed between transmembrane domains III and VII in the tachykinin NK1 receptor." Molecular Pharmacology 58(2): 263-270.

Horvath, G. (2000). "Endomorphin-1 and endomorphin-2: pharmacology of the selective endogenous mu-opioid receptor agonists." Pharmacology & Therapeutics 88(3): 437-463.

Houghten, R. A., C. T. Dooley, *et al.* (2006). "In vitro and direct in vivo testing of mixture-based combinatorial libraries for the identification of highly active and specific opiate ligands." Aaps Journal 8(2): E371-E382.

Houghten, R. A., C. Pinilla, *et al.* (1999). "Mixture-based synthetic combinatorial libraries." J. Med. Chem. 42(19): 3743-3778.

Houghten, R. A., C. Pinilla, *et al.* (2008). "Strategies for the use of mixture-based synthetic combinatorial libraries: Scaffold ranking, direct testing, in vivo, and enhanced deconvolution by computational methods." J. Comb. Chem. 10(1): 3-19.

Hruby, V. and R. S. Agnes (1999). "Conformation-activity relationships of opioid peptides with selective activities at opioid receptors." Biopolymers 51: 391-410.

Hubbell, W. L., C. Altenbach, *et al.* (2003). "Rhodopsin structure, dynamics, and activation: A perspective from crystallography, site-directed spin labeling, sulfhydryl reactivity, and disulfide cross-linking." Membrane Proteins 63: 243-290.

Inturrisi, C. (2002). "Clinical pharmacology of opioids for pain." Clinical Journal of Pain 18: S3-S13.

Jaakola, V. P., M. T. Griffith, *et al.* (2008). "The 2.6 Angstrom Crystal Structure of a Human A(2A) Adenosine Receptor Bound to an Antagonist." Science 322(5905): 1211-1217.

Karnik, S. S., C. Gogonea, *et al.* (2003). "Activation of G-protein-coupled receptors: a common molecular mechanism." Trends in Endocrinology and Metabolism 14(9): 431-437.

Knapp, R. J., E. Malatynska, *et al.* (1995). "Molecular-biology and pharmacology of cloned opioid receptors." Faseb Journal 9(7): 516-525.

Kobilka, B. and G. F. X. Schertler (2008). "New G-protein-coupled receptor crystal structures: insights and limitations." Trends in Pharmacological Sciences 29(2): 79-83.

Kolinski, M. and S. Filipek (2008). "Molecular dynamics of μ opioid receptor complexes with agonists and antagonists." The Open Structural Biology Journal 2: 8-20.

Lahti, R. A., M. M. Mickelson, *et al.* (1985). "[^{3}H]U-69593 a highly selective ligand for the opioid κ-receptor." European Journal of Pharmacology 109(2): 281-284.

Lau, P. W., A. Grossfield, *et al.* (2007). "Dynamic structure of retinylidene ligand of rhodopsin probed by molecular simulations." Journal of Molecular Biology 372(4): 906-917.

Leighton, G. E., M. A. Johnson, *et al.* (1987). "Pharmacological profile of PD-117302, a selective kappa-opioid agonist." British Journal of Pharmacology 92(4): 915-922.

Li, J. H., S. J. Han, *et al.* (2007). "Distinct structural changes in a g protein-coupled receptor caused by different classes of agonist ligands." Journal of Biological Chemistry 282(36): 26284-26293.

Li, Y., A. Yongye, *et al.* (2009). "Synthesis of Cyclic Peptides through Direct Aminolysis of Peptide Thioesters Catalyzed by Imidazole in Aqueous Organic Solutions." Journal of Combinatorial Chemistry 11(6): 1066-1072.

Lin, S. W. and T. P. Sakmar (1996). "Specific tryptophan UV-absorbance changes are probes of the transition of rhodopsin to its active state." Biochemistry 35(34): 11149-11159.

López-Vallejo, F., T. Caulfield, *et al.* (2011). "Integrating virtual screening and combinatorial chemistry for accelerated drug discovery." Comb. Chem. High Throughput Screening 14(6): 475-487.

Maldonado, R., S. Negus, *et al.* (1992). "Precipitation of morphine-withdrawal syndrome in rats by administration of mu-selective, delta-selective and kappa-selective opioid antagonists." Neuropharmacology 31(12): 1231-1241.

Mansour, A., H. Khachaturian, *et al.* (1988). "Anatomy of CNS opioid receptors." Trends in Neuroscience 11: 308.

Martinez-Mayorga, K., J. L. Medina-Franco, *et al.* (2008). "Conformation-opioid activity relationships of bicyclic guanidines from 3D similarity analysis." Bioorg. & Med. Chem. 16(11): 5932-5938.

Martinez-Mayorga, K., M. C. Pitman, *et al.* (2006). "Retinal counterion switch mechanism in vision evaluated by molecular simulations." J. Am. Chem. Soc. 128: 16502-16503.

Martini, L. and J. L. Whistler (2007). "The role of mu opioid receptor desensitization and endocytosis in morphine tolerance and dependence." Current Opinion in Neurobiology 17(5): 556-564.

Medina-Franco, J. L., K. Martínez-Mayorga, *et al.* (2009). "Characterization of Activity Landscapes Using 2D and 3D Similarity Methods: Consensus Activity Cliffs." J. Chem. Inf. Model. 49(2): 477-491.

Meng, E. C. and H. R. Bourne (2001). "Receptor activation: what does the rhodopsin structure tell us?" Trends in Pharmacological Sciences 22(11): 587-593.

Metcalf, M. D. and A. Coop (2005). "Kappa opioid antagonists: Past successes and future prospects." Aaps Journal 7(3): E704-E722.

Musafia, B. and H. Senderowitz (2010). "Biasing conformational ensembles towards bioactive-like conformers for ligand-based drug design." Expert Opinion on Drug Discovery 5(10): 943-959.

Pak, Y., B. F. Odowd, *et al.* (1997). "Agonist-induced desensitization of the mu opioid receptor is determined by threonine 394 preceded by acidic amino acids in the COOH-terminal tail." Journal of Biological Chemistry 272(40): 24961-24965.

Palczewski, K., T. Kumasaka, *et al.* (2000). "Crystal structure of rhodopsin: A G protein-coupled receptor." Science 289(5480): 739-745.

Pan, Z. Z. (1998). "mu-opposing actions of the kappa-opioid receptor." Trends in Pharmacological Sciences 19(3): 94-98.

Parnot, C., S. Miserey-Lenkei, *et al.* (2002). "Lessons from constitutively active mutants of G protein-coupled receptors." Trends in Endocrinology and Metabolism 13(8): 336-343.

Pasternak, G. W. (1993). "Pharmacological mechanisms of opioid analgesics." Clinical Neuropharmacology 16(1): 1-18.

Pert, C. B., G. Pasternak, *et al.* (1973). "Opiate agonists and antagonist discriminated by receptor binding in brain." Science 182(4119): 1359-1361.

Pinilla, C., J. R. Appel, *et al.* (2003). "Advances in the use of synthetic combinatorial chemistry: mixture-based libraries." Nat. Med. 9(1): 118-122.

Pogozheva, I. D., A. L. Lomize, *et al.* (1998). "Opioid receptor three-dimensional structures from distance geometry calculations with hydrogen bonding constraints." Biophysical Journal 75: 612-634.

Pogozheva, I. D., M. J. Przydzial, *et al.* (2005). "Homology modeling of opioid receptor-ligand complexes using experimental constraints." The AAAPS Journal 7(2): E434-E448.

Prisinzano, T. E. and R. B. Rothman (2008). "Salvinorin A analogs as probes in opiold pharmacology." Chemical Reviews 108(5): 1732-1743.

Qiu, Y., P. Y. Law, *et al.* (2003). "mu-opioid receptor desensitization - Role of receptor phosphorylation, internalization, and resensitization." Journal of Biological Chemistry 278(38): 36733-36739.

Reilley, K., M. A. Giulianotti, *et al.* (2010). "Identification of Two Novel, Potent, Low-Liability Antinociceptive Compounds from the Direct In Vivo Screening of a Large Mixture-Based Combinatorial Library." AAAPS J. 12: 318-329.

Reisine, T. and G. Pasternak (1996). Opioid analgesics and antagonists, In: *Goodman and Gilman's The Pharmacological Basis of Therapeutics*. Hardman J.G., Limbird L.E., pp 521-555, McGraw-Hill, New York.

Ridge, K. D. and K. Palczewski (2007). "Visual rhodopsin sees the light: Structure and mechanism of G protein signaling." Journal of Biological Chemistry 282(13): 9297-9301.

Roth, B. L., K. Baner, *et al.* (2002). "Salvinorin A: A potent naturally occurring nonnitrogenous kappa opioid selective agonist." Proceedings of the National Academy of Sciences of the United States of America 99(18): 11934-11939.

Rutherford, J. M., J. Wang, *et al.* (2008). "Evidence for a mu-delta opioid receptor complex in CHO cells co-expressing mu and delta opioid peptide receptors." Peptides 29(8): 1424-1431.

Schmauss, C. and T. L. Yaksh (1984). "*In vivo* studies on spinal opiate receptor systems mediating antinociception. 2. Pharmacological profiles suggesting a differential association of mu-receptor, delta-receptor and kappa-receptor with visceral chemical and cutaneous thermal stimuli in the rat." Journal of Pharmacology and Experimental Therapeutics 228(1): 1-12.

Sharma, S. K., W. A. Klee, *et al.* (1975). "Dual regulation of adenylate cyclase accounts for narcotic dependence and tolerance." Proceedings of the National Academy of Sciences of the United States of America 72(8): 3092-3096.

Shim, J., A. Coop, *et al.* (2011). "Consensus 3D Model of mu-Opioid Receptor Ligand Efficacy Based on a Quantitative Conformationally Sampled Pharmacophore." Journal of Physical Chemistry B 115(22): 7487-7496.

Stevens, W. C., R. M. Jones, *et al.* (2000). "Potent and Selective Indolomorphinan Antagonists of the Kappa-Opioid Receptor." J. Med. Chem. 43(14): 2759-2769.

Struts, A. V., G. F. J. Salgado, *et al.* (2011). "Retinal dynamics underlie its switch from inverse agonist to agonist during rhodopsin activation." Nature Structural & Molecular Biology 18(3): 392-394.

Swaminath, G., T. W. Lee, *et al.* (2003). "Identification of an allosteric binding site for ZN(2+) on the beta(2) adrenergic receptor." Journal of Biological Chemistry 278(1): 352-356.

Swaminath, G., Y. Xiang, *et al.* (2004). "Sequential binding of agonists to the beta(2) adrenoceptor - Kinetic evidence for intermediate conformational states." Journal of Biological Chemistry 279(1): 686-691.

Volpe, D. A., G. A. M. Tobin, *et al.* (2011). "Uniform assessment and ranking of opioid Mu receptor binding constants for selected opioid drugs." Regulatory Toxicology and Pharmacology 59(3): 385-390.

von Voigtlander, P. F., R. A. Lahti, *et al.* (1983). "U-50,488: a selective and structurally novel non-*mu*-(*kappa*)-opioid agonist." Journal of Pharmacology and Experimental Therapeutics 224(1): 7-12.

Waldhoer, M., S. E. Bartlett, *et al.* (2004). "Opioid receptors." Annual Review of Biochemistry 73: 953-990.

Waldhoer, M., J. Fong, *et al.* (2005). "A heterodimer-selective agonist shows in vivo relevance of G protein-coupled receptor dimers." Proceedings of the National Academy of Sciences of the United States of America 102(25): 9050-9055.

Whistler, J. L., H. H. Chuang, *et al.* (1999). "Functional dissociation of mu opioid receptor signaling and endocytosis: Implications for the biology of opiate tolerance and addiction." Neuron 23(4): 737-746.

Witt, K. A., T. J. Gillespie, *et al.* (2001). "Peptide drug modifications to enhance bioavailability and blood-brain barrier permeability." Peptides 22(12): 2329-2343.

Wolf, R., T. Koch, *et al.* (1999). "Replacement of threonine 394 by alanine facilitates internalization and resensitization of the rat mu opioid receptor." Molecular Pharmacology 55(2): 263-268.

Wollemann, M., S. Benyhe, *et al.* (1993). "The kappa-opioid receptor: evidence for the different subtypes." Life Sciences 52(7): 599-611.

Xu, W., A. Sanz, *et al.* (2008). "Activation of the mu opioid receptor involves conformational rearrangements of multiple transmembrane domains." Biochemistry 47(40): 10576-10586.

Yamaotsu, N. and S. Hirono (2011). "3D-pharmacophore identification for κ-opioid agonists using ligand-based drug-design techniques." Topics in Current Chemistry 299: 277-307.

Yongye, A. B., J. R. Appel, *et al.* (2009). "Identification, structure-activity relationships and molecular modeling of potent triamine and piperazine opioid ligands." Bioorg. & Med. Chem. 17(15): 5583-5597.

Yongye, A. B., A. Bender, *et al.* (2010). "Dynamic clustering threshold reduces conformer ensemble size while maintaining a biologically relevant ensemble." J. Comput. Aided. Mol. Des. 24: 675-686.

Yongye, A. B., Y. M. Li, *et al.* (2009). "Modeling of peptides containing D-amino acids: implications on cyclization." J. Comp.-Aid. Mol. Des. 23(9): 677-689.

Yongye, A. B., C. Pinilla, *et al.* (2011). "Integrating computational and mixture-based screening of combinatorial libraries." Journal of Molecular Modeling 17: 1473-1482.

Zadina, J. E., L. Hackler, *et al.* (1997). "A potent and selective endogenous agonist for the mu-opiate receptor." Nature 386(6624): 499-502.

Zhu, Y. X., M. A. King, *et al.* (1999). "Retention of supraspinal delta-like analgesia and loss of morphine tolerance in delta opioid receptor knockout mice." Neuron 24(1): 243-252.

4

Creation of New Local Anesthetics Based on Quinoline Derivatives and Related Heterocycles

Igor Ukrainets
National University of Pharmacy
Ukraine

1. Introduction

Pain is a widely spread symptom and one of the most common causes making people seek medical attention. Though at present, different methods of pain control such as general narcosis, acupuncture, hypnosis, electroanaesthesia, homeopathy, etc., are known, nothing is better for safety and reliability than local anaesthesia. More often it is an effective alternative to general narcosis and promotes decreasing and even eliminating the use of narcotic analgesics in surgery. Dentists, dermatologists and other medical professionals apply it in their work. Unfortunately, an "ideal" local anesthetic has not been created yet, and all current medicines of the given pharmacological group have some drawbacks. The most serious disadvantages are high neuro- and cardiotoxicity, as well as tendency to cause allergy. Thus, the search for new, more effective and safe local anesthetics is ongoing and scientists all over the world continue to work on this problem.

Quinolines are the interesting compounds for research in this area. Numerous derivatives of this azaheterocycle are widely distributed in nature. Some of them are well-known to man and used for curative purposes from ancient times. For example, alkaloids cinchonine (**1a**, R = H) and quinine (**1b**, R = OMe, Figure 1) with antimalarial properties are isolated from *Cinchona* L. The utility of the majority of other natural quinolines prospects are to be determined. However, recently there has been a noticeable progress toward a solution of this problem. Natural compounds themselves more often attract the attention of scientists working in different fields of science and engineering. The stimulating motive for their research is the widely spread conviction that the living nature does nothing without purpose and everything it synthesizes is important at all events for life and, therefore, for man (Bochkov & Smith, 1987). This conviction finds the experimental confirmation constantly, as a result, at present the spectrum of biological properties of natural quinolines has expanded significantly (Kartsev, 2007).

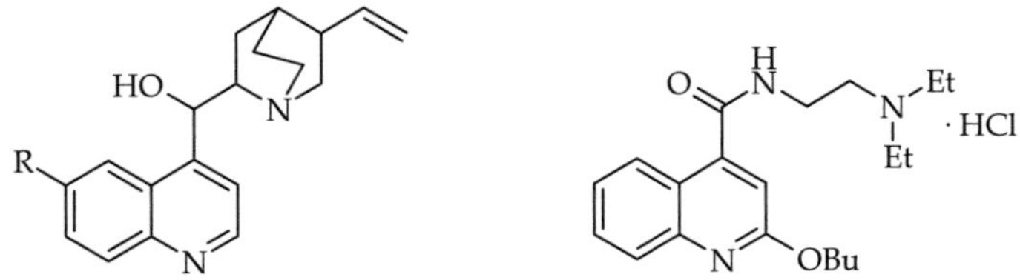

1a,b **2**

Fig. 1. Natural antimalarial drugs and the first synthetic local anesthetic of the quinoline group

Hence the increased interest in quinolines by synthetic chemists becomes clear. Their belonging to natural metabolites, as well as practically unlimited possibilities for chemical transformations make this molecular system, especially its hydroxyanalogues, rather convenient matrices for fixing various structural elements-pharmacophores on them. It allows making systematic changes into the structure of the finished products and thus to purposefully change their physical and chemical, as well as biological properties. Finally one can succeed in obtaining new substances corresponding to high requirements for medicines. So, in particular, the first local anesthetic of the quinoline group - Cinchocaine (**2**, Figure 1) was synthesized; though it was created 85 ago (Kleemann & Engel, 2001), it has been applied successfully in medical practice nowadays (Tomoda et al., 2009; Kang & Shin, 2010; Douglas et al., 2011).

2. 1-R-4-Hydroxy-2-oxo-1,2-dihydroquinoline-3-carboxamides as a source of new privileged structures with the local anesthetics activity

When systematically studying the biological properties of 1-R-4-hydroxy-2-oxo-1,2-dihydroquinoline-3-carboxamides we repeatedly noted the opportunity of creating new potential medicines with various effects on a living organism on their basis, including local anesthetics (Ukrainets, 1992; Ukrainets et al., 1994). After the experimental study of anaesthetic properties of a large group of compounds of this chemical range, our attention was paid to the most active of them. Hydrochlorides of (2-diethylaminoethyl)amides of 1-ethyl- (**3a**, R = Et) and, especially, 1-propyl- (**3b**, R = Pr) substituted 4-hydroxy-2-oxo-1,2-dihydroquinoline-3-carboxylic acids (Figure 2), were superior the known local anesthetic Lidocaine by the specific activity possessing at the same time the lower toxicity.

Later (Gorokhova, 1993) in the same range one more compound - hydrochloride of 1-ethyl-4-hydroxy-2-oxo-1,2-dihydroquinoline-3-carboxylic acid (2-morpholin-4-ylethyl)amide (**4**) was found. By the level of infiltration anaesthesia this amide had some more activity than its 1-N-ethyl analogue **3a**, but it was noticeably inferior to 1-N-propyl derivative **3b**. However, after the primary screening it was also included into the list of candidates for profound research as it possessed another important for future medicine property - a relatively low toxicity. By this parameter amide **4** prevailed over its acyclic analogues **3a,b** by a factor of almost 2.

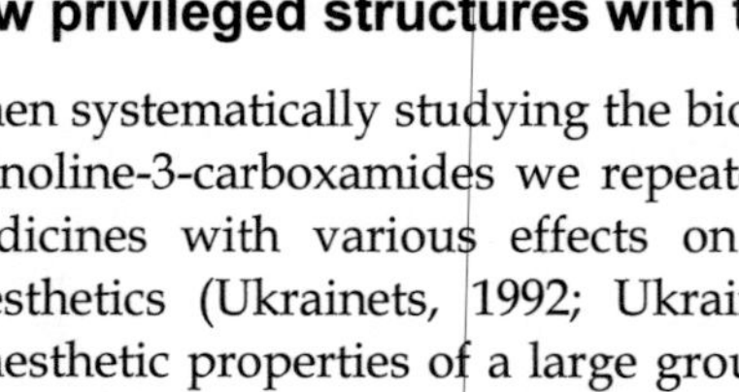

3a,b

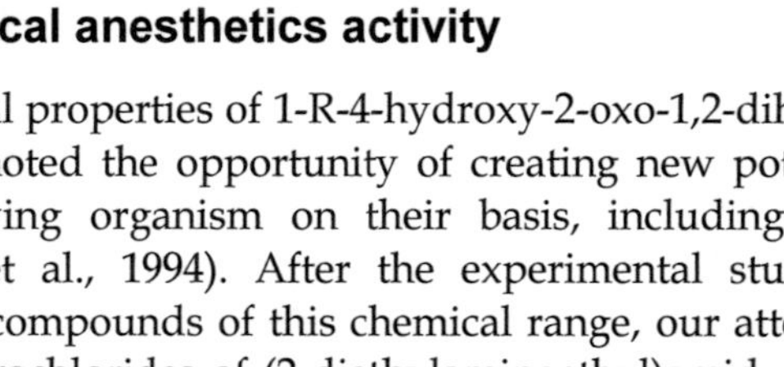

5

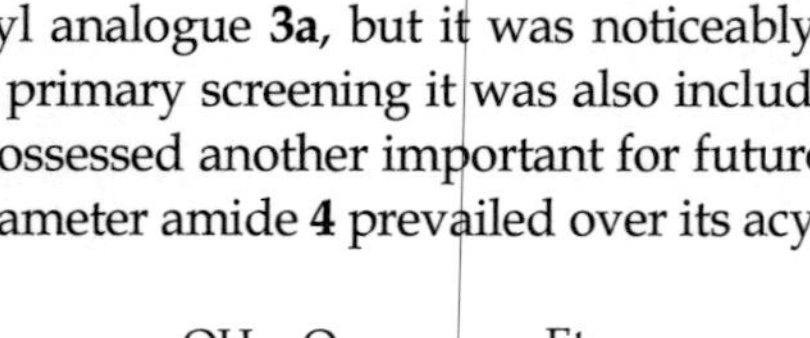

4

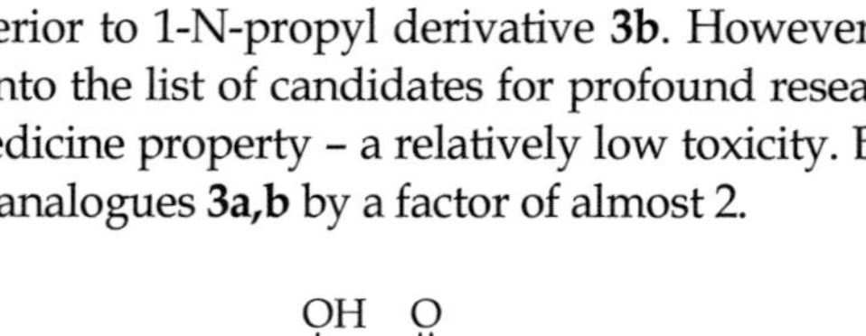

6

Fig. 2. Biologically active 4-hydroxy-2-oxo-1,2-dihydroquinoline-3-carboxamides

And recently (Davidenko, 2011) a new pharmacological property - the ability to block opioid receptors - has been revealed in 4-hydroxy-2-oxo-1,2-dihydroquinoline-3-carboxamides. It has also been found that substances closely related in structure can reveal quite opposite biological effects. Hydrochloride of 1-allyl-4-hydroxy-6,7-dimethoxy-2-oxo-1,2-dihydroquinoline-3-carboxylic acid (3-morpholin-4-ylpropyl)amide (**5**) in the dose of 1 mg/kg completely eliminates the analgesic effect of Tramadol and its homologue - (2-morpholin-4-yl-ethyl)amide **6** - prolongs the analgesic effect significantly. This fact requires further research and is doubtless of interest for researchers engaged in searching not only new opioid receptors antagonists, but highly effective pain-killers as well.

3. Chemical modification of Chinoxicaine by its transformation into pro-drugs

All compounds that passed the stage of primary pharmacological screening were subjected to more profound and thorough analysis in pre-clinical trials. To evaluate the local anaesthetic properties a greater number of parameters were taken into account; these parameters characterized the main specific manifestations of the biological effect: potency of local anaesthesia, the rate of its onset and duration. Additionally at this stage some experimental models, such as repeated infiltration and additional conduction anaesthesia, epidural and surface anaesthesia, were involved. The local irritant properties of the compounds, as well as their acute and chronic toxicity were studied.

From the experiments, only one compound emerged - hydrochloride of 4-hydroxy-2-oxo-1-propyl-1,2-dihydroquinoline-3-carboxylic acid (2-diethylaminoethyl)amide (**3b**), which further was studied as a privileged structure under the name of Chinoxicaine and was transferred to the next level of investigations. This amide causes a rapid, deep and long local anaesthesia on all models studied and has a low toxicity. It has been found that prolonged introduction of Chinoxicaine to the experimental animals does not produce any statistically significant changes in the activity of central nervous and cardio-vascular systems and does not cause negative reactions of the liver and gastrointestinal tract. The medicine does not produce nephrotoxic action and, thus, it can be used safely by the patients with renal pathology. While using Chinoxicaine, there were no cases of blood pressure decrease, which is its beneficial advantage over many known anesthetics. Additional advantages of Chinoxicaine are that together with the high specific activity it shows clear antiarrhythmic, antimicrobial, antioxidant, and fungicidal effects.

Simultaneously with the pharmacological studies, diversified synthetic research to find the most available method for obtaining Chinoxicaine substance was carried out. As the result, principally different synthetic schemes providing a high quality of the final product have been suggested (Ukrainets et al., 1998; Ukrayinecz & Bezuhliy, 2002; Romanov & Ukrainets, 2006).

Unfortunately, the "Chinoxicaine" project faced some problems. For example, possessing a unique set of pharmacological properties Chinoxicaine appeared to be surprisingly poorly soluble in water. Its solubility is only 13.85 g in 100 ml of water at 20°C, and this caused great difficulty when preparing a stable medicinal form for injections. We solved this problem rather rapidly, though water had to be replaced by the combined solvent.

At the later stages of introduction of a new local anesthetic into medical practice, namely at the stage of clinical trials, one more serious drawback was revealed. In some patients, Chinoxicaine solution in the site of injection caused a transient feeling of burning. Though this undesirable effect lasted less than one minute, further work with the medicine practically lost any progress without its removal. Theoretically a rather simple and effective solution of the problem has been found. The irritant action of Chinoxicaine is completely eliminated by addition such substances as adrenaline in insignificant concentrations in its solution.

However, we tried to solve the problem by structure modification well known in the art to modern researchers (Kubinyi, 2006).

For example, on the basis of structural biological regularities previously revealed a quite new analogue of Chinoxicaine with the improved properties can be synthesized. But is should be taken into account that in such case all complex of biological and pharmaceutical trials have to be carried out in a full volume. Besides to achieve the aim is quite unreal as a result of synthesis of only one new substance. Most likely, to solve the task successfully is possible only after the study of the series of new compounds.

Taking this into account we began to improve pharmaceutical properties of Chinoxicaine from the most rational variant - creation of pro-drugs on its basis. Biologically active source in this approach remains the same, that is why both the terms of development and costs for its implementation are greatly reduced.

However, the practical realization of the method is linked with certain difficulties. In particular, to increase the water solubility, as a rule, it is necessary to introduce additional ionizing groups into the structure of the modified compounds, while to eliminate the irritant action the same ionizing groups in the molecule should be masked (Kuznetsov et al., 1991). In other words, theoretically possible methods of elimination of the revealed drawbacks of Chinoxicaine mutually exclude each other.

Most likely the irritant action of Chinoxicaine is related to the presence of 4-OH-group in its structure, which accounts for the marked acid properties in 1-R-4-hydroxy-2-oxo-1,2-dihydroquinoline-3-carboxamides (Ukrainets, 1988). However, it has been noted (Gorokhova, 1993) that the potency of the given side effect to a great extent depends on the structure of the amide fragment as well. For example, hydrochloride of 4-hydroxy-2-oxo-1-propyl-1,2-dihydroquinoline-3-carboxylic acid (2-morpholin-4-ylethyl)amide (**7**, Figure 3) and its 1-N-ethyl analogue **4** mentioned above do not yield to Chinoxicaine in the specific activity, but they do not practically render the irritant action. This fact was the foundation for performing bioreversible chemical modification of Chinoxicaine by the tertiary amino group (Ukrainets et al., 2009).

One of the obvious solutions of the target trasformation of the Chinoxicaine molecule is trasformation into quaternary ammonium salts, which is simple in its performance. It should be noted here that common alkyl halides are not suitable for such transformation since they form with the medicine - tertiary amine - the stable compounds, which are almost not subjected to metabolism and are excreted from the organism unchanged (Kuznetsov et al., 1991). Carboxylic acid haloalkyl esters are more interesting. They allow to transform tertiary amines in quaternary ammonium salts with labile grouping $N^{+}-C-O$, which is capable of relatively easily to be splitted by hydrolysis and release the initial medicine in the form of the corresponding hydrohalide (Kuznetsov et al., 1991; Vinogradova et al., 1980). One of this reagents is commercially available bromomethylacetate, by its interaction with (2-diethylaminoethyl)amide of 4-hydroxy-2-oxo-1-propyl-1,2-dihydro-quinoline-3-carboxylic acid (**8**) in the anhydrous acetonitrile medium the target bromo-acetoxymethylate **9** was obtained (Figure 3).

The biological screening has demonstrated that quaternization conducted eliminated the irritant action of Chinoxicaine almost completely, unlike it bromoacetoxy-methylate **9** in the form of 2% aqueous solution which causes only insignificant hyperemia of conjunctiva of the rabbit's eye. At the same time in spite of expectations, dissolution in water decreased significantly (up to 8.86 g per 100 ml), but usually it increases sharply in pro-drugs of this type in 1-2 thresholds comparing to hydrohalides (Vinogradova et al., 1980). Significantly there is almost a threefold shortening of the duration of the surface anesthesia by the bromoacetoxymethylate **9** and this is evidently due to the low rate of liberation of the starting tertiary amine.

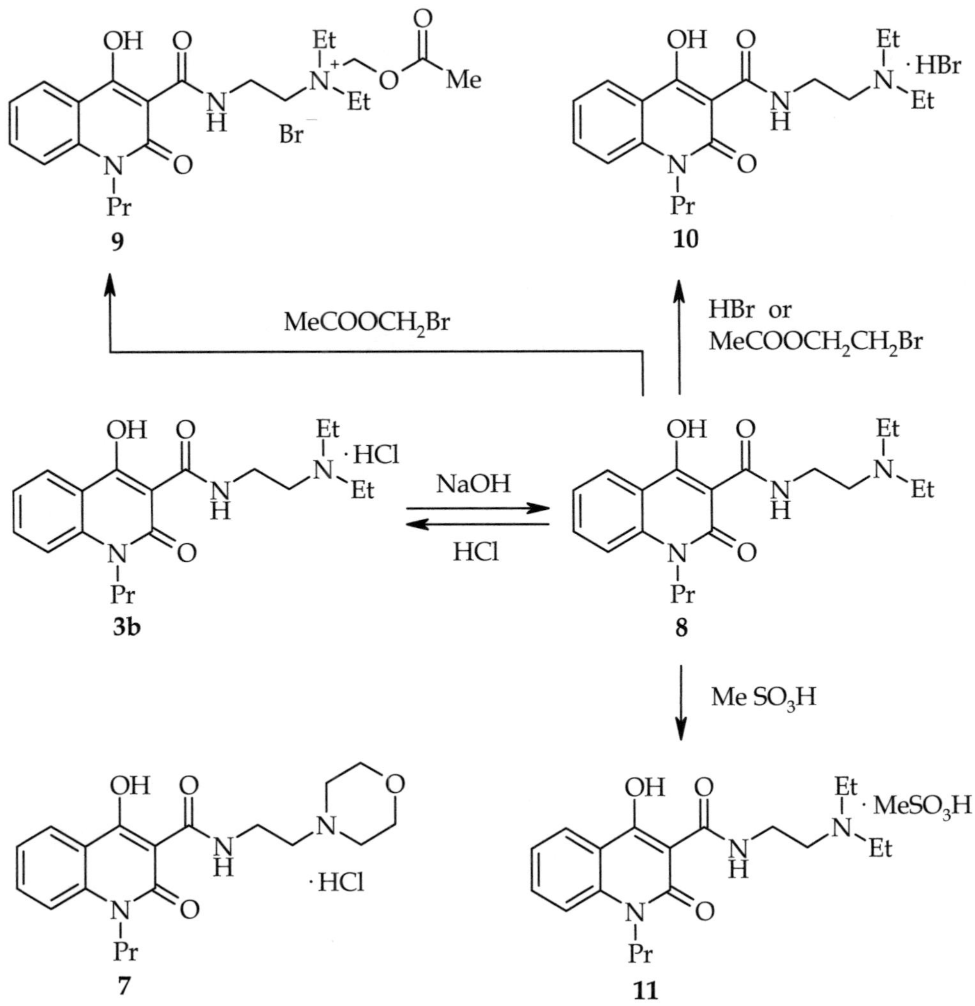

Fig. 3. Modification of Chinoxicaine into pro-drugs

The attempt to optimize the value by substitution of 2-bromomethyl acetate with 2-bromoethyl failed. Under the action of amide **8** the reagent is dehydrobrominated, as a result, instead of bromoacetoxyethylate hydrobromide **10** was isolated, it could be also obtained by neutralization of the tertiary amino group of amide **8** by hydrobromic acid. Though salt formation is not accompanied with the change of number, character and location of covalent bonds, it is widely used as an individual type of chemical modification of medicinal substances in medical chemistry. Hence, hydrobromide **10** can be considered as an original pro-drug of Chinoxicaine. However, there was no positive results due to transfer of hydrochloride to hydrobromide. Absolutely all the parameters worsened: solubility decreased to 3.40 g in 100 ml of water, the irritant action increased considerably, and the local anaesthetic activity decreased.

The substitution of hydrogen chloride as a salt-forming reagent of methanesulfonic acid, which forms methanesulfonate **11** practically with the quantitative yield reacting with amide **8** in the anhydrous diethyl ester medium, was more successful.

According to the X-ray structural data, in the symmetrically independent part of the unit cell of the methanesulfonate **11** there is a molecule of the 4-hydroxy-2-oxo-1-propyl-1,2-dihydroquinoline-3-carboxylic acid (2-diethylaminoethyl)amide protonated at atom $N_{(19)}$ and the methanesulfonic acid anion (see Figure 4).

The dihydroquinolone fragment is planar within 0.02 Å. The deviations of atoms $C_{(11)}$ and $C_{(15)}$ from the mean square plane of the dihydropyridine ring are 0.067 and 0.022 Å respectively. A marked deviation of atom $C_{(11)}$ from the ring plane is explained by the presence of a shortened intramolecular contact $H_{(9)}\cdots H_{(11B)}$ of 1.986 Å. The amide fragment is virtually coplanar with the dihydroquinolone (torsional angle $C_{(4)}$-$C_{(3)}$-$C_{(15)}$-$O_{(15)}$ = 4°). Such an orientation is stabilized by two intramolecular hydrogen bonds: $O_{(4)}$-$H_{(4)}\cdots O_{(15)}$ (H···O 1.74 Å, O-H···O 155°) and $N_{(16)}$-$H_{(16)}\cdots O_{(2)}$ (H···N 1.91 Å, N···H-O 140°).

The $O_{(4)}$-$C_{(4)}$ 1.319(3), $N_{(16)}$-$C_{(15)}$ 1.313(3), and $C_{(2)}$-$C_{(3)}$ 1.451(3) Å bonds in the compound studied are shortened (mean values 1.331, 1.334, and 1.464 Å respectively) but the $O_{(15)}$-$C_{(15)}$ 1.264(3) and $C_{(3)}$-$C_{(4)}$ 1.379(3) Å bonds are lengthened (mean values 1.231 and 1.363 Å respectively).

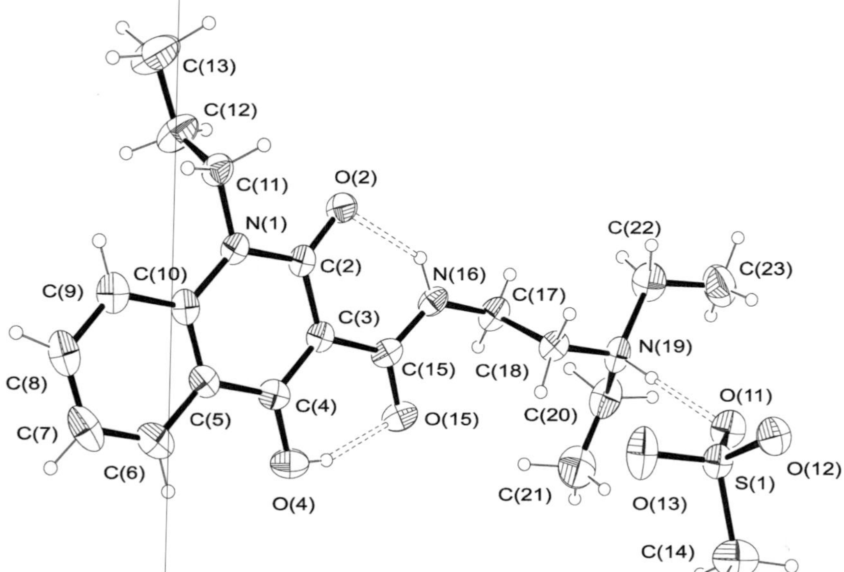

Fig. 4. The structure of the methanesulfonate **11** molecule with atomic numbering. The dotted lines indicate the intra- and intermolecular hydrogen bonds

Atom $N_{(1)}$ has a planar trigonal configuration. The substituents at atoms $N_{(1)}$ and $N_{(16)}$ have an *anti*-periplanar conformation (torsional angles $N_{(1)}$-$C_{(11)}$-$C_{(12)}$-$C_{(13)}$ and $N_{(16)}$-$C_{(17)}$-$C_{(18)}$-

$N_{(19)}$ 176.2 and 176.3° respectively). The plane of the carbon atoms of the propyl group on the $N_{(1)}$ atom is virtually perpendicular to the mean-square plane of the dihydropyridine ring, the angle between them being 89.1°.

In the crystal the molecules of the methanesulfonate **11** form dimers *via* stacking interactions between the dihydroquinolone fragments, the benzene rings being situated over the dihydropyridines. The distance between the ring centroids is 3.54 Å and the mean-square planes of the dihydropyridine and benzene fragments form a dihedral angle of 2.2°.

The cation and anion are mutually bonded by an intermolecular hydrogen bond $N_{(19)}$–$H_{(19)}\cdots O_{(11)}$ (H···O 1.88 Å, N-H···O 176°).

The biological screening has shown that methanesulfonate **11** demonstrates a significant improvement of all pharmaceutical properties comparing to the initial hydrochloride **3b** (Chinoxicaine). In particular, the local irritant action was successfully decreased to the level of bromoacetoxymethylate **9**. Dissolution in water increased in more than six times - up to 85.72 g per 100 ml, and it has eliminated the problem of choosing a solvent for preparation of a stable medicinal form for injections. Finally, there are also some positive aspects of revealing the specific activity: the rate of anaesthesia onset remains the same, but the total duration of the surface anaesthesia and the deep anaesthetization phase increased.

4. Synthesis of conformation stable forms of quinolones as an attempt to improve pharmaceutical properties of Chinoxicaine

In modern medical chemistry several standard methods are successfully applied for improving the privileged structures chosen according to the results of preliminary pharmacological trials. Recently with accumulation of information about the spatial structure of active binding sites for many types of receptors a greater attention has been paid to methodology of conformation restrictions (Chen et al., 2010; Watanabe et al., 2010; Nirogia et al., 2011). In general, this method of the structural transformation of a molecule suggests the preservation of all functional groups contacting with a biological target in their original form and at the same time it is directed to fixing of some of them in "active" conformation.

One of the most wide-spread ways of practical realization of the method is cyclization, which allows transformation of the open side chains of the initial molecule in endo- or exo-cyclic fragments, making possible the change of the pharmaceutical and (or) pharmacokinetic properties. Taking into account the given data it is quite logical to study N-R-amides of 1-hydroxy-3-oxo-5,6-dihydro-3H-pyrrolo- (**12a-m**) and 1-hydroxy-3-oxo-6,7-dihydro-3H,5H-pyrido- (**13a-m**) [3,2,1-*ij*]quinoline-2-carboxylic acids as potential local anesthetics (Figure 5).

The interest of these compounds is caused by the fact that they are very similar to Chinoxicaine (**3b**) and its 1-N-ethyl analogue **3a** by their structure. At the same time amides **12-13a-m** have a principally important structural difference: though their 1-N-alkyl substituents contain the same two-three carbon atoms, they are situated not in the open alkyl chains, but are included in the composition of pyrrole or tetrahydropyridine cycles annelation with the quinolone nucleus. Such modification is known to lead to the essential spatial trasformation of the molecule. In particular, in 1-propylsubstituted 4-hydroxy-quinolones-2 the ethyl fragment is placed perpendicular the plane of the quinolone nucleus, as a result the terminal methyl group is far from the bicycle more than 3 Å (Ukrainets et al., 2009). And on the contrary, the tricyclic pyrido[3,2,1-*ij*]quinoline system is much compact – in spite of the *sofa* conformation of the tetrahydropyridine ring, $C_{(6)}$ atom deviates from its relative plane only in 0.56 Å (Ukrainets et al., 2008). Unlike 1-N-ethylsubstituted 4-hydroxyquinolones-2, in which the methyl group of ethyl substituent is never located in the quinolone cycle plane (Baumer et al., 2004; Ukrainets et al., 2007), tricyclic pyrrolo[3,2,1-*ij*]- quinoline system is practically flat (Ukrainets et al., 2006a). It is clear that transfer from 1-N-ethyl- and 1-N-propylsubtituted **3a,b** to conformation limited pyrrolo- and pyridoquinolines **12-13** should be obligatory reflected to the biological properties. The answer to the question about this influence has been found in one of the recent investigations (Kravtsova, 2011).

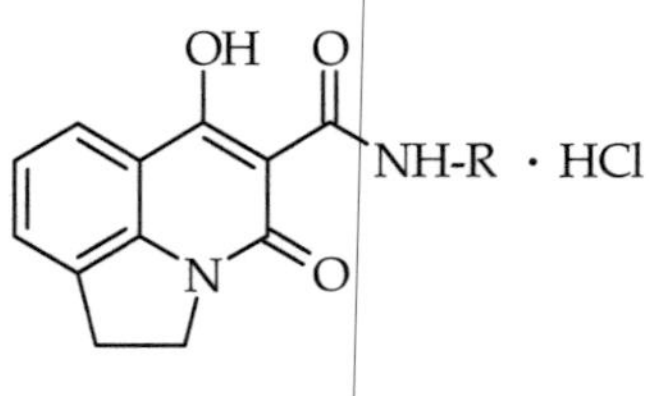

12a-m

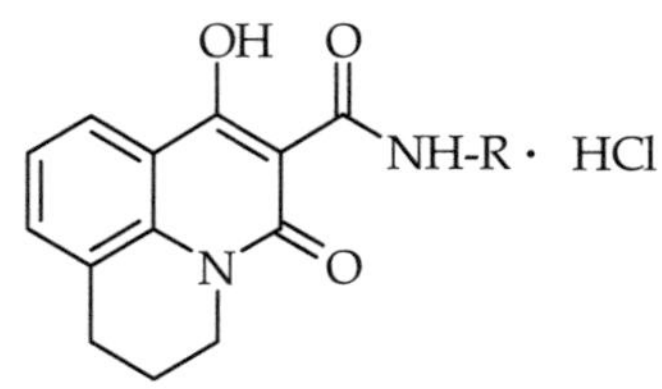

13a-m

12-13: **a** R = 2-aminoethyl; **b** R = 3-aminopropyl; **c** R = 4-aminobutyl; **d** R = 6-aminohexyl; **e** R = 2-ethylaminoethyl; **f** R = 2-(2-hydroxyethylamino)ethyl; **g** R = 2-dimetylaminoethyl; **h** R = 2-diethylaminoethyl; **i** R = 3-dimethylaminopropyl; **j** R = 3-diethylaminopropyl; **k** R = 2-piperazin-1-ylethyl; **l** R = 2-morpholin-4-ylethyl; **m** R = 3-morpholin-4-ylpropyl

Fig. 5. Tricyclic analogues of Chinoxicaine

Testing of the samples synthesized has been carried out on the infiltration anaesthesia model by Buelbring-Yueid method (Table 1).

Analysis of the experimental data obtained demonstrates that compounds with the primary amino groups, i.e. amides **12-13a-d**, do not practically show the anesthetic properties. The weak activity (the anaesthesia lasts for not more 5 min, and the phase of complete sensitivity loss has not come) has appeared in monoalkylaminoalkylamides **12-13e,f**. And only when the second alkyl residue is introduced into the terminal amino group (amides **12-13g-m**), the local anaesthetic action increases noticeably, but though in this case its duration remains rather short. For example, for the most active diethylaminoethyl derivative **13h** this index is approximately 40 min, though the infiltration anaesthesia index reaches the maximum possible value. As compared, Chinoxicaine in the similar conditions causes total anaesthesia lasting for approximately 75 min (with the general duration of anaesthesia of 4 hours), and its 1-N-ethyl analogue **3a** – approximately 60 min (with the general duration of anaesthesia of 2 hours).

It is interesting to note that the irritant action of 2% aqueous solutions of tricyclic amides **12-13,** determined by the rabbit's eye cornea according to the simplified modification of Setnikar method, is absent in most examples at all or decreases significantly comparing to its bicyclic prototypes **3a,b**. And it is in spite of the fact that acidity of enolic OH-groups in 1-hydroxy-3-oxo-5,6-dihydro-3H-pyrrolo[3,2,1-*ij*]quinoline-2-carboxylic acid and its 1-N-ethyl analogue is practically the same, and in 1-hydroxy-3-oxo-6,7-dihydro-3H,5H-pyrido[3,2,1-*ij*]-quinoline-2-carboxylic acid is similar with its 1-N-propyl analogue (pKa^{OH} = 13,44-13,48).

In general, based on the biological trials conducted, it can be stated that the structural transformation of the molecule, which accompanies the transfer from 1-alkylsubstitued 4-hydroxyquinolin-2-ones to conformation limited tricyclic pyrrolo- or tetrahydropyrido-quinolones, allows to decrease the irritant action of compounds of this class, but at the same time it has a strong negative effect on the local anesthetic properties and that is why it can be considered as unperspective.

Compound	Infiltration anaesthesia			Irritative effect, points
	The start of anaesthesia, min	Index	Duration of total anaesthesia, min	
12a	4.32 ± 0.28	1.1	Undetermined	0
12b	3.81 ± 0.21	2.7	Undetermined	0
12c	4.60 ± 0.33	2.0	Undetermined	0
12d	4.93 ± 0.39	1.2	Undetermined	0
12e	3.27 ± 0.30	5.1	Undetermined	0
12f	3.66 ± 0.27	3.5	Undetermined	0
12g	2.82 ± 0.31	12.2	10.64 ± 1.20	2
12h	2.05 ± 0.17	36.0	39.82 ± 2.37	1
12i	3.09 ± 0.28	9.8	9.27 ± 1.33	2
12j	2.91 ± 0.32	14.2	15.92 ± 1.24	1
12k	3.87 ± 0.45	6.4	5.30 ± 1.45	1
12l	2.24 ± 0.26	27.0	25.56 ± 1.62	0
12m	3.04 ± 0.34	16.2	14.75 ± 1.18	0
13a	5.26 ± 0.44	2.8	Undetermined	0
13b	4.32 ± 0.35	3.9	Undetermined	0
13c	4.63 ± 0.41	4.2	Undetermined	0
13d	5.65 ± 0.48	2.3	Undetermined	0
13e	3.72 ± 0.33	7.6	Undetermined	0
13f	4.08 ± 0.29	5.4	Undetermined	0
13g	3.26 ± 0.30	16.7	13.51 ± 1.81	1
13h	2.23 ± 0.23	36.0	40.24 ± 3.06	1
13i	3.92 ± 0.22	14.1	8.83 ± 1.26	1
13j	3.10 ± 0.25	17.3	11.48 ± 2.55	1
13k	4.05 ± 0.36	9.7	6.63 ± 1.14	0
13l	2.64 ± 0.23	21.4	28.96 ± 3.73	0
13m	3.22 ± 0.31	15.8	15.37 ± 2.02	0
3a	1.84 ± 0.10	36.0	58.92 ± 4.11	2
Chinoxicaine	1.61 ± 0.13	36.0	74.79 ± 4.71	2

Table 1. Biological properties of tricyclic compounds **12-13**

5. Application of the bioisosteric replacements methodology for optimization of the Chinoxicaine molecule

The term „isosters" was introduced by Irwing Langmuir at the beginning of the 20th century. By his definition, isosters are molecules or ions containing the same number of atoms, as well as the same number and arrangement of electrons. Therefore, "isosteric replacements" in the created drugs are replacement of an atom or the group to the similar one by size or valency. If the physiological activity remains at the same time, then such replacement is called "bioisosteric". After a while the term "bioisoster" has been referred to compounds obtained by replacement of quite "unsimilar" groupings, but with preserving their biological properties (King, 2002). As a result, the concept of bioisosteric replacements at present has become one of the most powerful means for creating effective and safe medicines (Devereux & Popelier, 2010; Wassermann & Bajorath, 2011; Large et al., 2011). Its application allows not only to optimise the known biologically active substances, but to reveal new structures with the similar or related properties and, thus, to increase the patent protection of a future medicine.

5.1 Hydrochlorides of 4-hydroxy-2-oxo-1,2,5,6,7,8-hexahydroquinoline-3-carboxylic acids N-R-amides

The first attempt to optimize the Chinoxicaine molecule by the method of bioisosteric replacements was replacement of its 1,2-dihydroquinoline nucleus by 1,2,5,6,7,8-hexahydroquinoline. We did it expecting that such transformation may appear to be bioisosteric. With this aim a large group of hydrochlorides of 4-hydroxy-2-oxo-1,2,5,6,7,8-hexahydroquinoline-3-carboxylic acids N-R-amides **14a-y** has been synthesized by the method developed earlier (Kolisnyk, 2009) (Figure 6).

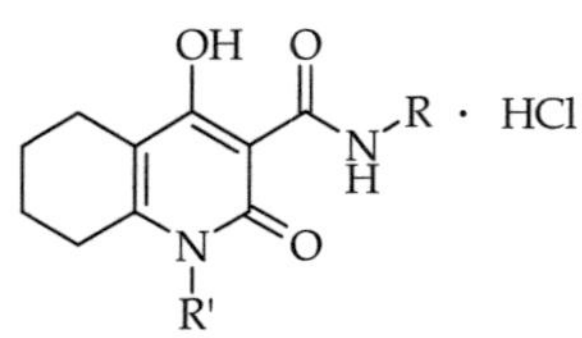

14a-y

14: R' = H: **a** R = 2-aminoethyl; **b** R = 3-aminopropyl; **c** R = 4-aminobutyl; **d** R = 6-aminohexyl; **e** R = 2-ethylaminoethyl; **f** R = 2-(2-hydroxyethylamino)ethyl; **g** R = 2-dimetylaminoethyl; **h** R = 2-diethylaminoethyl; **i** R = 3-dimethylaminopropyl; **j** R = 3-diethylaminopropyl; **k** R = 1-ethylpyrrolidin-2-ylmethyl; **l** R = 2-morpholin-4-ylethyl; **m** R = 3-morpholin-4-ylpropyl; **o** R = 3-piperidin-1-ylpropyl; **p** R = 3-(4-methylpiperazin-1-yl)propyl; **q** R = 4-diethylamino-1-methylbutyl

R' = Pr: **r** R = 2-diethylaminoethyl; **s** R = 3-diethylaminopropyl

R' = *cyclo*-Pr: **t** R = 2-ethylaminoethyl; **u** R = 2-(2-hydroxyethylamino)ethyl; **v** R = 2-dimetylaminoethyl; **w** R = 2-diethylaminoethyl; **x** R = 3-dimethylaminopropyl; **y** R = 3-diethylaminopropyl

Fig. 6. Hydrogenated analogues of Chinoxicaine

The biological screening conducted allow to state that reduction of the benzene part of the quinolone ring, unfortunately, leads to practically complete loss of local anaesthetic properties and that is why such modification should be considered unsuccessful. In other words, there is no reason to declare 4-hydroxy-2-oxo-1,2-dihydroquinoline and 4-hydroxy-2-oxo-1,2,5,6,7,8-hexahydroquinoline molecular systems to be bioisosteric (at least, in relation to local anaesthesia).

5.2 1-R-3-(2-Diethylaminoethyl)-1H-quinazoline-2,4-diones hydrochlorides

All ways of modification of Chinoxicaine molecule considered by us previously could not remove the local irritant action completely, therefore, it can be assumed that this drawback had been stipulated mainly by the presence of 4-OH-group. Thus, the next step of potentially bioisosteric transformation of Chinoxicaine was the synthesis of compounds known to be without groupings with acid properties. One of the examples of such substances were 1-R-3-(2-diethylaminoethyl)-1H-quinazoline-2,4-diones hydrochlorides **15a-f** (Figure 7). We considered various variants of obtaining compounds of this class allowing to choose the most suitable of them depending on the structure of the target product (Ukrainets et al., 2010)

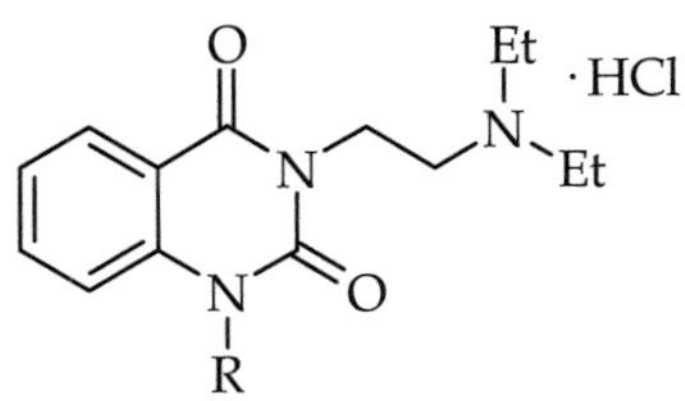

15: **a** R = H; **b** R = Me; **c** R = Et; **d** R = Pr; **e** R = Bu; **f** R = *i*-Bu

Fig. 7. Derivatives of 1H-quinazoline-2,4-dione

The study of the local irritant action of 1-R-3-(2-diethylaminoethyl)-1H-quinazoline-2,4-diones hydrochlorides **15** conducted in rabbits by the method of Lebo and Camage, has shown that the substances under research in the form of aqueous solutions with 2% concentration do not cause any reactive changes on the surface of the skin of the experimental animals. It should be worth mentioning that in similar conditions Chinoxicaine also does not reveal the irritating effect. That is why other, more sensitive, models should be involved in further research.

The ability of 2% aqueous solutions of the compounds synthesized to cause infiltration anaesthesia of the skin and subcutaneous cellulose has been studied in guinea pigs (Buelbring-Yueid method). Simultaneously several parameters characterizing the basic specific manifestations of the pharmacological effect such as the rate of anaesthesia onset, its depth (potency) and duration were taken into account. The data given in Table 2 shows that all 1-R-3-(2-diethylaminoethyl)-1H-quinazoline-2,4-diones hydrochlorides **15**, without exception, possess the local anaesthetic properties in some degree. In most cases anaesthesia occurs rather quickly and in some minutes after injection, the phase of deep anaesthesia begins. However, in spite of high values of the infiltration anaesthesia index, sometimes reaching the duration of the total anaesthesia caused by quinazolones **15** remains comparatively short and they yield to Chinoxicaine and Lidocaine greatly by this parameter. However, unlike the reference drugs the most active of the compounds synthesized – hydrochlorides **15a,e,f** – reveal a number of new properties, which can be considered as useful in the complex of the short, but powerful local anaesthetic action. They are sedation as well as movement disorder or motor block on the site of introduction of the substance examined. The motor block was estimated on the "peak" of the local anesthesia by 5 point scale: 0 points - the tail root tone preserved, movements preserved in full; 1 point - weakening of the tail root tone; 2 points - the weak tail root tone, sluggish movement, the animal sitting more; 3 points - lowering of the tail root tone and possible slight movement of the animal during stimulation of the skin section not occurring in the anesthetized zone, slight inhibition of the animal; 4 points - general atonia of the tail root, appearance of some inhibition of movement in response to stimulation, overall inhibition of the animal; 5 points

- the state of general atonia of the tail root without movement upon pain or electrical stimulation of the skin outside the area of anesthesia, the animal lying on side.

Compound	Infiltration anaesthesia			Motor block, points	Sedative effect, points
	The start of anaesthesia, min	Index	Duration of total anaesthesia, min		
15a	1.14 ± 0.16	36.0	32.35 ± 1.38	4	1
15b	1.53 ± 0.19	35.8	30.19 ± 0.75	0	0
15c	4.46 ± 0.29	18.5	15.74 ± 1.05	0	1
15d	2.97 ± 0.32	35.7	29.82 ± 0.59	0	0
15e	2.82 ± 0.43	36.0	36.46 ± 2.53	5	1
15f	1.59 ± 0.25	34.2	29.20 ± 1.43	5	3
Chinoxicaine	1.50 ± 0.04	36.0	75.61 ± 4.54	0	0
Lidocaine	2.12 ± 0.19	36.0	52.80 ± 3.76	0	0

Table 2. Biological properties of the quinazoline-2,4-diones hydrochlorides **15**

The sedative effect was estimated in the following way: 0 points - absent, the animal moving independently in cage; 1 point - the animal calm, sitting more, moving around the cage only when disturbed by the researcher; 2 points - the animal slowed down, sitting in the corner of the cage, anxiety with the researcher significantly set aside and again sitting, often closing eyelids, sleep onset; 3 points - the animal sleeping, lying on side, not responsive to stimulation by the researcher or to needle stick.

In general, the combination of analgesic, sedative and immobile extremities effects rendering by hydrochlorides **15a,e,f** can be used in creating medicines on their basis that are available for practical application in tiny surgical interventions, for example, in veterinary medicine. Thus, it can be stated confidently that 1-R-quinazoline-2,4-dionic cycle is bioisoster of 4-hydroxy-2-oxo-1,2-dihydroquinoline nucleus.

5.3 The irreversible chemical modification of Chinoxicaine at position 4 of the quinolone nucleus

The complex research described by us above has shown convincingly that 4-OH-group is the main cause of the local irritant properties of Chinoxicaine. Therefore, after its blocking one can expect the elimination of the undesired side effect. Meanwhile, we have not even considered alkylation or acylation of 4-OH-group as the most obvious variant of another bioreversible modification of Chinoxicaine. The reason is quite simple. Within a rather limited choice of pharmacologically available protective groups, neither 4-O-alkyl, nor 4-O-acyl derivatives of 4-hydroxyquinolin-2-ones have a high chemical stability. It is the tendency to hydrolysis that is a serious obstacle when synthesizing such compounds, as well as when further preparing sterile solutions for injections on their basis.

Taking it into account we tried to modify 4-OH-group of Chinoxicaine not by means of forming pro-drugs, but by using the same method of bioisosteric replacements, i.e. by its irreversible replacement with the groupings similar not by sizes or volume, but having the same physical and chemical properties and that is why inducing the similar pharmacological effect (King, 2002).

The first example of such transformation was 4-chloro-2-oxo-1-propyl-1,2-dihydroquinoline-3-carboxylic acid (2-diethylaminoethyl)amide hydrochloride **16** (Figure 8).
A high reactivity of the chlorine atom in 1-R-4-chloro-3-ethoxycarbonyl-2-oxo-1,2-dihydroquinolines in relation to nucleophilic reagents allows to transform them easily into 4-methyl-2-oxo-1,2-dihydroquinoline-3-carboxylic acids, one being the basis for synthesis of one more bioisoster of Chinoxicaine – 4-methyl substituted analogue **17**.
N-R-Amides of 2-oxo-1,2-dihydroquinoline-3-carboxylic acid with a primary amino group in position 4 of the quinolone ring exist in the 2-hydroxy-4-imino form rapidly hydrolyzed by mineral acids to 4-hydroxy-2-quinolones (Ukrainets et al., 2006b). Proceeding from it as the next object for pharmacological screening we deliberately obtained hydrochloride of 4-diethylamino-2-oxo-1-propyl-1,2-dihydroquinoline-3-carboxylic acid (2-diethylaminoethyl)-amide **18** as chemically more stable product. Amides **19a-d** containing no substituents at position 4 are of particular interest, in spite of the fact that due to the absence of these substituents they cannot be considered to be classical bioisosters of Chinoxicaine.
The study of local irritant action of the compounds synthesized, the ability to cause infiltration anaesthesia of the skin and subcutaneous cellulose, as well as the evaluation of the motor block and the sedative effect were carried out by standard methods previously described in detail by us (Ukrainets et al., 2010). It has been determined that all substances tested in the form of aqueous solutions with 2% concentration do not cause any reactive changes on the skin surface of the experimental animals.
From the data presented in Table 3 it follows that bioisosteric replacement of 4-OH-group to the chlorine atom – amide **16** – leads to significant decrease of all pharmacological indexes and, therefore, it is unsuccessful.

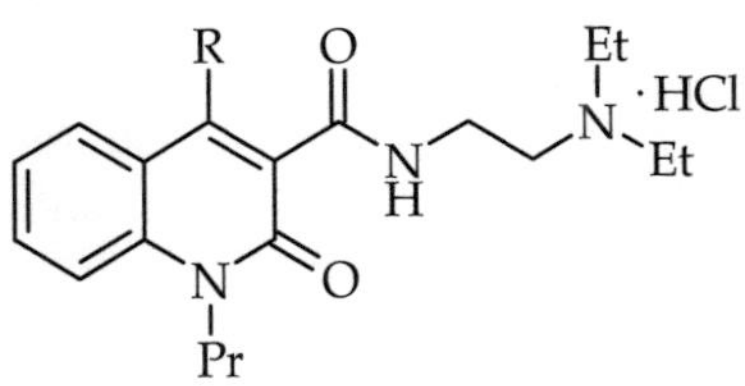

16 R = Cl
17 R = Me
18 R = $N(Et)_2$

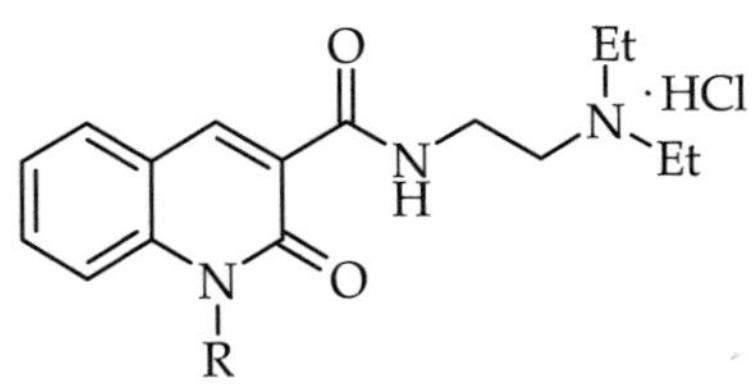

19: a R = Et; **b** R = Pr; **c** R = Bu; **d** R = *i*-Bu

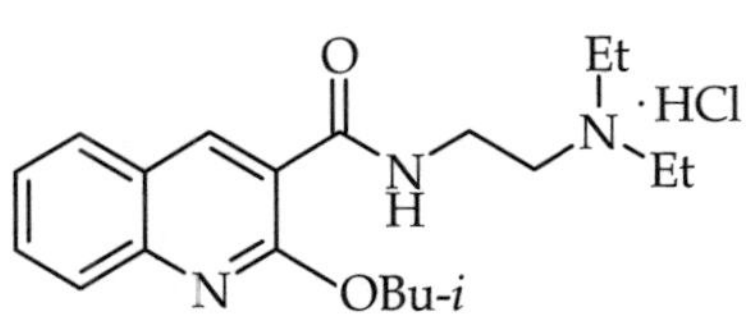

20

Fig. 8. Modification of 4-OH-group of Chinoxicaine

More interesting was the replacement of the hydroxyl group to the methyl one. From all substances of the last series 4-methyl-substituted amide **17** possesses the most rapid development of the biological effect (less than 2 min after injection). The infiltration anaesthesia index reaches the maximum possible value, and the total anaesthesia or the time of absence of pain and all types of sensitivity (tactile, temperature, etc.), during which the surgical intervention can be made (the section of tissues, wound suture, etc.), last approximately 55 min. These data prove the sufficient high activity of amide **17**, which are comparable to the reference drugs - Chinoxicaine and Lidocaine. However, amide **17** yields them significantly in the total duration of anaesthesia, i.e. time when the sensitivity increases gradually and then restores completely.

Compound	Infiltration anaesthesia				Motor block, points	Sedative effect, points
	The start of anaesthesia, min	Index	The total anaesthesia, min	The general duration of anaesthesia, min		
16	3.96 ± 0.42	26.3	14.25 ± 1.11	24.72 ± 2.18	0	0
17	1.94 ± 0.21	36.0	55.33 ± 2.74	68.38 ± 2.68	0	0
18	2.28 ± 0.31	36.0	37.51 ± 2.83	67.85 ± 2.37	0	0
19a	4.52 ± 0.32	19.3	13.20 ± 1.00	21.01 ± 1.67	0	0
19b	4.50 ± 0.36	35.5	27.89 ± 1.89	32.34 ± 2.92	0	0
19c	3.03 ± 0.28	36.0	39.04 ± 2.12	58.26 ± 2.81	5	2
19d	2.71 ± 0.37	36.0	53.77 ± 1.93	83.28 ± 2.05	5	3
20	2.82 ± 0.44	35.6	47.56 ± 1.74	85.48 ± 2.33	5	3
Chinoxicaine	1.62 ± 0.13	36.0	74.74 ± 4.71	236.89 ± 9.34	0	0
Lidocaine	2.34 ± 0.20	36.0	51.26 ± 3.45	140.27 ± 6.20	0	0

Table 3. Biological properties of 4-OH-modified derivatives of Chinoxicaine

A special attention should be paid to 4-diethylamine derivative **18**, not only for its high anaesthetic properties, but for the perspective to perform further modifications of such type easily and practically in unlimited quantity as well and to reach the result required.

From the series of non-substituted amides **19** at position 4 it is worth mentioning only compounds with butyl and *iso*-butyl substituents at the cyclic nitrogen atom (amides **19c** and **19d** respectively). Both are characterized by a rather rapid onset of action and high values of infiltration anaesthesia indexes. The distinctive feature of the first one is the signs of drowsiness, inertia in animals in 10-15 min after the injection and complete sleepiness can occur at 15-20 min. The motor block with the strength of 5 points lasts for approximately 20 min on the site of introduction of the substance examined. In the case of amide **19d** already by 7-10 min after injection the animals had the state of deep sleep: they slept on their side without the reaction to the active stimulation by the needle (tactile, pain and temperature sensitivity is absent). In 15-20 min the animals awoke, but they were drowsy and motionless for approximately 20 min and then began to move their paws. Therefore, one can speak about the deep and prolonged motor block and the marked sedative effect, which can be very useful properties of local anesthetic while conducting a number of short-termed surgical interventions, especially when rendering aid to patients with the increased excitability and possible fear before any surgical manipulations.

The study of hydrochloride of 2-isobutoxyquinoline-3-carboxylic acid (2-diethylamino-ethyl)amide **20** is of particular interest. This compound has been specially synthesized by us as an aromatic analogue of the most active of 1,2-dihydro derivatives, i.e. amide **19d**. A comparative analysis of biological properties of these isomers demonstrates that with transfer to the aromatic structure some parameters decrease, and others, vice versa, intensify. For example, amide **20** differs with the later start of anaesthesia, decrease of the index and reduction of duration of the deep anaesthesia phase. At the same time the general duration of anaesthesia increases a little, as well as duration of the sedative effect. Unfortunately, transfer of the isobutyl substituent from the nitrogen atom to the oxygen atom is accompanied by appearance of undesirable properties - unlike amide **19d** its aromatic isomer **20** has been found to have the irritant action, though a transient one.

6. Conclusion

The research carried out by us gives reason to suppose that 4-hydroxy-2-oxo-1,2-dihydroquinoline-3-carboxylic acids are of great interest as a base in creating new effective medicines to eliminate pain. Such medicines can be not only local anesthetics possessing the unique complex of pharmacological properties, but, as it has been found quite recently, non-narcotic analgesics with high activity and low toxicity as well. The rich arsenal of structural and biological regularities accumulated, as well as practically unlimited synthetic potential of 4-hydroxyquinolin-2-ones allow to change the character of impact of such compounds on a living organism easily and in the required direction, and thus, to provide their direct practical value and a great perspective.

7. Acknowledgment

We appreciate the assistance of professor V.I. Mamchur (Dnepropetrovsk State Medical Academy, Ukraine) in studying biological properties of the compounds synthesized and useful comments while discussing the results obtained.

8. References

Bochkov, A.F. & Smit, V.A. (1987). *Organic Synthesis. Purposes, Methods, Tactics, Strategy* [in Russian], Nauka, Moscow, Russia

Kartsev, V.G. (Ed.). (2007). *Selected Methods for Synthesis and Modification of Heterocycles. Vol. 6. Quinolines: Chemistry and Biological Activity* [in Russian], International charitable foundation "Scientific Partnership Foundation" (ICSPF), ISBN 978-5-903078-10-3, Moscow, Russia

Kleemann, A. & Engel J. (2001). *Pharmaceutical Substances: Syntheses, Patents, Applications,* Thieme Medical Publishers, ISBN 1588900312, Stuttgart, Germany

Tomoda, K.; Asahiyama, M.; Ohtsuki, E.; Nakajima, T.; Terada, H.; Kanebako, M.; Inagi, T. & Makino, K. (2009). Preparation and Properties of Carrageenan Microspheres Containing Allopurinol and Local Anesthetic Agents for the Treatment of Oral Mucositis. *Colloids and Surfaces. B, Biointerfaces,* Vol.71, No.1, pp. 27-35, ISSN 0927-7765

Kang, C. & Shin, S.C. (2010). Preparation and Evaluation of Bioadhesive Dibucaine Gels for Enhanced Local Anesthetic Action. *Archives of Pharmacal Research,* Vol.33, No.8, pp. 1277-1283, ISSN 0253-6269

Douglas, H.A.; Callaway, J.K.; Sword, J.; Kirov, S.A. & Andrew, R.D. (2011). Potent Inhibition of Anoxic Depolarization by the Sodium Channel Blocker Dibucaine. *Journal of Neurophysiology,* Vol.105, No.4, pp. 1482-1494, ISSN 0022-3077

Ukrainets, I.V. (1992). Synthesis, Chemical Transformation and Biological Properties of Alkyl(aryl)amides of Malonic Acid Derivatives [in Russian]. *Thesis for Doctor Degree in Chemistry in speciality 15.00.02 – Pharmaceutical Chemistry and Pharmacognosy,* Manuscript, Kharkov, Ukraine

Ukrainets, I.V.; Gorokhova, O.V.; Taran, S.G.; Bezugly, P.A.; Filimonova, N.I. & Turov, A.V. (1994). 4-Hydroxy-2-Quinolones. 24. Improved Synthesis and Biological Properties of 1-Alkyl-4-Hydroxy-2-Quinoline-3-Carboxylic Acid β-Dialkylaminoalkylamide Hydrochlorides. *Chemistry of Heterocyclic Compounds,* Vol.30, No.10, pp. 1214-1219, ISSN 0009-3122

Gorokhova, O.V. (1993). Synthesis, Chemical and Biological Properties of Alkyl- and Arylamides of Malonic Acid Derivatives [in Russian]. *Thesis for Candidate Degree in Chemistry in speciality 15.00.02 – Pharmaceutical Chemistry and Pharmacognosy,* Manuscript, Kharkov, Ukraine

Davidenko, O.O. (2011). Synthesis, Physical, Chemical Properties and Biological Activity of Substituted 4-Hydroxy-2-Oxo-1,2-Dihydroquinoline-3-Carboxylic Acids and Their Derivatives [in Ukrainian]. *Thesis for Candidate Degree in Pharmacy in speciality 15.00.02 – Pharmaceutical Chemistry and Pharmacognosy,* Manuscript, Kharkov, Ukraine

Ukrainets, I.V.; Bezugly, P.A.; Gorokhova, O.V.; Taran, S.G. & Treskach, V.I. (1998). Method for Preparing 1-Propyl-2-Oxo-4-Hydroxyquinoline-3-Carboxylic Acid Diethylaminoethylamide Hydrochloride (Chinoxycaine). *Patent Ukraine 24967,* Available from http://base.ukrpatent.org/searchINV/

Ukrayinecz, I.V. & Bezuhliy, P.A. (2002). Injectable Anesthetic. *Patent USA 6340692,* Available from http://worldwide.espacenet.com/searchResults?NUM=US6340692&DB=EPODOC&locale=en_EP&ST=number&compact=false

Romanov, I.V. & Ukrainets, I.V. (2006). Method for Preparing 1-Propyl-2-Oxo-4-Hydroxyquinoline-3-Carboxylic Acid Diethylaminoethylamide Hydrochloride (Chinoxycaine). *Patent Russia 2285692,* Available from http://worldwide.espacenet.com/searchResults?NUM=RU2285692&DB=EPODOC&locale=en_EP&ST=number&compact=false

Kubinyi, H. (2006). In Looking ups of the New Compounds-leaders for Creation of Drugs [in Russian]. *Russian Chemical Journal,* Vol.L, No.2, pp. 5-17, ISSN 0373-0247, Available from http://www.chem.msu.su/rus/journals/jvho/2006-2/5.pdf

Kuznetsov, S.G.; Chigareva, S.M. & Ramsh, S.M. (1991). Pro-drugs. Chemical Aspect. *Summaries in Science and Technology. Organic Chemistry* [in Russian], VINITI, ISSN 0137-0251, Moscow, Russia

Ukrainets, I.V. (1988). Synthesis and Research of New Biological Active Derivatives of Malonic Acid 2-Carboxyphenylamide [in Russian]. *Thesis for Candidate Degree in Pharmacy in speciality 15.00.02 – Pharmaceutical Chemistry and Pharmacognosy,* Manuscript, Kharkov, Ukraine

Ukrainets, I.V.; Kravtzova, V.V.; Tkach, A.A. & Rybakov, V.B. (2009). 4-Hydroxy-2-Quinolones. 155. Bioreversible Chemical Modification of Chinoxycaine at the Tertiary Amino Group as a Method of Improving its Pharmaceutical Activity. *Chemistry of Heterocyclic Compounds,* Vol.45, No.6, pp. 698-704, ISSN 0009-3122

Vinogradova, N.D.; Kuznetsov, S.G. & Chigareva, S.M. (1980). Quaternary Ammonium Salts with Labile N+-C Bonds as Drug Precursors. *Pharmaceutical Chemistry Journal,* Vol.14, No.9, pp. 604-609, ISSN 0091-150X

Chen, H.; Gong, Y.; Gries, R.M. & Plettner, E. (2010). Synthesis and Biological Activity of Conformationally Restricted Gypsy Moth Pheromone Mimics. Bioorganic and Medicinal Chemistry, Vol.18, No.8, pp. 2920-2929, ISSN 0968-0896

Watanabe, M.; Hirokawa, T.; Kobayashi, T.; Yoshida, A.; Ito, Y.; Yamada, S.; Orimoto, N.; Yamasaki, Y.; Arisawa, M. & Shuto, S. (2010). Investigation of the Bioactive Conformation of Histamine H3 Receptor Antagonists by the Cyclopropylic Strain-based Conformational Restriction Strategy. Journal of Medicinal Chemistry, Vol.53, No.9, pp. 3585-93, ISSN 0022-2623

Nirogia, R.V.; Kambhampati, R.; Daulatabad, A.V.; Gudla, P.; Shaikh, M.; Achanta, P.K.; Shinde, A.K. & Dubey, P.K. (2011). Design, Synthesis and Pharmacological Evaluation of Conformationally Restricted N-Arylsulfonyl-3-Aminoalkoxy Indoles as a Potential 5-HT(6) Receptor Ligands. *Journal of Enzyme Inhibition and Medicinal Chemistry,* Vol.26, No.3, pp. 341-349, ISSN 1475-6366

Ukrainets, I.V.; Tkach, A.A. & Grinevich, L.A. (2008). 4-Hydroxy-2-Quinolones. 148. Synthesis and Anti-tubercular Activity of 1-Hydroxy-3-Oxo-6,7-Dihydro-3H,5H-Pyrido-[3,2,1-*ij*]quinoline-2-Carboxylic Acid N-R-Amides. *Chemistry of Heterocyclic Compounds,* Vol.44, No.8, pp. 956-966, ISSN 0009-3122

Baumer, V.N.; Shishkin, O.V.; Ukrainets, I.V.; Sidorenko, L.V. & El Kayal, S.A. (2004). 1-Ethyl-4-Hydroxyquinolin-2(1H)-one. *Acta Crystallographica Section E,* Vol.60, No.12, pp. o2356-o2358, ISSN 1600-5368

Ukrainets, I.V.; Gorokhova, O.V.; Sidorenko, L.V. & Bereznyakova, N.L. (2007). 4-Hydroxy-2-Quinolones. 111. Simple Synthesis of 1-Substituted 4-Methyl-2-Oxo-1,2-Dihydroquino-line-3-Carboxylic Acids. *Chemistry of Heterocyclic Compounds,* Vol.43, No.1, pp. 58-62, ISSN 0009-3122

Ukrainets, I.V.; Sidorenko, L.V.; Gorokhova, O.V.; Mospanova, E.V. & Shishkin, O.V. (2006a). 4-Hydroxy-2-Quinolones. 94. Improved Synthesis and Structure of 1-Hydroxy-3-Oxo-5,6-Dihydro-3H-Pyrrolo[3,2,1-*i,j*]quinoline-2-Carboxylic Acid Ethyl Ester. *Chemistry of Heterocyclic Compounds,* Vol.42, No.5, pp. 631-635, ISSN 0009-3122

Kravtsova, V.V. (2011). The Search of New Local Anesthetics in the Range of Amide Derivatives of Oxoquinoline-3-Carboxylic Acids [in Ukrainian]. *Thesis for Candidate Degree in Pharmacy in speciality 15.00.02 – Pharmaceutical Chemistry and Pharmacognosy,* Manuscript, Kharkov, Ukraine

King, F.D. (Ed.). (2002). *Medicinal Chemistry: Principles and Practice,* Royal Society of Chemistry, ISBN 0854046313, Cambridge, UK

Devereux, M. & Popelier, P.L. (2010). In Silico Techniques for the Identification of Bioisosteric Replacements for Drug Design. *Current Topics in Medicinal Chemistry,* Vol.10, No.6, pp. 657-668, ISSN 1568-0266

Wassermann, A.M. & Bajorath, J. (2011). Large-scale Exploration of Bioisosteric Replacements on the Basis of Matched Molecular Pairs. *Future Medicinal Chemistry,* Vol.3, No.4, pp. 425-36, ISSN 1756-8919

Large, J.M.; Torr, J.E.; Raynaud, F.I.; Clarke, P.A.; Hayes, A.; Stefano, F.; Urban, F.; Shuttleworth, S.J.; Saghir, N.; Sheldrake, P.; Workman, P. & McDonald, E. (2011). Preparation and Evaluation of Trisubstituted Pyrimidines as Phosphatidylinositol 3-Kinase Inhibitors. 3-Hydroxyphenol Analogues and Bioisosteric Replacements. Bioorganic and Medicinal Chemistry, Vol.19, No.2, pp. 836-851, ISSN 0968-0896

Kolisnyk, O.V. (2009). Synthesis, Physical, Chemical and Biological Properties of 4-Hydroxy-2-Oxo-1,2,5,6,7,8-Hexahydroquinoline-3-Carboxylic Acids Amidation Derivatives. [in Ukrainian]. *Thesis for Candidate Degree in Pharmacy in speciality 15.00.02 – Pharmaceutical Chemistry and Pharmacognosy,* Manuscript, Kharkov, Ukraine

Ukrainets, I.V., Kravtsova, V.V., Tkach, A.A., Mamchur, V.I. & Kovalenko, E.Yu. (2010). 4-Hydroxy-2-Quinolones. 173. 1-R-3-(2-Diethylaminoethyl)-1H-Quinazoline-2,4-Dione Hydrochlorides as Potential Local Anesthetic Agents. *Chemistry of Heterocyclic Compounds,* Vol.46, No.1, pp. 96-105, ISSN 0009-3122

Ukrainets, I.V.; Sidorenko, L.V.; Gorokhova, O.V. & Jaradat, N.A. (2006b). 4-Hydroxy-2-Quinolones. 93. Synthesis and Biological Properties of 2-Hydroxy-4-Imino-1,4-Dihydroquinoline-3-Carboxylic Acid N-R-Amides. *Chemistry of Heterocyclic Compounds,* Vol.42, No.4, pp. 475-487, ISSN 0009-3122

5

Neuroprotection and Pain Management

Kambiz Hassanzadeh and Esmael Izadpanah
Kurdistan University of Medical Sciences, Sanandaj
Iran

1. Introduction

Pain, as a sub modality of somatic sensation, has been defined as a complex constellation of unpleasant sensory, emotional and cognitive experiences provoked by real or perceived tissue damage and manifested by certain autonomic, psychological, and behavioral reactions. The benefit of these unpleasant sensations, however, is underscored by extreme cases: patients lacking the ability to perceive pain due to hereditary neuropathies often maintain unrealized infections; self mutilate, and have curtailed life spans. Normally, nociception and the perception of pain are evoked only at pressures and temperatures extreme enough to potentially injured tissues and by toxic molecules and inflammatory mediators. As opposed to the relatively more objective nature of other senses, pain is highly individual and subjective and the translation of nociception into pain perception can be curtailed by stress or exacerbated by anticipation (Woolf).

Chronic pain is estimated to affect millions of people worldwide and is one of the most common reasons for physician visits (Scascighini et al. 2008). Inflammation may cause direct painful stimuli as well as sensitize nociceptors to stimulation (McMahon et al. 2005). Thus, there are multiple points along the pain pathway that represent opportunities for therapeutic intervention. Despite this, there are only a limited number of mechanisms through which current pain medications work. Major classes of analgesics include opioids, non-steroidal anti-inflammatory drugs, antidepressants, and anticonvulsants. Although these treatments provide relief, the effects are often incomplete and complicated by serious side effects and/or tolerance. Thus, therapeutics with novel mechanisms of actions are desperately needed (Finnerup et al. 2005).

What exactly, from a neurobiological perspective, is pain? Pain is actually three quite different things, although it is difficult to make the distinction; nociceptive pain, inflammatory pain and neuropathic pain. Nociceptive pain is not a clinical problem, except in the specific context of surgery and other clinical procedures that necessarily involve noxious stimuli, where it must be suppressed by local and general anesthetics or high-dose opioids (Woolf).

Nociception involves multiple steps from the peripheral receptor, the afferent nerve transmitting the impulse to the spinal cord, the signal processing in the dorsal horn, with inhibitory and facilitatory elements and finally transmission to higher cerebral centers where the peripheral nociceptive stimulus is perceived as pain (Arendt-Nielsen and Sumikura 2002).

The second kind of pain is also adaptive and protective. By heightening sensory sensitivity after unavoidable tissue damage, this pain assists in the healing of the injured body part by creating a situation that discourages physical contact and movement. Pain hypersensitivity, or tenderness, reduces further risk of damage and promotes recovery, as after a surgical wound or in an inflamed joint, where normally innocuous stimuli now elicit pain. This pain is caused by activation of the immune system by tissue injury or infection, and is therefore called inflammatory pain.

Finally, there is the pain that is not protective, but maladaptive, resulting from abnormal functioning of the nervous system. This pathological pain, which is not a symptom of some disorder but rather a disease state of the nervous system, can occur after damage to the nervous system (neuropathic pain), but also in conditions in which there is no such damage or inflammation (dysfunctional pain) (Woolf).

The incidence of pain rises as people get older and women are more likely to be in pain than men. Pain management strategies include pain relieving medications, physical or occupational therapy and complementary therapies (such as acupuncture and massage).

Pharmacologic therapies are the foundation of chronic pain management. These therapies include nonopioids, opioids, and adjuvant analgesics, physical techniques physical measures, such as physical activity, physical and occupational therapy, orthotics, and assistive devices can serve as adjuncts to analgesics in the management of chronic pain (Paice and Ferrell).

On the other hand in recent years, we and others have focused on the relationship between neuroprotection and pain mechanism and management. Thus in this chapter we will review recent progress related to neuronal mechanism for using neuroprotective agents alone or in combination with antinociceptive drugs to reduce the pain. In addition we will focus on the effect of neuroprotective agents on prevention of tolerance to the analgesic effect of opiates.

2. Neuroprotection

Neuroprotection is the mechanism and strategies used to protect against neural injury or degeneration in the central nervous system (CNS). There is a wide range of neuroprotective products available or under investigation. Some products with neuroprotective effects are grouped into the following categories:

- Free radical scavengers
- Anti excitotoxic agents
- Anti apoptotic agents
- Anti inflammatory agents
- Neurotrophic factors

To better understand, we first discuss the mechanism by which neurotoxins induce toxicity.

3. Glutamate

Glutamate is a neurotransmitter with roles such as long-term potentiation and synaptic plasticity of the brain (Harris et al. 1984) and is also a exitotoxin whose neurotoxicity has been associated with numerous neurodegenerative diseases, such as Alzheimer disease (AD), (Kihara et al. 2002) vascular dementia, (Martinez et al. 1993) Parkinson disease (Greenamyre 2001) and amyotrophic lateral sclerosis (Cid et al. 2003).

Glutamatergic synapses are the key excitatory synapses within the brain, and mechanisms of both hyperglutamatergic and hypoglutamatergic functioning have been implicated in the pathophysiology of CNS disorders (Olney et al. 1999).

Glutamatergic receptors include both iontropic and metabotropic receptor subtypes. The iontropic receptors include N-Methyl-D-Aspartat (NMDA), α-amino-3-hydroxy-5-methyl-4-isoxazole propionic acid (AMPA), and kainate receptors. Binding of glutamate to these receptors causes Ca^{2+} and Na^{+} entry into neurons, resulting in excitatory postsynaptic potentials and membrane depolarization. In addition, increased intracellular Ca^{2+} levels activate a number of signaling cascades (Berridge 1998). The NMDA receptor forms a channel allowing for ion influx, whereas the AMPA and kainate receptors open voltage-sensitive ion channels on the cell membrane. The NMDA receptor is voltage-gated and is blocked by magnesium and modulated by two coagonists, glycine and d-serine, as well as by several intracellular and extracellular mediators (Millan 2005)). It has been proposed that NMDA receptor hypofunction may lead to excessive stimulation of other iontropic receptors, causing a cascade of excitotoxic events including oxidative stress and apoptosis (Deutsch et al. 2001). Dysregulation of glutamateric functioning has been observed across many components of the glutamate neurotransmission system.

The mechanism of glutamate-induced neuronal death has been extensively studied: glutamate induces neuronal death *via* stimulation of NMDA receptor through which Ca^{2+} enters the cell and activates Ca^{2+}-dependent nitric oxide (NO) synthase, resulting in excessive nitric oxide formation, production of radicals, mitochondrial dysfunction and cell death (Kaneko et al. 1997). It has been shown that glutamate induces neuronal death associated with necrosis and apoptosis. Necrosis is caused by catastrophic cell damage and is characterized by cell swelling, injury to cytoplasmic organelles and rapid collapse of internal homeostasis, leading to the lysis of membranes and the release of cellular contents, resulting in inflammation. On the other hand, apoptosis is a process characterized by cell shrinkage, membrane blebbing, nuclear pyknosis, chromatin condensation and genomic fragmentation (Kerr et al. 1972; Schulte-Hermann et al. 1992; Takada-Takatori et al. 2009).

In rodents, blocking of NMDA receptors is associated with increased release of glutamate within the cerebral cortex (Moghaddam et al. 1997), (Adams and Moghaddam 1998) and nucleus accumbens (Razoux et al. 2007). However, elevations in glutamate within the prefrontal cortex of rodents occurs during short-term administration of NMDA antagonists, whereas long-term administration over 7 consecutive days actually results in a trend for lower basal levels and lower dialysate levels of glutamate upon challenge (Zuo et al. 2006). Thus, excitotoxic events associated with NMDA antagonists may be reflected by initial increases in glutamatergic neurotransmission that are followed subsequently and chronically by lower levels.

4. Apoptosis and *N*-Methyl-*D*-Aspartate antagonist-induced neurodegeneration

As noted before glutamate can induce apoptosis via NMDA receptor activation. Apoptosis or programmed cell death is a process normally associated with the elimination of redundant neurons during neurodevelopment (Johnson et al. 1995). Apoptosis involves the regulation of a complex molecular cascade controlling the activation of a family of cysteine proteases known as caspase proteins (Glantz et al. 2006). Caspases are responsible for breaking down important structural and functional proteins, leading to cellular degradation and eventually death. Apoptosis results from a cascade of gene activation and involves genes that both promote (i.e., Bax) (Schlesinger et al. 1997), (Gross et al. 1998) and oppose

the process (i.e., Bcl-2) (Craig 1995), (Schlesinger et al. 1997), (Adams and Cory 1998). In a study we showed that there is a relation between glutamate increase and apoptosis promotion and increase in proapoptotic agent activity in both cerebral cortex and lumbar spinal cord of rat (Hassanzadeh et al.).
A vast array of stimuli can activate apoptosis in neurons (Sastry and Rao 2000). Many of these stimuli have been implicated in the pathophysiology of opioid-induced tolerance including glutamate excitotoxicity, increased calcium flux and mitochondria dysfunction and these mechanisms are discussed in detail later in this chapter.

5. Neuroactive steroids are neuroprotective

Neuroactive steroids are endogenous neuromodulators synthesized either within the brain (neurosteroids) or in the periphery by the adrenal glands and gonads. In addition to the classic effect of steroids on gene transcription via binding to intracellular steroid receptors, neuroactive steroids can alter neuronal excitability via nongenomic effects by acting at inhibitory Gama Amino Butiric Acid A ($GABA_A$) receptors and/or excitatory NMDA receptors, among others (Shulman and Tibbo 2005), (Marx et al. 2006). There is also evidence for a potential role of these neurosteroids in controlling GABA and glutamate release. Neuroactive steroids have also been implicated in neuroprotection, myelination, and modulation of the stress response. A number of neuroactive steroids are present in human postmortem brain at physiologically relevant nanomolar concentrations and serve as allosteric modulators of the $GABA_A$ receptor (Marx et al. 2006). Neuroactive steroids that are effective modulators of $GABA_A$ and/or T-type Ca2+ channels are promising tools for studying the role of these channels in peripheral pain perception. They appear to be very effective in alleviating peripheral Nociception in rat models of acute and chronic pain (Jevtovic-Todorovic et al. 2009).

6. Acetyl Choline Receptors (AChRs) and neuroprotection

Agonists and antagonist selective for AChR subtypes have been used in experimental and clinical research. Some of those compounds are potential candidates for the treatment of neurodegenerative disease such as Alzheimer's disease, Parkinson's disease and others. A growing list of *in vivo* and *in vitro* research suggest that AChRs modulators are gaining importance as clinically relevant neuroprotective drugs (Mudo et al. 2007).
The inhibition of α7 AChRs decreases the GABAergic tone causing increased ACh release into the synaptic cleft (Giorgetti et al. 2000), which then activates the α4β2 AChRs located post-synaptically. The selective α7 inhibitor methyllycaconitine (Ivy Carroll et al. 2007) mimics, at least in part, the neuroprotective effect of 4R (Ferchmin et al. 2003). Other i*n vivo* and *in vitro* studies confirm that α7 inhibition can be neuroprotective (de Fiebre and de Fiebre 2005), (Laudenbach et al. 2002), (Martin et al. 2004).
Protection of neurons from neuronal damage and cell death in neurodegenerative disease is a major challenge in neuroscience research. Donepezil, galantamine and tacrine are acetylcholinesterase inhibitors used for the treatment of Alzheimer's disease, and were believed to be symptomatic drugs whose therapeutic effects are achieved by slowing the hydrolysis of acetylcholine at synaptic termini. However, recent accumulated evidence strongly suggests that these acetylcholinesterase inhibitors also possess neuroprotective properties whose mechanism is independent of acetylcholinesterase inhibition. It has been

shown that acetylcholinesterase inhibitors protect neurons from glutamate-induced neurotoxicity in the primary culture of rat cortical neurons.
The long-standing belief was that acetylcholinesterase inhibitors are symptomatic agents that ameliorate cholinergic deficits by slowing the hydrolysis of acetylcholinesterase at synaptic nerve termini; however, recent studies have shown that acetylcholinesterase inhibitors have other pharmacological properties, for example, neuroprotection against toxic insults, such as glutamate and up-regulation of nicotinic receptors (Akaike 2006), (Takada-Takatori et al. 2009).
Several reports have indicated that activation of cholinergic neurons in the central nervous system produces antinociception and analgesia in a variety of animals, including humans (Harte et al. 2004) provide evidence supporting the involvement of the intralaminar thalamus in muscarinic induced antinociception. Pharmacological experiments have shown that the microinjection of acetylcholine or carbachol into specific brainstem nuclei can produce antinociception and can be reversed by muscarinic receptor antagonists (Brodie and Proudfit 1984), (Yaksh et al. 1985). Meanwhile some other types of receptors or drugs produce analgesia by mediation of ACh. Sumatriptan (5- HT1agonist) is able to induce antinociception by increasing cholinergic neurotransmission (Ghelardini et al. 1997). D2 antagonist prochlorperazine exerts an antinocicptive effect mediated by a central cholinergic mechanism (Ghelardini et al. 2004), (Yang et al. 2008). In addition, more recently we showed that an acethylcolinesterase inhibitor, donepezil, could prevent tolerance to the analgesic effect of morphine (unpublished data).

7. Cannabinoids, pain and neuroprotection

Pain severely impairs quality of life. Currently available treatments, generally opioids and anti-inflammatory drugs, are not always effective for certain painful conditions. The discovery of the cannabinoid receptors in the 1990s led to the characterization of the endogenous cannabinoid system in terms of its components and numerous basic physiologic functions. Cannabinoid$_1$ (CB1) receptors are present in nervous system areas involved in modulating nociception and evidence supports a role of the endocannabinoids in pain modulation. Cannabinoids have antinociceptive mechanisms different from that of other drugs currently in use, which thus opens a new line of promising treatment to mitigate pain that fails to respond to the pharmacologic treatments available, especially for neuropathic and inflammatory pains (Manzanares et al. 2006).
Cannabis extracts and synthetic cannabinoids are still widely considered illegal substances. The Cannabis sativa plant has been exploited for medicinal, agricultural and spiritual purposes in diverse cultures over thousands of years. Cannabis has been used recreationally for its psychotropic properties, while effects such as stimulation of appetite, analgesia and anti-emesis have lead to the medicinal application of cannabis. Indeed, reports of medicinal efficacy of cannabis can been traced back as far as 2700 BC, and even at that time reports also suggested a neuroprotective effect of the cultivar (Scotter et al.).
Preclinical and clinical studies have suggested that they may result useful to treat diverse diseases, including those related with acute or chronic pain. The discovery of cannabinoid receptors, their endogenous ligands, and the machinery for the synthesis, transport, and degradation of these retrograde messengers, has equipped us with neurochemical tools for novel drug design. Agonist-activated cannabinoid receptors, modulate nociceptive thresholds, inhibit release of pro-inflammatory molecules, and display synergistic effects

with other systems that influence analgesia, especially the endogenous opioid system. Cannabinoid receptor agonists have shown therapeutic value against inflammatory and neuropathic pains, conditions that are often refractory to therapy. Although the psychoactive effects of these substances have limited clinical progress to study cannabinoid actions in pain mechanisms, preclinical research is progressing rapidly.

There has been anecdotal and preliminary scientific evidence of cannabis affording symptomatic relief in diverse neurodegenerative disorders. These include multiple sclerosis, Huntington's, Parkinson's and Alzheimer's diseases, and amyotrophic lateral sclerosis. This evidence implied that hypofunction or dysregulation of the endocannabinoid system may be responsible for some of the symptomatology of these diseases.

In Huntington's disease, Alzheimer's disease, as well as in ALS, pathologic changes in endocannabinoid levels and CB2 expression are induced by the inflammatory environment.

CB1 activation has been shown to be effective in limiting cell death following excitotoxic lesions, while CB2 is involved in dampening inflammatory immune cell response to disease. These two targets may therefore work together to provide both neuroprotection to acute injury and immune suppression during more chronic responses (Scotter et al.).

During the last two decades, a large number of research papers have demonstrated the efficacy of cannabinoids and modulators of the endocannabinoid system in suppressing neuropathic pain in animal models. Cannabinoids suppress hyperalgesia and allodynia (i.e. mechanical allodynia, mechanical hyperalgesia, thermal hyperalgesia and, where evaluated, cold allodynia), induced by diverse neuropathic pain states through CB1 and CB2-specific mechanisms (Rahn and Hohmann 2009).

On the other hand, responses to cannabinoid (CB) receptor activation include opening of potassium channels, inhibition of calcium currents, and stimulation of various protein kinases (Deadwyler et al. 1995; Gomez del Pulgar et al. 2000; Galve-Roperh et al. 2002; Karanian et al. 2005b; Molina-Holgado et al. 2005; Karanian et al. 2007). Some of the many such signaling elements activated by endocannabinoids play important roles in neuronal maintenance (Bahr et al. 2006; Galve-Roperh et al. 2008). CB receptor transmission elicits modulatory effects on calcium channels, resulting in reduced neurotransmitter (e.g., GABA, glutamate) release (Hajos et al. 2000; Kreitzer and Regehr 2001; Wilson et al. 2001). One particular mitogen-activated protein kinase, extracellular signal-regulated kinase (ERK), is involved in cannabinergic signaling, as are focal adhesion kinase (FAK) and phosphatidylinositol 3'-kinase (PI3K). These signaling elements appear to play key roles in the neuroprotective nature of the endocannabinoid system, and the associated signaling pathways are disrupted by blocking CB receptor activation (Hwang et al.; Wallace et al. 2003; Khaspekov et al. 2004; Karanian et al. 2005a; Karanian et al. 2005b).

Together, these studies indicate that the neuroprotectant cannabinoids have antinociceptive properties.

8. Neuroprotection and tolerance to the analgesic effect

8.1 Opioid tolerance

Many types of neuronal cells and brain nuclei have the property of changing, acutely or chronically, their regular behavior by the action of pharmacological agents, such as psychoactive drugs. Acute changes, those that cease in a short time, would not be important to the chronic altered behavior if the cell recovered its original drug-free state, but it is observed that some adaptation occurs that impairs such a recovery. In fact, the disturbed cell under the influence of a drug tries to compensate for its acute effects by promoting changes in the opposite direction, transiently restoring its homeostasis. However, when the acute action of the drug is finished, the cell is imbalanced by its own reactive response(Sharma SK et al. 1975). As a consequence, the phenomenon of tolerance develops, that is, the need for an increased dose of the drug to produce the same effect (McQuay 1999). After tolerance is established, the withdrawal of the drug may produce physical or psychological symptoms opposed to the acute pharmacological actions of the drug itself. Opioid drugs are used clinically as unsurpassed analgesic agents but are also illegally abused on the street to induce a sense of well-being and euphoria. Tolerance to opioids, defined as a loss of effect following repeated treatments such that a higher dose is required for equivalent effect, limits the analgesic efficacy of these drugs and contributes to the social problems surrounding recreational opioid abuse.

In order to safely use morphine in clinic, we need to know how morphine tolerance and dependence are developed and what kinds of medicines could inhibit or prevent such mechanisms. In line with this, various approaches have been attempted to clarify the mechanisms underlying morphine tolerance and dependence. Here we summarize various proposed hypotheses and introduce our new approaches in this area.

8.2 Mechanisms for acute morphine tolerance

Prolonged and repeated exposures to opioid agonists reduce the responsiveness of G protein coupled opioid receptors. This reduction in receptor function is hypothesized to contribute to opioid tolerance, dependence, and addiction in humans (Nestler 1992). Substantial experimental evidence has divided this reduced function into separate but correlated receptor traffickings, 1) desensitization, 2) internalization, 3) sequestration/recycling, 4) down regulation (Law et al. 2000). The molecular events underlying opioid tolerance are currently discussed in relation to all these receptor trafficking mechanisms. According to current understanding, opioid receptors are desensitized on the cell surface through a phosphorylation process in the C-terminal (Afify et al. 1998) and/or third intracellular loop. On the other hand, receptor internalization or receptor disappearance from the cell surface, is now believed to contribute to resensitization through dephosphorylation during endosomal stages (Krueger et al. 1997; Zhang et al. 1997). Down-regulation is a loss of receptor protein in cells through increased degradation or decreased synthesis of the receptor. Little is known, however, regarding the regulation of this mechanism and involvement in opioid tolerance. Thus, much research has been done on the molecular basis of events in receptor phosphorylation in the membranes and internalization. Recent studies revealed that cAMP-dependent protein kinase A (PKA) (Harada et al. 1990), protein kinase C (PKC) (Ueda et al. 1995), Ca^{2+}/calmodulin-dependent protein kinases (Koch et al. 1997), G protein-coupled receptor kinases (GRKs) (Zhang et al. 1998), and mitogen-activated protein kinase (Polakiewicz et al. 1998) have roles in opioid receptor phosphorylation. PKC and GRK mechanisms are likely candidates for opioid desensitization and internalization (Ueda et al. 1995; Zhang et al. 1998).

8.3 PKC hypothesis

A number of reports have demonstrated that PKC is involved in the opioid tolerance or desensitization. Most of recent reports have demonstrated that PKC activators or inhibitors modulate opioid signaling in cells expressing opioid receptors. A series of reports have demonstrated the involvement of PKC in opioid tolerance by correlating both in vitro and in vivo studies.

8.4 Mechanisms for chronic morphine tolerance and dependence

Clear difference between acute morphine tolerance and chronic one has not been demonstrated for a long time. In algogenic-induced nociceptive flexion (ANF) test in mice the peripheral morphine analgesia developed the acute tolerance by 4 h pretreatment with morphine (Ueda et al. 2001). However, the peripheral analgesia had no change in mice that were given morphine for 5 days, a treatment which caused a marked chronic tolerance to systemic morphine analgesia (Ueda and Inoue 1999). Thus, it is evident that acute morphine tolerance mediates distinct mechanisms from the chronic one, and chronic tolerance is likely mediated through a complicated neuronal network present in the central nervous system.

8.5 cAMP hypothesis

Since the report by Sharma et al. (1975), it has been accepted that cAMP may play a key role in the morphine tolerance and dependence. According to this so-called cAMP hypothesis, a morphine-induced decrease in cAMP production is getting disappeared during long-period exposure to morphine (Sharma SK et al. 1975). As the naloxone application causes an abrupt increase in cAMP production, some unidentified mechanisms are supposed to mediate an increase in cAMP production through specific gene expressions during chronic morphine treatment. A candidate could be a cAMP-responsive element binding protein (CREB), which is involved in the gene expression of adenylyl cyclase. In vivo study using knockout mice demonstrates that CREB plays roles in the development of morphine dependence (Maldonado et al. 1996). Although several compounds possessing the antagonistic activity are reported to inhibit morphine tolerance and dependence, they have serious side effects at the same time (Trujillo and Akil 1991; Mao et al. 1992; Trujillo 1995; Mao 1999; Habibi-Asl and Hassanzadeh 2004; Habibi-Asl 2005; Asl et al. 2008).

8.6 Anti-opioid hypothesis

In addition to mechanisms at the single cellular level, the plasticity through neuronal networks would be involved in the development of morphine tolerance and dependence, as above-mentioned. One of approaches to cut in the mechanisms is based on the view that enhanced anti-opioid neuronal activity during chronic morphine treatments might suppress the acute morphine actions. The candidates include cholecystokinin (Mitchell et al. 2000), neuropeptide FF (Lake et al. 1992), nociceptin (Ueda et al. 2000) and glutamate, as an NMDA receptor ligand (Ueda et al. 2000; Mao and Mayer 2001). Among them the nociceptin (N/OFQ) system has been extensively characterized to be involved in the development of morphine tolerance and dependence. NMDA receptor has been long supposed to play important roles in the development of morphine tolerance and dependence (Trujillo and Akil 1991). Although several compounds possessing the antagonistic activity are reported to inhibit morphine tolerance and dependence, they have serious side effects at the same time (Trujillo and Akil 1991; Mao et al. 1992; Trujillo 1995; Mao 1999; Habibi-Asl and Hassanzadeh 2004; Habibi-Asl 2005; Asl et al. 2008).

8.7 Apoptosis hypothesis

Apoptosis, or programmed cell death, is an active process of normal cell death during development and also occurs as a consequence of the cytotoxic effect of various neurotoxins (e.g., MPTP/MPP+, MDMA, ethanol and cocaine) (Sastry and Rao 2000). Among the drugs of abuse, cocaine has been shown to cause a direct cytotoxic effect on the foetal rat heart, and to induce apoptosis in foetal rat myocardial cells in a dose-dependent manner (Xiao et al. 2000).

The induction of apoptosis in neurons has been demonstrated to share the same basic mechanisms with all other cell types (Sastry and Rao 2000). In vitro studies also indicate that exposure to μ- and/or κ-opioid receptor agonists of neuronal cultures from embryonic chick brain (Goswami et al. 1998) and specific cell lines (Dawson et al. 1997; Singhal et al. 1998; Singhal et al. 1999) increases their vulnerability to death by apoptotic mechanisms. The molecular mechanisms of apoptosis (i.e., the detailed cascade of events from the cell surface to final changes in the nucleus) have not been established yet, but various key proteins are involved in the regulation of programmed cell death (Sastry and Rao 2000). Some members of the Bcl-2 family of proteins, such as Bcl-2 and Bcl-xL, suppresses apoptosis, while the expression of other, such as the homologues Bax and Bak, are pro-apoptotic (Adams and Cory 1998). Specifically, the Bcl-2 oncoprotein, localized mainly to the mitochondrial membranes, has been shown to play an important role in protecting neurons from apoptotic cell death (Hockenbery et al. 1990), probably by preventing the release of cytochrome c (induced by Bax) and the subsequent activation of specific proteases termed caspases, the proteolytic enzymes which are crucial for the execution of nuclear fragmentation and apoptosis (Adams and Cory 1998; Sastry and Rao 2000). In fact, Bax mRNA and Bax protein are increased in the substantia nigra of MPTP-treated mice (degeneration of dopamine neurons by apoptosis) (Hassouna et al. 1996), and the release of cytochrome c from the mitochondria and the subsequent activation of caspases-3/9 was shown to play a key role in cocaine-induced apoptosis in foetal rat myocardial cells (Xiao et al. 2000). The results of our studies demonstrated that chronic morphine administration in rat, induced apoptosis; decrease in Bcl-2 and increase in caspase3 activity in both cerebral cortex and lumbar spinal cord in rat (Hassanzadeh et al.). Another key element involved in the regulation of apoptosis is the Fas glycoprotein (also known as CD95 or Apo1), a cell surface receptor that belongs to the tumor necrosis factor receptor family (death receptors) and that is expressed abundantly in various tissues (Nagata 1999). In contrast to Bcl-2 mitochondrial protein, the Fas receptor triggers cell apoptosis when it binds to its ligand, Fas, and Fas-mediated death bypasses the usual long sequence of signaling enzymes and immediately activates a pre-existing caspase cascade (Nagata 1999). In the context of the induction of aberrant apoptosis in opioid addiction, it was of great interest the in vitro study demonstrating the ability of morphine to increase, through a naloxone-sensitive mechanism, the expression (mRNA) of the pro-apoptotic receptor Fas in mouse splenocytes and in human blood lymphocytes (Yin et al. 1999). A relevant consequence of the morphine-induced potentiation of apoptosis in lymphocytes (Singhal et al. 1999; Yin et al. 1999) is the reduction of the immune response (and the increase in recurrent infections) observed in heroin addicts (Govitrapong et al. 1998).

On the other hand, over a decade, the NMDA receptor (NMDAR), a subgroup of glutamate receptors, has been implicated in the development of opioid tolerance (Trujillo and Akil 1991; Mao et al. 1994). Activation of NMDARs can lead to neurotoxicity under many circumstances (Rothman and Olney 1986; Moncada et al. 1992; Catania et al. 1993) For instance, peripheral nerve injury has been shown to activate spinal cord NMDARs, which results in not only intractable neuropathic pain but also neuronal cell death by means of apoptosis (Mao et al. 1997; Whiteside and Munglani 2001). Furthermore, cross talk between the cellular mechanisms of opioid tolerance and neuropathic pain has been proposed, suggesting that a common cellular mechanism may be involved in both neuropathic pain and opioid tolerance (Mayer et al. 1999). Thus, it is possible that the cellular process leading to the development of opioid tolerance may also cause neurotoxic changes in response to prolonged opioid administration. More recently, we examined the hypothesis that neurotoxicity in the form of apoptotic cell death would be induced in association with the development of morphine tolerance. In confirmation of Mao et al. findings, we demonstrated that chronic opioid injection leads to apoptosis in the CNS which was in association with the development of tolerance to the analgesic effect (Habibi-Asl et al. 2009a). Figure1 shows the possible mechanisms of opioid-induced neuronal apoptosis and its association with opioid tolerance.

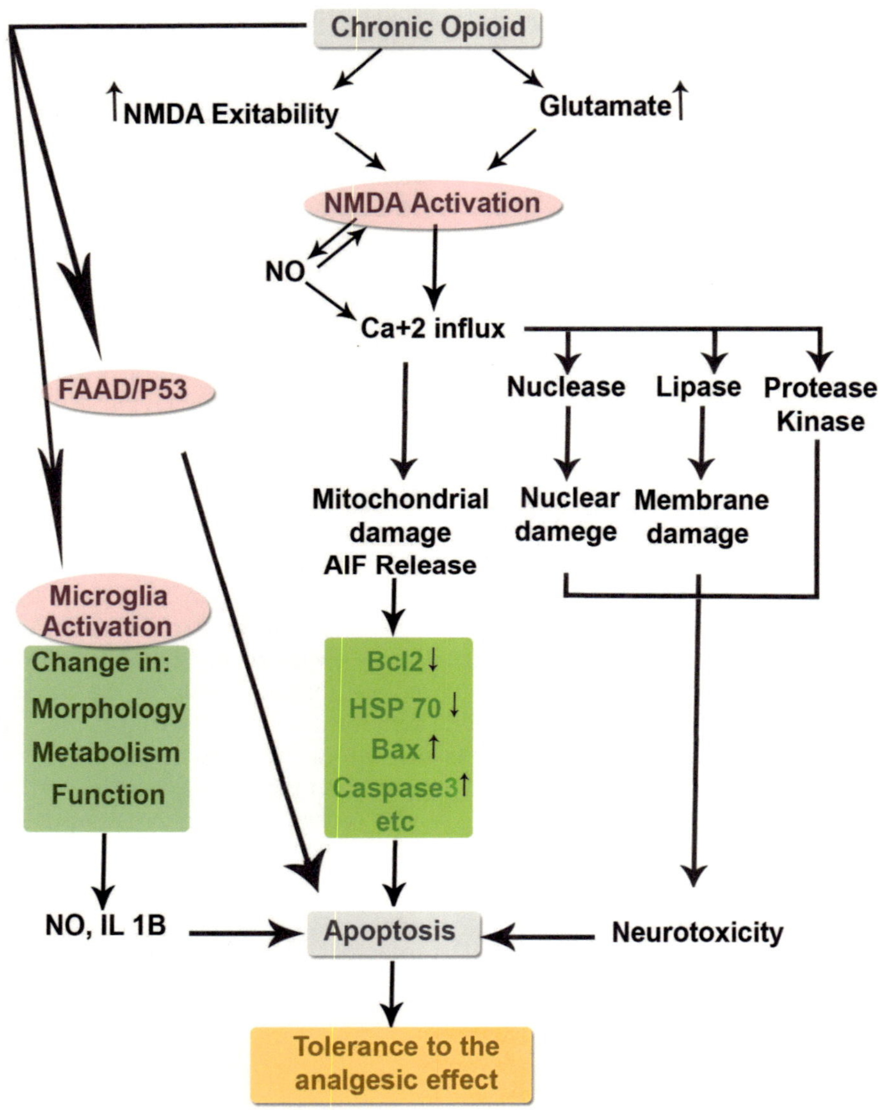

Fig. 1. Schematic diagram illustrating the possible mechanisms of opioid-induced neuronal apoptosis and tolerance. The results of before studies suggest that chronic opioid administration may induce NMDAR, microglia, FAAD/P53,… activation resulting in intracellular positive apoptosis regulators induction. The resultant apoptosis contributes to the cellular mechanism of opioid tolerance. NMDA: N-Methyl-D-Aspartate, NO: Nitric Oxide, AIF: Apoptosis-Inducing Factor, FADD: Fas-Associated Death Domain,

Opioid tolerance manifests as a loss of agonist potency and as a shift of the dose-response curve to the right. During the past decades, many studies have focused on excitatory amino acid receptors to investigate the role which they play in the development of tolerance to the antinociceptive action of opiates. This idea was suggested by Trujillo and Akil who reported that the NMDA receptor antagonist, MK801 (dizocilpine), inhibited the development of tolerance to the antinociceptive effect of morphine and morphine physical dependence (Trujillo and Akil 1991).

Using behavioral studies, we and others have shown that a variety of NMDA receptor antagonists have the ability to inhibit the development of opiate tolerance and dependence (Trujillo and Akil 1991; Trujillo 1995; Habibi-Asl and Hassanzadeh 2004; Asl et al. 2008; Habibi-Asl et al. 2009b). There are also several lines of evidence which suggest that activation of NMDARs leads to removing the magnesium blockade (Begon et al. 2001) in the calcium channel and toxic calcium influx, which activates numerous enzymes, including neuronal nitric oxide (NO) synthase (NOS). In our unpublished data we observed that nitric oxide donors such as nitroglycerin or nicorandil increased the tolerance to the analgesic effect of morphine. On the other hand the nitric oxide synthase inhibitor, N-Nitro-L-Arginine Methyl Ester (LNAME) could prevent the tolerance. It has been demonstrated that Magnesium (Mg)-deficient rats develop a mechanical hyperalgesia which is reversed by a N-Methyl-D-Aspartate (NMDA) receptor antagonist (Begon et al. 2001). Our study in agreement with those studies showed that systemic administration of magnesium sulfate could attenuate morphine tolerance to the analgesic effect (Habibi-Asl 2005; Habibi-Asl et al. 2009b). Also we showed that selenium with similar mechanism appeared to have a weaker effect than magnesium (Charkhpour M et al. 2009).

Our recently published finding, indicated that riluzole (2- amino-6-[trifluoromethoxy] benzothiazole), an antiglutamatergic agent, decreases the development of tolerance, shifting the first day of established tolerance from the 8th day in the control group to the 13th day (Habibi-Asl et al. 2009a). Riluzole interferes with responses mediated by excitatory amino acids, even though it does not interact with any known binding sites on the NMDA, kainate or AMPA glutamate receptors (Debono et al. 1993). The neuroprotective effect of riluzole, which has been shown both in vivo and in vitro, is believed to be beneficial in various neurodegenerative diseases and amelioration of trauma and stroke (Doble 1999; Albo et al. 2004).

The results indicated that there was a significant shift to the right in the dose-response curve as well as an increase in the antinociceptive 50% effective dose (ED50) of morphine for animals who received morphine also compared with those that received morphine and riluzole. On the other hand, co-administration of riluzole delayed the onset of morphine-induced apoptosis and significantly decreased the average number of TUNEL-positive cells ($p < 0.01$). This finding is in line with our recent results concerning the lumbar region of the spinal cord (Hassanzadeh et al.). In addition, we found that the group that received morphine and riluzole for 13 days had developed tolerance; they showed an increase in the number of apoptotic cells, as under control conditions. This result indicates that after the completion of tolerance in both the control and the treated groups, apoptosis had already developed. Previous studies have indicated that certain addictive drugs, such as morphine, could induce apoptosis in cultured neuronal cell lines as well as human cells (Singhal et al. 1998; Singhal et al. 1999). More recently, it has been shown that in vivo neuronal apoptosis occurs in the rat's spinal cord dorsal horn after chronic morphine treatment that was associated with the expression of activated caspase- 3 and the involvement of mitogen-activated protein kinase (MAPK) (Mao et al. 2002), suggesting that chronic morphine may lead to changes within the central nervous system.

Our more recent studies demonstrated that prolonged morphine administration induces up-regulation of proapoptotic elements such as caspase-3 and down regulation of the anti-apoptotic factors Bcl-2 and HSP70 in the rat cerebral cortex and spinal cord (Hassanzadeh et al.; Hassanzadeh et al.; Tikka and Koistinaho 2001; Gabra et al. 2005; Hassanzadeh K et al. 2011). Importantly, up-regulation of caspase-3 and Bax was inhibited when morphine was co-administered with the noncompetitive NMDAR antagonist MK-801, thereby supporting a link between NMDAR activation and intracellular changes in caspase-3 and Bax in response to prolonged morphine administration (Jordan et al. 2007).

Interestingly, our results demonstrated that neuroprotective agents such as serotonin$_{1A}$ receptor agonist, minocycline (Habibi-Asl 2009; Habibi-Asl et al. 2009a), selegiline,... could prevent morphine induced tolerance and apoptosis. The stimulation of serotonin$_{1A}$ (5HT1A) receptors induces a variable level of neuroprotection in different animal models of central nervous system injury such as ischemia, (Prehn et al. 1993; Semkova et al. 1998; Schaper et al. 2000; Kukley et al. 2001; Torup et al. 2000) N-methyl-D-aspartate (NMDA) excitotoxicity, (Oosterink et al. 1998; Oosterink et al. 2003) acute subdural hematoma, (Alessandri et al. 1999) and traumatic brain injury (Kline et al. 2001). Furthermore, in vitro evidence indicates that 5HT1A agonists are able to protect neurons from apoptosis induced by staurosporine (Suchanek et al. 1998), glutamate (Semkova et al. 1998), or serum deprivation (Ahlemeyer and Krieglstein 1997; Ahlemeyer et al. 1999). There are different hypotheses on the mechanisms involved in 5HT1A-mediated neuroprotection, including neuronal membrane hyperpolarization that reduces excitability,(Ahlemeyer and Krieglstein 1997; Krüger et al. 1999), reduced glutamate release, (Mauler et al. 2001) and blockade of voltage-sensitive Na channels (Melena et al. 2000).

Other neuroprotective mechanisms have also been proposed for 5HT1A agonists such as stimulation of the anti-apoptotic proto-oncogene B-cell lymphoma protein 2 (BCL-2) expression through the mitogen-activated protein kinase (MAPK/ERK) signaling pathway (Kukley et al. 2001) and suppression of the proapoptotic protein caspase-3 in a MAPK- and protein kinase C alfa-dependent manner (Adayev et al. 2003).

More recently we examined the effect of 8-OH-DPAT, a specific 5-HT1A receptor agonist, on morphine induced tolerance to an analgesic effect in rat. We found that Intra-dorsal raphe nucleus (DRN) administration of the 5-HT1A receptor agonist, 8-OH-DPAT, prevented morphine-induced apoptosis after tolerance to the analgesic effect. On the other hand, the total analgesic effect of morphine significantly increased in animals treated with morphine and 8-OH-DPAT in comparison with the control group. In addition, the results indicated that administration of both 5HT1 agonist (8-OH-DPAT) and antagonist (NAN-190) together with morphine prevent the antiapoptotic activity of the 5HT1A agonist. This means that after antagonizing the 5HT1A receptor, the apoptosis process has already developed. Another mechanism contributes to the morphine tolerance is microglial activation. Studies showed that NMDA-induced neuronal death involved proliferation and activation of microglial cells and that neuroprotective agents such as minocycline completely prevented NMDA toxicity and the preceding activation and proliferation of microglial cells. These results support the notion that microglial activation contributes to excitotoxic neuronal death, which can be inhibited by anti- inflammatory compounds, such as minocycline (Tikka and Koistinaho 2001). The mechanism underlying the role of glial cells in the effects of morphine on naive mice is unclear. It is possible that morphine acts directly on microglia,

triggering alterations in their morphology, metabolism, and function (Watkins et al. 2005). Mika et al. concluded that the effect of minocycline on morphine tolerance is related to microglia. Their results provide evidence that systemic administration of minocycline in mice influences morphine's effectiveness and delays the development of morphine tolerance by attenuating microglial activation and its markers (Mika et al. 2009).
In summary, we believe that adding the neuroprotective agents to analgesic drugs specially opioids, increase the analgesic effect and prevents the hyperalgesia and tolerance to their analgesic effects.

9. References

Adams B, Moghaddam B. Corticolimbic dopamine neurotransmission is temporally dissociated from the cognitive and locomotor effects of phencyclidine. J Neurosci 1998;18(14):5545-5554.
Adams JM, Cory S. The Bcl-2 protein family: arbiters of cell survival. Science 1998;281(5381):1322-1326.
Adayev T, Ray I, Sondhi R, Sobocki T, Banerjee P. The G protein-coupled 5-HT1A receptor causes suppression of caspase-3 through MAPK and protein kinase Calpha. Biochim Biophys Acta 2003;1640(1):85-96.
Afify EA, Law PY, Riedl M, Elde R, Loh HH. Role of carboxyl terminus of mu-and delta-opioid receptor in agonist-induced down-regulation. Brain Res Mol Brain Res 1998;54(1):24-34.
Ahlemeyer B, Glaser A, Schaper C, Semkova I, Krieglstein J. The 5-HT1A receptor agonist Bay x 3702 inhibits apoptosis induced by serum deprivation in cultured neurons. Eur J Pharmacol 1999;370(2):211-216.
Ahlemeyer B, Krieglstein J. Stimulation of 5-HT1A receptor inhibits apoptosis induced by serum deprivation in cultured neurons from chick embryo. Brain Res 1997;777(1-2):179-186.
Akaike A. Preclinical evidence of neuroprotection by cholinesterase inhibitors. Alzheimer Dis Assoc Disord 2006;20(2 Suppl 1):S8-11.
Albo F, Pieri M, Zona C. Modulation of AMPA receptors in spinal motor neurons by the neuroprotective agent riluzole. J Neurosci Res 2004;78(2):200-207.
Alessandri B, Tsuchida E, Bullock RM. The neuroprotective effect of a new serotonin receptor agonist, BAY X3702, upon focal ischemic brain damage caused by acute subdural hematoma in the rat. Brain Res 1999;845(2):232-235.
Arendt-Nielsen L, Sumikura H. From pain research to pain treatment: role of human pain models. J Nihon Med Sch 2002;69(6):514-524.
Asl BH, Hassanzadeh K, Khezri E, Mohammadi S. Evaluation the effects of dextromethorphan and midazolam on morphine induced tolerance and dependence in mice. Pak J Biol Sci 2008;11(13):1690-1695.
Bahr BA, Karanian DA, Makanji SS, Makriyannis A. Targeting the endocannabinoid system in treating brain disorders. Expert Opin Investig Drugs 2006;15(4):351-365.
Begon S, Pickering G, Eschalier A, Mazur A, Rayssiguier Y, Dubray C. Role of spinal NMDA receptors, protein kinase C and nitric oxide synthase in the hyperalgesia induced by magnesium deficiency in rats. Br J Pharmacol 2001;134(6):1227-1236.
Berridge MJ. Neuronal calcium signaling. Neuron 1998;21(1):13-26.
Brodie MS, Proudfit HK. Hypoalgesia induced by the local injection of carbachol into the nucleus raphe magnus. Brain Res 1984;291(2):337-342.

Catania MV, Hollingsworth Z, Penney JB, Young AB. Phospholipase A2 modulates different subtypes of excitatory amino acid receptors: autoradiographic evidence. J Neurochem 1993;60(1):236-245.

Charkhpour M, Habibi Asl B, Yagobifard S, Hassanzadeh K. Evaluation the effect of co-administration of gabapentin and sodium selenite on the development of tolerance to morphine analgesia and dependence in mice. Pharmaceutical Sciences 2009;14(4):209-217.

Cid C, Alvarez-Cermeno JC, Regidor I, Salinas M, Alcazar A. Low concentrations of glutamate induce apoptosis in cultured neurons: implications for amyotrophic lateral sclerosis. J Neurol Sci 2003;206(1):91-95.

Craig RW. The bcl-2 gene family. Semin Cancer Biol 1995;6(1):35-43.

Dawson G, Dawson SA, Goswami R. Chronic exposure to kappa-opioids enhances the susceptibility of immortalized neurons (F-11kappa 7) to apoptosis-inducing drugs by a mechanism that may involve ceramide.

J Neurochem 1997;68(6):2363-2370.

de Fiebre NC, de Fiebre CM. alpha7 Nicotinic acetylcholine receptor knockout selectively enhances ethanol-, but not beta-amyloid-induced neurotoxicity. Neurosci Lett 2005;373(1):42-47.

Deadwyler SA, Hampson RE, Mu J, Whyte A, Childers S. Cannabinoids modulate voltage sensitive potassium A-current in hippocampal neurons via a cAMP-dependent process. J Pharmacol Exp Ther 1995;273(2):734-743.

Debono MW, Le GJ, Canton T, Doble A, Pradier L. Inhibition by riluzole of electrophysiological responses mediated by rat kainate and NMDA receptors expressed in Xenopus oocytes. Eur J Pharmacol 1993;235(2-3):283-289.

Deutsch SI, Rosse RB, Schwartz BL, Mastropaolo J. A revised excitotoxic hypothesis of schizophrenia: therapeutic implications. Clin Neuropharmacol 2001;24(1):43-49.

Doble A. The role of excitotoxicity in neurodegenerative disease: implications for therapy. Pharmacol Ther 1999;81(3):163-221.

Ferchmin PA, Perez D, Eterovic VA, de Vellis J. Nicotinic receptors differentially regulate N-methyl-D-aspartate damage in acute hippocampal slices. J Pharmacol Exp Ther 2003;305(3):1071-1078.

Finnerup NB, Otto M, McQuay HJ, Jensen TS, Sindrup SH. Algorithm for neuropathic pain treatment: an evidence based proposal. Pain 2005;118(3):289-305.

Gabra BH, Afify EA, Daabees TT, Abou Zeit-Har MS. The role of the NO/NMDA pathways in the development of morphine withdrawal induced by naloxone in vitro. Pharmacol Res 2005;51(4):319-327.

Galve-Roperh I, Aguado T, Palazuelos J, Guzman M. Mechanisms of control of neuron survival by the endocannabinoid system. Curr Pharm Des 2008;14(23):2279-2288.

Galve-Roperh I, Rueda D, Gomez del Pulgar T, Velasco G, Guzman M. Mechanism of extracellular signal-regulated kinase activation by the CB(1) cannabinoid receptor. Mol Pharmacol 2002;62(6):1385-1392.

Ghelardini C, Galeotti N, Nicolodi M, Donaldson S, Sicuteri F, Bartolini A. Involvement of central cholinergic system in antinociception induced by sumatriptan in mouse. Int J Clin Pharmacol Res 1997;17(2-3):105-109.

Ghelardini C, Galeotti N, Uslenghi C, Grazioli I, Bartolini A. Prochlorperazine induces central antinociception mediated by the muscarinic system. Pharmacol Res 2004;50(3):351-358.

Giorgetti M, Bacciottini L, Giovannini MG, Colivicchi MA, Goldfarb J, Blandina P. Local GABAergic modulation of acetylcholine release from the cortex of freely moving rats. Eur J Neurosci 2000;12(6):1941-1948.

Glantz LA, Gilmore JH, Lieberman JA, Jarskog LF. Apoptotic mechanisms and the synaptic pathology of schizophrenia. Schizophr Res 2006;81(1):47-63.

Gomez del Pulgar T, Velasco G, Guzman M. The CB1 cannabinoid receptor is coupled to the activation of protein kinase B/Akt. Biochem J 2000;347(Pt 2):369-373.

Goswami R, Dawson SA, Dawson G. Cyclic AMP protects against staurosporine and wortmannin-induced apoptosis and opioid-enhanced apoptosis in both embryonic and immortalized (F-11kappa7) neurons. J Neurochem 1998;70(4):1376-1382.

Govitrapong P, Suttitum T, Kotchabhakdi N, Uneklabh T. Alterations of immune functions in heroin addicts and heroin withdrawal subjects. J Pharmacol Exp Ther 1998;286(2):883-889.

Greenamyre JT. Glutamatergic influences on the basal ganglia. Clin Neuropharmacol 2001;24(2):65-70.

Gross A, Jockel J, Wei MC, Korsmeyer SJ. Enforced dimerization of BAX results in its translocation, mitochondrial dysfunction and apoptosis. Embo J 1998;17(14):3878-3885.

Habibi-Asl B, Alimohammadi, B., Charkhpour, M., Hassanzadeh, K. Evaluation the Effects of Systemic Administration of Minocycline and Riluzole on Tolerance to Morphine Analgesic effect in rat. . Pharmaceutical Sciences (Journal of Faculty of Pharmacy, Tabriz University of Medical Sciences) 2009;15:205-212.

Habibi-Asl B, Hassanzadeh K. Effects of ketamine and midazolam on morphine induced dependence and tolerance in mice. DARU 2004;12:101-105.

Habibi-Asl B, Hassanzadeh K, Charkhpour M. Central administration of minocycline and riluzole prevents morphine-induced tolerance in rats. Anesth Analg 2009a;109(3):936-942.

Habibi-Asl B, Hassanzadeh K, Vafai H, Mohammadi S. Development of morphine induced tolerance and withdrawal symptoms is attenuated by lamotrigine and magnesium sulfate in mice. Pak J Biol Sci 2009b;12(10):798-803.

Habibi-Asl B, Hassanzadeh, K., Moosazadeh, S. Effects of ketamine and magnesium on morphine induced tolerance and dependence in mice. DARU 2005;13:110-115.

Hajos N, Katona I, Naiem SS, MacKie K, Ledent C, Mody I, Freund TF. Cannabinoids inhibit hippocampal GABAergic transmission and network oscillations. Eur J Neurosci 2000;12(9):3239-3249.

Harada H, Ueda H, Katada T, Ui M, Satoh M. Phosphorylated mu-opioid receptor purified from rat brains lacks functional coupling with Gi1, a GTP-binding protein in reconstituted lipid vesicles. Neurosci Lett 1990;113(1):47-49.

Harris EW, Ganong AH, Cotman CW. Long-term potentiation in the hippocampus involves activation of N-methyl-D-aspartate receptors. Brain Res 1984;323(1):132-137.

Harte SE, Hoot MR, Borszcz GS. Involvement of the intralaminar parafascicular nucleus in muscarinic-induced antinociception in rats. Brain Res 2004;1019(1-2):152-161.

Hassanzadeh K, L R, Habibi-asl B, Farajnia S, Izadpanah E, Nemati M, Arasteh M, Mohammadi S. Riluzole prevents morphine-induced apoptosis in rat cerebral cortex. Pharamacol Rep 2011;63:697-707.

Hassanzadeh K, Habibi-asl B, Farajnia S, Roshangar L. Minocycline prevents morphine-induced apoptosis in rat cerebral cortex and lumbar spinal cord: a possible mechanism for attenuating morphine tolerance. Neurotox Res;19(4):649-659.

Hassanzadeh K, Habibi-asl B, Roshangar L, Nemati M, Ansarin M, Farajnia S. Intracerebroventricular administration of riluzole prevents morphine-induced apoptosis in the lumbar region of the rat spinal cord. Pharmacol Rep;62(4):664-673.

Hassouna I, Wickert H, Zimmermann M, Gillardon F. Increase in bax expression in substantia nigra following 1-methyl-4-phenyl-1,2,3,6-tetrahydropyridine (MPTP) treatment of mice. Neurosci Lett 1996;204(1-2):85-88.

Hockenbery D, Nuñez G, Milliman C, Schreiber RD, Korsmeyer SJ. Bcl-2 is an inner mitochondrial membrane protein that blocks programmed cell death. Nature 1990;348(6299):334-336.

Hwang J, Adamson C, Butler D, Janero DR, Makriyannis A, Bahr BA. Enhancement of endocannabinoid signaling by fatty acid amide hydrolase inhibition: a neuroprotective therapeutic modality. Life Sci;86(15-16):615-623.

Ivy Carroll F, Ma W, Navarro HA, Abraham P, Wolckenhauer SA, Damaj MI, Martin BR. Synthesis, nicotinic acetylcholine receptor binding, antinociceptive and seizure properties of methyllycaconitine analogs. Bioorg Med Chem 2007;15(2):678-685.

Jevtovic-Todorovic V, Covey DF, Todorovic SM. Are neuroactive steroids promising therapeutic agents in the management of acute and chronic pain? Psychoneuroendocrinology 2009;34 Suppl 1:S178-185.

Johnson EM, Jr., Greenlund LJ, Akins PT, Hsu CY. Neuronal apoptosis: current understanding of molecular mechanisms and potential role in ischemic brain injury. J Neurotrauma 1995;12(5):843-852.

Jordan J, Fernandez-Gomez FJ, Ramos M, Ikuta I, Aguirre N, Galindo MF. Minocycline and cytoprotection: shedding new light on a shadowy controversy. Curr Drug Deliv 2007;4(3):225-231.

Kaneko S, Maeda T, Kume T, Kochiyama H, Akaike A, Shimohama S, Kimura J. Nicotine protects cultured cortical neurons against glutamate-induced cytotoxicity via alpha7-neuronal receptors and neuronal CNS receptors. Brain Res 1997;765(1):135-140.

Karanian DA, Brown QB, Makriyannis A, Bahr BA. Blocking cannabinoid activation of FAK and ERK1/2 compromises synaptic integrity in hippocampus. Eur J Pharmacol 2005a;508(1-3):47-56.

Karanian DA, Brown QB, Makriyannis A, Kosten TA, Bahr BA. Dual modulation of endocannabinoid transport and fatty acid amide hydrolase protects against excitotoxicity. J Neurosci 2005b;25(34):7813-7820.

Karanian DA, Karim SL, Wood JT, Williams JS, Lin S, Makriyannis A, Bahr BA. Endocannabinoid enhancement protects against kainic acid-induced seizures and associated brain damage. J Pharmacol Exp Ther 2007;322(3):1059-1066.

Kerr JF, Wyllie AH, Currie AR. Apoptosis: a basic biological phenomenon with wide-ranging implications in tissue kinetics. Br J Cancer 1972;26(4):239-257.

Khaspekov LG, Brenz Verca MS, Frumkina LE, Hermann H, Marsicano G, Lutz B. Involvement of brain-derived neurotrophic factor in cannabinoid receptor-dependent protection against excitotoxicity. Eur J Neurosci 2004;19(7):1691-1698.

Kihara T, Shimohama S, Sawada H, Honda K, Nakamizo T, Kanki R, Yamashita H, Akaike A. Protective effect of dopamine D2 agonists in cortical neurons via the phosphatidylinositol 3 kinase cascade. J Neurosci Res 2002;70(3):274-282.

Kline AE, Yu J, Horváth E, Marion DW, Dixon CE. The selective 5-HT(1A) receptor agonist repinotan HCl attenuates histopathology and spatial learning deficits following traumatic brain injury in rats. Neuroscience 2001;106(3):547-555.

Koch T, Kroslak T, Mayer P, Raulf E, Höllt V. Site mutation in the rat mu-opioid receptor demonstrates the involvement of calcium/calmodulin-dependent protein kinase II in agonist-mediated desensitization.
J Neurochem 1997;69(4):1767-1770.
Kreitzer AC, Regehr WG. Retrograde inhibition of presynaptic calcium influx by endogenous cannabinoids at excitatory synapses onto Purkinje cells. Neuron 2001;29(3):717-727.
Krueger KM, Daaka Y, Pitcher JA, Lefkowitz RJ. The role of sequestration in G protein-coupled receptor resensitization. Regulation of beta2-adrenergic receptor dephosphorylation by vesicular acidification. J Biol Chem 1997;272(1):5-8.
Krüger H, Heinemann U, Luhmann HJ. Effects of ionotropic glutamate receptor blockade and 5-HT1A receptor activation on spreading depression in rat neocortical slices. Neuroreport 1999;10(12):2651-2656.
Kukley M, Schaper C, Becker A, Rose K, Krieglstein J. Effect of 5-hydroxytryptamine 1A receptor agonist BAY X 3702 on BCL-2 and BAX proteins level in the ipsilateral cerebral cortex of rats after transient focal ischaemia. Neuroscience 2001;107(3):405-413.
Lake JR, Hebert KM, Payza K, Deshotel KD, Hausam DD, Witherspoon WE, Arcangeli KA, Malin DH. Analog of neuropeptide FF attenuates morphine tolerance. Neurosci Lett 1992;146(2):203-206.
Laudenbach V, Medja F, Zoli M, Rossi FM, Evrard P, Changeux JP, Gressens P. Selective activation of central subtypes of the nicotinic acetylcholine receptor has opposite effects on neonatal excitotoxic brain injuries. Faseb J 2002;16(3):423-425.
Law PY, Wong YH, Loh HH. Molecular mechanisms and regulation of opioid receptor signaling. Annu Rev Pharmacol Toxicol 2000;40:389-430.
Maldonado R, Blendy JA, Tzavara E, Gass P, Roques BP, Hanoune J, Schütz G. Reduction of morphine abstinence in mice with a mutation in the gene encoding CREB. Science 1996;273(5275):657-659.
Manzanares J, Julian M, Carrascosa A. Role of the cannabinoid system in pain control and therapeutic implications for the management of acute and chronic pain episodes. Curr Neuropharmacol 2006;4(3):239-257.
Mao J. NMDA and opioid receptors: their interactions in antinociception, tolerance and neuroplasticity. Brain Res Brain Res Rev 1999;30(3):289-304.
Mao J, Mayer DJ. Spinal cord neuroplasticity following repeated opioid exposure and its relation to pathological pain. Ann N Y Acad Sci 2001;933(175-84).
Mao J, Mayer DJ, Hayes RL, Lu J, Price DD. Differential roles of NMDA and non-NMDA receptor activation in induction and maintenance of thermal hyperalgesia in rats with painful peripheral mononeuropathy Brain Res 1992;598:271–278.
Mao J, Price DD, Mayer DJ. Thermal hyperalgesia in association with the development of morphine tolerance in rats: roles of excitatory amino acid receptors and protein kinase C. J Neurosci 1994;14(4):2301-2312.
Mao J, Price DD, Zhu J, Lu J, Mayer DJ. The inhibition of nitric oxide-activated poly(ADP-ribose) synthetase attenuates transsynaptic alteration of spinal cord dorsal horn neurons and neuropathic pain in the rat. Pain 1997;72(3):355-366.
Mao J, Sung B, Ji RR, Lim G. Neuronal apoptosis associated with morphine tolerance: evidence for an opioid-induced neurotoxic mechanism. J Neurosci 2002;22(17):7650-7661.
Martin SE, de Fiebre NE, de Fiebre CM. The alpha7 nicotinic acetylcholine receptor-selective antagonist, methyllycaconitine, partially protects against beta-amyloid1-42 toxicity in primary neuron-enriched cultures. Brain Res 2004;1022(1-2):254-256.

Martinez M, Frank A, Diez-Tejedor E, Hernanz A. Amino acid concentrations in cerebrospinal fluid and serum in Alzheimer's disease and vascular dementia. J Neural Transm Park Dis Dement Sect 1993;6(1):1-9.

Marx CE, Stevens RD, Shampine LJ, Uzunova V, Trost WT, Butterfield MI, Massing MW, Hamer RM, Morrow AL, Lieberman JA. Neuroactive steroids are altered in schizophrenia and bipolar disorder: relevance to pathophysiology and therapeutics. Neuropsychopharmacology 2006;31(6):1249-1263.

Mauler F, Fahrig T, Horváth E, Jork R. Inhibition of evoked glutamate release by the neuroprotective 5-HT(1A) receptor agonist BAY x 3702 in vitro and in vivo. Brain Res 2001;888(1):150-157.

Mayer DJ, Mao J, Holt J, Price DD. Cellular mechanisms of neuropathic pain, morphine tolerance, and their interactions. Proc Natl Acad Sci U S A 1999;96(14):7731-7736.

McMahon SB, Cafferty WB, Marchand F. Immune and glial cell factors as pain mediators and modulators. Exp Neurol 2005;192(2):444-462.

McQuay H. Opioids in pain management. Lancet 1999;353:2229-2232.

Melena J, Chidlow G, Osborne NN. Blockade of voltage-sensitive Na(+) channels by the 5-HT(1A) receptor agonist 8-OH-DPAT: possible significance for neuroprotection. Eur J Pharmacol 2000;406(3):319-324.

Mika J, Wawrzczak-Bargiela A, Osikowicz M, Makuch W, Przewlocka B. Attenuation of morphine tolerance by minocycline and pentoxifylline in naive and neuropathic mice. Brain Behav Immun 2009;23(1):75-84.

Millan MJ. N-Methyl-D-aspartate receptors as a target for improved antipsychotic agents: novel insights and clinical perspectives. Psychopharmacology (Berl) 2005;179(1):30-53.

Mitchell JM, Basbaum AI, Fields HL. A locus and mechanism of action for associative morphine tolerance. Nat Neurosci 2000 3(1):47-53.

Moghaddam B, Adams B, Verma A, Daly D. Activation of glutamatergic neurotransmission by ketamine: a novel step in the pathway from NMDA receptor blockade to dopaminergic and cognitive disruptions associated with the prefrontal cortex. J Neurosci 1997;17(8):2921-2927.

Molina-Holgado F, Pinteaux E, Heenan L, Moore JD, Rothwell NJ, Gibson RM. Neuroprotective effects of the synthetic cannabinoid HU-210 in primary cortical neurons are mediated by phosphatidylinositol 3-kinase/AKT signaling. Mol Cell Neurosci 2005;28(1):189-194.

Moncada C, Lekieffre D, Arvin B, Meldrum B. Effect of NO synthase inhibition on NMDA- and ischaemia-induced hippocampal lesions. Neuroreport 1992;3(6):530-532.

Mudo G, Belluardo N, Fuxe K. Nicotinic receptor agonists as neuroprotective/neurotrophic drugs. Progress in molecular mechanisms. J Neural Transm 2007;114(1):135-147.

Nagata S. Fas ligand-induced apoptosis. Annu Rev Genet 1999;33:29-55.

Nestler EJ. Molecular mechanisms of drug addiction. Journal of Neuroscience 1992;12(7):2439-2450.

Olney JW, Newcomer JW, Farber NB. NMDA receptor hypofunction model of schizophrenia. J Psychiatr Res 1999;33(6):523-533.

Oosterink BJ, Harkany T, Luiten PG. Post-lesion administration of 5-HT1A receptor agonist 8-OH-DPAT protects cholinergic nucleus basalis neurons against NMDA excitotoxicity. Neuroreport 2003;14(1):57-60.

Oosterink BJ, Korte SM, Nyakas C, Korf J, Luiten PGM. Neuroprotection against N-methyl-D-aspartate-induced excitotoxicity in rat magnocellular nucleus basalis by the 5-HT1A receptor agonist 8-OH-DPAT. Eur J Pharmacol 1998;358(2):147-152.

Paice JA, Ferrell B. The management of cancer pain. CA Cancer J Clin;61(3):157-182.
Polakiewicz RD, Schieferl SM, Dorner LF, Kansra V, Comb MJ. A mitogen-activated protein kinase pathway is required for mu-opioid receptor desensitization. J Biol Chem 1998;273(20):12402-12406.
Prehn JH, Welsch M, Backhauss C, Nuglisch J, Ausmeier F, Karkoutly C, Krieglstein J. Effects of serotonergic drugs in experimental brain ischemia: evidence for a protective role of serotonin in cerebral ischemia. Brain Res 1993;630(1-2):10-20.
Rahn EJ, Hohmann AG. Cannabinoids as pharmacotherapies for neuropathic pain: from the bench to the bedside. Neurotherapeutics 2009;6(4):713-737.
Razoux F, Garcia R, Lena I. Ketamine, at a dose that disrupts motor behavior and latent inhibition, enhances prefrontal cortex synaptic efficacy and glutamate release in the nucleus accumbens. Neuropsychopharmacology 2007;32(3):719-727.
Rothman SM, Olney JW. Glutamate and the pathophysiology of hypoxic--ischemic brain damage. Ann Neurol 1986;19(2):105-111.
Sastry PS, Rao KS. Apoptosis and the nervous system. J Neurochem 2000;74(1):1-20.
Scascighini L, Toma V, Dober-Spielmann S, Sprott H. Multidisciplinary treatment for chronic pain: a systematic review of interventions and outcomes. Rheumatology (Oxford) 2008;47(5):670-678.
Schaper C, Zhu Y, Kouklei M, Culmsee C, Krieglstein J. Stimulation of 5-HT(1A) receptors reduces apoptosis after transient forebrain ischemia in the rat. Brain Res 2000;883(1):41-50.
Schlesinger PH, Gross A, Yin XM, Yamamoto K, Saito M, Waksman G, Korsmeyer SJ. Comparison of the ion channel characteristics of proapoptotic BAX and antiapoptotic BCL-2. Proc Natl Acad Sci U S A 1997;94(21):11357-11362.
Schulte-Hermann R, Bursch W, Kraupp-Grasl B, Oberhammer F, Wagner A. Programmed cell death and its protective role with particular reference to apoptosis. Toxicol Lett 1992;64-65 Spec No:569-574.
Scotter EL, Abood ME, Glass M. The endocannabinoid system as a target for the treatment of neurodegenerative disease. Br J Pharmacol;160(3):480-498.
Semkova I, Wolz P, Krieglstein J. Neuroprotective effect of 5-HT1A receptor agonist, Bay X 3702, demonstrated in vitro and in vivo. Eur J Pharmacol 1998;359(2-3):251-260.
Sharma SK, Klee WA, Nirenberg M. Dual regulation of adenylate cyclase accounts for narcotic dependence and tolerance. Proc Natl Acad Sci U S A 1975;72(8):3092-3096.
Shulman Y, Tibbo PG. Neuroactive steroids in schizophrenia. Can J Psychiatry 2005;50(11):695-702.
Singhal PC, Kapasi AA, Reddy K, Franki N, Gibbons N, Ding G. Morphine promotes apoptosis in Jurkat cells. J Leukoc Biol 1999;66(4):650-658.
Singhal PC, Sharma P, Kapasi AA, Reddy K, Franki N, Gibbons N. Morphine enhances macrophage apoptosis. J Immunol 1998;160(4):1886-1893.
Suchanek B, Struppeck H, Fahrig T. The 5-HT1A receptor agonist BAY x 3702 prevents staurosporine-induced apoptosis. Eur J Pharmacol 1998;355(1):95-101.
Takada-Takatori Y, Kume T, Izumi Y, Ohgi Y, Niidome T, Fujii T, Sugimoto H, Akaike A. Roles of nicotinic receptors in acetylcholinesterase inhibitor-induced neuroprotection and nicotinic receptor up-regulation. Biol Pharm Bull 2009;32(3):318-324.
Tikka TM, Koistinaho JE. Minocycline provides neuroprotection against N-methyl-D-aspartate neurotoxicity by inhibiting microglia. J Immunol 2001;166(12):7527-7533.

Torup L, Møller A, Sager TN, Diemer NH. Neuroprotective effect of 8-OH-DPAT in global cerebral ischemia assessed by stereological cell counting. Eur J Pharmacol 2000;395(2):137-141.

Trujillo KA. Effects of noncompetitive N-methyl-D-aspartate receptor antagonists on opiate tolerance and physical dependence. Neuropsychopharmacology 1995;13(4):301-307.

Trujillo KA, Akil H. Inhibition of morphine tolerance and dependence by the NMDA receptor antagonist MK-801. Science 1991;251(4989):85-87.

Ueda H, Inoue M. Peripheral morphine analgesia resistant to tolerance in chronic morphine-treated mice. Neurosci Lett 1999;266(2):105-108.

Ueda H, Inoue M, Matsumoto T. Protein kinase C-mediated inhibition of mu-opioid receptor internalization and its involvement in the development of acute tolerance to peripheral mu-agonist analgesia. J Neurosci 2001;21(9):2967-2973.

Ueda H, Inoue M, Takeshima H, Iwasawa Y. Enhanced spinal nociceptin receptor expression develops morphine tolerance and dependence. J Neurosci 2000;20(20):7640-7647.

Ueda H, Miyamae T, Hayashi C, Watanabe S, Fukushima N, Sasaki Y, Iwamura T, Misu Y. Protein kinase C involvement in homologous desensitization of delta-opioid receptor coupled to Gi1-phospholipase C activation in Xenopus oocytes. J Neurosci 1995;15(11):7485-4799.

Wallace MJ, Blair RE, Falenski KW, Martin BR, DeLorenzo RJ. The endogenous cannabinoid system regulates seizure frequency and duration in a model of temporal lobe epilepsy. J Pharmacol Exp Ther 2003;307(1):129-137.

Watkins LR, Hutchinson MR, Johnston IN, Maier SF. Glia: novel counter-regulators of opioid analgesia. Trends Neurosci 2005;28(12):661-669.

Whiteside GT, Munglani R. Cell death in the superficial dorsal horn in a model of neuropathic pain. J Neurosci Res 2001;64(2):168-173.

Wilson RI, Kunos G, Nicoll RA. Presynaptic specificity of endocannabinoid signaling in the hippocampus. Neuron 2001;31(3):453-462.

Woolf CJ. What is this thing called pain? J Clin Invest;120(11):3742-3744.

Xiao Y, He J, Gilbert RD, Zhang L. Cocaine induces apoptosis in fetal myocardial cells through a mitochondria-dependent pathway. J Pharmacol Exp Ther 2000;292(1):8-14.

Yaksh TL, Dirksen R, Harty GJ. Antinociceptive effects of intrathecally injected cholinomimetic drugs in the rat and cat. Eur J Pharmacol 1985;117(1):81-88.

Yang XF, Xiao Y, Xu MY. Both endogenous and exogenous ACh plays antinociceptive role in the hippocampus CA1 of rats. J Neural Transm 2008;115(1):1-6.

Yin D, Mufson RA, Wang R, Shi Y. Fas-mediated cell death promoted by opioids. Nature 1999;397(6716):218.

Zhang J, Barak LS, Winkler KE, Caron MG, Ferguson SS. A central role for beta-arrestins and clathrin-coated vesicle-mediated endocytosis in beta2-adrenergic receptor resensitization. Differential regulation of receptor resensitization in two distinct cell types. J Biol Chem 1997;272(43):27005-27014.

Zhang J, Ferguson SS, Barak LS, Bodduluri SR, Laporte SA, Law PY, Caron MG. Role for G protein-coupled receptor kinase in agonist-specific regulation of mu-opioid receptor responsiveness. Proc Natl Acad Sci U S A 1998;95(12):7157-7162.

Zuo DY, Zhang YH, Cao Y, Wu CF, Tanaka M, Wu YL. Effect of acute and chronic MK-801 administration on extracellular glutamate and ascorbic acid release in the prefrontal cortex of freely moving mice on line with open-field behavior. Life Sci 2006;78(19):2172-2178.

6

Reduced Antinociceptive Effect of Repeated Treatment with a Cannabinoid Receptor Type 2 Agonist in Cannabinoid-Tolerant Rats Following Spinal Nerve Transection

Matthew S. Alkaitis[1,2], Christian Ndong[1,3], Russell P. Landry III[1,3], Joyce A. DeLeo[1,3,4] and E. Alfonso Romero-Sandoval[1,3,4]
[1]*Neuroscience Center at Dartmouth, Dartmouth Medical School,*
[2]*Nuffield Department of Clinical Laboratory Sciences, John Radcliffe Hospital,*
[3]*Department of Anesthesiology, Dartmouth-Hitchcock Medical Center,*
[4]*Department of Pharmacology and Toxicology, Dartmouth-Hitchcock Medical Center,*
[1,3,4]*USA*
[2]*UK*

1. Introduction

In both preclinical and clinical studies, agents that activate cannabinoid receptors type 1 (CB1) and 2 (CB2) have shown promise in the treatment of pain (Wade et al., 2004; Romero-Sandoval and Eisenach, 2007). Cannabinoids are licensed for the clinical treatment of cancer chemotherapy-associated nausea and vomiting (USA and Canada), immunodeficiency syndrome-associated loss of appetite and weight loss (USA and Canada), multiple sclerosis-associated spasticity (United Kingdom and Canada) and neuropathic pain (Canada). However, clinical use of cannabinoid compounds is limited both by undesirable neurological side effects and by induction of tolerance. In animal models, neurological side effects have been shown to be dependent on CB1 receptor but not CB2 receptor activation (Romero-Sandoval and Eisenach, 2007). Furthermore, sustained spinal or subcutaneous administration of the CB1 receptor agonist, WIN 55,212-2 has been shown to induce hypersensitivity and antinociceptive tolerance in naive mice and rats. In contrast, we (Romero-Sandoval and Eisenach, 2007; Romero-Sandoval et al., 2008a) and others (Yao et al., 2009) have shown that spinal CB2 receptor agonists (such as JWH015) relieve postoperative and neuropathic pain in rodent models without inducing neurological side effects or antinociceptive tolerance. Despite advancements in the molecular mechanisms involved in cannabinoid tolerance (Martini et al., 2010), a better understanding of the respective roles of CB1 and CB2 receptors is required to design effective therapies that do not induce tolerance. Further advances in this area may also guide clinical treatment of patients who have already developed tolerance through prior exposure to non-selective cannabinoid agonists for recreational or medical purposes.

Using the L5 nerve transection (L5NT) rodent model of chronic neuropathic pain, this study was designed to test: 1) whether a non-selective cannabinoid agonist (CP55940) induces tolerance following repeated intrathecal (i.t.) administration in a model of neuropathic pain; 2) whether this antinociceptive tolerance could be reversed by the cessation of drug exposure; and 3) whether sustained spinal administration of the non-selective cannabinoid CP55940 affects antinociception induced by a CB2 receptor agonist (JWH015). To determine the site of action of these agonists we additionally examined expression levels and cellular localization of CB1 and CB2 receptors in the spinal cord of rats receiving either L5NT or sham surgery.

2. Materials and methods

2.1 Animals and surgical procedures

These studies were performed in accordance with the Guidelines for Animal Experimentation of the International Association for the Study of Pain (IASP) and after approval by the Institutional Animal Care and Use Committee at Dartmouth College (Dartmouth Medical School, Hanover, New Hampshire). Male Sprague-Dawley rats weighing 200–250 g (Harlan, Indianapolis, IN) at the start of surgery underwent L5NT surgery as previous described (Tanga et al., 2005). Briefly, rats were anesthetized with 2% isoflurane in oxygen and a small incision to the skin overlying L5–S1 was made followed by retraction of the paravertebral musculature from the vertebral transverse processes. The L6 transverse process was then partially removed to expose the L4 and L5 spinal nerves. The L5 spinal nerve was identified, lifted slightly, and transected. The wound was irrigated with saline and sutured in two layers. Sham surgeries were performed in other group of rats following the same procedure but without manipulating or injuring the nerves. The surgeries and anesthesia exposure lasted 15 - 20 minutes. Animals were housed individually and maintained in a 12:12 hr light/dark cycle with *ad libitum* access to food and water. Efforts were made to limit animal distress and to use the minimum number of animals necessary to achieve statistical significance.

2.2 Tissue preparation, immunohistochemistry, imaging and image analysis

After being anesthetized with 2-4% isoflurane in oxygen, rats were perfused transcardially with phosphate buffered saline (0.01 M, 150 ml) followed by 4% formaldehyde (350 ml) at room temperature. The L5 spinal cord section was collected and placed in 30% sucrose for 48–72 hr at 4 °C. The tissue was then frozen in O.C.T. Compound (Sakura Finetek, Torrance, CA) and stored at -80 °C. To determine the expression of spinal CB2 receptor immunohistochemistry was performed on transverse 20-µm L5 spinal cord free-floating sections by using the Vector ELITE ABC (Vector Labs, Burlingame, CA), avidin-biotin complex technique and a goat polyclonal antibody against the C-terminus of CB2 receptor (1:150, Santa Cruz biotechnology, Santa Cruz, CA, sc10076) as we have previously described (Romero-Sandoval et al., 2008a). Immunofluorescence was performed to determine the spinal CB1 receptor expression level using a rabbit polyclonal antibody (1:200, Cayman, Ann Arbor, MI) and a Alexa-Fluor™ 488 Goat anti-Rabbit IgG1 secondary antibody (Molecular Probes, Eugene, Oregon). For CB1 receptor and CB2 receptor expression quantification, the sections were examined with an Olympus microscope, and images were captured with a Q-Fire cooled camera (Olympus, Melville, NY). We quantified the CB1 receptor or CB2 receptor expression, blinded to experimental conditions, as the number of pixels above a preset intensity threshold using SigmaScan Pro 5 as previously described (Romero-Sandoval and Eisenach, 2007; Romero-Sandoval et al., 2008b). For both CB1 receptor and CB2 receptor expression, the staining intensity was examined in a standardized area of superficial laminae (I-II) and deep laminae (III-V) of the L5 dorsal horn in 3–4 slices examined per animal.

Immunofluorescence was also used for dual labeling with specific cell markers and CB1 receptor or CB2 receptor. All sections were blocked in 5% Normal Goat Serum (NGS) and 0.01% Triton-X-100 for 1 hour at 4 °C. Sections were incubated in the appropriate primary antibody or antibodies diluted in a buffer composed of 1% NGS and 1% Triton-X-100 in PBS overnight at 4 °C. To determine the cellular localization of CB1 receptor or CB2 receptor we co-labeled antibodies for CB1 receptor and CB2 receptor with the following cellular markers (antibodies): rabbit polyclonal anti-Iba-1 for microglia (1:1000, Wako Pure Chemical Industries, Richmond, VA), mouse polyclonal anti-GFAP for astrocytes (1:400, Sigma, Saint Louis, Missouri), mouse polyclonal antibody anti- ED2/CD163 for perivascular cells (1:150, Serotec, Raleigh, NC), mouse polyclonal anti-Neuronal Nuclei, NeuN for neurons (1:10,000, Chemicon, Billerica, Massachusetts).

The following secondary antibodies were used as indicated in table 1: Alexa-Fluor™ 488 Goat anti-Rabbit IgG1 (Molecular Probes, Eugene, Oregon), Alexa-Fluor™ 488 Goat anti-Mouse IgG1 (Molecular Probes, Eugene, Oregon), Alexa-Fluor™ 555 Goat anti-Mouse IgG (Molecular Probes, Eugene, Oregon) and Alexa-Fluor™ 555 Donkey anti-Goat IgG (Molecular Probes, Eugene, Oregon).

To avoid cross-reactivity between the secondary antibodies in the CB_2 receptor co-localization experiments, sections were first incubated in Alexa-Fluor™ 555 Donkey anti-Goat IgG (Molecular Probes, Eugene, Oregon) as described above, washed 2 times in PBS and then incubated in the appropriate Alexa-Fluor™ 488 secondary antibody as described above. This protocol modification prevented binding of the Alexa-Fluor™ 555 Donkey anti-Goat IgG to the goat-derived Alexa-Fluor™ 488. The specificity of each antibody was tested by omitting the primary antibody on 1-3 additional sections. To avoid cross-reactivity when co-staining with primary antibodies against Iba-1 and CB_1 receptors that are both rabbit-derived, a TSA Signal Amplification Kit was used following the manufacturer instructions (PerkinElmer LifeSciences Inc, Boston, MA). On the first day, normal immunofluorescence protocol was followed except that sections were incubated only in anti-CB_1 receptor antibody at a concentration of 1:10,000. On the second day sections were washed 2 times for 5 minutes in PBS then incubated in a biotinylated Goat α Rabbit secondary antibody for 1 hour at 4 °C. Sections were then subjected to another wash, incubated in SA-HRP (1:100) for 1 hour at 4 °C, washed again and incubated in the TSA fluorophore (1:250) for 10 minutes at 4 °C. Sections were then washed again and incubated overnight in the Iba-1 primary antibody (1:1000). The next day sections were subjected to normal day 2 immunofluorescence protocol to visualize Iba-1 (described above). One control was included with only the anti-CB_1 receptor primary antibody (1:10,000) and the Alexa 555 Goat α Rabbit secondary antibody to control for any cross-reactivity that might cause CB_1 receptor expression to appear in red. A second control included only the anti-CB_1 receptor primary antibody and the TSA kit in order to visualize the staining achieved in the absence of the co-stain. Finally, a third control included the TSA kit, Iba-1 primary and the Alexa 555 Goat α Rabbit secondary antibody but excluded the anti-CB_1 receptor primary antibody. This third control provided visualization of the non-specific background staining produced by the kit alone. All controls confirmed the specificity of the co-stain.

Antigen (Co-stain)	Primary	Secondary	Fluorophore optimal excitation (nm)
CB1	Rabbit	Goat α Rabbit	488
Iba1 (CB1)	Rabbit (Rabbit)	Goat α Rabbit (TSA Signal Amplification Kit)	488 (555)
GFAP (CB1)	Mouse (Rabbit)	Goat α Mouse (Goat α Rabbit)	488 (555)
ED2 (CB1)	Mouse (Rabbit)	Goat α Mouse (Goat α Rabbit)	488 (555)
Iba1 (CB2)	Rabbit (Goat)	Goat α Rabbit (Donkey α Goat)	488 (555)
GFAP (CB2)	Rabbit (Goat)	Goat α Rabbit (Donkey α Goat)	488 (555)
ED2 (CB2)	Mouse (Goat)	Goat α Mouse (Donkey α Goat)	488 (555)
NeuN (CB2)	Mouse (Goat)	Goat α Mouse (Donkey α Goat)	488 (555)

Table 1. Details of antibody selections for all immunofluorescense experiments, CB1: Cannabinoid receptor type 1, CB2: Cannabinoid receptor type 2, ED2: Perivascular cell marker, GFAP: Glial Fibrillary Acidic Protein, Iba-1: Ionized Calcium-Binding Adapter Molecule 1, NeuN: Neuronal Nuclei.

Stained sections were examined with an Olympus fluorescence microscope, and images were captured with a Q-Fire cooled camera (Olympus, Melville, NY). Confocal microscopy was also performed using a Zeiss LSM 510 Meta confocal microscope (Carl Zeiss AG, Oberkochen, Germany; Englert Cell Analysis Laboratory, Dartmouth). Merged color images were processed using Adobe Photoshop 7.0 (Adobe Systems, San Jose, CA).

2.3 Behavioral testing

Mechanical allodynia was evaluated by measuring the 50% withdrawal threshold using an up-down statistical method (Chaplan et al., 1994) and calibrated von Frey filaments (1 - 60 g, Stoelting, Wood Dale, IL). At each time point, two measurements were made on the paw ipsilateral to surgery in 5-10 min intervals, and the average of these values was used for data analyses. As an internal control, withdrawal thresholds were also measured in the paw contralateral to surgery (uninjured side). The withdrawal threshold was determined for each animal before surgery, 4 days after surgery (immediately before any pharmacological treatment), and after drug administration (different time points for different paradigms, see below). The investigator was blinded to drug treatment in all behavioral tests.

2.4 Drugs and treatments

Drugs were administered by intrathecal (i.t.) injection by means of lumbar puncture under brief inhalational anesthesia (2-4% isoflurane in oxygen) using a Hamilton syringe and a 28-

gauge 5/8-inch hypodermic needle. The needle was inserted intrathecally, on the midline between the fourth and fifth lumbar vertebrae. The correct injection site was confirmed with the stimulation of nerves in the cauda equina when the lumbar needle penetrated the dura and produced a brief but obvious movement of the tail and/or the hind paws. The animals regained consciousness 2–3 min after the discontinuation of anesthesia. Drugs were diluted in dimethylsulfoxide and saline in a ratio of 1:1 and administered in a volume of 15 μl as previously described (Romero-Sandoval et al., 2008a). The drugs used were: the dual (CB1 receptor and CB2 receptor) cannabinoid receptor agonist CP55940 (5-(1,1-Dimethylheptyl)-2-[5-hydroxy-2-(3-hydroxypropyl) cyclohexyl]phenol; Sigma Chemical Co., St. Louis, MO); the CB2 receptor agonist JWH015 ((2-Methyl-1-propyl-1*H*-indol-3-yl)-1-naphthalenylmethanone), the CB1 receptor antagonist AM281 (1-(2,4-Dichlorophenyl)-5-(4-iodophenyl)-4-methyl-*N*-4-morpholinyl-1*H*-pyrazole-3-carboxamide) and the CB2 receptor antagonist AM630 (6-Iodo-2-methyl-1-[2-(4-morpholinyl)ethyl]-1*H*-indol-3-yl](4-methoxyphenyl)methanone), purchased from Tocris, Ellisville, MI.

2.5 Repeated CP55940 administration and monitoring of behavioral effects

Beginning four days after surgery, CP55940 (100 μg/injection, n=18) or vehicle (n=17) was administered in single daily injections (8:00-9:00 AM) for five days. This dose and i.t. administration method were chosen based on our previous study using CP55940 in the same model of neuropathic pain (Romero-Sandoval and Eisenach, 2007), and on a previous study that demonstrated induction of antinociceptive tolerance with another non-selective cannabinoid agonist WIN 55,212-2 (Gardell et al., 2002) at a dose of 100 μg twice daily. Drugs and vehicle were administered i.t. based on previous evidence that spinal cord mechanisms drive induction of cannabinoid tolerance (Gardell et al., 2002). Two hours after each injection, mechanical withdrawal thresholds in both ipsilateral and contralateral hind-paws were evaluated as described above.

2.6 Evaluation of response to acute CP55940 dose escalation in tolerant and non-tolerant animals

CP55940 was acutely administered i.t. in 30-min interval escalating doses: 0.4, 2, 10 and 50 μg in L5NT animals 24 hr before and 24 hr after the repeated (5 day) treatment with CP55940 (n=5) or vehicle (n=6). As a control, vehicle was administered i.t. using the same dose escalation paradigm in animals that had previously received L5NT followed by repeated (5 days) treatment with CP55940 (n=8). The antinociceptive effect of escalating doses of CP55940 was evaluated 15 min after every injection. The effectiveness and potency of CP55940 were calculated using these dose responses and were compared in both repeated CP55940 and repeated vehicle treatment groups. To determine whether cannabinoid-mediated tolerance was reversed following the discontinuation of sustained CP55940 administration, the antinociceptive response to escalating doses of CP55940 were also measured two weeks after the last day of repeated CP55940 treatment (washout period). In summary, responses to acute CP55940 dose escalation (or vehicle) was evaluated in the following cases: 1) prior to any additional treatment, 2) 24 hours after repeated (5-day) treatment with CP55940, 3) 24 hours after repeated (5-day) treatment with vehicle, and 4) 2 weeks (washout period) after repeated (5-day) treatment with CP55940. To confirm that CP55940 induced its effects via CB1 receptor and CB2 receptor as we have previously demonstrated (Romero-Sandoval and Eisenach, 2007; Romero-Sandoval et al., 2008a), we administered CP55940 at a dose of 50 µg in combination with vehicle, the CB1 receptor antagonist AM281 at a dose of 50 µg or the CB2 receptor antagonist AM630 at a dose of 50 µg in a separate group of rats. Mechanical withdrawal threshold was determined 2 hr after treatments.

2.7 Evaluation of response to acute JWH015 dose escalation in tolerant and non-tolerant animals

JWH015, a CB2 receptor agonist, was acutely administered i.t. in 30-min interval escalating doses: 0.4, 2, 10 and 50 µg in L5NT animals that had previously received repeated (5 days) treatment with CP55940 (n=8) or vehicle (n=8). Vehicle was acutely administered i.t. using the same dose escalation paradigm in animals that had previously received L5NT followed by repeated (5 days) treatment with CP55940 (n=8). The antinociceptive effect of escalating doses of JWH015 was evaluated 15 min after every injection and its efficacy and potency were quantified. The first set of experiments was performed 24 hr after the last day of repeated CP55940 administration to test whether the cannabinoid-mediated tolerance influenced the antinociceptive effects of a CB2 receptor agonist administered acutely. The second set of experiments was performed two weeks after the last day of repeated CP55940 treatment (washout period) to test whether the potency and/or efficacy of the CB2 receptor agonist, JWH015 improves following the discontinuation of sustained CP55940 treatment. In summary, responses to acute JWH015 dose escalation (or vehicle) were evaluated in the following cases: 1) 24 hours after repeated (5-day) treatment with CP55940 or vehicle and 2) 2 weeks (washout period) after repeated (5-day) treatment with CP55940 or vehicle.

To confirm that JWH015 induced its effects via CB2 receptors as we have previously demonstrated (Romero-Sandoval and Eisenach, 2007; Romero-Sandoval et al., 2008a), we administered JWH015 at a dose of 50 µg in combination with the CB2 receptor antagonist AM630 at a dose of 50 µg or vehicle in a separate group of animals. Mechanical withdrawal threshold was determined 2 hr after treatments.

2.8 Evaluation of response to repeated JWH015 administration in tolerant and non-tolerant animals

Following the washout period (two weeks after repeated administration of CP55940 or vehicle), JWH015 (50 µg/injection, n=9) or vehicle (n=8) was administered in single daily injections (8:00-9:00 AM) for four days. Behavioral testing were performed before and 2 hr after each injection. Antinociceptive tolerance was evaluated by testing mechanical withdrawal thresholds in the paw ipsilateral or contralateral to surgery.

2.9 Assessment of neurological side effects

Based on our previous studies (Romero-Sandoval and Eisenach, 2007; Romero-Sandoval et al., 2008a) righting and placing-stepping tests were used to evaluate motor reflexes; the bar test was used to evaluate catalepsy; vocalization was used as a sign of irritability or discomfort to manipulation and exploratory activity was used as a measure of awareness. These parameters were evaluated before, 20 minutes and 2.5 hr after each injection (following behavioral mechanical hypersensitivity testing). The placing-stepping reflex was tested by placing the rostral aspect of the hind paws on the edge of a table and was quantified as the seconds in which the animals put the paws up and forward into a position to walk. A cut-off of 60 s was used. The bar test consists of placing the forelimbs on a bar of

~1 cm of diameter and 10 cm above and parallel to a table, leaving the hind paws resting on the table. A cataleptic animal will stay in that position longer than a normal animal. The time in which the animal puts its forelimb on the table was recorded, using a cut off time of 60 s. The righting test consists of placing the animal supine and recording the ability to right itself. Righting was scored on a scale of 0-3, 0 indicating normal righting reflex (an immediate and coordinated twisting of the body to an upright position), 1 indicating mild impairment (ability to completely right, but slowly), 2 indicating moderate impairment (ability to right the forelimbs slowly followed by the hind limbs with more difficulty) and 3 indicating severe impairment (inability to right in 20 sec). Vocalization was rated on a scale of 0-3, 0 indicating absent vocalization, 1 indicating some vocalization when manipulated, 2 indicating consistent vocalization when manipulated and 3 indicating vocalization even light touch. Exploratory activity was rated on a scale of 0-3 with 0 indicating normal activity, 1 indicating only head movements without vertical and/or horizontal exploration, 2 indicating no spontaneous movements and 3 indicating splayed posture with no spontaneous movements. All behavioral measures were performed twice and the average used for analyses.

2.10 Statistical analyses

The effects of L5NT surgery and drug injections on bar test, placing-stepping test and withdrawal thresholds were examined using the repetitive measurements one-way analysis of variance. If significant effects were found, Tukey's multiple comparison or Dunnett's test was conducted. Differences between groups were examined using two-way analysis of variance. If differences were found, the Bonferroni post test was used. In the acute antinociceptive effect studies, acute i.t. JWH015 50% of maximum efficacy (ED50) and its 95% confidence limits were calculated and compared between repeated CP55940 and repeated vehicle groups using Student's *t* test. ED50s were calculated using the baseline and after-surgery withdrawal thresholds as maximum and minimum effect values respectively. Vocalization, righting test and exploratory activity data following treatment were compared using the Friedman Repeated Measures Analysis of Variance on Rank test. If significant effects were found, non-parametric Wilcoxon signed ranks tests were conducted comparing each time point to the baseline value (before surgery). Between group differences were compared at each time period using the Kruskal-Wallis test. Significant effects were further evaluated using the Mann-Whitney U test comparing only the novel treatment to control or agonist group. The effects of CP55940 in acute antinociception vs. CP55940 in the presence of CB1 receptor or CB2 receptor antagonist was evaluated by one-way ANOVA followed by Dunnett's post-test. The effects of JWH015 in acute antinociception in the presence of the CB2 receptor antagonist was evaluated by unpaired Student's t-test. Data are presented as mean ± SEM. In all cases a *P* value less than 0.05 was considered significant. SigmaStat and GraphPad inStat software were used for statistical analyses.

3. Results

3.1 Spinal cord CB1 and CB2 receptor expression and cellular localization

Compared to rats receiving sham surgery, rats receiving L5NT surgery demonstrated significantly higher CB1 receptor expression in the L5 dorsal horn on postoperative days 4 and 7 (Figure 1). The changes in CB1 receptor expression were primarily apparent in the deeper laminae (III-V) of the dorsal horn in rats that had received L5NT surgery. CB1 receptor expression on day 1 after surgery was not significantly different between groups.

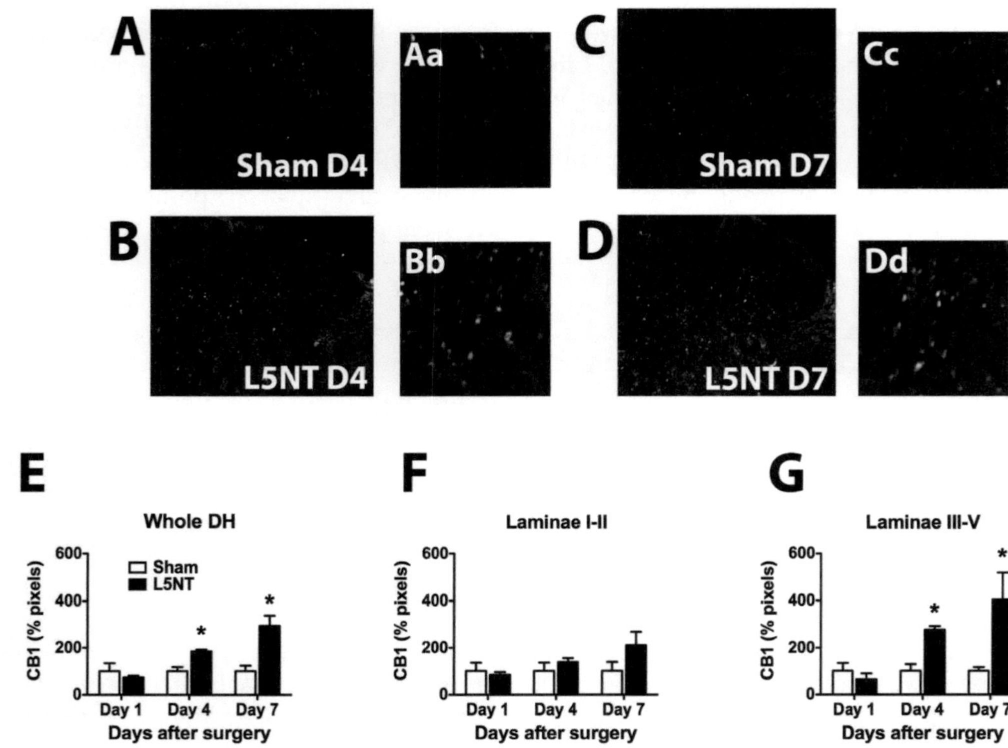

Fig. 1. CB1 receptor expression is increased on days 4 and 7 after L5 nerve transection. Representative images (A-D) show CB1 receptor expression at postoperative days 4 (D4) and 7 (D7) in the L5 dorsal horn of rats receiving sham surgery or L5 nerve transection. Details of the deep laminae (III-IV) of the dorsal horn of these spinal cord tissues are shown next to each original image (Aa-Dd). CB1 expression was quantified in the ipsilateral whole dorsal horn (E), laminae I-II (F) and laminae III-IV (G) of rats receiving sham surgery or L5 nerve transection at postoperative days 1, 4 and 7. Receptor expression was quantified as the number of pixels above a set threshold per total pixels in the selected area and normalized to percent of each control, sham group. *$p<0.05$ vs. respective sham group by t test. N=3 for all groups.

Compared to the sham surgery group, rats receiving L5NT also demonstrated significantly higher spinal CB2 receptor expression on postoperative day 4 (Figure 2). This increased CB2 receptor expression was mainly observed in the superficial laminae (I-II) of the dorsal horn in animals with L5NT surgery. No significant changes in CB2 receptor expression were observed on postoperative days 1 or 7 following nerve injury compared to the sham surgery group.

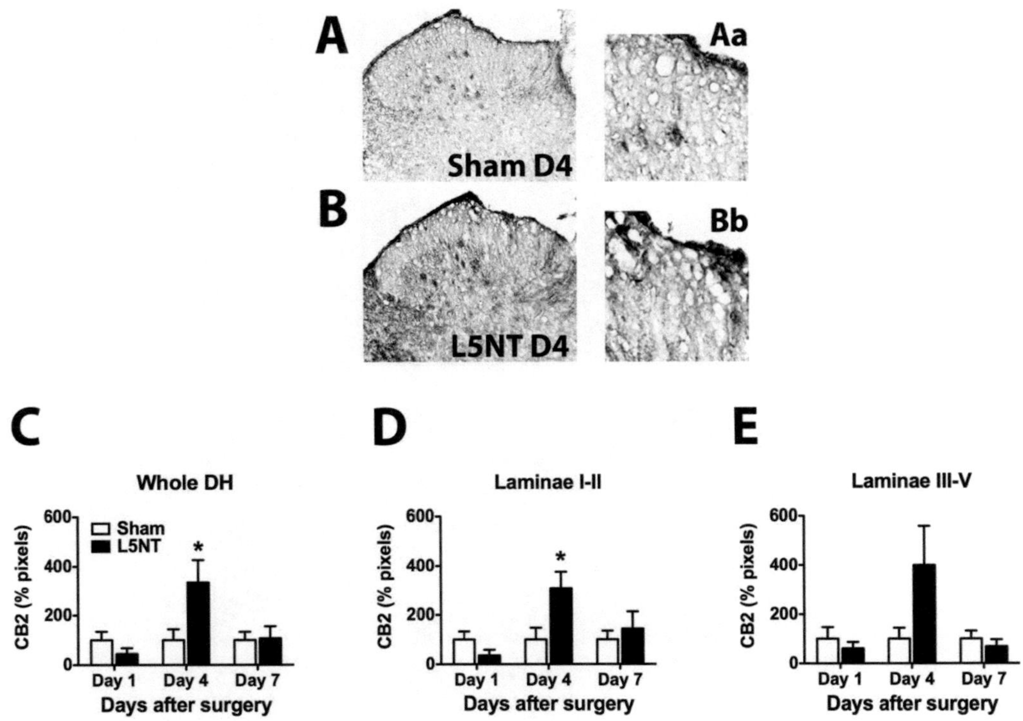

Fig. 2. CB2 receptor expression is increased on day 4 following L5 nerve transection. Representative images (A-B) show CB2 receptor expression at postoperative day 4 (D4) in the L5 dorsal horn of rats receiving sham surgery or L5 nerve transection. Details of the superficial laminae (II-III) of the dorsal horn of these spinal cord tissues are shown next to each original image (Aa and Bb). CB2 expression was quantified in the ipsilateral whole dorsal horn (C), laminae I-II (D) and laminae III-IV (E) of rats receiving sham surgery or L5 nerve transection at postoperative days 1, 4 and 7. Receptor expression was quantified as the number of pixels above a set threshold per total pixels in the selected area and normalized to percent of each control, sham group. *$p<0.05$ vs. respective sham group by t test. N=3 for all groups.

Using confocal microscopy, we observed that spinal CB1 receptors were primarily expressed on NeuN-positive neurons in the dorsal horns of animals receiving L5NT surgery (Figure 3). Occasionally, CB1 receptors expression co-localized with the astrocyte marker GFAP (Figure 3). CB1 receptor expression did not co-localize with Iba-1-positive microglia or ED2/CD163-positive perivascular cells at any observed time point following L5NT (Figure 3). However, cells expressing CB1 receptor were in close proximity to Iba-1-positive microglia and perivascular cells.

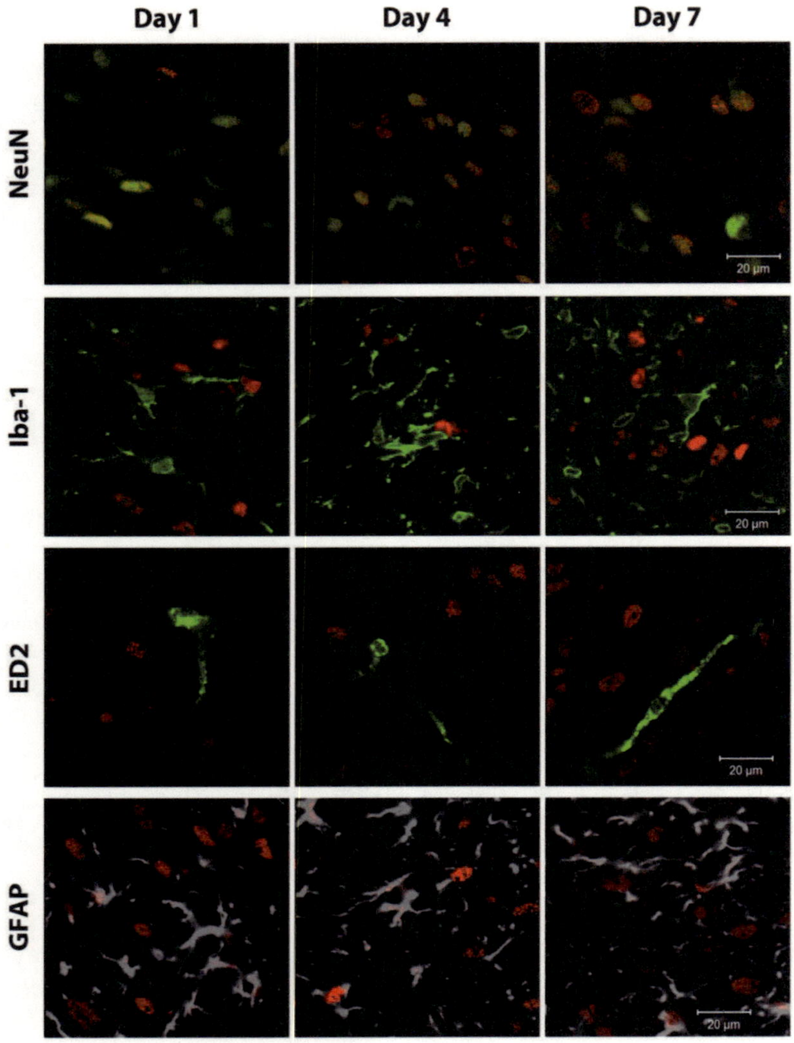

Fig. 3. CB1 receptor is expressed primarily in neurons. Representative confocal images show CB1 receptor cell localization in the ipsilateral L5 dorsal horn of rats at days 1, 4 and 7 after L5 nerve transection. CB1 receptor staining appears in red. NeuN (marker for neurons), Iba-1 (marker for microglia) and ED2/CD163 (ED2, marker for perivascular microglia) appear in green, and GFAP (marker for astrocytes) appears in grey. In the images of CB1 receptors and Iba-1, Iba-1 (originally in red) was changed to green, and CB1 receptor (originally in green) was changed to red to consistently show CB1 receptors in red in all images. GFAP color (originally in green) was changed to grey to obtain a better visualization of occasional expression of CB1 receptors on GFAP-positive cells. The colocalization of CB1 receptors with NeuN appears in yellow.

Microglia (Iba-1 positive cells) and perivascular cells (ED2/CD163 positive cells) displayed localized areas of CB2 receptor expression (Figure 4). Diffuse, punctate CB2 receptor expression was occasionally observed on NeuN-positive neuronal somata (Figure 4). Even though GFAP-positive spinal cord astrocytes did not demonstrate CB2 receptor expression, these cells were in close proximity to cells that expressed CB2 receptor (Figure 4).

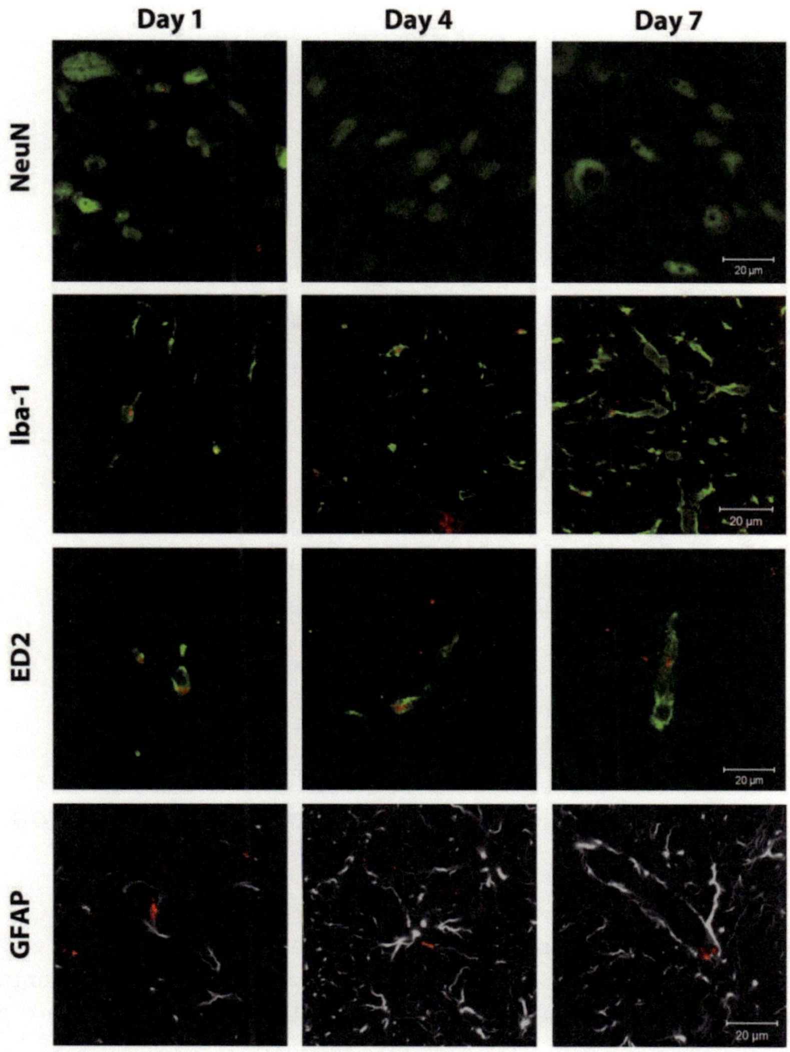

Fig. 4. CB2 receptors are mainly expressed in microglial cells. Representative confocal images show CB2 receptor cell localization in the ipsilateral L5 dorsal horn of rats at days 1, 4 and 7 after L5 nerve transection. CB2 receptor appears in red. NeuN (marker for neurons), Iba-1 (marker for microglia) and ED2/CD163 (ED2, marker for perivascular microglia) appear in green, and GFAP (marker for astrocytes) appears in grey. GFAP color (originally in green) was changed to grey to obtain a better visualization of this specific marker and any potential expression of CB2 receptors. The colocalization of CB2 receptors with the other cellular markers is visualized in yellow.

3.2 CP55940 antinociceptive tolerance

Mechanical withdrawal thresholds on the uninjured side (paw contralateral to L5NT) were not affected by surgery (26.7±1.4 g vs. 23.1±1.1 g, before and after surgery respectively), nor were they significantly different at any observed time point during the five subsequent days of intrathecal vehicle or CP55940 administration (Figure 5). In the paw ipsilateral to L5NT surgery, withdrawal thresholds were significantly reduced after surgery (26.6±1.3 g vs. 5.4±0.5 g, before and after surgery respectively, $p<0.05$).

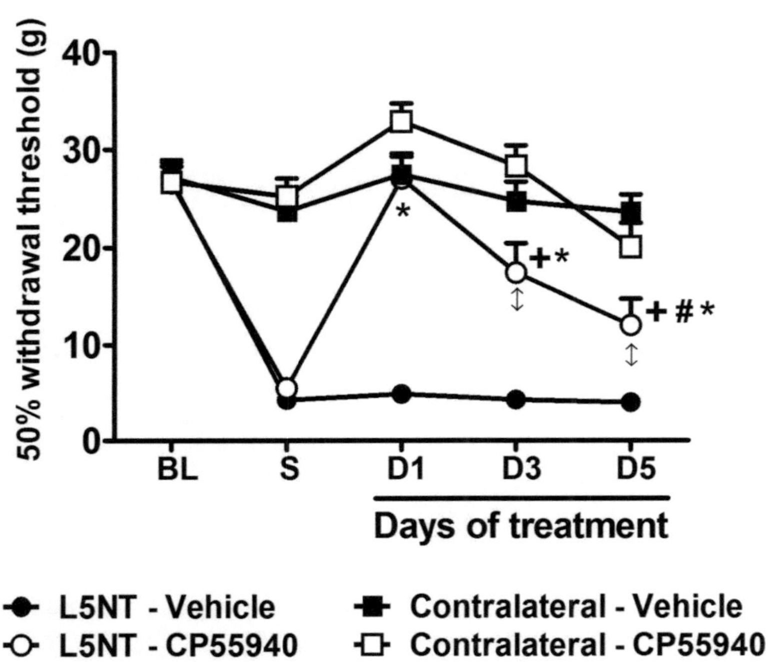

Fig. 5. Antinociceptive effects of repeated i.t. administration of CP55940. Paw withdrawal thresholds indicate responses to von Frey stimulation ipsilateral to L5NT or contralateral to surgery (uninjured side) before surgery (base line = BL), four days after surgery (S), and 2 hr after i.t. injections of vehicle (n=17) or CP55940 (n=18) on days 1, 3 and 5. Withdrawal thresholds on day 1 (D1), day 3 (D3) and day 5 (D5) vs. after surgery data significantly differ by repeated measures one way ANOVA; *$p<0.05$ vs. after surgery, +$p<0.05$ vs. D1 L5NT-CP55940, # $p<0.05$ vs. D3 L5NT-CP55940 by repeated measures one way ANOVA followed by Tukey's multiple comparison test. Groups significantly differ by two way ANOVA; ↕$p<0.05$ compared to vehicle and both contralateral groups by two way ANOVA followed by Bonferroni post tests.

Administration of vehicle (i.t.) on each of the subsequent 5 days did not significantly alter this L5NT-induced hypersensitivity at any time point observed (Figure 5). In contrast, administration of the non-selective cannabinoid agonist CP55940 (100 μg, i.t.) resulted in significantly higher withdrawal thresholds (measured 2 hours following injection) compared to vehicle-treated controls on each day observations were made (Figure 1). However, ipsilateral withdrawal thresholds in animals treated with CP55940 were significantly lower at 2 hr after injection on days 3 - 5 compared to day 1 values (Figure 1). Additionally, the anti-allodynic effect of CP55940 was significantly lower at 2 hr after injection on day 5 compared to day 3 (Figure 5).

In order to test the efficacy and potency of CP55940 before and after its repeated administration, we performed an acute dose escalation with i.t. CP55940. CP55940 reduced L5NT-induced hypersensitivity in a significant and dose-dependent manner before and 24 hr after the 5-day course of daily CP55940 administration (Figure 6). Compared to acute i.t. vehicle treatment, the minimum effective dose of CP55940 was 10 μg, and its maximum effective dose (dose that induced a return to base line values) was 50 μg (the maximum dose tested) before and after its repeated administration. However, CP55940 displayed an approximately 2-fold higher efficacy ($p<0.05$, Table 2) and an approximately 7-fold higher potency ($p<0.05$, Table 2) in untreated animals (Figure 6A) than in animals previously treated with CP55940 for five days (repeated CP55940 group, Figure 6B). The higher efficacy and potency of CP55940 observed in untreated animals were similar to the ones observed in animals previously treated for five days with vehicle (repeated vehicle group, Figure 6C, Table 2). We then evaluated the effects of acute CP55940 two weeks after repeated treatment with CP55940 was discontinued (washout period). Even though acute CP55940 was still effective (at 10 and 50 μg doses vs. vehicle) following 2 weeks of washout period, its efficacy and potency were significantly lower than in animals that had not received repeated CP55940 treatment (Figure 6D, Table 2). The acute antinociception induced by CP55940 50 μg (plus vehicle, 32.9 ± 2.1 g, n=6) in the L5NT group was blocked by either the CB1 receptor antagonist AM281 50 μg (14.5 ± 4.3 g, n=4, $P<0.05$) or the CB2 receptor antagonist AM630 50 μg (15.2 ± 4.3 g, n=4, $P<0.05$), confirming that the activity of this compound depends on activation of both CB1 and CB2 receptors.

	50% w.t. for the 50 μg dose (efficacy in g)		ED50 (95% confidence limits)	
	CP55940	JWH015	CP55940	JWH015
L5NT no previous treatment	32.9±1.94		14.7 (10.91-19.9)	
24 hr after repeated vehicle	29.7±2.85	17.0±2.7	11.9 (7.6-18.6)	26.4 (13.8-50.5)
24 hr after repeated CP55940	14.9±1.12 *	16.3±3.9	112.6 (21.2-596.6) *	37.4 (26.7-52.5)
2 weeks after repeated CP55940	15.7±4.8 *	14.2±2.5	162.6 (5.7-4567) *	32.5 (1.2-872)

Table 2. Effect of the highest dose (50 μg) and ED50 (95% confidence limits) of acute i.t. administration of CP55940 and JWH015 in L5NT, *$P<0.05$ vs. L5NT no previous treatment and 24 hr after repeated vehicle groups. Withdrawal threshold = w.t.

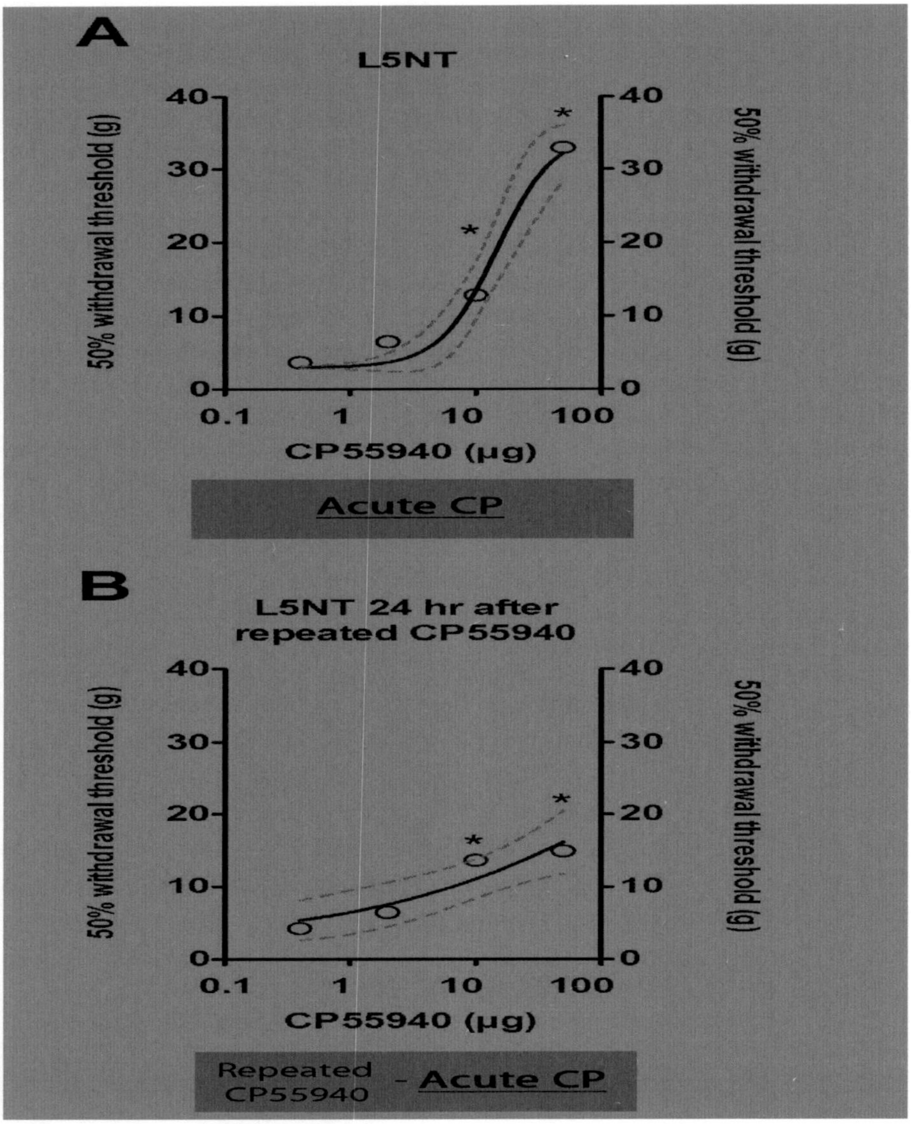

Fig. 6. Antinociceptive effects of acute i.t. administration of CP55940. Withdrawal thresholds (95% confidence limits, doted lines) indicate responses to von Frey stimulation ipsilateral to L5NT surgery 15 min after escalating doses (0.4, 2, 10 and 50 µg) of i.t. CP55940 in animals receiving no additional treatment (A, n=5), 24 hr after the discontinuation of repeated treatment (5 days) with CP55940 i.t., 100 µg (B, n=6) or vehicle (C, n=6) and 2 weeks (washout period) after the discontinuation of repeated treatment (5 days) with CP55940 100 µg (D, n=5). Withdrawal thresholds in response to dose escalation of CP55940 significantly differ from after-surgery values by repeated measures one way ANOVA, *$p<0.05$ vs. after surgery by repeated measures one way ANOVA followed by Tukey's multiple comparison test. Groups significantly differ by two way ANOVA; $p<0.05$ L5NT or L5NT 24 hr after repeated vehicle groups vs. L5NT 24 hr after repeated CP55940 or L5NT 2 weeks after repeated CP55940 groups for 50 µg by two way ANOVA followed by Bonferroni post tests.

3.3 CP55940 neurological side effects

In order to investigate the neurological side effects of CP55940 administration, we evaluated the place-stepping reflex, vocalization, exploratory activity and the bar test. Repeated vehicle injection did not significantly affect any of these behaviors at any time point observed. CP55940 significantly impaired the placing-stepping reflex (Figure 7A), induced vocalization (Figure 7B) and reduced exploratory activity (Figure 7C) on days 1, 2 and 3 compared to vehicle group, and induced catalepsy (Figure 7D) on days 1, 2, 3 and 4

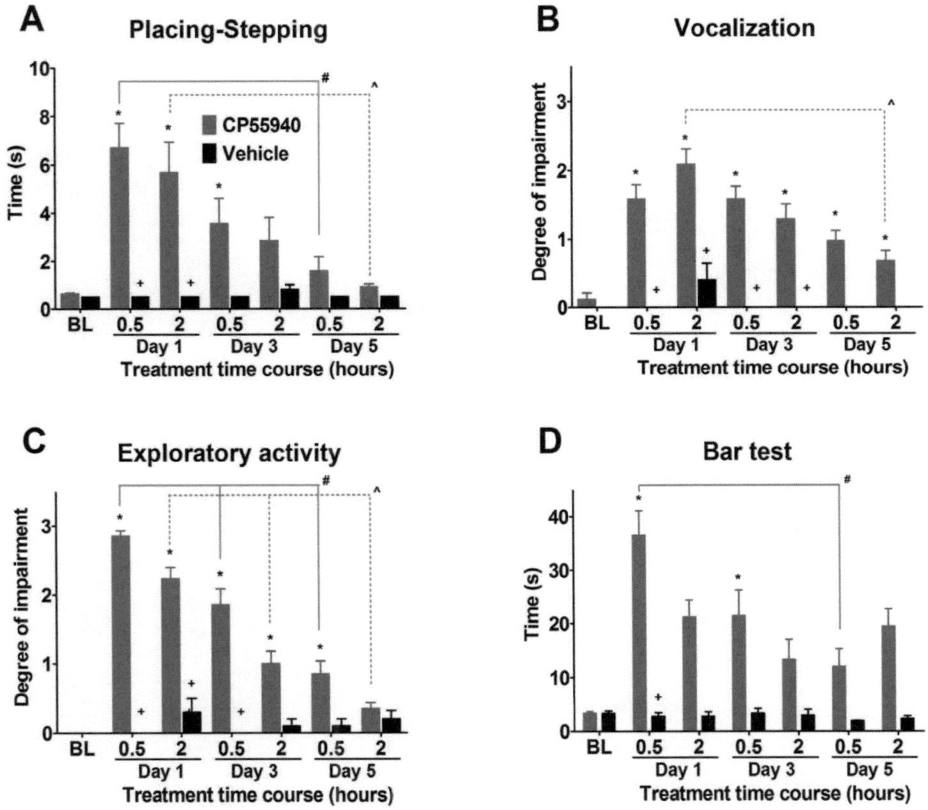

Fig. 7. Neurological side effects in response to repeated treatment with CP55940. Placing-stepping (A), vocalization (B), exploratory activity (C) and bar test (C) scores are shown from before the first injection (base line = BL), and 0.5, 2 and 24 hr after each i.t. injection (days 1 - 5) of vehicle (n=8) or CP55940 (n=13) during five consecutive days. Withdrawal thresholds on days 1, 3 and 5 in placing-stepping and bar test vs. base line data significantly differ by repeated measures one way ANOVA, *p<0.05 vs. base line, #p<0.05 vs. 0.5 hr, ^p<0.05 vs. 2 hr by repeated measures one way ANOVA followed by Tukey's multiple comparison test. Groups differ in placing-stepping and bar test by repetitive measurements two-way ANOVA, +p<0.05 vs. CP55940 group by two way ANOVA followed by Bonferroni post tests. Days 1, 3 and 5 values in vocalization and exploratory activity vs. base line significantly differ by Friedman test, *p<0.05 vs. base line, #p<0.05 vs. 0.5 hr, ^p<0.05 vs. 2 hr by Friedman test followed by Wilcoxon test. Groups in vocalization and exploratory activity significantly differ by Kruskal-Wallis test; +p<0.05 vs. CP55940 by Kruskal-Wallis test followed by Mann-Whitney U test.

compared to vehicle group. The magnitude of these neurological side effects decreased over the 5-day course of daily CP55940 injections until they were not significantly different compared to vehicle group on days 4 and 5 (except for catalepsy, 2 hr after CP55940 injection on day 4 vs. vehicle group, $p<0.05$). The righting reflex was significantly impaired by CP55940 compared to base line on days 1 and 3 (30 min and 2 hr after injections, data not shown). The effects of CP55940 on placing-stepping reflex, vocalization and bar test on day 1 were significantly higher compared to its effects on days 4 and 5. The effects of CP55940 on exploratory activity on day 1 were significantly higher compared to its effects on days 3, 4 and 5. For clarity, only the data obtained on days 1, 3 and 5 of treatment are shown.

3.4 Acute antinociceptive effect of JWH015 in CP55940-tolerant animals

JWH015, a selective CB2 receptor agonist, reduced mechanical hypersensitivity ipsilateral to surgery in a dose-dependent fashion when administered i.t. in cumulative, escalating doses in animals previously exposed to CP55940 or vehicle (Figure 8A). The minimum and

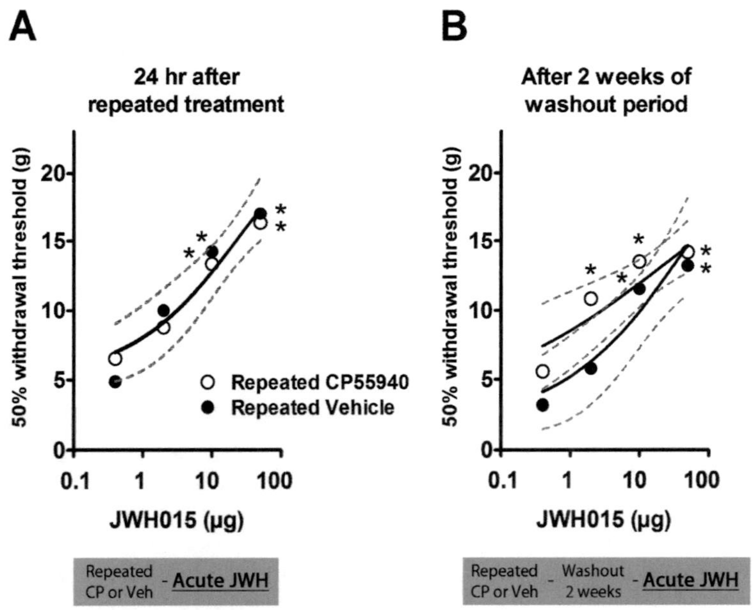

Fig. 8. Antinociceptive effects of acute i.t. administration of JWH015 in CP55940-mediated tolerant animals. Withdrawal thresholds (95% confidence limits, doted lines) indicate responses to von Frey stimulation ipsilateral to L5NT surgery 15 min after escalating doses (0.4, 2, 10 and 50 μg) of i.t. JWH015 administered 24 hr (A) or two weeks (washout period, B) after the discontinuation of repeated treatment with CP55940 100 μg (Repeated CP55940) or vehicle (Repeated Vehicle). Groups did not differ by two-way ANOVA. Withdrawal thresholds after each dose vs. after surgery values significantly differ by repeated measures one way ANOVA, *$p<0.05$ vs. after surgery by repeated measures one way ANOVA followed by Tukey's multiple comparison test. Twenty-four hr after repeated treatment cessation: Repeated CP55940 n=8, Repeated Vehicle n=8, Repeated CP55940-washout period n=6 and Repeated Vehicle-washout period n=5.

maximum effective doses of JWH015 in the repeated CP55940 group were 10 and 50 µg respectively (50 µg was the highest dose used). JWH015 was equally effective in both repeated CP55940 and vehicle groups since no significant difference in withdrawal thresholds was observed between groups in any dose tested. As a result, the ED50 value [95% confidence limits] of JWH015 was not significantly different in animals previously treated with repeated CP55940 compared to animals previously treated with vehicle (Table 1 and Figure 8A). Vehicle (same paradigm as cumulative JWH015) did not modify the withdrawal thresholds ipsilateral to surgery (3.5±0.6 vs. 5.3±1.4 g before and 15 min after the last injection respectively, n=6) 24 hr after repeated treatment with vehicle.

JWH015 was also effective in reversing the L5NT-induced hypersensitivity when it was administered in a cumulative manner two weeks after the cessation of CP5940 treatment (washout period). In this case, the minimum and maximum effective dose of JWH015 were 2 and 50 µg respectively in animals previously exposed to CP55940 (repeated CP55940 group), and 10 and 50 µg respectively in animals previously treated with vehicle (repeated vehicle group). Similar efficacy and potency of JWH015 were observed in both repeated CP55940 and vehicle groups (Table 2). No significant difference in withdrawal thresholds was observed between groups in any dose tested (Figure 8B). Vehicle (same paradigm as cumulative JWH015) did not modify the withdrawal thresholds ipsilateral to surgery in the repeated vehicle group after the two-week washout period (3.5±0.6 vs. 3.6±0.7 g before and 15 min after the last injection respectively, n=6). The acute antinociception induced by JWH015 50 µg (plus vehicle, 17 ± 2.7 g, n=8) in the L5NT group was completely blocked by the CB2 receptor antagonist AM630 50 µg (2.4 ± 0.4 g, n=4, $P<0.05$).

3.5 Antinociceptive effect of a CB2 receptor agonist administered repeatedly in CP55940 tolerant animals studies

JWH015 injected i.t. for four consecutive days induced similar antinociceptive effects on all days tested in animals previously exposed to repeated i.t. vehicle treatment (for 5 days) and a washout period of two weeks. However, JWH015 injected i.t. for four consecutive days induced antinociception only on days 1 and 4 in animals previously exposed to sustained spinal CP55940 administration (for 5 days) and a washout period of two weeks. Repeated i.t. JWH015 was significantly less effective on the last three days of treatment in animals previously exposed to repeated CP55940 when compared to those previously exposed to repeated vehicle (Figure 9A). The JWH015 repeated treatment did not modify the mechanical withdrawal threshold in the contralateral paw in the repeated vehicle or CP55940 group, and the effects of repeated JWH015 did not differ between groups, except on day 3 when the withdrawal threshold was significantly higher in the repeated vehicle group than the CP55940 one (Figure 9B). Vehicle (same paradigm as repeated JWH015) did not modify the withdrawal thresholds ipsilateral (n=6) or contralateral (n=6) to surgery in the repeated CP55940 group after the two-week washout period (data not shown).

4. Discussion

The main findings of our study are: 1) the repeated administration of a non-selective cannabinoid agonist (CP55940) induces antinociceptive tolerance and tolerance to cannabinoid-induced neurological side effects in a rat model of neuropathic pain; 2) CP55940 tolerance persists two weeks after the discontinuation of cannabinoid administration; 3) prior induction of CP55940 tolerance reduced the antinociceptive effect of repeated administration of a CB2 receptor agonist (JWH015), but did not alter the antinociceptive response to acute JWH015 dose escalation.

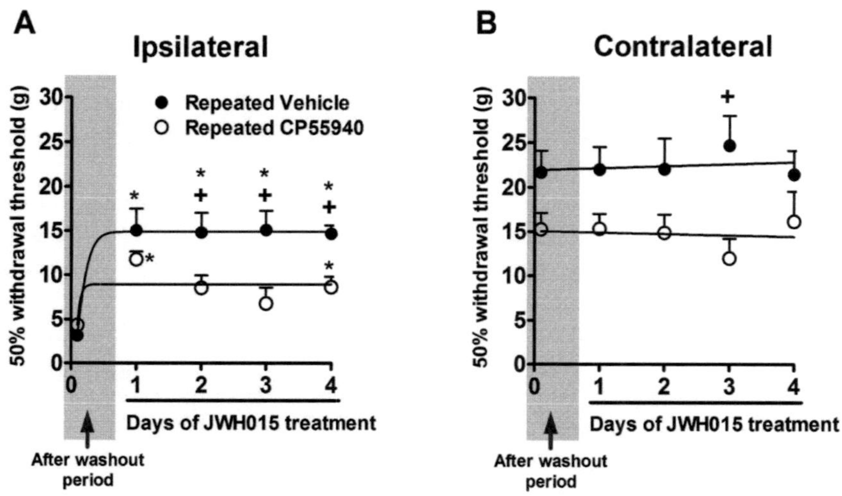

Fig. 9. Antinociceptive effects of repeated i.t. administration of JWH015 in CP55940-mediated tolerant animals. Paw withdrawal thresholds indicate responses to von Frey stimulation ipsilateral to L5NT (A) or contralateral to surgery (uninjured side, B) two weeks after the cessation of repeated CP55940 or vehicle administration (After washout period), and 2 hr after each i.t. injection of JWH015 during four consecutive days. Withdrawal thresholds on days 1-4 vs. after washout period data significantly differ by repeated measures one way ANOVA, $^*p<0.05$ after washout period by repeated measures one way ANOVA followed by Tukey's multiple comparison test. Groups significantly differ by two way ANOVA; $^+p<0.05$ compared to vehicle group by two way ANOVA followed by Bonferroni post tests.

We demonstrate that a non-selective cannabinoid agonist administered repeatedly at a concentration that induces neurological side effects (such as the effects that regular cannabis users seek for recreational purposes) is sufficient to produce a long lasting antinociceptive tolerance that persists weeks after the cessation of drug exposure. In agreement with these findings, diminished psychotropic effects (D'Souza et al., 2008) and analgesic tolerance to delta-9-tetrahydrocannabinol (Clark et al., 1981) have been demonstrated in frequent users of cannabis. This hypothesis has been further supported by a double-blind, placebo-controlled study demonstrating evidence of dronabinol tolerance in regular marijuana users (Bedi et al., 2010). It has also been shown that repeated administration of CB1 receptor agonists results in antinociceptive tolerance in naïve mice and rats (Gardell et al., 2002; Hama and Sagen, 2009), and that this tolerance is dependent on spinal cord mechanisms (Gardell et al., 2002). In contrast, we have previously shown that i.t. administration of the CB2 receptor agonist JWH015 effectively reverses L5 nerve transection-induced behavioral hypersensitivity without antinociceptive tolerance through at least five days of treatment (Romero-Sandoval and Eisenach, 2007). Similar findings have been described with another CB2 receptor agonist, A-836339 (Yao et al., 2009). Taken together, these previous findings suggest that CB1 rather than CB2 receptor agonism is responsible for the antinociceptive tolerance observed in response to CP55940 administration in the current study. Repeated administration of CP55940 also induced tolerance to a range of neurological side effects. We have previously observed that CP55940-induced neurological side effects are dependent on CB1 receptor activation, but not on CB2 receptor activation in rat postoperative and neuropathic pain models (Romero-Sandoval and Eisenach, 2007; Romero-Sandoval et al., 2008a). While these findings support the potential role of CB1 receptors in cannabinoid induced tolerance in our neuropathic pain model, CB1 receptor agonism does not induce antinociceptive tolerance in a spinal cord injury model (Hama and Sagen, 2009). Therefore, agonism of both CB1 and CB2 receptors may be required to induce antinociceptive tolerance to cannabinoid therapies in animals or patients with peripheral or central nerve injury.

CB1 receptor-dependent cross-tolerance among cannabinoids has recently been described between delta-tetrahydrocannabinol (the active ingredient of cannabis) and anandamide (one of the major endocannabinoids) (Falenski et al., 2010), and between 2-arachidonylglycerol (another major endocannabinoid) and the CB1 receptor agonist WIN55,212-2 (Schlosburg et al., 2010). This cross-tolerance is thought to be CB1-dependent (Falenski et al., 2010). However, we demonstrate in our current study that repeated administration of JWH015 exhibited reduced efficacy in rats with peripheral nerve injury that have been previously exposed to a non-selective cannabinoid agonist. This finding directly contrasts with our previous observation that repeated JWH015 reduces L5NT-induced hypersensitivity without signs of tolerance in the same rat model of neuropathic pain (Romero-Sandoval et al., 2008a). Taken together, these findings indicate that cannabinoid antinociceptive tolerance to non-selective cannabinoid agonists affects subsequent responsiveness of both CB1 and CB2 receptors. We also observed that CB1 receptors are predominantly expressed in neurons and that CB2 receptors are predominantly expressed in microglia in the spinal cord of both sham surgery and L5NT groups. Therefore, neuronal and glial interactions may contribute to the effects of CP55940-induced tolerance on JWH015's antinociceptive effectiveness.

Cannabinoid tolerance depends on CB receptor availability (Tappe-Theodor et al., 2007; Martini et al., 2010) and/or sensitivity (Jin et al., 1999; Selley et al., 2004). These receptor properties may change following peripheral insults such as paw incision (Alkaitis et al., 2010), peripheral nerve injury (Lim et al., 2003) or sustained activation by endogenous (Falenski et al., 2010; Schlosburg et al., 2010) or exogenous cannabinoids (Gardell et al., 2002; Hama and Sagen, 2009). In accordance with our findings, others have shown that a single intracerebroventricular dose of CB1 receptor agonists (WIN55,212-2 or ACEA) induces antinociceptive tolerance that lasts for more than 14 days through actions on the pertussis toxin-insensitive G proteins, Gz (Garzon et al., 2009). The mechanisms involved in long lasting CB1 receptor-mediated tolerance may also include the persistent cellular internalization or degradation of CB1 receptor (Sim-Selley et al., 2006). These data suggest that cannabinoid responsiveness and tolerance are shaped by a number of factors including type of pain or injury, exposure to endogenous or exogenous cannabinoids and receptor expression and sensitivity.

5. Conclusion

We demonstrate that a non-selective cannabinoid drug induces tolerance under neuropathic pain conditions, that this tolerance persists several weeks after the suspension of the treatment and that this tolerance affects the antinociceptive effects of repeated administration of a CB2 receptor agonist. These findings suggest that potential future analgesic drugs based on selective actions on CB2 receptor may not be a good alternative for long-term treatment in patients previously exposed to chronic cannabinoids. These results build on previous published data demonstrating that central CB1 receptor-mediated tolerance enhances tolerance to opioids (Trang et al., 2007; Garzon et al., 2009) and non-steroidal anti-inflammatory agents (Anikwue et al., 2002). Further research is needed to determine the mechanisms for this broad cross-tolerance among distinct drug classes. Additional studies are also warranted to determine whether patients with histories of cannabis or cannabinoid-based drug use for recreational or medical purposes demonstrate tolerance to common analgesic therapies.

6. Acknowledgements

Supported in part by grants DA025211 (AR-S) and DA11276 (JAD) from the National Institutes of Health (Bethesda, MD), and the American Pain Society Future Leaders in Pain Research grant. The authors declare that there are no conflicts of interest.

7. References

Alkaitis, MS., Solorzano, C., Landry, RP., Piomelli, D., DeLeo, JA., & Romero-Sandoval, EA. (2010). Evidence for a role of endocannabinoids, astrocytes and p38 phosphorylation in the resolution of postoperative pain. *PLoS One*, Vol. 5:e10891

Anikwue, R., Huffman, JW., Martin, ZL., & Welch, SP. (2002). Decrease in efficacy and potency of nonsteroidal anti-inflammatory drugs by chronic delta(9)-tetrahydrocannabinol administration. *J Pharmacol Exp Ther*, Vol. 303, No. 1, pp. 340-46

Bedi, G., Foltin, RW., Gunderson, EW., Rabkin, J., Hart, CL., Comer, SD., Vosburg, SK., & Haney, M. (2010). Efficacy and tolerability of high-dose dronabinol maintenance in HIV-positive marijuana smokers: a controlled laboratory study. *Psychopharmacology (Berl)*, Vol. 212, No. 4, pp. 675-86

Chaplan, SR., Bach, FW., Pogrel, JW., Chung, JM., & Yaksh, TL. (1994). Quantitative assessment of tactile allodynia in the rat paw. *J Neurosci Methods*, Vol. 43, No. 1, pp. 55-63

Clark, WC., Janal, MN., Zeidenberg, P., & Nahas, GG. (1981). Effects of moderate and high doses of marihuana on thermal pain: a sensory decision theory analysis. *J Clin Pharmacol*, Vol 21, pp. 299S-310S

D'Souza, DC., Ranganathan, M., Braley, G., Gueorguieva, R., Zimolo, Z., Cooper, T., Perry, E., & Krystal, J. (2008). Blunted Psychotomimetic and Amnestic Effects of Delta-9-Tetrahydrocannabinol in Frequent Users of Cannabis. *Neuropsychopharmacology*, Vol 33, No. 10, pp. 2505-16

Falenski, KW., Thorpe, AJ., Schlosburg, JE., Cravatt, BF., Abdullah, RA., Smith, TH., Selley, DE., Lichtman, AH., & Sim-Selley, LJ. (2010). FAAH-/- mice display differential tolerance, dependence, and cannabinoid receptor adaptation after delta 9-tetrahydrocannabinol and anandamide administration. *Neuropsychopharmacology*, Vol 35, No. 8, pp. 1775-1787

Gardell, LR., Burgess, SE., Dogrul, A., Ossipov, MH., Malan, TP., Lai, J., & Porreca, F. (2002). Pronociceptive effects of spinal dynorphin promote cannabinoid-induced pain and antinociceptive tolerance. *Pain*, Vol. 98, pp. 79-88

Garzon, J., de la Torre-Madrid, E., Rodriguez-Munoz, M., Vicente-Sanchez, A., & Sanchez-Blazquez, P. (2009). Gz mediates the long-lasting desensitization of brain CB1 receptors and is essential for cross-tolerance with morphine. *Mol Pain*, Vol. 5, No. 11

Hama, A., & Sagen, J. (2009). Sustained antinociceptive effect of cannabinoid receptor agonist WIN 55,212-2 over time in rat model of neuropathic spinal cord injury pain. *J Rehabil Res Dev*, Vol. 46, No. 1, pp. 135-143

Jin, W., Brown, S., Roche, JP., Hsieh, C., Celver, JP., Kovoor, A., Chavkin, C., & Mackie, K. (1999). Distinct domains of the CB1 cannabinoid receptor mediate desensitization and internalization. *J Neurosci*, Vol. 19, No. 10, pp. 3773-3780

Lim, G., Sung, B., Ji, RR., & Mao, J. (2003). Upregulation of spinal cannabinoid-1-receptors following nerve injury enhances the effects of Win 55,212-2 on neuropathic pain behaviors in rats. *Pain*, Vol. 105, pp. 275-283

Martini, L., Thompson, D., Kharazia, V., & Whistler, JL. (2010). Differential regulation of behavioral tolerance to WIN55,212-2 by GASP1. *Neuropsychopharmacology*, Vol. 35, No. 6, pp. 1363-1373

Romero-Sandoval, A., & Eisenach, JC. (2007). Spinal cannabinoid receptor type 2 activation reduces hypersensitivity and spinal cord glial activation after paw incision. *Anesthesiology*, Vol. 106, No. 4, pp. 787-794

Romero-Sandoval, A., Nutile-McMenemy, N., & DeLeo, JA. (2008a). Spinal microglial and perivascular cell cannabinoid receptor type 2 activation reduces behavioral hypersensitivity without tolerance after peripheral nerve injury. *Anesthesiology*, Vol. 108, No. 4, pp. 722-734

Romero-Sandoval, A., Chai, N., Nutile-McMenemy, N., & DeLeo, JA. (2008b). A comparison of spinal Iba1 and GFAP expression in rodent models of acute and chronic pain. *Brain Research*, Vol. 1219, pp. 116-26

Schlosburg, JE., Blankman, JL., Long, JZ., Nomura, DK., Pan, B., Kinsey, SG., Nguyen, PT., Ramesh, D., Booker, L., Burston, JJ., Thomas, EA., Selley, DE., Sim-Selley, LJ., Liu, QS., Lichtman, AH., & Cravatt, BF. (2010). Chronic monoacylglycerol lipase blockade causes functional antagonism of the endocannabinoid system. *Nat Neurosci*, Vol. 13, No. 9, pp. 1113-1119

Selley, DE., Cassidy, MP., Martin, BR., & Sim-Selley, LJ. (2004). Long-term administration of Delta9-tetrahydrocannabinol desensitizes CB1-, adenosine A1-, and GABAB-mediated inhibition of adenylyl cyclase in mouse cerebellum. *Mol Pharmacol*, Vol. 66, No. 5, pp. 1275-1284

Sim-Selley, LJ., Schechter, NS., Rorrer, WK., Dalton, GD., Hernandez, J., Martin, BR., & Selley, DE. (2006). Prolonged recovery rate of CB1 receptor adaptation after cessation of long-term cannabinoid administration. *Mol Pharmacol*, Vol. 70, No. 3, pp. 986-996

Tanga, FY., Nutile-McMenemy, N., & DeLeo, JA. (2005). The CNS role of Toll-like receptor 4 in innate neuroimmunity and painful neuropathy. *Proc Natl Acad Sci U S A*, Vol. 102, No. 16, pp. 5856-5861

Tappe-Theodor, A., Agarwal, N., Katona, I., Rubino, T., Martini, L., Swiercz, J., Mackie, K., Monyer, H., Parolaro, D., Whistler, J., Kuner, T., & Kuner, R. (2007). A molecular basis of analgesic tolerance to cannabinoids. *J Neurosci*, Vol. 27, No. 15, pp. 4165-4177

Trang, T., Sutak, M., & Jhamandas, K. (2007). Involvement of cannabinoid (CB1)-receptors in the development and maintenance of opioid tolerance. *Neuroscience*, Vol. 146, No. 3, pp. 1275-1288

Wade, DT., Makela, P., Robson, P., House, H., & Bateman, C. (2004). Do cannabis-based medicinal extracts have general or specific effects on symptoms in multiple sclerosis? A double-blind, randomized, placebo-controlled study on 160 patients. *Mult Scler*, Vol. 10, No. 4, pp. 434-441

Yao, BB., Hsieh, G., Daza, AV., Fan, Y., Grayson, GK., Garrison, TR., El Kouhen, O., Hooker, BA., Pai, M., Wensink, EJ., Salyers, AK., Chandran, P., Zhu, CZ., Zhong, C., Ryther, K., Gallagher, ME., Chin, CL., Tovcimak, AE., Hradil, VP., Fox, GB., Dart, MJ., Honore, P., & Meyer MD. (2009). Characterization of a cannabinoid CB2 receptor-selective agonist, A-836339 [2,2,3,3-tetramethyl-cyclopropanecarboxylic acid [3-(2-methoxy-ethyl)-4,5-dimethyl-3H-thiazol-(2Z)-ylidene]-amide], using in vitro pharmacological assays, in vivo pain models, and pharmacological magnetic resonance imaging. *J Pharmacol Exp Ther*, Vol. 328, No. 1, pp. 141-151

7

Applied Radiologic Science in the Treatment of Pain: Interventional Pain Medicine

Kevin L. Wininger[1,2]
[1]*Orthopaedic & Spine Center, Columbus, Ohio*
[2]*Otterbein University, Westerville, Ohio*
USA

1. Introduction

Accompanied by the work from innovative physician researchers and biomedical engineers who introduced new techniques and devices to expand armamentariums in interventional pain medicine in the 1990s and 2000s, the first decade of the 21st century resulted in a significant rise in the number of interventional procedures performed for pain management. For example, data from the Centers for Medicare and Medicaid Services shows a 518% increase from 1997 through 2006 in the Medicare population receiving spinal cord stimulation therapy (Manchikanti et al., 2009). Other examples include the efforts to design radiofrequency probes to target the sacroiliac joint and subsequently denervate this relatively complex but biomechanically unique structure with as little local tissue trauma as possible (Wininger, 2010); or the application of novel neuromodulation techniques to treat challenging cases of headache (Deshpande & Wininger, 2011).

The use of ionizing radiation for image construction (x-ray imaging) continues to be the standard in image guidance at many interventional pain medicine centers. Hence, the competent use of x-radiation not only benefits patients as well as physicians and ancillary staff in close proximity to the patient at the time of treatment—but from a health physics point of view also yields benefits for the general population given that recent evidence points to an overall increase in the use of radiation in medicine (Fazel et al., 2009; U.S. National Academy of Sciences, 2006). As of 2007, for example, medical sources of radiation represented the primary source of radiation exposure in the United States. Comparatively speaking, natural sources accounted for 3.0 mSv of the total dose, whereas medical sources accounted for 3.2 mSv (which was 5.9 times higher when compared to benchmark figures from 1980). The increase was primarily due to increased use of computed tomography (CT) and nuclear medicine studies. Note that medical sources were delineated as follows: 1.5 mSv from CT, 0.7 mSv from nuclear medicine, 0.6 mSv from radiography, and 0.4 mSv from interventional radiology (Johnston et al., 2011).

This chapter is intended to serve as a reference to help guide interventional pain physicians in their decision-making process concerning radiation risk management. In this context, the subject matter goes beyond the traditional emphasis placed solely on the cardinal rules of radiation safety (i.e., time, distance, and shielding) to render a systematic review of the different interventional imaging modalities used in the treatment of pain, namely fluoroscopy, CT, and ultrasound. Notably, we will center our discussion on the so-called "imaging (or 'viewing') chain" of each modality, and thus the issues surrounding image quality and signal processing relative to radiation exposure (or the lack thereof in the case of ultrasound imaging). Moreover, to develop a fundamental understanding of signal processing, key physical and mathematical concepts will be explored.

While this chapter is well-motivated allowing each section to stand alone, the subject matter is presented in such a way to promote continuity from one section to the next. We begin by focusing on fluoroscopic guidance; here analysis has been included to help establish benchmark radiation exposure for spinal cord stimulation procedures as first reported by Wininger et al. (2010). We then look closely at interventional approaches in pain medicine that utilize CT. Throughout these sections, ways to mitigate radiation dose will be considered, including recent steps to improve the shielding afforded by radiation protection apparel. Next, we provide an overview on ultrasound-guided pain medicine; here the tradeoff between spatial resolution and achievable depth of imaging is highlighted. Finally, future directions in image guidance for pain management will be surveyed, including non-ionizing radiation emitting modalities such as ultrasound imaging beyond regional anesthesia and interventional magnetic resonance imaging.

2. Fluoroscopy and interventional pain medicine

2.1 The fluoroscopic imaging chain

Overall radiographic quality is based on two principal properties, photographic quality (i.e., visibility of detail) and geometric quality (i.e., sharpness of detail) (Carlton & Adler, 2006; Bushong, 2004). Photographic quality is determined by density and contrast, whereas geometric quality is governed by recorded detail (i.e., resolution) and image distortion. In fluoroscopic image acquisition, the term "density" (a term derived from static film-based radiography) is replaced by the term "brightness" to be congruent with the language used to describe the visibility of images on a display monitor. The notion of an imaging chain makes reference to highly integrated instrumentation (together with the patient), regardless of the modality of interest. The fluoroscopic imaging chain denotes the x-ray generator, x-ray tube, collimator and filtration, table and patient, grid, image intensifier, optical coupler, and the image viewing system (Schueler, 2000). To this end, while each link in the chain is of equal importance, an understanding of fluoroscopic image quality relative to the image intensifier will be emphasized. The image intensifier functions as a "pass-through" device by converting x-rays to light (fluorescence) and then to electrons by way of its input phosphor-screen with adjoined photocathode backing (see Figure 1). This design effectively and efficiently reduces overall radiation exposure (Wang & Blackburn, 2000), and at the same time, allows physicians to dynamically view anatomy with a relatively high degree of resolution due to the total brightness gain. It is the ability to view dynamically with excellent image resolution—that underpins the role of fluoroscopy in many of the modern disciplines of medicine.

The potential for x-rays to penetrate an object (i.e., soft tissue or bone) and create an image is related to the quality of the x-ray beam as a result of the operating kilovoltage (kV) at the x-ray tube, and may simply be referred to as the "x-ray tube intensity," "tube intensity," or "tube potential." The amount of x-rays produced is related to tube current (in milliamperage (mA)) and time (in seconds (s)). Whereas the operator presets these factors in static film-based radiography, producing kilovoltage peak (kVp) and milliamperage seconds (mAs) upon exposure, this is not commonplace in fluoroscopic imaging due to automatic brightness control and real-time intended-use. Automatic brightness control is a type of automated "negative feedback" commonly set by most operators to ensure a proper amount of x-rays in order to image patients with thin to average body types. Because of its real-time imaging capability, extended exposure times are possible when operating fluoroscopy systems, and thus, the amount of tube current is substantially less compared to that used in static film-based radiography, 1 to 5 mA versus 100 to 500 mA, respectively (Carlton & Adler, 2006; Bushong, 2004). However, the physician has likely encountered degradation of recorded detail while using fluoroscopy due to a blotchy or grainy appearance that is directly related to an insufficient amount of radiation to create a uniform image (a phenomenon common to all electromagnetic imaging modalities) (Carlton & Adler, 2006). This is referred to as quantum noise or quantum mottle, as "quantum" means counted or measured. According to Carlton and Adler (2006):

> With fluoroscopy, the time factor is controlled by the length of time the eye can integrate, or accumulate, light photons from the fluoro imaging chain. Because this period is 0.2 seconds, fluoroscopy must provide sufficient photons, through mA, to avoid mottle. Quantum mottle is also a large part of video noise and is a special problem during fluoroscopy because the units operate with the minimum number of photons possible to activate the fluoro screen. The factors that influence mottle are those that affect the total number of photons arriving at the retina of the eye. This includes radiation output, beam attenuation by the subject, the conversion efficiency of the input screen, minification gain, flux gain, total brightness gain, viewing system, and the distance of the eye from the viewing system. Increasing the efficiency of any of these factors can assist in reducing quantum mottle, but the most common solution is to increase the fluoro tube mA.

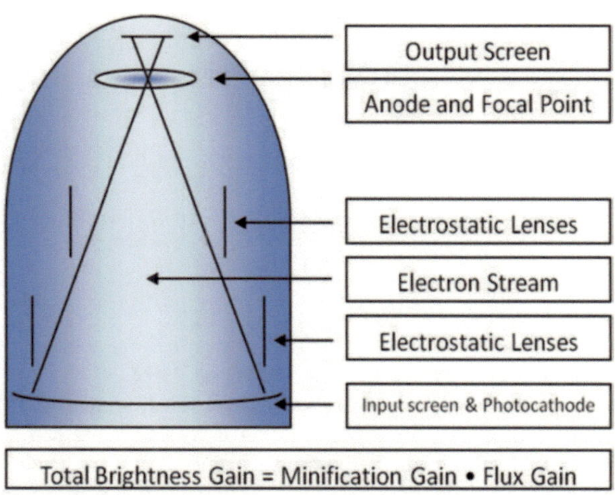

Fig. 1. Inside the image intensifier tube, x-rays photons are converted to light photons at the input screen and then to electrons at the photocathode. Flowing through the image intensifier tube the electron stream is repelled by the negatively charged electrostatic lenses and is attracted to the positively charged anode. Electrons are converted back to light at the output screen in order to proceed to the image viewing system. The output quantity of light photons is significantly greater than the input quantity of x-ray photons due to total brightness gain.

Image degradation from quantum mottle not only presents patient safety concerns due to challenges surrounding needle placement, particularly in patients with hypersthenic body habitus, but can also be a concern to the interventional pain physician and staff members inside the fluoroscopy suite, especially when team members are standing near the patient. We turn to x-ray attenuation physics to help us better understand this (McKetty, 1998). We see that in most fluoroscopically-guided pain procedures, the primary beam is directed at bony structures (i.e., material with a large content of calcium atoms, atomic number-20, which efficiently attenuates the beam) as opposed to soft tissues (i.e., material containing more atoms of carbon, oxygen, and hydrogen, producing an effective atomic number-7.4 and thus allowing more of the beam to transmit to the image intensifier). Moreover, Table 1 lists differences in the atomic numbers and densities of matter found in the makeup of the human body. It follows that in order to compensate for the attenuated beam within the field-of-view for bony imaging compared to soft tissue imaging, radiation output ramps up either as a result of adjustments to technique factors via automatic brightness control or by means of manual technique adjustments or activation of high-fluoro/boost mode by the operator. It is also important to note that most manufacturers incorporate an increase in mA during pulsed fluoroscopy to maintain equivalent image perception (Mahesh, 2001). With this in mind, a study on perceptual comparison between pulsed and continuous fluoroscopy concluded that the average absolute differences in the equivalent-perception dose is approximately 3% (Aufrichtig et al., 1994), where the equivalent-perception dose is defined as the dose of radiation in pulsed mode needed to give the visual equivalence in continuous mode. Thus, we find, importantly, an average radiation dose savings of 22%, 38%, and 49% for pulsed-15 frames per second, pulsed-10 frames per second, and pulsed-7.5 frames per second, respectively (Aufrichtig et al., 1994).

Matter	Effective Atomic Number	Density (kg/m^3)
Air	7.78	1.29
Fat	6.46	916.
Soft Tissue	7.40	n/a
*Water	7.51	1000.
Muscle	7.64	1040.
Spongy Bone	12.31	1650.
Compact Bone	13.80	1850.
Calcium	20.00	n/a

Adapted from Johns & Cunningham, 1983, and Dowd & Tilson, 1999.
*Note: x-ray output relative to the density of water serves as a baseline measure of x-ray output in the original design and calibration of x-ray producing systems as well as many radiation dose models, and may still be used to check system standards during annual physics acceptance testing. To this point, CT systems assign the number zero to water when calculating voxel/pixel brightness values (see Figure 6, CT Numbers and Hounsfield Units).

Table 1. Differences between matter in the makeup of the human body.

2.2 The physics of fluoroscopy

2.2.1 Primary radiation

When the x-ray tube is activated, electrons are "boiled off" from the wire element (i.e., a thin filament of tungsten) to form an electron cloud (see Figure 2). The wire element is strategically located opposite from the spinning target anode as part of a built-in concavity (of which the rim is slightly more negatively charged to concentrate the electrons in the cloud) on the cathode. The number of electrons boiled off is directly related to the tube current. Occurring nearly simultaneously with tube activation, the electrons in the electron cloud are forcefully attracted to the target anode due to the potential difference between the cathode and anode. The rate of speed and the efficiency of attraction are dependent on the potential difference across the tube. When high-speed (incident) electrons strike the target, the change in kinetic energy produces only less than 1% of x-rays, with most of the change occurring in the form of heat production (99% or greater) (Dowd & Tilson, 1999). More specifically, x-rays are generated by two processes. The first process involves the interaction of electrons with the nucleus of an atom of tungsten in which the incident electron slows down to change direction (called bremsstrahlung, or "braking radiation"). Bremsstrahlung radiation is emitted from zero to the maximum energy (operating kV). The second process is a collision of the incident electron and an outer shell electron of the tungsten atom. The collision knocks the outer shell electron out of orbit (producing characteristic radiation). Characteristic radiation is the term used to reference the fact that the x-ray energy produced is related to the binding energy between the outer shell electron and the nucleus of the target atom, and is always the same for a specific target atom (again, tungsten in the case of x-ray production in fluoroscopy) (Dowd & Tilson, 1999).

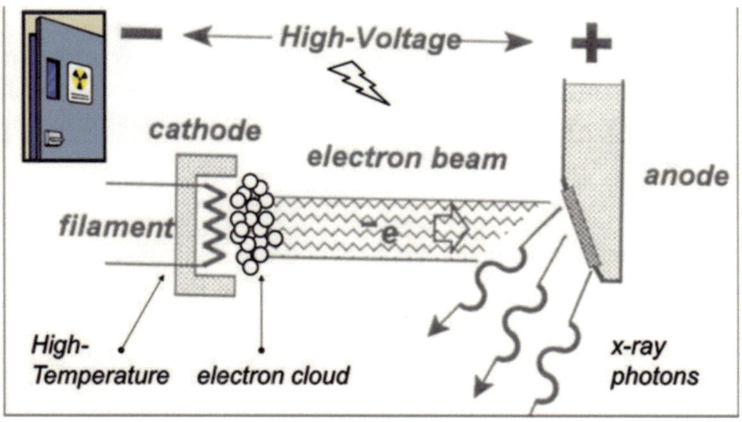

Fig. 2. A closer look inside the x-ray tube. When **tube current** is applied the filament heats up to boil off electrons into a cloud. X-rays are produced as the **tube potential** forces the incident (free) electrons to strike the target on the anode at a high-speed.

2.2.2 Secondary radiation—the patient as the point source

When x-ray photons in the primary beam pass through matter, they either pass unaltered (transmission) or undergo attenuation. Moreover, attenuated x-ray photons are either absorbed (all energy lost and the photon "dies") or scattered (some energy lost and the photon changes direction). The x-ray photons which are absorbed are primarily responsible for patient radiation exposure (via the photoelectric effect) and those photons which scatter are responsible for occupational radiation exposure (via Compton scattering). Note: when tube potential increases the photoelectric effect decreases *greatly* and the percentage of Compton interactions decreases *slightly*. (Dowd & Tilson, 1999). We will further elucidate the significance of the patient as the point source when discussing radiation risk management in fluoroscopy (or otherwise briefly stated, the occupational exposure due to secondary radiation emanating from the patient due to the interactions between the primary beam and the patient).

2.3 Fluoroscopically-guided pain medicine procedures

Nearly all interventional pain treatments and techniques evolved using fluoroscopic guidance. This was, in part, due to the capability of fluoroscopy systems to render high resolution images of bony anatomy (and adjacent tissues) to target pain generators. Today, with the versatility afforded by mobile C-arms (Tuohy et al., 1997), together with continued fidelity of the images rendered, the fluoroscope remains the principal modality for pain medicine image guidance. As a resulting consequence of this history, the literature not only contains several articles on the pros and cons of imaging techniques (for example, see Kapural and Goyle, 2007), but also contains multiple and diverse reports on radiation exposure associated with interventional pain procedures.

Notably, data collected on fluoroscopy time (the traditional metric used for clinical radiation management) serves to benchmark performance (Balter, 2006). While this parameter (fluoroscopy time) plays an essential role in the development of suitable registries to catalog radiation exposure levels according to the different pain procedures being performed, it may also be said that it is simply an awareness of this parameter by the physician that is inherent to optimization strategies in health physics (Shahabi, 1999). Table 2 presents the fluoroscopy times reported for the more common interventional pain medicine procedures using mobile multi-directional fluoroscopy systems (i.e., the conventional mobile C-arm). Other data noteworthy to collect includes: dose settings employed (operator chosen) and patient body mass. It is this additional information along with fluoroscopy time which may be used to calculate patient radiation dose received (i.e., entrance skin exposure). Table 3 shows fluoroscopy time as well as radiation dose using mobile multi-directional systems or biplanar systems for vertebral augmentation procedures.

Botwin **2001 2002 2003**	*Wininger **2010**	Zhou **2003**	Manchikanti **2002**	Manchikanti **2003a**	Manchikanti **2003b**	
–	–	–	13.2	8.9	12.5	Per Procedure
–	–	–	7.7	4.9	7.5	Per Patient
–	–	81.5	–	4.5	5.8	Facet Nerve Blocks
–	–	–	5.9	–	–	Cervical
–	–	–	5.5	–	–	Thoracic
–	–	–	5.7	–	–	Lumbar
–	–	50.6	–	–	7.5	Sacroiliac Joint Blocks
–	–	46.6	3.75	2.7	3.7	Epidurals
–	–	–	–	–	–	Interlaminar
12.6	–	–	–	–	–	Caudal
–	–	–	8.8	–	–	TFESI - Cervical
15.2	–	–	10.9	–	–	TFESI - Lumbar
–	–	–	12.7	–	–	Medial Branch Block
57.2	–	146.8	–	–	–	Discography
–	133.4	–	–	–	–	Spinal Cord Stimulation

*Wininger et al. also reported calculations on entrance skin exposure.

Table 2. Fluoroscopy time (in seconds) using mobile multi-directional systems.

Kallmes **2003**	Boszczyk **2006**	**Perisinakis **2004**	***Villavicencio **2005**	***Izadpanah **2009**	Thoracic Spine
522	216	609	81.3	175	Total Fluoroscopy Time
–	100	203	–	–	Total Patient *ESE*
–	32	–	–	–	*ESE* - AP Imaging
–	68	–	–	–	*ESE* - Lateral Imaging
–	–	3598	–	1245	Total DAP
–	–	2294	–	–	DAP - AP Imaging
–	–	1304	–	–	DAP - Lateral Imaging
–	–	–	–	–	Effective Dose/Minute
236	–	–	–	–	Physician Hand

**without or ***with 3D navigation in vertebroplasty or kyphoplasty procedures.
Fluoroscopy time (in seconds); patient entrance skin exposure (*ESE*) and dose area product (DAP, a calculation of stochastic risk for the patient [Vano et al., 2001]) (in centiGray); physician total and hand exposure (in microSieverts/minute).

Table 3. Radiation exposure associated with biplanar systems or multi-directional systems.

Inter-procedural variance compared to fluoroscopy times observed in Tables 2 and 3 may be attributed to differences in procedural techniques, level of experience, and/or physician preferences in imaging assistance, as well as attenuation physics relative to image quality. To illustrate this last point, we consider spinal imaging. During spinal imaging, two common challenges associated with image quality exist: 1) highly radiolucent vertebral bodies, particularly against the imaged lung field, creating excess image brightness in the region of interest, and 2) large body habitus with resultant poor image quality. In the former, tight collimation with the paired leaves shutters drawn close to the spine and continuous-mode imaging may help compensate for poor contrast resolution due to the vertebral bodies lacking enough cortical bone density to effectively attenuate the beam (i.e., low beam attenuation) (Johns & Cunningham, 1983). Subsequently, overriding automatic brightness control by manually ramping down tube current (mA) during tightly collimated bony imaging can help improve image resolution, especially for extremely radiolucent vertebral bodies. Alternatively, a manual adjustment to monitor/display window contrast may effectively improve image quality. To compensate for poor image quality secondary to large body habitus (i.e., a highly attenuated beam with resultant image granularity), it too may be necessary to operate the fluoroscope in continuous mode to increase the overall radiation at the image intensifier rather than disengaging the low dose feature. This strategy may improve image contrast while limiting patient exposure if a "manual beam on/off" operator technique is used, e.g., while panning or moving the C-arm between anteroposterior/oblique positioning to keep region of interest in the field of view.

2.4 Radiation risk management/safety

In recent years the assessment of radiation dose has received increased scrutiny; notably, the evaluation of deterministic effects, for which the severity of effects will vary according to the dose received and for which dose thresholds usually exist (e.g., radiation induced skin injuries) (Balter, 2006 & 2008). Moreover, dose assessment has seemingly evolved from an academic enterprise to a clinical endeavour. Direct influence on clinical practice is appreciated by The Joint Commission's recent decision to add unexpectedly prolonged fluoroscopic exposure to its list of reviewable sentinel events, as well as their suggestion to follow-up qualifying events with a period of over six-months to one-year to monitor cumulative skin dose (The Joint Commission, n.d.). While fluoroscopy time alone provides inadequate skin dose estimates (Balter, 2006; Balter, 2008), the evaluation of incident air kerma (x-ray exposure to the skin, previously referred to as entrance skin exposure) is possible by simplistic modeling (Balter, 2008; American Association of Physicists in Medicine (AAPM), 2001; Bushong, 2004).

In part with its approach to minimally invasive treatments and therapeutic procedures, interventional medicine is the one branch of medicine which, in its practice, is riddled with concepts that stem from physics. It may be further stated that physicians, even interventionally-trained physicians, may feel as though they are not able to translate applicable literature into everyday practice without possessing a doctorate in the physical sciences. For example, radiation dose models can be complicated as there exists many nuances when talking about dose, and the units of measure are not intuitive. However, both radiation safety and radiation protection are fundamental considerations for the interventional pain physician, and are equally paramount responsibilities in the interventional pain practice. In the view of the author, physicians who utilize fluoroscopic guidance will find that keeping radiation exposure, and therefore radiation dose, as low as reasonably achievable (given the acronym ALARA) is a challenge that is not insurmountable. This goal is achieved by exploitation of the principles unique to image acquisition in fluoroscopy, together with radiologic physics and applied radiobiology (Dowd & Tilson, 1999), and a suitable quality assurance program. Thus, by first laying out the conversion between the basic units of measure in radiation physics,

$$1\,R \approx 1\,rad = 10\,mGy = 10\,mSv$$

this section will strive to provide the interventional pain physician with information on radiation risk management which may be readily acted on and implemented.

Entrance skin exposure is the radiation exposure to the skin measured in Roentgen (R) or milliRoentgen (mR) at the point of skin entrance for the nominal patient (i.e., 30 cm from the image intensifier). The measurement is made without the contributions from scatter radiation. In compliance with physics acceptance testing, the fluoroscopic tube potentials (kVp) under automatic brightness control should operate at/or between 70 and 90 kVp with 3.8 cm of aluminum (~15 cm of water or acrylic plastic) attenuation material. This produces measured fluoroscopic exposure rates in the range of 1.0 to 4.0 R/minute for all magnification modes (fields of view) for continuous mode in the normal dose setting (AAPM, 2001; Bushong, 2004). The lower portion of the exposure range accounts for the largest field of view (least magnification), and the upper portion of the exposure range accounts for the smallest field of view (most magnification). The name of the quantity which corresponds to entrance skin exposure and which is recognized by the International Commission on Radiation Units and Measurements is incident air kerma (Balter, 2008), and the unit of measurement is milligray (mGy). (Note: 1 R = 1 Roentgen = 2.58×10^{-4} coulombs/kg-m of air at standard temperature and pressure, and 1 R = 8.76 mGy [milligray].)

The dedicated use of the low dose setting (which provides 40% or more dose reduction compared to the normal dose setting, Smiddy et al., 1996; Davies et al., 2006), when paired with pulsed fluoroscopy (which provides 50% dose reduction at 7.5 frames per second, Aufrichtig et al., 1994) promotes optimal radiation risk management. This impact is best observed by a closer inspection of the work by Wininger et al. (2010) on radiation exposure in spinal cord stimulation [trialing] procedures. The authors point out that although pulsed fluoroscopy was utilized differently during cases #3 and #43, the fluoroscopy time for each case was recorded as 198.9 seconds. Analysis between actual settings used and hypothetical use variances for the low dose setting and the pulsed mode feature, based on simplistic modeling, illustrated how fluoroscopy time alone may lead to inadequate skin dose assessments. In other words, analysis of incident air kerma derived from the actual settings revealed that case #43 incurred 39.4% more skin exposure than case #3. Hypothetically, if neither the low dose feature nor pulsed fluoroscopy had been utilized, the resultant incident air kerma (i.e., 38.7 mGy) would have approximated the actual estimates derived for fluoroscopy times greater than 300 seconds (i.e., approximately double) for this procedure (i.e., 25.7–43.7 mGy). However, because the earliest deterministic threshold is 2.0 Gy, the level associated with transient erythema (Geleijns & Wondergem, 2005), research indicates that induction of deterministic insults (such as skin injuries) is highly unlikely during interventional pain medicine procedures. *Rather, in interventional pain medicine, the prime objective is to safeguard to the degree possible (i.e., ALARA) against low doses of x-radiation (U.S. National Academy of Sciences, 2006; Little et al., 2009).*

With respect to quality assurance programs for fluoroscopy systems, it is important to address mechanical and electrical safety in addition to radiation safety and image quality. Moreover, such programs are particularly important for mobile systems due to the various uses and locations in which these units are intended to perform. Given that mobile units are often the more commonly utilized systems in pain management applications, a quality assurance protocol is essential. However, due to differences between mobile systems from the various manufacturers, as well the different regulations overseeing radiologic licensure in the various jurisdictions the reader finds him- or herself in, an outline of such program is beyond the scope of this chapter. The reader is, therefore, referred to Tuohy et al. (1997) who tackled these issues and made several key recommendations.

Reports on occupational incurred dose from scatter radiation are typically based on radiation exposure to standardized phantoms, thus representing the symmetrical ideal "small lumbar" spine. This methodology, however, may potentially underestimate the amount of occupational radiation exposure since body habitus does not always lend itself to symmetry and body size varies from patient to patient. Hence, Whitworth (n.d.) performed scatter radiation vector analysis on the lumbar spines of five cadavers to better parallel the general experience of the interventional pain physician and those team members inside the fluoroscopy suite. The study employed an OEC 9800 mobile C-arm with automatic brightness control engaged. Radiation exposure was recorded using Geiger Mueller techniques (measurements are shown in Table 4).

OEC 9800	mrem/hour	kV	mA
High Level/Boost Fluoro	204	71	3.9
Normal Dose	111	70	2.2
Low Dose	56	72	0.76
Low Dose + Collimation	15	74	0.82
Pulsed-8 frames per second	7	76	0.86

Meter set at 17 inches above the floor and 12 inches lateral to the image intensifier.

Table 4. Scatter radiation measurements: imaging the lumbar spine of a cadaver with 21.5 body mass index.

Four important concepts were drawn from the resulting data set, as follows:

- Scatter radiation is exponential with increasing kilovoltage (kV) and linear with increasing mA;
- Collimation reduces scatter radiation by 50% or more;
- Use of low dose reduces scatter radiation by 50-75%; use of pulsed mode reduces scatter radiation by 65-90%; and
- Scatter radiation drops 50% every 6 inches away from the image intensifier.

It is interesting to pair the data set obtained by Whitworth with a law in radiophysics which aptly describes the phenomenon of scatter radiation in a meaningful way: as kilovoltage increases the photoelectric effect decreases *greatly* and the percentage of Compton interactions decreases *slightly*. Thus, Whitworth actually observed the following. As tube potential (kVp) increases, fewer x-rays interact with tissue, and therefore less scatter is created. However, the scatter that is created has higher energy and is more likely to reach the image intensifier [or nearby dosimeter(s)] than to interact with the patient's body. This makes increased kVp a radiation protection tool that must be counterbalanced with image concerns (Dowd & Tilson, 1999). See Table 5.

Tube Potential Kilovoltage (kVp)	**Secondary Radiation** (The Patient as the Point Source)		**Total Number of Interactions in 1mm Tissue**
	Total Number of Photoelectric Effects	Total Number of Compton Scatter/ Coherent Interactions	
50	500 (50%)	500 (50%)	1000
90	165 (33%)	335 (67%)	500

Adapted from Dowd & Tilson, 1999.

Table 5. Effects of x-ray tube potential (kilovoltage) on secondary radiation generated.

In many interventional pain suites, "lead aprons" are the principal shield for radiation protection of personnel. In addition, it should be noted that a table skirt substantially decreases occupational radiation levels—since the majority of scatter radiation is produced under the fluoroscopy table (for fluoroscopes/C-arms with under-table x-ray tubes) in the form of backscatter. Thus, significant reduction to scatter radiation is gained from the combined pair, as each scattering incidence results in x-radiation energy levels of only 1/1000 of that prior to the episode (Dowd & Tilson, 1999). Moreover, largely as a consequence of complaints of back pain over time from the wearers of lead aprons (Christodoulou et al., 2003), lead equivalent aprons became the apron-of-choice among interventionalists, and recently, "lead free" aprons have emerged in the marketplace. Such alternative materials include tin, iodine, barium, and antimony, or any combination thereof. Such "lead free" alternatives offer significant weight reduction, compared to primarily-leaded aprons, and equivalent radiation protection (Finnerty, 2005) (see Table 6). As part of an occupation radiation safety program, it is suggested that the reader ensure annual inspections of aprons are performed and rejection criteria established. Practical rejection criteria have been offered by Stam and Pillay (2008).

It is know that the dominant hand of the interventionalist receives the highest dose of radiation. It is interesting to note that a new type of sterilizable, radiation protection glove (primarily composed of tungsten) was recently tested among surgeons during a variety of cases, including micro-discectomy (Back et al., 2004). In terms of radiation protection, results revealed that the glove was superior to all other gloves in the marketplace, attenuating 90% of x-rays (see Table 6), and radiation dose to the dominant hand was reduced to less than the dose received by the non-dominant hand.

Aprons (0.25 mm)		**Aprons (0.50 mm)**			
Pure lead	Lead equivalent	Pure lead	Lead equivalent	"Lead-free"	
Attenuation at 70 kVp					
95%	92% 89-95%	99%	98-99%	n/a 98.1-98.3%	Mean Range
Transmission at 70 kVp					
	8% 5-11%		1% 1-2%		Mean Range
Attenuation at 100 kVp					
85%	83% 79-87%	95%	95% 93-96%	n/a 93.2-93.9%	Mean Range
Transmission at 100 kVp					
	17% 13-31%		5% 4-7%		Mean Range
Gloves - supplier or *type, and quoted decrease at 80 kVp					
*Tungsten		Henleys Medical (3 STAR)	Henleys Medical (2 STAR)	Henleys Medical (1 STAR)	F&L Medical Products Co.
90%		65%	57%	32%	25%

Adapted from Back et al., 2005; Christodoulou et al., 2003; and Clasper & Pinks, 1995.

Table 6. Radiation protection apparel.

Risks of cataract development due to radiation exposure to the eyes have been investigated in interventionalists, with no conclusive evidence to date. However, the use of lead-based glasses is advocated, especially when the risk of "rescatter" (radiation which emanates from within the interventionalist's head, or so-called tertiary exposure) is considered (Cousin et al. 1987). As pointed out in a review on exposure risks of interventional pain physicians, studies demonstrate a decrease in transmission rates of 70-90% with appropriate eyewear ("lead" glasses) (Fish et al., 2011). Moreover, because it is the patient that is the point source of occupational radiation risk coupled with the proximity of the interventional pain physician to the patient, positioning the monitor to require the interventionalist to look 90° (from the patient) with eyewear with side shields could further help reduce eye exposure. As stated by Fish et al. (2011), "...It is extremely vital for the interventionalist to be cognizant of his/her surroundings. This reiterates the importance of increasing the distance between the physician and the source of the radiation, it also emphasizes decreasing the amount of exposure time, which can both drastically reduce unnecessary radiation via scatter."

2.5 Special report: Radiation exposure during spinal cord stimulation mapping: A new data set

Summary of Background Data: The increase in exposure to low-dose radiation from the growing use of medical imaging has raised concerns about cumulative dose among the general population (Fazel et al., 2009; U.S. National Academy of Sciences, 2006; Little et al., 2009), and accordingly, dose assessment has received increased scrutiny (Balter, 2008). Conversely, unique among implantable devices, some spinal cord stimulation systems utilize integrated technology to perform "electronic fluoroscopy" to assess device orientation (i.e., the leads) without irradiation (Kosek et al., 2006). Recently, however, a first look at radiation exposure from spinal cord stimulation [trialing] procedures was published to help benchmark radiation exposure reference levels for this procedure (Wininger et al., 2010). Although estimated exposure was negligible, data on patient size was unavailable and the source-to-skin distance (SSD) was not taken into account due to simplistic modeling.

Objective: To address the aforementioned limitations, radiation exposure was reexamined by the author for a new patient population.

Methods: 106 dual parallel lead spinal cord stimulation trialing procedures [using either multiple-independent current-controlled systems or constant-voltage systems] in the non-university, outpatient setting, from October 2008 to October 2009, were studied prospectively. Body mass index (BMI) measurements were retrieved. The *fluoroscopy system automatically tabulated total fluoro-time (in seconds) per case, and partitioned the absolute time- and the percentage of time allocated to- pulsed and continuous-mode imaging. High dose fluoroscopy, or "boost" mode, was not used. A study specific ‡personal dosimeter was worn by the physician. For the dose model, radiation output was measured with a §dosimeter/ion chamber located 30 cm from the image intensifier, along the central axis of an anteroposterior projected beam, and calculated based on the following equation.

$$ESE_{pat} = ESE_{pha} \bullet \left[\frac{O_{pha}}{O_{pat}} \bullet \left(\frac{SSD_{pat}}{SSD_{pha}} \right)^2 \right] \bullet t_{flu}$$

Where ESE_{pat} and ESE_{pha} are skin exposure to the patient and †phantom; O_{pha} and O_{pat} are radiation output for phantom and patient exposure (in Röentgens); SSD_{pat} and SSD_{pha} are the distances from the x-ray source to the skin for the patient and phantom; and t_{flu} is fluoro-time (converted to minutes). Note: incident air kerma is measured in milligray (mGy) and is converted from ESE_{pat} by applying a factor of 8.76 mGy to 1 Röentgen. Incident air kerma estimates were stratified according to SSD and low dose mode engaged/disengaged.

Results:

Total fluoroscopy time:

Mean: 71.7 seconds
(standard deviation: 34.9 seconds)
Range: 19.5 seconds to 166.6 seconds

Percentage pulsed imaging:
    Mean: 33.4%
    Range: 1.80% to 75.2%
    Mode: 55.4% (compiled % most frequent)
Source-to-skin distance:
    Mean: not reported
    Range: 43 cm to 50 cm
Body mass index:
    n = 54 females
    Mean: 31.54 kg/m^2
    Range: 18.46-53.32 kg/m^2
    n = 52 males
    Mean: 29.65 kg/m^2
    Range: 17.03-42.45 kg/m^2
Incident air kerma:
    Mean: 8.33 mGy
    Range: 1.53 mGy to 32.0 mGy
Physician dosimeter:
Whole body cumulative dose: 73 mrem

Discussion:

1. Figure 3 shows the descriptive statistical summary for fluoroscopy time. Seven outliers were identified in each data set. Notably, less variance around the median value occurred with the new data (i.e., the interquartile range was reduced by 47.4%).
2. Accounting for outliers, total fluoroscopy time was normally distributed.
   - Figure 4 compares the grouped subsets—based on one minute intervals.
3. Mean total fluoroscopy time was 46.3% less (71.7 seconds compared to 133.4 seconds). However, it is noted that outliers from the previous data set had not been removed in the reporting of that data, and thus mean total fluoroscopy time for the previous data set was artificially inflated.
4. Percentage pulsed imaging was equivalent.
5. Patient radiation exposure was reduced: 1.53—32.0 mGy compared to 1.8—43.7 mGy.
6. Patient size ranged from mildly underweight to morbidly obese according to BMI (as defined by the World Health Organization, n.d.). The mean BMI, by gender, bordered pre-obese and obese.
   - Note: trending increase in body weight among the U.S. population paired with concern about cumulative dose trends (Yanch et al., 2009; Fazel et al., 2009) underscore the need to obtain accurate reference levels on radiation exposure, as such exposure will, in general, be higher for patients with greater body mass.
7. Estimates for incident air kerma were stratified according to various SSDs, see Figure 5.

Conclusions:

Radiation exposure from spinal cord stimulation trialing procedures remains negligible despite the likelihood, as suggested here, for this therapy to be used in a patient population with a greater risk for increased irradiation based on BMI valuations.

Acknowledgements:

The author thanks Siva Gopal, PhD, Otterbein University, for his constructive instruction in descriptive statistical methods.

Footnotes:

*OEC 9800 Super-C, GE Healthcare, Salt Lake City, UT, USA.

†Phantom: 3.8 cm of aluminum.

‡Badge report, study specific: Luxel, optically stimulated luminescence dosimetry, LANDAUER, Glenwood, IL, USA.

§Radiation meter - Model 1515 with converter model 1050U and ion chamber model 10X6-6M, Radcal Co., Monrovia, CA, USA.

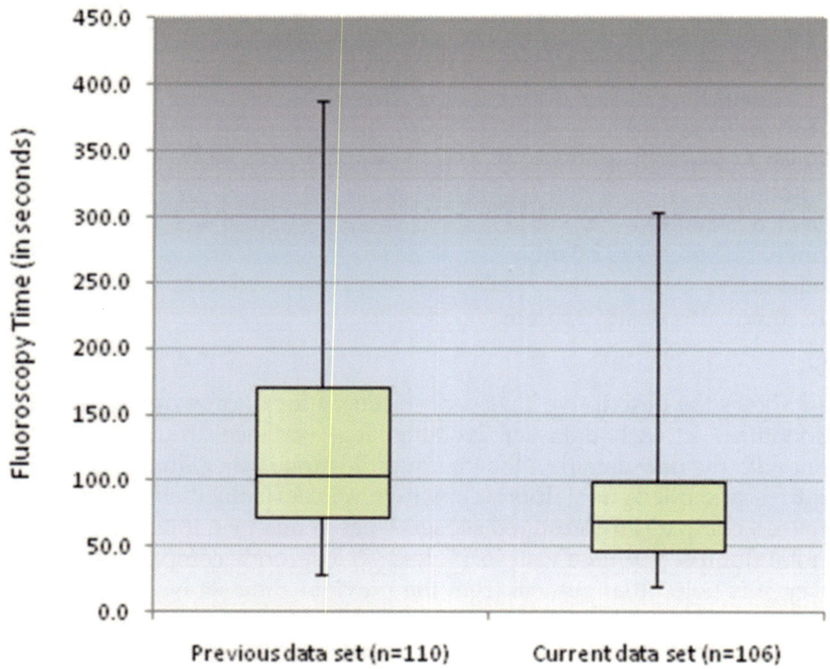

	Previous data set (n=110)	Current data set (n=106)
Interquartile Range	98.9	52.0
Lower Fence	-76.6	-30.8
Upper Fence	319.1	177.2
Outliers	321.1	208.9
	329.3	217.7
	336.2	236.3
	343.8	239.4
	373.1	294.0
	387.2	299.7
	387.4	304.0

Fig. 3. Box plots comparing previous and current fluoroscopy time data sets for spinal cord stimulation mapping procedures. Note: Because all data (both sets) were obtained from the same interventional spine team, inter- and intra- procedural variability was minimized.

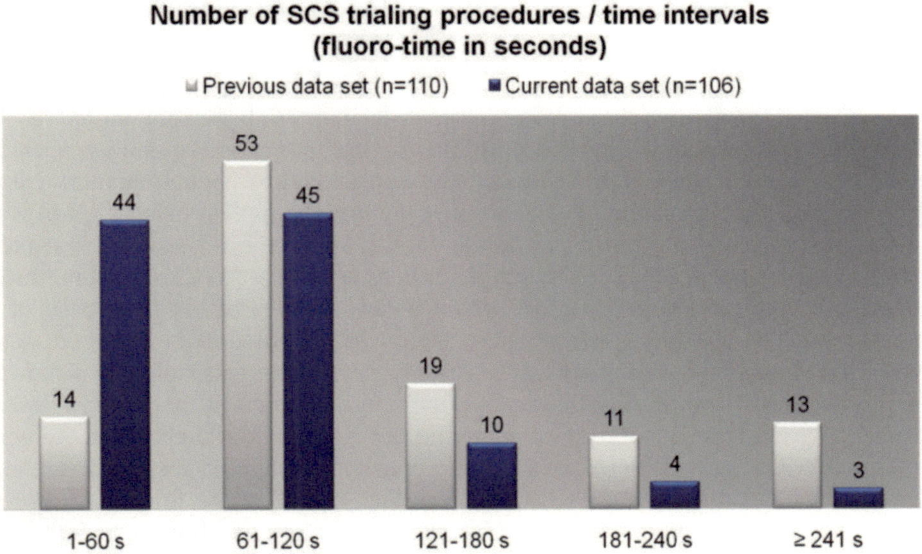

Fig. 4. Bar chart comparing the prior and new data sets with respect to fluoroscopy time during percutaneous spinal cord stimulation mapping procedures.

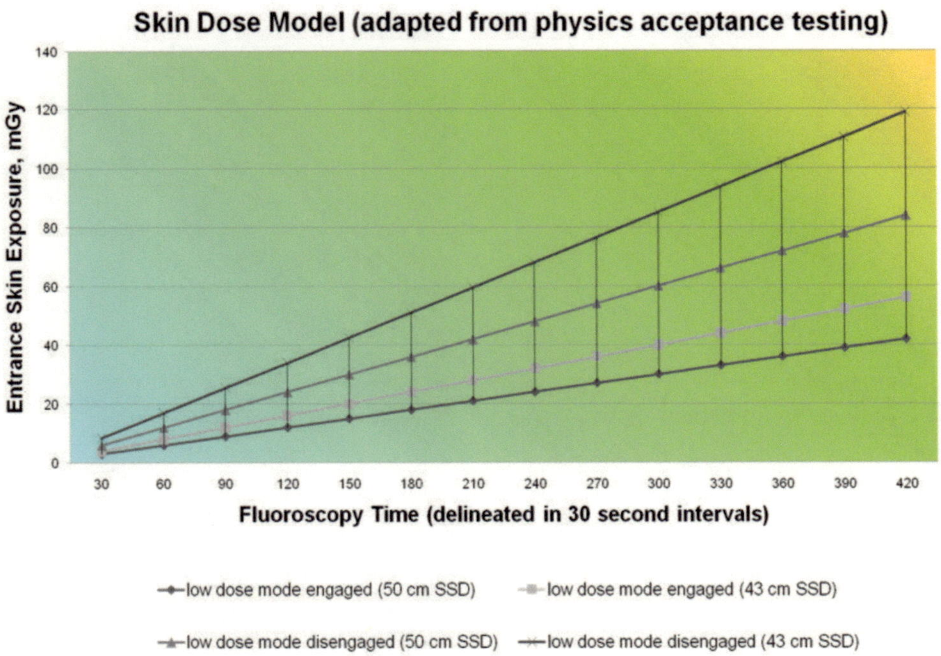

Fig. 5. ESE_{pat} to anterior chest: 50 kg. adult patient accounting for one dose reduction feature, i.e., the low dose mode, either "on" or "off" for stratified SSDs (either 43 cm or 50 cm) in percutaneous spinal cord stimulation mapping. (Note: valuations represent continuous-mode imaging, no beam collimation.)

3. Computed Tomography (CT) and interventional pain medicine

3.1 The CT imaging chain

Although the underlying physical concepts are, for the most part, the same (such as x-ray production), the CT imaging chain offers a higher level of sophistication compared to the imaging chain of fluoroscopy. This is exemplified by the application of mathematical filters selected for a desired level of image reconstruction to control signal/quantum noise to optimize image quality (Sprawls, 1992), and most commonly applied using high-pass filters to control edge artifacts. According to Barnes (1992), while the CT scanner is capable of dividing its measurement of tissue attenuation into a range of 4,096 CT numbers, the eye is not capable of distinguishing this much detail in an image. The image display of a CT scanner represents only 256 levels of gray, which must therefore be mapped onto the portion of the Hounsfield scale that is to be displayed. Adjustments called "window level" and "window width" are used to define this mapping. Selection of the window level (i.e., brightness) specifies the CT number for centering the gray scale, and choice of the window width (i.e., contrast) defines the range of CT numbers over which the gray scale is to extend. These adjustments can be thought of as defining the "slope" of the gray scale. When the gray scale is placed at a window level of 100 and the window width is set at 500, the gray scale permits display of CT numbers from -150 to +350. All CT numbers below the lower limit of the window width are displayed as black, and all those above the upper limit are displayed as white on the image (see Figure 6).

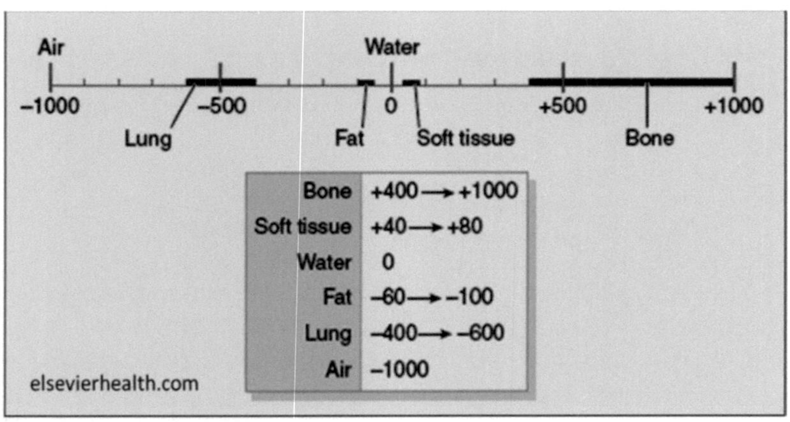

Fig. 6. CT Numbers = Hounsfield Units.

3.2 The mathematics of CT physics

The language of mathematics not only permeates all scientific study, but the very application of mathematics itself allows exploration to occur at the limits-of-discovery to find answers to questions that vex human nature. To this end, it is through a mathematical framework that physicists talk about dosimetry—with various selected examples on dosimetric methods in CT given in Table 7. Moreover, computational models for CT scanning enable testing of quality control algorithms to ultimately help reduce overexposure errors (Ferreira et al., 2010). This section will serve as a mathematical primer to highlight the physics behind image acquisition/signal processing of CT scanning to allow interventional pain physicians to gain deeper insight into this modality, and through this appreciation, demystify the process of CT imaging.

First Author	Title of Article	Citation: Journal	Year;Volume:Page
Balter	Why (Continue to) Study Physics?	Radiographics	1992;12:609
Rothenberg	Radiation Dose in CT	Radiographics	1992;12:1225
McNitt-Gray	Topics in CT: Radiation Dose in CT?	Radiographics	2002;22:1541
Bauhs	CT Dosimetry: Comparison of Measurement Techniques and Devices	Radiographics	2008;28:245
Huda	Converting Dose-Length Products to Effective Dose at CT	Radiology	2008;248:995

Table 7. Select references on the physics of CT appearing in the journals of the Radiological Society of North America.

Although the subject matter on this topic is diverse, no truly rigorous mathematical justification of a tomographic algorithm exists (Shepp & Kruskal, 1978). For this reason a generalized derivation (that of inverting the Radon transform, as this is the widely accepted technique to describe how we recapture the information lost to attenuated x-ray photons) will be described in plain mathematical language. In addition, where noted, Wolfram *Mathematica*—the online computational engine, Wolfram|Alpha™—was used to plot the traditional representative line equations of the x-ray photons. It is also important to note that in order to simplify the derivation the following three constraints will be made. First, we will ignore the playoff between Cartesian and polar coordinate representations, i.e., the 2-dimensional xy-plane versus spherical or circular symmetry. Second, we will not account for adjustments in the derivation for cone beam and/or fan-beam CT constructs due to their mathematical complexities (Note: the fan-beam third generation CT scanner, see Figure 7, is the most commonly utilized type of scanner.) Finally, discrete numerical analysis will not be

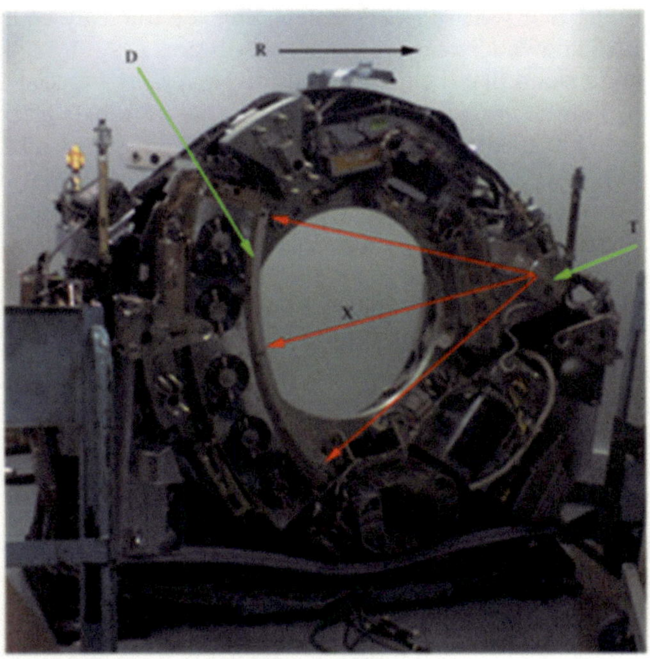

Fig. 7. Third generation "fan-beam" CT scanner.

addressed. To this end, the steps necessary to invert the Radon transform with respect to the parallel beam model (and thus most enthusiastically applicable to first and second generation CT scanners will constitute the balance of this section. It is the hope that such insight will complement the physician's knowledge-base when carrying out CT-guided pain procedures.

The set up

The underlying theme in this mathematical application is a signal processing challenge, and the set up for the analysis is straightforward. We have a 2-dimensional slice of a region of variable density (the patient), and the goal as applied to CT scanning is to reconstruct the resulting x-ray signal (the image) after repeatedly passing x-rays through the region at different angles of initial projection (the CT gantry). More concisely stated, we are measuring the resultant signal at different trajectory lines by accumulating (integrating) the signal after projecting x-ray photons through the region. Hence, the approach reconstructs the densities of the materials interacting with the x-ray photons (Johns & Cunningham, 1983), to ultimately assign density values according to the Hounsfield unit scale of CT numbers for data acquisition/image processing (Jackson & Thomas, 2004). Such modeling serves as an engineering template for trouble-shooting in the event of errors, such as equipment failure or computer algorithm failures, which may lead to radiation overdose of the patient.

Given that the approach resolves signal processing by means of calculating line integrals to recover the intensity of the x-ray signal (i.e., capture the data lost to attenuated or scattered x-rays), a comparison may be made to the inverse square law which estimates beam intensity from known initial conditions, the intensity of- and distance from- the beam (Carlton & Adler, 2006). However, the comparison is rudimentary at best because the central and interesting feature of the model applicable here, i.e., the Radon transform and its inverse, lies in the fact that we are *strictly* calculating the intensity of the exit/secondary beam based *solely* on a known intensity of the primary beam.

It is important to understand that the Radon transform refers to a special case of the Fourier transform; and the Fourier transform is a limiting case of the Fourier series (Boyce & DiPrima, 2005; Bracewell, 1986). This means whereas a Fourier series is the mathematical instrument used when evaluating periodic phenomena (Boyce & DiPrima, 2005), a Fourier transform is reserved for the study of phenomena that is nonperiodic (Bracewell, 1986). Thus, the choice of the application of a "transform" is an intuitively simple decision, given that x-ray photons in the exit beam strike the image receptor in burst-like impulses that are mostly nonperiodic rather than periodic in fashion. In mathematical terms, burst-like physical phenomena that are almost periodic are known as line impulses. *The concept of the line impulse will be a key point expanded upon below.*

The derivation of the mathematical model can be relatively easy to follow since the steps involved are pragmatic to imaging tasks carried out in the CT suite. We begin by a detailed inspection of representative x-ray trajectories relative to the CT gantry (i.e., the family of parallel lines), and then compare the suitability of two different proposed coordinate systems for the model.

Lines/family of lines

Refer to Figure 8 for a depiction of the CT gantry with the x-ray beam drawn as a family of parallel lines though the region. Each representative x-ray trajectory (i.e., the parallel lines) can be written in the slope-intercept form of a line.

$$y = mx + b \qquad -\infty < b < \infty\ , \qquad 0 \leq m < \infty$$

In this form, the coordinates of the lines in the xy-plane are the points (m,b), "m" the slope of the line and "b" the y-intercept. However, this coordinate system breaks down as "m" and "b" vary because the formula is not valid for vertical lines, such that a vertical slope is not defined (Larson et al., 2007). Therefore, a more suitable coordinate system is required to parameterize a line (and all families of parallel lines), and therefore, it is interesting to look at what a family of parallel lines may have in common (see Figure 9).

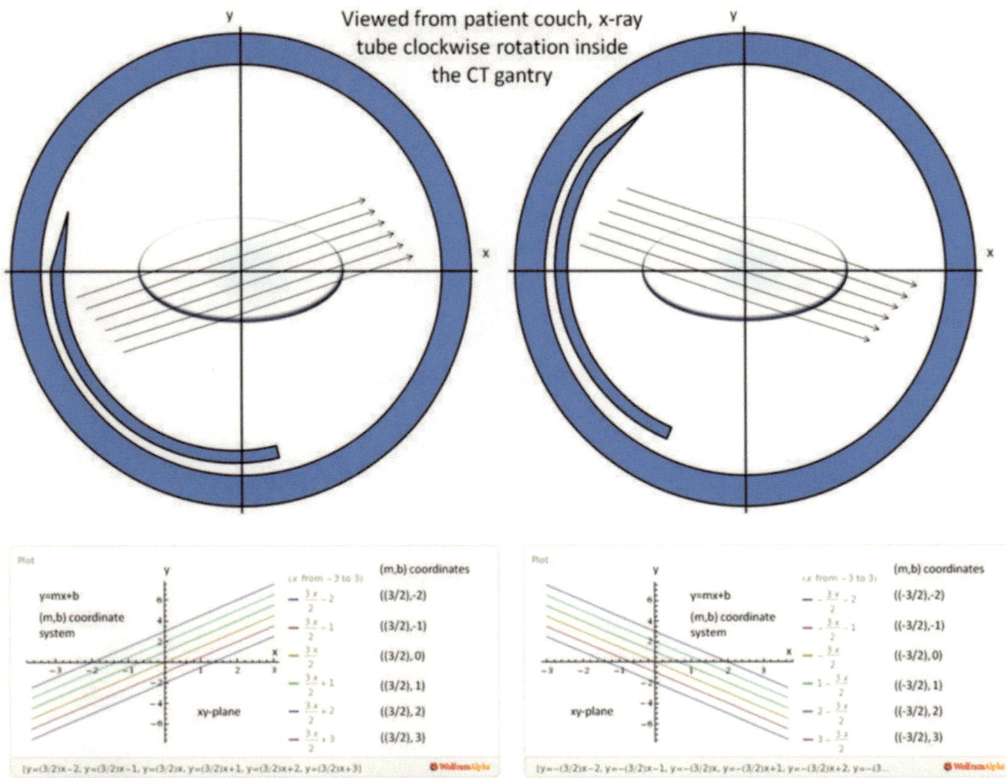

Fig. 8. (Top left) Gantry of CT scanner showing trajectories of x-rays [long arrows] emitted as lines/family of parallel lines. (Top right) Illustrated clockwise rotation of the x-ray tube inside the gantry. (Bottom left/right) Representative, corresponding line equations written in the slope-intercept form y=mx+b in the xy-plane. The (m,b) coordinates are given by the line equations.

Referring to Figure 9, one such identified commonality is that each line has the same angle to the horizontal axis, the x_1-axis. Thus, we will call this angle, the angle φ (phi). Specifically, it is the normal vectors of these lines that have the same angle to the x_1-axis. However, to better identify locations of lines, we need more than just the angle to the x_1-axis. To single-out a line we look at its distance ρ (rho) from the line passing through the origin (see Figure 9). Thus, with these parameters, the distance ρ (rho) and the angle φ (phi), we have successfully established an unambiguous coordinate system that is not flawed by the non-existence issue of a vertical slope. The *Cartesian equation of the line for the model,* is now specified by a given coordinate pair (ρ,φ) in the form:

$$\boldsymbol{x} \cdot \boldsymbol{n} = x_1 \cos\varphi + x_2 \sin\varphi = \rho$$

where both **x** and **n** are vectors, each defined in the following way, **x**=‹x_1,x_2› and **n**=‹cos(φ),sin(φ)›, and the line equation is derived by vector multiplication, in this case by using the dot product method, where it is said that **x** is dotted with **n**.

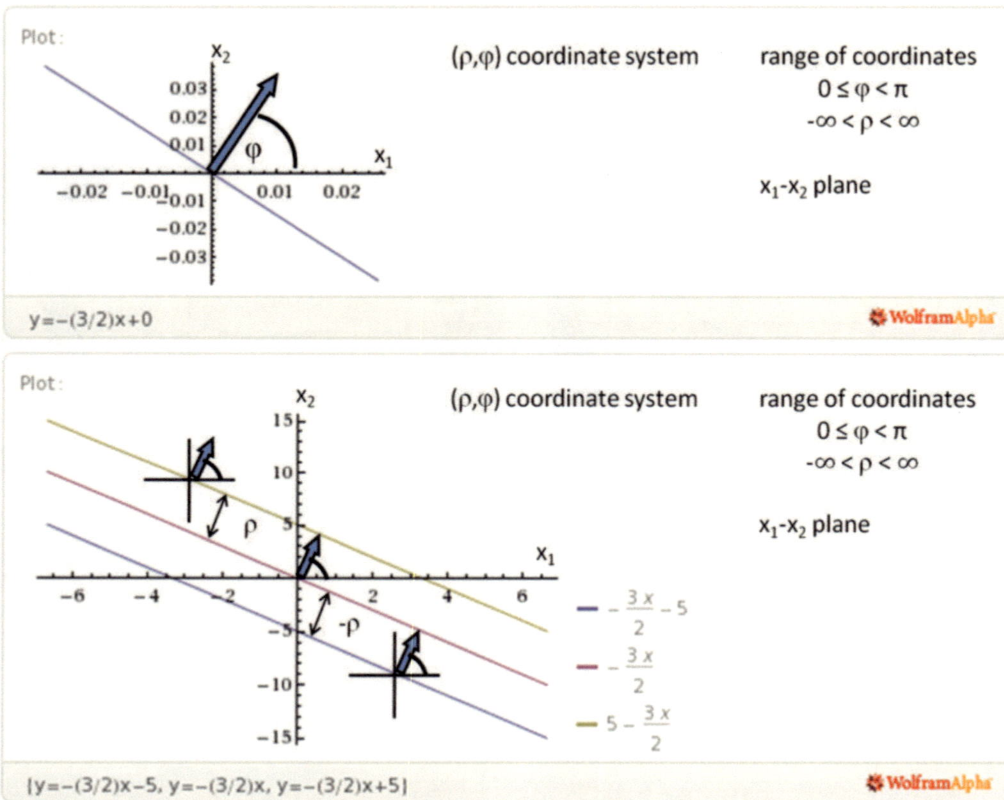

Fig. 9. A better-suited coordinate system (ρ,φ) for the model. (Top panel) Arrow demonstrating the unit normal vector associated with the line passing through the origin, and oriented with an angle phi (φ) to the x_1-axis in the x_1-x_2 plane. (Bottom panel) A family of 3-parallel lines and their unit normal vectors [arbitrarily placed on the lines] showing signed distances rho (ρ) from the origin [double ended arrows]. By convention, distances are positive [i.e., positive rho (ρ)] when measured *in the direction of the normal vector from the line passing through the origin to associated parallel lines.* In a similar fashion, distances are negative [i.e., negative rho (-ρ)] when measured *from the line passing through the origin to parallel lines spatially existing opposite to the direction established for the normal vector.* Rho (ρ) is zero at the line passing through the origin. (Note: the unit normal vectors are not drawn to scale, and when compared to Figure 8, the xy-plane has been renamed the x_1-x_2 plane.)

Line impulse

Accordingly, it is necessary to account for the nonperiodic nature of the signal concentrated along each trajectory taken by the x-ray photons, and this is accomplished by considering the line impulse (Bracewell, 1986). The line impulse describes the physical phenomena of x-ray photons striking the image receptor in the CT gantry. To define the line impulse mathematically, we first need to set the *Cartesian equation of the line for the model* to zero as shown.

$$\rho = x_1 \cos\varphi + x_2 \sin\varphi \xrightarrow[\textit{set to zero}]{} \rho - x_1 \cos\varphi - x_2 \sin\varphi = 0$$

The resultant equation, specifically the left hand side of the new equation above, then becomes a function of delta, denoted by δ, on the right hand side (Bracewell, 1986).

$$\rho - x_1 \cos\varphi - x_2 \sin\varphi \xrightarrow{\textit{becomes}} \delta(\rho - x_1 \cos\varphi - x_2 \sin\varphi)$$

The delta function δ, is the classical way to approach the line impulse, and has advantageous implications for dimensionality and integration of a line (Figure 10) (Bracewell, 1986). Such line integrals have a domain of infinity on the line and zero off the line (Bracewell, 1986).

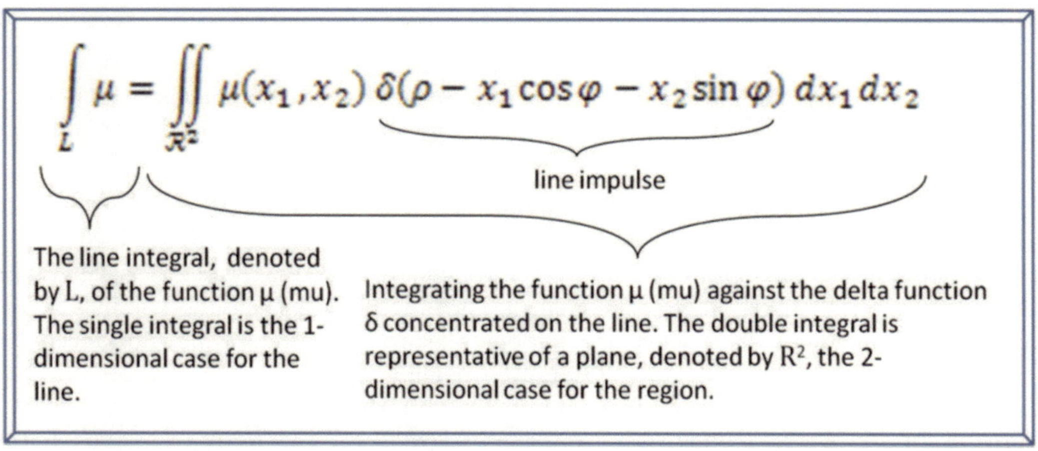

Fig. 10. Expansion of the line integral to an integral of a plane (2-dimensional space) containing the line impulse. The above notations of the integrals, L and R^2, are understood to have domains or "boundaries" from negative infinity (-∞) to infinity (∞).

The Radon transform

Equipped with a suitable coordinate system and having addressed the line integral with respect to the line impulse, we are ready to introduce the computational steps central to the mathematical model, inverting the Radon transform. As we do this, it is important to first point out what is varying as we work through the computations, i.e., to identify the variables associated with the integrand (those terms being integrated).

As shown below in Figure 11, superimposition of the useful/suitable coordinate system (as described earlier) onto a representative cross-sectional image (the region of interest) will help identify the variable.

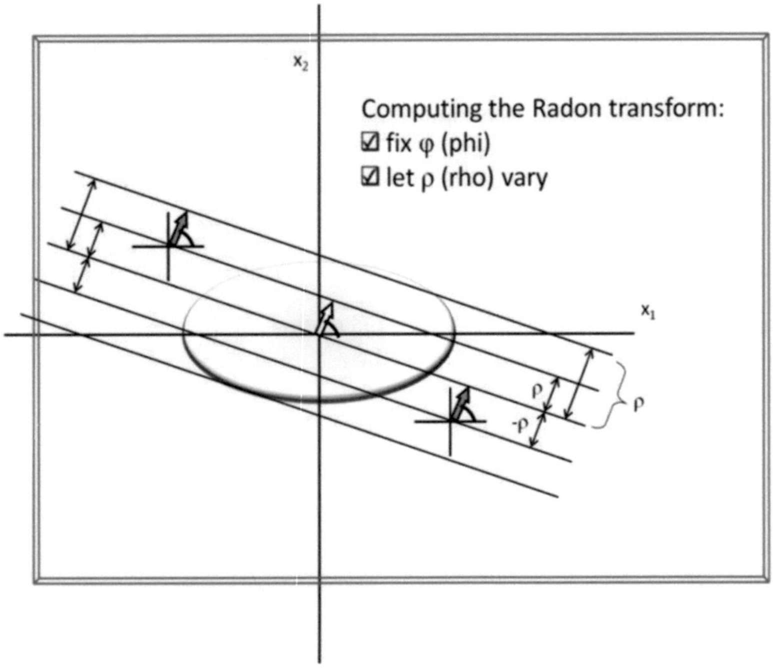

Fig. 11. Notice what this family of parallel lines has in common, each line has the same angle φ (phi) to the x_1-axis. Thus, the variable to use with respect to integrating the constituent integrals of the Radon transform (and those integrals contributing to the Fourier transform) is the distance ρ (rho) of a line from the line passing through the origin.

Looking at Figure 11, think in terms of what it means to fix φ (phi) and let ρ (rho) vary. This means the family of parallel lines will be defined by the angle made with the x_1-axis, and only the distance of a line from the line going through the origin will be of concern. In other words, the angle is fixed, it does not change, allowing ρ (rho) to be the variable as we accumulate (integrate) data. Thus, the Radon transform R can now be introduced by rewriting the equation from Figure 10 in greater detail (Bracewell, 1986), in relation to the signal/function μ (mu), where μ (mu) is a function of ρ (rho) and φ (phi), as shown below. ***Note: in this and the remaining sections, the x-ray signal will be written as the function μ (mu).***

$$\mathcal{R}\mu(\rho,\varphi) = \int_{L(\rho,\varphi)} \mu = \int_{-\infty}^{\infty}\int_{-\infty}^{\infty} \mu(x_1, x_2)\, \delta\,(\rho - x_1\cos\varphi - x_2\sin\varphi)\, dx_1\, dx_2$$

Accordingly, both the line integral L and the double integral above are more concisely expressed here than that seen in Figure 10. With respect to the line integral, it is now written as a function of ρ (rho) and φ (phi), and the limits of integration (-∞ to ∞) are explicitly stated for the double integral.

As discussed earlier the Radon transform is a special case of the Fourier transform, thus it is accurate to write the Fourier transform F with respect to ρ (rho) (denoted by the subscript ρ) as a function of the Radon transform R, as seen in the following notation (Bracewell, 1986).

$$\mathcal{F}_\rho(\mathcal{R}\mu(\rho,\varphi)) = \int_{-\infty}^{\infty} e^{-2\pi i r \rho} (\mathcal{R}\mu(\rho,\varphi))\, d\rho$$

The significance of this step is that we are now accounting for the spatial domain, denoted by the letter "r" in the complex exponential, $e^{-2\pi i r\rho}$ (Boyce & DiPrima, 2005). In reality, the derivation for this mathematical application (as we strive to understand it in the context of CT) is concerned with two domains, the spatial domain and the frequency domain, and moreover, both are present/available in the complex exponential, $e^{-2\pi i r\rho}$.

$$\mathcal{F}_\rho(\mathcal{R}\mu(\rho,\varphi)) = \int_{-\infty}^{\infty} e^{-2\pi i r\rho} (\mathcal{R}\mu(\rho,\varphi))\, d\rho$$

$$= \int_{-\infty}^{\infty} e^{-2\pi i r\rho}\left(\int_{-\infty}^{\infty}\int_{-\infty}^{\infty} \mu(x_1,x_2)\,\delta(\rho - x_1\cos\varphi - x_2\sin\varphi)\, dx_1\, dx_2\right) d\rho$$

The right hand side of the Fourier transform $\mathcal{F}$ equality (top equation) contains the Radon transform $\mathcal{R}$ (underscored). It is subsequently rewritten (underscored) as the function μ (mu), as seen in Figure 3, to evaluate **the line impulse delta function δ (i.e., bursts of x-ray phenomena)**. Then, the selected (boxed) terms are switched to rearrange the order of integration and evaluate the single integral first (illustrated below).

$$= \int_{-\infty}^{\infty}\int_{-\infty}^{\infty} \mu(x_1,x_2)\left(\int_{-\infty}^{\infty} e^{-2\pi i r\rho}\,\delta(\rho - x_1\cos\varphi - x_2\sin\varphi)\, d\rho\right) dx_1\, dx_2$$

With the terms now rearranged and grouped together, the equation is set up to integrate the 1-dimensional Fourier transform (the single integral in parentheses), in order that we may later deal with the 2-dimensional Fourier transform (the double integral) to recover the densities contained in the function μ (mu), along the line/family of lines (i.e., the information concentrated in the trajectories of the x-rays in the exit beam). **Note: the delta function δ remains in place, ready to be integrated.**

Fig. 12. Illustrative drawing to explain the way in which the dimensionality of the model is handled as the mathematical derivation unfolds.

Refer to Figure 12 which shows the critical steps on how dimensionality is dealt with in the model. The 1-dimensional component is evaluated first, as described in Figure 12, and is rewritten below in bold type face for emphasis, note the left hand side of the equation below.

$$\int_{-\infty}^{\infty} \boldsymbol{e^{-2\pi i r\rho}\,\delta\,(\rho - (x_1\cos\varphi + x_2\sin\varphi))\,d\rho} = e^{-2\pi i r(x_1\cos\varphi + x_2\sin\varphi)}$$

We see that the integral equates to the complex exponential, $e^{-2\pi i r(x_1\cos\varphi + x_2\sin\varphi)}$, which is rewritten after distributing the "r".

$$e^{-2\pi i r(x_1 \cos\varphi + x_2 \sin\varphi)} = e^{-2\pi i(x_1 r \cos\varphi + x_2 r \sin\varphi)}$$

To finish simplifying the complex exponential, we introduce the concept of dual variables, in that (x_1 is paired with ξ_1) and (x_2 is paired with ξ_2), where ξ_1 and ξ_2 are each constants defined in the following way:

$$\xi_1 = r\cos\varphi \quad \text{and} \quad \xi_2 = r\sin\varphi$$

Although it is noted that each of these equalities above suggest implementation of polar coordinates (the coordinate system employed for spherical/circular symmetry), they are not intended to do so in this derivation. The equalities merely serve as a means to express the complex exponential more simply with dual variables, as follows:

$$= e^{-2\pi i(x_1\xi_1 + x_2\xi_2)}$$

It is now important to emphasize what has been derived thus far, and what computational steps remain. The above result is the answer to the evaluation of the 1-dimensional integral described in Figure 12 (that integral involving the line impulse, which has now been computed). The remaining computational steps involve the actual processes to recover the values of the densities μ (mu), i.e., to reconstruct the densities from the region, by inverting the Radon transform as a function of the Fourier transform over 2-dimensional region.

Inverting the Radon transform

To invert the Radon transform, we first plug the result of the 1-dimensional integral (as derived above and in bold type face below) back into the original Fourier transform which we set up earlier. This is shown below. We now have the 2-dimensional Fourier transform of μ (mu), i.e., the double integral, set up to integrate first with respect to dx_1 and then with respect to dx_2.

$$\mathcal{F}_\rho(\mathcal{R}\mu(\rho,\varphi)) = \int_{-\infty}^{\infty}\int_{-\infty}^{\infty} \mu(x_1, x_2)\, \boldsymbol{e^{-2\pi i(x_1\xi_1 + x_2\xi_2)}}\, dx_1\, dx_2$$

Hence, to best convey the details of the final computation step, it is of certain benefit to pause in order to recapitulate the entire mathematical derivation up to this point.

1. A suitable coordinate system (ρ,φ) was found.
2. φ (phi) was fixed to let ρ (rho) vary, where φ (phi) is the angle that each line in the family of parallel lines makes with the x_1-axis, and ρ (rho) represents the values of distances of these lines from the line passing through the origin.
3. The 1-dimensional Fourier transform of the corresponding Radon transform was found with respect to ρ (rho), resulting in the 2-dimensional Fourier transform of μ (mu).
    a. In principle the problem is solved. We have measured the Radon transform, i.e., the line integral of μ (mu) along the family of parallel lines.
    b. Because we know the 1-dimensional transform expression and the values which emerge, those associated with [$e^{-2\pi i(x_1\xi_1 + x_2\xi_2)}$], we can now compute the Fourier transform with respect to ρ (rho) (Bracewell, 1986).

By computing the Fourier transform with respect to ρ (rho), we get the 2-dimensional Fourier transform with respect to μ (mu). This means that we can find μ (mu) by taking the inverse of the 2-dimensional Fourier transform of what was found:

$$\mathcal{F}\mu(\xi_1,\xi_2) = \mathbb{G}(\xi_1,\xi_2) \xrightarrow{recovers\ \mu} \mu = \mathcal{F}^{-1}\mathbb{G}(\xi_1,\xi_2)$$

where $\mathbb{G}(\xi_1,\xi_2)$ equals ($e^{-2\pi i(x_1\xi_1+x_2\xi_2)}$), the known values of the 1-dimensional Fourier transform. By taking the inverse of the signal/function μ (mu) (we recover the lost data contained in the trajectory lines of the x-ray photons passing through the region of interest), and we are able to reconstruct the densities of the region (Bracewell, 1986). That is to say, we now have μ (mu). *In turn, this enables the CT scanner to assign density values according to the Hounsfield unit scale of CT numbers for data acquisition/image processing* (Jackson & Thomas, 2004).

In summary, the goal of this section was to familiarize interventional pain physicians with the equations that ultimately underscore quality control algorithms for CT scanners and provide a footprint to build quality assurance protocols for CT scanning to help reduce risks of radiation overexposure. Accordingly, the derivation presented here represents the mathematical framework employing the parallel beam model. Ideally, to make the model practical, and to implement it numerically, discrete versions need to be rooted in the steps above, and certain computation issues, such as the playoff between Cartesian and polar coordinate representations, need to be dealt with.

Acknowledgements: The author thanks Stanford University Engineering for open access to EE261 The Fourier Transform and Its Applications as taught by Brad Osgood, PhD, as well as acknowledges John Labowsky for his technical critique of this section.

3.3 Triplanar imaging in pain medicine procedures: Conventional-CT guidance and CT-fluoroscopy

In the 1990s conventional-CT guidance began to be used by interventionally-trained pain physicians for chronic benign spinal pain (Aguirre et al., 2005; Gangi et al., 1998). During this period, algorithms were also developed to establish CT-fluoroscopy, which introduced a real-time feature to this modality (Daly & Templeton, 1999). Accordingly, CT-fluoroscopy has become a powerful imaging tool (Meleka, 2005). To this point, interventional pain techniques have been proposed and studied under this imaging technique, such as treatment of coccydynia by targeting the ganglion impar (Datir et al., 2010) or the efficacy of lumbar sympathetic blocks (Schmid, 2006). Interestingly, the literature remains sparse for pain procedure-specific dosimetry reports relative to CT, although Table 8 highlights the work in this area by Wagner (2004a, 2004b). In this light, the interested reader performing CT-guided pain procedures (or interested in being trained for such procedures) may wish to initiate dosimetry studies, since all radiologic based procedures should be evaluated specifically and the knowledge gained disseminated to help follow ALARA principles for patients and personnel radiation exposure (and hence, optimize health physics strategies).

3.4 Radiation risk management/safety

While CT-fluoroscopy may decrease patient absorbed dose by 94% compared to conventional CT (Meleka et al., 2005), others argue that the radiation exposure may not be justified, especially when other modalities can be used which eliminate the need for such exposure altogether, such as CT-guided (Thoumas et al., 1999) versus ultrasound-guided (Gruber & Bodner, 2004) pudendal nerve blocks. In cases were CT guidance has shown to be clearly beneficial, the lower doses associated with CT-fluoroscopy have been attributed to intermittent exposure techniques and/or exposure parameters, such as lower tube current (Meleka et al., 2005). Moreover, strategies have also emerged to help reduce occupational radiation dose. For example, the use of lead shields, or as previously discussed, the use of lead aprons. In addition, the use of needle holders, when feasible during the procedure, avoids physician hand placement directly into the x-ray beam (Kato, 1996).

Kato **1996**	Wagner **2004a**	Wagner **2004b**	CT-Fluoroscopy
			• Lumbar Selective Nerve Root Block
–	2	–	CT-Fluoroscopy Time
–	7.3	–	o Patient Effective Dose
–	390	–	o Effective Dose (Total) Physician
			• Lumbar Epidural
		Not specified	CT-Fluoroscopy Time
–	–	> 1	o Effective Dose (Physician/Procedure)
–	–	75	o Effective Dose (Total) Physician
			• Effective Dose (given in microSieverts per second)
1140	–	–	o Physician Hand

Key: CT-Fluoroscopy time (in seconds); effective dose (in microSieverts).

Table 8. CT-Fluoroscopy exposure metrics.

4. Ultrasound and interventional pain medicine

4.1 The ultrasound imaging chain

Continued research in the area of medical imaging has led to the development of compact and durable ultrasound scanners with improved imaging capabilities. Nevertheless, the basic instrumentation and underlying principles of this modality remain the same. The ultrasound imaging chain is considered a "closed" loop made up of the following links: a transmitter, a transducer, a receiver, and the image viewing system (Aldrich, 2007). Note that the physical phenomenon behind image creation is the piezoelectric effect, or stated more explicitly it is the effect on and induced by deformations of piezoelectric crystals embedded within materials housed inside the transducer which enables mechanical energy to be transformed into ultrasonic impulses—and vice versa for signal processing.

Upon interaction with tissue, ultrasonic waveforms may be 1) transmitted through the tissue, 2) undergo reflection (echo) or refraction (bending) at tissue boundaries, or 3) the acoustic energy may be attenuated. Surfaces that **reflect** these sound waves are classified as either *specular reflectors* or *scattering reflectors*. An example of the former is the needle, whereas an example of the latter is the interface between neural and adjacent tissues. Thus, it is the reflected sound waves (i.e., the available energy contained in the echoes collected at the transducer) which contribute to a meaningful image. **Refracted** sound waves are those which change direction due to slight differences at the boundary (i.e., edge) between two tissue types. We note that such waves may not contribute to successful imaging if a significant amount of the propagated waveform is lost. Finally, with similarities which evoke comparisons to the attenuated x-ray beam, the attenuation of sound beams conveys a loss of energy as the ultrasonic waveforms are absorbed by the tissue. According to Sites et al. (2007):

> While attenuation can have a profound negative impact on image quality, there are two important adjustments that can be made on the ultrasound machine that help to overcome

some of the effects of attenuation. First, most machines allow the operator to artificially increase (or decrease) the signal intensity of the return echoes from all points in the displayed field. This is accomplished by adjusting the gain control higher to increase the overall brightness. Second, most machines offer the operator the ability to control gain independently at specified depth intervals. This is known as time gain compensation. The time gain compensation should be progressively increased as the depth of penetration increases in order to compensate for the corresponding loss of signal intensity.

It is also interesting to note that *attenuation is inversely related to waveform frequency*, and that this relationship is nontrivial with respect to image resolution (i.e., recorded detail or the ability to distinguish between objects) and ultrasound physics. In the following subsection, which highlights the physics behind ultrasound imaging, we will further explore this relation to better understand the clinical impact of sound wave attenuation.

4.2 Waveform propagation in tissue: The physics of ultrasound

Based on waveform physics, that is, frequency, amplitude, and wavelength, the principles of ultrasound are unified by the foregoing description. A pulse of sound is emitted from a source (i.e., the transducer) and travels outward through a medium. If an object reflects the wave, then acoustic energy travels back to the source and is detected as an echo at the source. Thus, at a known speed (the speed of sound of the surrounding medium), the waveform travels a distance equal to twice the distance from the source to the reflected object (Kane, 2009). The basic equation follows:

$$L = (V_S \cdot T)/2$$

where L is twice the distance from the source to the object, V_S is the speed of sound of the surrounding medium, and T is time. Note: the average value of V_S in soft tissue is 1540 m/s. The ultrasound scanner records the time required for each pulse to return, and then uses the speed of sound to calculate the distance of the object. See Figure 13. Echo intensity is indicated by plotting a variety of intensities on the monitor subsequent to a gray-scale (white to gray to black). Thus, brightness is a consequence of a mapping of echo intensity versus position; hence this viewing algorithm/mode is named B-scan, where "B" means brightness.

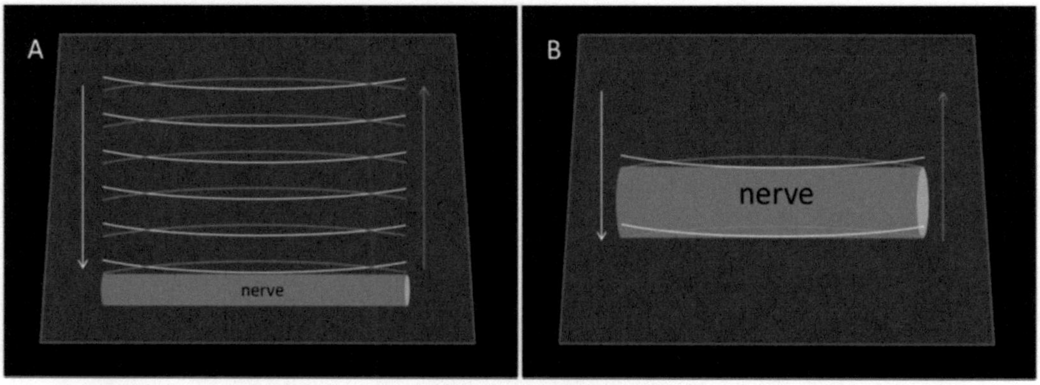

Fig. 13. Panel-A shows a target nerve (or scattering reflector) and direction of travel of incident sound waves (white) and echoes (blue). Panel-B shows a zoomed-in view of the same nerve to more closely exhibit the reflection of sound waves from near and far tissue borders (with respect to the transducer).

As emphasized in the above subsection, a nontrivial inverse relationship exists between attenuation and waveform frequency. We will now look more closely at this relation.
The most important aspects of ultrasound image resolution are those which govern axial, lateral, and temporal resolution—*in which all three together comprise spatial resolution.* **Axial resolution** is the ability to distinguish two structures at different depths, parallel to the direction of the ultrasound beam. Furthermore, it is approximately equal to one half of the ultrasound pulse length. In other words, if the distance between two objects is greater than one half of the pulse length, then the objects will appear as two distinct structures. It follows that higher waveform frequencies (short pulse lengths) produce the best axial resolution. However, because of the existing inverse relationship, higher frequency waveforms are more readily attenuated, and thus, tissue penetration is sacrificed. **Lateral resolution** is the ability to distinguish two structures at the same depth, perpendicular to the direction of the ultrasound beam. High frequency and focused ultrasound beams produce the narrowest beams, thus maximizing lateral resolution, but once again tissue penetration is sacrificed. Finally, **temporal resolution** relates to frame rate, and therefore, the ability to distinguish between real-time imaging and motion artifacts. During nerve blocks in regional anesthesia for example, motion artifacts occur with movement of the probe/transducer, or during needle insertion, or with injection of the anesthetic agent. Ultimately, temporal resolution is limited by the sweep speed (activation of the piezoelectric crystals) of the ultrasound beam, which in turn is limited by the speed of sound in tissue. Attempts to control temporal resolution consist of 1) increasing the sweep speed or 2) decreasing the scanning angle (applicable to phased array probes only). The first option decreases the lateral resolution, and the second option decreases the field of view. Thus, not only do we see an interconnected relationship with respect to image resolution, but at present, adjustments available to try to improve resolution are restrained by the laws of waveform physics. That is to say, despite the progress made in ultrasound equipment and technology (which we will highlight in the accompanying discussion on regional anesthesia), ultrasound imaging is, in reality, a tradeoff between spatial resolution and achievable depth of imaging (Sites et al., 2007).

4.3 Ultrasound guidance in pain medicine: Regional anesthesia

The use of ultrasound for image guidance in regional anesthesia has several practical benefits (Sites et al., 2009), the foremost being that ionizing radiation is not necessary for image production enabling ultrasound machines to be highly portable. Case series and small-scaled outcomes studies with respect to nerve blocks have purported shortened procedure times and faster block onset; increased patient satisfaction; and fewer block-related complications (Marhofer & Chan, 2007). As far as limitations, there are two primary considerations: 1) resolution and image quality vary inversely with depth of penetration, as previously discussed; and 2) needle tracking for in-plane needle entry is a challenge in part because the needle is not visible on the monitor (Marhofer & Chan, 2007). However, with respect to in-plane needle tracking, one company (SonoSite, Inc.) has developed an ultrasound system to remedy this problem. By sending out a "secondary beam" at a 45° angle from the transducer for perpendicular beam-to-needle alignment established outside the region of interest, needle visualization is optimized. This enables the physician to see the needle's approach to the target nerve within the field of view. In addition, to help improve therapeutic accuracy of ultrasound-guided pain medicine, the ultrasound characteristics of needles have been described (Maecken et al., 2007), "echo-friendly" needle designs have been developed (Deam, 2007), and the benefits of three-dimensional (3D) ultrasound imaging has been investigated (Feinglass et al., 2007; Foxall, et al., 2007). Moreover, cutting edge ultrasonic technological advances have introduced image-enhanced tissue staining to remotely palpate the target nerve of interest using acoustic radiation force imaging to both improve accuracy and limit variability in regional anesthesia (Palmeri et al., 2008; Nightingale et al., 2001).

4.4 Risk management: Ultrasound safety

While there are no known absolute contraindications in ultrasound imaging, the position of The U.S. Food and Drug Administration (FDA) (n.d.) concerning ultrasound safety follows.

> Ultrasound imaging has been used for over 20 years and has an excellent safety record. It is non-ionizing radiation, so it does not have the same risks as x-rays or other types of ionizing radiation. Even though there are no known risks of ultrasound imaging, it can produce effects on the body. When ultrasound enters the body, it heats the tissues slightly. In some cases, it can also produce small pockets of gas in body fluids or tissues (cavitation). The long-term effects of tissue heating and cavitation are not known.

For a more in-depth discussion on tissue sensitivity relative to interpreting risk from exposure to ultrasound imaging, the reader is encouraged to study the report on this topic issued by members of the World Federation for Ultrasound in Medicine and Biology Safety Committee (Barnett et al., 1997).

5. Future directions in interventional pain medicine

5.1 *The promise of real-time three-dimensional (3D) fluoroscopy

While CT-fluoroscopy offers unique viewing perspectives with overall imaging capabilities (as discussed in the earlier section, "Triplanar Imaging in Pain Medicine Procedures: Conventional-CT Guidance and CT-Fluoroscopy"), interestingly, real-time 3D imaging has not been reported. Conversely, although real-time 3D ultrasound has been show to be beneficial in regional anesthesia (as cited in the above section, "Ultrasound guidance in Pain Medicine: Regional Anesthesia"), ultrasound imaging does not offer the allure that fluoroscopy enjoys with respect to image resolution, particularly of bony anatomy.

Technology is currently available to fit mobile C-arm fluoroscopy systems with 3D imaging capabilities (Stübig et al., 2009; Izadpanah et al., 2009; Villavicencio et al., 2005). (Note: current fluoroscopy systems creating 3D imagery are limited to 150°—360° with mechanical orientation or manipulation or post-processing.) Notably, the limiting factor in the utility of these systems under most interventional pain protocols is image construction time. However, one company, Imaging3 Inc., claims to have developed signal processing algorithms to produce 3D high-resolution fluoroscopic images in *real-time* via its "Dominion" platform. (Note: at the time of this publication, this device has *not* received FDA clearance.) The design is built around a dedicated O-arm—a gantry similar to that used in CT—to allow continuous 360° rotation of the x-ray tube and scintillation detector with on-demand imaging of the patient under continuous or pulsed fluoroscopy. (See the earlier discussion on radiation risk management in fluoroscopy to review the advantages of pulsed fluoroscopy.) This approach is expected to allow imaging of the patient from any frame of reference or angulation. Intended use is anticipated by the company to be procedures in which multiple frames of reference are required. From a pain medicine perspective, real-time 3D fluoroscopic guidance may be possible for discography, vertebral augmentation, percutaneous lumbar decompression, facet rhizotomy, or intradiscal electrothermal therapy.

In addition, it is projected that the Dominion will offer a multi-modal feature to give physicians the ability to view cross-sectional anatomy by emulating CT, using a cone-beam CT model.
*Note: neither the author nor anyone known to the author has any relationship with any of the companies mentioned in this subsection. This includes but is not limited to financial, consulting, and business relationships. All information was obtained through company filings and/or press releases and/or marketing literature.

5.2 *Interventional magnetic resonance imaging (MRI)

This section presents a brief discussion on the concept of MRI-guided procedures. Whereas the use of MRI for this purpose is in its infancy, the intent of MRI-guided/interventional scanning is to assist physicians during intra-operative, and diagnostic and therapeutic procedures using magnetic-compatible instrumentation. The Fonar 360™ MRI unit represents the cutting edge in technology for this vision. The Fonar 360™ is a specialized MRI design with the field and gradient magnets encapsulated in the ceiling and floor of a dedicated, monolithic room. In this capacity, the enlarged room-sized magnet and the 360° access to the patient permits full-fledged medical teams to walk into the room (i.e., "inside the magnet") to interact with the patient. The first unit was installed at the Nuffield Orthopaedic Centre in Oxford, United Kingdom.
Another developer, MRI Interventions Inc., a medical device maker focusing on interventional MRI applications, has obtained FDA clearance on their ClearPoint® system which is designed to enable minimally invasive procedures in the brain—namely to facilitate image guidance for the introduction of deep brain stimulation leads—utilizing a hospital's existing MRI suite. On this note, although to date the use of deep brain stimulation for pain is limited due to lackluster outcomes (Levy et al., 1987; Coffey, 2001; Hamani et al., 2006), research is ongoing to find appropriate surgical candidates and areas in the brain conducive to long-term efficacy for conditions with a central pain aspect. Such targeted brain centers currently under investigation are the ventral capsule/ventral striatum in thalamic pain syndrome (U.S. National Institutes of Health [NIH], NCT 01072656). On another note, the introduction of deep brain stimulation systems with "steerable" field currents (the VANTAGE trial) (NIH, NCT 01221948) may ultimately prove clinically advantageous in such approaches to pain management.
Finally, our discussion on interventional MRI would be incomplete without reference made to patient care and concerns about biologic effects relative to exposure to MRI. Hence, we refer the reader to the collection of work by Frank Shellock. On this point, we encourage the reader to begin with Shellock and Cruse (2004) to gain an overview on tissue sensitivity associated with gradient magnetic fields, acoustic noise, and radiofrequency fields/radiation in MRI.
*Note: neither the author nor anyone known to the author has any relationship with any of the companies mentioned in this subsection. This includes but is not limited to financial, consulting, and business relationships. All information was obtained through company filings and/or press releases and/or marketing literature.

5.3 Ultrasound imaging: Beyond regional anesthesia

With ultrasound guidance for nerve blocks in regional anesthesia established, intriguing applications of this modality in pain medicine are beginning to surface. For example, ultrasound guidance for trigger point injection therapy has been shown to be comparable to electromyographic guidance (Botwin et al., 2008). One advantage of this technique is that in the cervicothoracic area, the physician can see the lungs in order to guard against inadvertent procedure-induced pneumothorax. In other applications, the use of ultrasound was also recently documented as the modality of choice to facilitate placement of percutaneous leads in two peripheral nerve stimulation trialing procedures to treat ilioinguinal neuralgia (Carayannopoulos et al., 2009). This marked a new era in ultrasound-guided pain medicine, as well as technical improvement and refinement of a surgical technique. Likewise, image guidance with ultrasound in pain procedures traditionally reserved for x-ray producing modalities (fluoroscopy) have been reported. The evidence for this is gleaned from reports on real-time ultrasound-guided epidural injections (Karmakar, 2009), and even the introduction of current procedural terminology codes for transforaminal epidural injections and paravertebral/facet injections.

However, more compelling evidence for the versatility of ultrasound in pain medicine is found in its utility in pain-related physical rehabilitation (a role for this modality which is in its infancy) (Peolsson & Brodin, 2009; Primack, 2010; Wininger, 2010). It is well recognized that when musculoskeletal injuries/syndromes induce pain, use of the involved body part (such as the shoulder for example) becomes limited, which may in turn cause more pain and more limited use and a vicious cycle is started, possibly leading to physical limitation that negatively influences the quality of life of the patient. Alternatively, qualitative and quantitative description of musculoskeletal tissue dynamics and coordination during real-time procedures is possible through ultrasound imaging via tissue velocity imaging. This technique may be used to scrutinize both intra-muscular and inter-muscular coordination patterns (Peolsson & Brodin, 2009). Dynamic imaging using ultrasound to assess shoulder impingement syndromes is another example of pain-related physical rehabilitation ultrasound use (Bureau et al., 2006). To this point, it is noteworthy to mention that researchers have looked into how the overall utility of musculoskeletal ultrasound imaging impacts MRI. It was discovered that selective substitution of musculoskeletal ultrasound for MRI can result in significant cost savings to the health care system, but issues related to accuracy, variability, education and competence need to be further addressed (Jacobson, 2009).

6. References

AAPM. Cardiac catheterization equipment performance. (2001). American Association of Physicists in Medicine. Report Series No. 70.

Aguirre DA, Bermudez S, & Diaz OM. (2005). Spinal CT-guided interventional procedures for management of chronic back pain. *J Vasc Interv Radiol*, vol. 16, no. 5, pp. 689-697.

Aldrich JE. (2007). Basic physics of ultrasound imaging. *Crit Care Med*, vol. 35, no. 5, pp. S131-S137.

Aufrichtig R, Xue P, Thomas CW, Gilmore GC, & Wilson DL. (1994). Perceptual comparison of pulsed and continuous fluoroscopy. *Med Phys*, vol. 21, no. 2, pp. 245-256.

Back DL, Hilton AI, Briggs TW, Scott J, Burns M, & Warren P. (2005). Radiation protection for your hands. *Injury*, vol. 36, no. 12, pp. 1416-1420.

Barnes JE. (1992). Characteristics and control of contrast in CT. *Radiographics*, vol. 12, no. 4, pp. 825-837.

Barnett SB, Rott HD, ter Haar GR. Ziskin MC, Maeda K. (1997). The sensitivity of biological tissue to ultrasound. *Ultrasound Med Biol*, vol. 23, no. 6, pp. 805-812.

Balter S. (2006). Methods for measuring fluoroscopic skin dose. *Pediatr Radiol*, vol. 36, suppl. 2, pp. 136-140.

Balter S. (2008). Capturing patient doses from fluoroscopically based diagnostic and interventional systems. *Health Phys*, vol. 95, no. 5, pp. 535-540.

Boszczyk BM, Bierschneider M, Panzer S, et al. (2006). Fluoroscopic radiation exposure of the kyphoplasty patient. *Eur Spine J*, vol. 15, no. 3, pp. 347-355.

Botwin KP, Freeman ED, Gruber RD, et al. (2001). Radiation exposure to a physician performing fluoroscopically guided caudal epidural steroid injections. *Pain Physician*, vol. 4, no. 4, pp. 343-348.

Botwin KP, Thomas S, Gruber RD, et al. (2002). Radiation exposure of the spinal interventionalist performing fluoroscopically guided transforaminal epidural steroid injections. *Arch Phys Med Rehabil*, vol. 83, no. 5, pp. 697-701.

Botwin KP, Fuoco GS, Torres FM, et al. (2003). Radiation exposure to the spinal interventionalist performing lumbar discography. *Pain Physician*, vol. 6, no. 3, pp. 295-300.

Botwin KP, Sharma K, Saliba R, & Patel BC. (2008). Ultrasound-guided trigger point injections in the cervicothoracic musculature: a new and unreported technique. *Pain Physician*, vol. 11, no. 6, pp. 885-889.

Boyce WE, DiPrima RC. (2005). *Elementary Differential Equations*. 8th ed. John Wiley & Sons, Inc; Hoboken, NJ.

Bracewell RN. (1986). *The Fourier Transform and Its Applications*. 3rd ed. McGraw Hill. Singapore.

Bureau NJ, Beauchamp M, Cardinal E, & Brassard P. (2006). Dynamic sonography evaluation of shoulder impingement syndrome. *AJR Am J Roentgenol*, vo. 187, no. 1, pp. 216-220.

Bushong SC. (2004). Radiation protection procedures. In: Bushong SC, ed. *Radiologic Science for Technologists: Physics, Biology, and Protection*. 8th ed. pp. 583-601, Mosby Inc., St. Louis, Mo.

Carayannopoulos A, Beasley R, & Sites B. (2009). Facilitation of percutaneous trial lead placement with ultrasound guidance for peripheral nerve stimulation trial of ilioinguinal neuralgia: a technical note. *Neuromodulation*, vol. 12, no. 4, pp. 296-301.

Carlton RR, Adler AM. (2006). *Principles of Radiographic Imaging: An Art and a Science*. 4th ed. Clifton Park, NY: Thomson Delmar.

Clasper JC, Pinks T. (1995). Technical note: an assessment of x-ray protective gloves. *Br J Radiol*, vol. 68, no. 812, pp. 917-919.

Christodoulou EG, Goodsitt MM, Larson SC, Darner KL, Satti J, & Chan HP. (2003). Evaluation of the transmitted exposure through lead equivalent aprons in a radiology department, including the contribution from backscatter. *Med Phys*, vol. 30, no. 6, pp. 1033-1038.

Coffey RJ. (2001). Deep brain stimulation for chronic pain: results of two multicenter trials and a structured review. *Pain Med*, vol. 2, no. 3, pp. 183-192.

Cousin AJ, Lawdahl RB, Chakraborty DP, & Koehler RE. (1987). The case for radioprotective eyewear/facewear. Practical implications and suggestions. *Invest Radiol*, vol. 22, no. 8, pp. 688-692.

Daly B, Templeton PA. (1999). Real-time CT fluoroscopy: evolution of an interventional tool. *Radiology*, vol. 211, no. 2, pp. 309-315.

Datir A, Connell D. (2010). CT-guided injection for ganglion impar blockade: a radiological approach to the management of coccydynia. *Clin Radiol*, vol. 65, no. 1, pp. 21-25.

Davies AG, Cowen AR, Kengyelics SM, et al. (2006). X-ray dose reduction in fluoroscopically guided electrophysiology procedures. *PACE*, vol. 29, no. 3, pp. 262-271.

Deam RK, Kluger R, Barrington MJ, & McCutcheon CA. (2007). Investigation of a new echogenic needle for use with ultrasound peripheral nerve blocks. *Anaesth Intensive Care*, vol. 35, no. 4, pp. 582-586.

Deshpande KK, Wininger KL. (2011). Feasibility of combined epicranial temporal and occipital neurostimulation: treatment of a challenging case of headache. *Pain Physician*, vol. 14, no. 1, pp. 37-44.

Dowd SB, Tilson ER. (1999). *Practical Radiation Protection and Applied Radiobiology*. 2nd ed. Philadelphia, Pa: Saunders.

Fazel R, Krumholz HM, Wang Y, et al. (2009). Exposure to low-dose ionizing radiation from medical imaging procedures. *N Eng J Med*, vol. 361, no. 9, pp. 849-857.

Feinglass NG, Clendenen SR, Torp KD, Wang RD, Castello R, & Greengrass RA. (2007). Real-time three-dimensional ultrasound for continuous popliteal blockade: a case report and image description. *Anesth Analg*, vol. 105, no. 1, pp. 272-274.

Ferreira CC, Galvão LA, Veira JW, Maia AF. (2010). Validation of an exposure computational model to computed tomography. *Brazilian Journal of Physics Médica*, vol. 4, no. 1, pp. 19-22.

Finnerty M, Brennan PC. (2005). Protective aprons in imaging departments: manufacturer stated lead equivalence values require validation. *Eur Radiol*, vol. 15, no. 7, pp. 1477-1484.

Fish DE, Kim A, Ornelas C, Song S, & Pangarkar S. The risks of radiation exposure to the eyes of the interventional pain physician. *Radiology Research and Practice*, vol. 2011. Article ID 609537, 5 pages, 2011. doi:10.1155/2011/609537.

Foxall GL, Hardman JG, Bedforth NM. (2007). Three-dimensional, multiplanar, ultrasound-guided, radial nerve block. *Reg Anesth Pain Med*, vol. 32, no. 6, pp. 516-521.

Gangi A, Dietemann JL, Mortazavi R, Pfleger D, Kauff C, & Roy C. (1998). CT-guided Interventional procedures for pain management in the lumbosacral spine. *Radiographics*, vol. 18, no. 3, pp. 621-633.

Geleijns J, Wondergem J. (2005). X-ray imaging and the skin: Radiation biology, patient dosimetry and observed effects. *Rad Prot Dos*, vol. 114, no. 1-3, pp. 121-125.

Kapural L, Goyle A. (2007). Imaging for provocative discography and minimally invasive percutaneous procedures for treatment of discogenic lower back pain. *Tech Reg Anesth Pain Manag*, vol. 11, no. 2, pp. 73-80.

Gruber H, Bodner G. (2004). Why CT guided? [comment]. *AJR Am J Roentgenol*, vol. 182, no. 3, p. 824.

Hamani C, Schwalb JM, Rezai AR, Dostrovsky JO, Davis KD, Lozano AM. (2006). Deep brain stimulation for chronic neuropathic pain: long-term outcome and the incidence of insertional effect. *Pain*, vol. 125, no. 1, pp. 188-196.

Izadpanah K, Konrad G, Südkamp NP, & Oberst M. (2009). Computer navigation in balloon kyphoplasty reduces the intraoperative radiation exposure. *Spine*, vol. 34, no. 12, pp. 1325-1329.

Jackson S, Thomas R. (2004). Introduction to CT physics. *Cross-Sectional Imaging Made Easy*. p. 7, Churchill Livingston; Edinburgh, Scotland. 2004.

Jacobson JA. (2009). Musculoskeletal ultrasound: focused impact on MRI. *AJR Am J Roentgenol*, vol. 193, no. 3, pp. 619-627.

Johns HE, Cunningham JR. (1983). The interaction of ionizing radiation with matter. In: *The Physics of Radiology*. 4th ed. pp. 133-164, Thomas, Springfield, IL.

Johnston J, Killion JB, Vealé B, & Comello R. (2011). U.S. technologists' radiation exposure perceptions and practices. *Radiol Technol*, vol. 82, no. 4, pp. 311-320.

Kallmes DF, O E, Roy SS, et al. (2003). Radiation dose to the operator during vertebroplasty: prospective comparison of the use of 1-cc syringes versus an injection device. *AJNR Am J Neuroradiol*, vol. 24, no. 6, pp. 1257-1260.

Kane SA. (2009). *Introduction to Physics in Modern Medicine.* 2nd ed. Boca Raton, Fl: CRC Press.

Karmaka MK, Li X, Ho AM, Kwok WH, & Chui PT. (2009). Real-time ultrasound-guided paramedian epidural access: evaluation of a novel in-plane technique. *Br J Anaesth*, vol. 102, no. 6, pp. 845-854.

Kato R, Katada K, Anno H, Suzuki S, Ida Y, Koga S. (1996). Radiation dosimetry at CT fluoroscopy: physician's hand dose and development of needle holders. *Radiology*, vol. 201, no. 2, pp. 576-578.

Kosek P, Morgan D, Dunn J, et al. Electronically generated lead (EGL) scan: report of first clinical use. [abstract]. *North American Neuromodulation Society*. Dec. 7-9, 2006.

Levy RM, Lamb S, & Adams JE. (1987). Treatment of chronic pain by deep brain stimulation: long term follow-up and review of the literature. *Neurosurgery*, vol. 21, no. 6, pp. 885-893.

Larson R, Hostetler B, & Edwards BH. (2007). Calculus: Early Transcendental Functions. 4th ed. Houghton Mifflin Company; Boston, MA.

Little MP, Wakeford R, Tawn EJ, Bouffler SD, & Berrington de Gonzalez A. (2009). Risks associated with low doses and low dose rates of ionizing radiation: why linearity may be (almost) the best we can do. *Radiology*, vol. 251, no. 1, pp. 6-12.

Maecken T, Zenz M, & Grau T. (2007). Ultrasound characteristics of needles for regional anesthesia. *Reg Anesth Pain Med*, vol. 32, no. 5, pp. 440-447.

Mahesh M. (2001). Fluoroscopy: patient radiation exposure issues. *Radiographics*, vol. 21, no. 4, pp. 1033-1045.

Manchikanti L, Cash KA, Moss TL, & Pampati V. (2002). Radiation exposure to the physician in interventional pain management. *Pain Physician*, vol. 5, no. 4, pp. 385-393.

Manchikanti L, Cash KA, Moss TL, & Pampati V. (2003a). Effectiveness of protective measures in reducing risk of radiation exposure in interventional pain management: a prospective study. *Pain Physician*, vol. 6, no. 3, pp. 301-305.

Manchikanti L, Cash KA, Moss TL, Rivera J, & Pampati V. (2003b). Risk of whole body radiation exposure and protection measures in fluoroscopically guided interventional techniques: a prospective evaluation. *BMC Anesthesiol*, vol. 3, no. 1, p. 2.

Manchikanti L, Singh V, Pampati V, Smith HS, & Hirsch J. (2009). Analysis of growth of interventional techniques in managing chronic pain in the Medicare population: A 10-year evaluation from 1997 to 2006. *Pain Physician*, vol. 12, no. 1, pp. 9-34.

Marhofer P, Chan VWS. (2007). Ultrasound-guided regional anesthesia: current concepts and future trends. *Anesth Analg*, vol. 104, no. 5, pp. 1265-1269.

McKetty MH. (1998). The AAPM/RSNA physics tutorial for residents. X-ray attenuation. *Radiographics*, vol. 18, no. 1, pp. 151-163.

Meleka S, Patra A, Minkoff E, & Murphy K. (2005). Value of CT fluoroscopy for lumbar facet blocks. *AJNR Am J Neuroradiol*, vol. 26, no. 5, pp. 1001-1003.

Nightingale KR, Palmeri ML, Nightingale RW, & Trahey GE. (2001). On the feasibility of remote palpation using acoustic radiation force. *J Acoust Soc Am*, vol. 110, no. 1, pp. 625-634.

Oritz AO, Natarajan V, Gregorius DR, & Pollack S. (2006). Significantly reduced radiation exposure to operators during kyphoplasty and vertebroplasty procedures: methods and techniques. *AJNR Am J Neuroradiol*, vol. 27, no. 5, pp. 989-994.

Palmeri ML, Dahl JJ, MacLeod D, Grant S, & Nightingale KR. Regional anesthesia guidance using acoustic radiation force imaging. [abstract]. Proceedings of the Seventh International Conference on the Ultrasonic Measurement and Imaging of Tissue Elasticity. Oct. 27-30, 2008.

Peolsson M, Brodin LA. (2009). Functional musculoskeletal ultrasound. *European Musculoskeletal Review*, vol. 4, no. 2, pp. 102-107.

Perisinakis K, Damilakis J, Theocharopoulos N, Papadokostakis G, Hadjipavlou A, & Gourtsoylannis N. (2004). Patient exposure and associated radiation risks from fluoroscopically-guided vertebroplasty or kyphoplasty. *Radiology*, vol. 232, no. 3, pp. 701-701.

Primack SJ. (2010). A physiatrist's perspective on musculoskeletal ultrasound. *Phys Med Rehabil Clin N Am*, vol. 21, no. 3, pp. 645-650.

Schmid MR, Kissling RO, Curt A, Jaschko G, & Hodler J. (2006). Sympathetic skin response: monitoring of CT-guided lumbar sympathetic blocks. *Radiology*, vol. 241, no. 2, pp. 595-602.

Schueler BA. (2000). The AAPM/RSNA physics tutorial for residents: general overview of fluoroscopic imaging. *Radiographics*, vol. 20, no. 4, pp. 1115-1126.

Sentinel Event Policy and Procedures. The Joint Commission website. http://www.jointcommission.org/assets/1/18/Radiation_Overdose.pdf. Accessed June 21, 2008.

Shahabi S. Radiation safety/protection and health physics. (1999). In: Dowd SB, Tilson ER, eds. *Practical Radiation Protection and Applied Radiobiology*. 2nd ed. pp. 167-196, Saunders, Philadelphia, Pa.

Shellock FA, Crues JV. (2004). MR procedures: biologic effects, safety, and patient care. *Radiology*, vol. 232, no. 3, pp. 635-652.

Shepp LA, Kruskal JB. (1978). Computerized tomography: the new medical x-ray technology. *Am Math Mon*, vol. 85, no. 6, pp. 420-439.

Sites BD, Brull R, Chan VWS, et al. (2007). Artifacts and pitfall errors associated with ultrasound-guided regional anesthesia. Part I: Understanding the basic principles of ultrasound physics and machine operations. *Reg Anesth Pain Med*, vol. 32, no. 5, pp. 412-418.

Sites BD, Chan VW, Neal JM, et al. (2009). The American Society of Regional Anesthesia and Pain Medicine and the European Society of Regional Anaesthesia and Pain Therapy joint committee recommendations for education and training in ultrasound-guided regional anesthesia. *Reg Anesth Pain Med*, vol. 34, no. 1, pp. 40-46.

Smiddy PF, Quinn AD, Freyne PJ, Marsh D, & Murphy JM. (1996). Dose reduction in double contrast barium enema by use of low fluoroscopic current. *Br J Radiol*, vol. 69, no. 825, pp. 852-854.

Sprawls P. AAPM tutorial. (1992). CT image detail and noise. *Radiographics*, vol. 12, no. 5, pp. 1041-1046.

Stam W, Pillay M. (2008). Inspection of lead aprons: a practical rejection model. *Health Phys*, vol. 95, suppl. 2, pp. S133-S136.

Stübig T, Kendoff D, Citak M, et al. (2009). Comparative study of different intraoperative 3-D image intensifiers in orthopedic trauma care. *J Trauma*, vol. 66, no. 3, pp. 821-830.

Thoumas D, Leroi AM, Mauillon J, et al. (1999). Pudendal neuralgia: CT-guided pudendal nerve block technique. *Abdom Imaging*, vol. 24, no. 3, pp. 309-312.

Tuohy B, Marsh DM, O'Reilly G, Dowling A, Cooney P, & Malone JF. (1997). Quality assurance programme applied to mobile C-arm fluoroscopy systems. *Eur Radiol*, vol. 7, no. 4, pp. 534-541.

U.S. Food and Drug Administration Radiation Emitting Products: Radiation Emitting Products and Procedures: Medical Imaging: Ultrasound Imaging: http://www.fda.gov/Radiation-EmittingProducts/RadiationEmittingProductsandProcedures/MedicalImaging/ucm115357.htm. n.d.

U.S. National Academy of Sciences, National Research Council, Committee to Assess Health Risks from Exposure to Low Levels of Ionizing Radiation. Health Risks from Exposure to Low Levels of Ionizing Radiation. BEIR VII Phase 2. Washington, DC: National Academies Press, 2006.

U.S. National Institutes of Health. Safety study of deep brain stimulation to manage thalamic pain syndrome. Identifier: NCT01072656. Clinical Trials website. http://clinicaltrials.gov. Accessed May 16, 2011

U.S. National Institutes of Health. Vercise implantable stimulator for treating Parkinson's disease (VANTAGE). Identifier: NCT01221948. Clinical Trials website. http://clinicaltrials.gov. Accessed May 16, 2011.

Vano E, Gonzalez L, Ten JI, et al. (2001). Skin dose and dose-area product values for interventional cardiology procedures. *Br J Radiol*, vol. 74, no. 877, pp. 48-55.

Villavicencio AT, Burneikiene S, Bulsara KR, & Thramann JJ. (2005). Intraoperative three-dimensional fluoroscopy-based computerized tomography guidance for percutaneous kyphoplasty. *Neurosurg Focus*, vol. 18, no. 3, p. E3.

Wagner AL. (2004a). Selective lumbar nerve root blocks with CT fluoroscopic guidance: technique, results, procedure time, and radiation dose. *AJNR Am J Neuroradiol*, vol. 25, no. 9, pp. 1592-1594.

Wagner AL. (2004b). CT fluoroscopy-guided epidural injections: techniques and results. *AJNR Am J Neuroradiol*, vol. 25, no. 10, pp. 1821-1823.

Wang J, Blackburn TJ. (2000). The AAPM/RSNA physics tutorial for residents: x-ray image intensifiers for fluoroscopy. *Radiographics*, vol. 20, no. 5, pp. 1471-1477.

Whitworth ML. Fluoroscopy scatter radiation studies of the lumbar spine. In: Interventional Spine. Volume 5, Issue 5. Kentfield, Ca: International Spine Intervention Society, n.d.

Wininger KL. (2010). The lumbosacral spine: kinesiology, physical rehabilitation, and interventional pain medicine. *Clinical Kinesiology*, vol. 64, no. 3, pp. 22-50.

Wininger KL, Deshpande KK, & Deshpande KK. (2010). Radiation exposure in percutaneous spinal cord stimulation mapping: a preliminary report. Pain Physician, vol. 13, no. 1, pp. 7-18.

World Health Organization. The WHO Global Database on Body Mass Index. BMI Classification website. http://apps.who.int/bmi/index.jsp?introPage=intro_3.html. n.d.

Yanch JC, Behrman RH, Hendricks MJ, & McCall JH. (2009). Increased radiation dose to overweight and obese patients from radiographic examinations. *Radiology*, 2009, vol. 252, no. 1, pp. 128-139.

Zhou Y, Singh N, Abdi S, Wu J, Crawford J, Furgang FA. (2005). Fluoroscopy radiation safety for spine interventional pain procedures in university teaching hospitals. *Pain Physician*, vol. 8, no. 1, pp. 49-53.

Part 2

Acute Pain

8

Local Anesthetic Agents in Arthroscopy

Joseph Baker
Cappagh National Orthopaedic Hospital
Ireland

1. Introduction

Arthroscopy is performed with increasing frequency on a number of joints. In the lower limb the role of knee arthroscopy is well established with procedures enabling more accurate diagnosis and treatment of a myriad of conditions including but not being limited to meniscal injury and articular surface defects. Hip and ankle arthroscopy are less widely performed. However, despite this their use can be expected to increase as indications are better developed and techniques honed.

While surgical technique often determines outcome in the long-term, analgesic control can significantly affect the patient's satisfaction following a procedure as well as the overall acceptability of a procedure. Arthroscopic procedures in particular have enabled many procedures to be performed on a day case basis where as more traditional surgical interventions may have required at least an overnight hospital stay. This trend toward day case surgery also emphasizes the importance of optimum analgesic control.

Traditionally intra-articular analgesic agents have been used following arthroscopic procedures as an augment to post-operative pain control. Classically these include the typical local anesthetic agents but also alternatives such as morphine. Recently however, the potential for deleterious effects of the intra-articular analgesics on the articular cartilage has been reported in a number of experimental studies, which has caused concern among practicing arthroscopic surgeons. The purpose of this chapter is to review the potential intra-articular analgesic agents used for pain control following lower limb arthroscopy and to also provide an up-to-date review of the evidence for the potential chondrotoxic effect of these agents.

2. Analgesic agents

Classical local anesthetic agents can be classified into the esters and amides. Amides including lignocaine and bupivacaine among others have commonly been used in arthroscopy. Local anesthetics block action potential initiation and propagation along sensory pathways by blocking the sodium channel transmembrane pores. Their activity is increased in alkaline conditions and this enables them to penetrate the nerve sheath and axonal membrane.

Other agents to have been trialed as intra-articular agents include opiates or opiate related substances (e.g. morphine, tramadol), non-steroidal anti-inflammatory medications, benzodiazepines and NMDA-receptor antagonists (e.g. magnesium sulfate) among others.

2.1 Hip and ankle arthroscopy

Numerous studies have assessed the ability of local anesthetic agents to provide pain control following arthroscopic procedures in the lower limb. A vast majority of these have focused on the knee and only a few have reported the use of local anaesthetic following hip and ankle arthroscopy(Middleton et al., 2006, Baker et al., 2011c).

Of these two studies both found that intra-articular local anaesthetic was superior to either placebo or local anesthetic infiltrated around the arthroscopic portals (Table 1). The paucity of data here reflects the relative infancy of hip and ankle arthroscopy compared to knee arthroscopy and highlights the need for further work - hip arthroscopy in particular requires significant force to overcome the intra-articular negative pressures and can result in significant post-operative pain(Baker et al., 2011a).

Author	Setting	Number	Key findings
(Baker et al., 2011c)	RCT	73	Intra-articular bupivacaine superior to peri-portal bupivacaine at controlling pain following HIP arthroscopy
(Middleton et al., 2006)	RCT	35	Intra-articular bupivacaine was superior to saline placebo in reducing post-operative VAS pain scores and need for supplemental analgesia following ANKLE arthroscopy

Table 1. Studies assessing the benefit of intra-articular analgesic agents following hip and ankle arthroscopy

2.2 Knee arthroscopy

Numerous studies have attempted to establish the ideal intra-articular analgesic for pain control following knee arthroscopy (for a summary of these studies see Table2). The studies selected for inclusion here predominantly include those that use an intra-articular analgesic following surgery in a bolus dose fashion. Some studies that use it prior to surgery are also included for comparison sake particularly where comparison is later made with a bolus given following surgery. This section focuses on intra-articular analgesia given as an augment following surgery performed under general anesthesia or spinal anesthesia.

Although many studies have found that classical local anesthetic agents are of benefit following knee arthroscopy a randomized controlled trial reported by Townsend et al noted that intra-articular bupivacaine was no more effective that bupivacaine infiltrated around the portal sites(Townshend et al., 2009). This equivalence takes on even more importance with the reported potential for the toxic effect on articular cartilage of bupivacaine and other similar agents.

In general local anesthetics have been shown to be effective compared to placebo although this is not necessarily the case if the surgery is performed under spinal anesthetic when it appears the additional use of an intra-articular agent is negated by the spinal block(Santanen et al., 2001).

Non-steroidal anti-inflammatory medications have been trialed as intra-articular agents but are not in wide spread use. A single study has found that tenoxicam was superior to bupivacaine following surgery but this was only with regards analgesic consumption - the reported pain scores were still similar(Cook et al., 1997). It was similarly found that lornoxicam resulted in lower pain scores than did bupivacaine in a randomized controlled trial of 40 patients(Fagan et al., 2003). The use of an anti-inflammatory into the joint cavity may play a role in pain control particularly when a significant inflammatory component to the intra-articular pathology is found(Izdes et al., 2003).

When compared to opiate type analgesics ropivacaine was shown in one study to provide quicker onset of analgesia but was not significantly better at 24 hours after surgery(Franceschi et al., 2001). The benefit of morphine as an intra-articular analgesic is questionable however as noted later and this perhaps reflects poorly on ropivacaine.

Combinations of amide local anesthetics with other agents have been tried and this may represent the optimum way to control pain although at this point in time it is unknown. A combination of magnesium sulfate and bupivacaine was shown to be superior to either agent in isolation, which were again superior to placebo with regard pain scores following knee arthroscopy(Elsharnouby et al., 2008). These findings are supported by another study that also included morphine in the intra-articular cocktail but again found that a combination of agents was superior to any of the agents given in isolation(Farouk and Aly, 2009). A combination of bupivacaine with fentanyl was shown to be superior to bupivacaine in isolation following knee arthroscopy in a randomized trial including 33 patients(Jawish et al., 1996). Despite these promising reports in combinations of an amide local anesthetic and an opiate type agent others have failed to find this multimodal approach any better than placebo alone(Aasbo et al., 1996). While pain intensity or pain scale score is a frequent measure in these studies, the actual need for additional analgesia is a limiting factor with regard the ability to perform a procedure as a day case or not and may reflect a more practical end-point for further research.

Despite a small number of studies suggesting that morphine provides adequate analgesic control following knee a recent review of these studies has suggested that of the higher quality studies, most had a negative finding not in favor of its use as an intra-articular analgesic agent(Rosseland, 2005, Drosos et al., 2002). The key point of this review was that post-operative pain intensity was no less in the morphine treated groups than the placebo treated groups in the well-designed studies. This review is supported by a study by the same author group that found only those with intense pain after arthroscopy had any benefit from intra-articular morphine(Rosseland et al., 1999).

Other agents have been studied in with some success including midazolam (increased the time to first analgesia after surgery compared to placebo), clonidine (additive effect with bupivacaine compared to bupivacaine alone) and neostigmine (more effective when compared to morphine)(Batra et al., 2008, Tamosiunas et al., 2005, Yang et al., 1998). Unfortunately these agents have been studies in a very limited capacity and a clear conclusion in unable to be drawn as their effectiveness.

Author	Setting	Number	Key findings
(Aasbo et al., 1996)	RCT	107	Patients randomised to receive either: **bupivacaine** (20ml of 2.5mg/ml) + **morphine** (3mg); **bupivacaine** (20ml of 2.5mg/ml) alone; **morphine** (3mg) alone; or isotonic saline – no differences between the groups with regard analgesic requirement post-surgery
(Al-Metwalli et al., 2008)	RCT	60	Intra-articular **dexmedetomidine** (α-2-adrenergic agonist) given via the intra-articular route resulted in less post-operative pain and analgesic requirement than either **dexmedetomidine** given intravenously or intra-articulat and intravenous placebo (saline)
(Alagol et al., 2004)	RCT	210	Intra-articular **tramadol** at doses 50-100mg provided good post-operative analgesia with the higher doe more effectuve. The intra-articular route was more effective than the intravenous route.
(Batra et al., 2008)	RCT	60	Intra-articular **midazolam** (50 or 75μg/kg) provided superior, albeit briefly, analgesic control compared to saline placebo. Time to first analgesic requirement was 4.7 and 4.6 hours compared to 0.7.

Author	Setting	Number	Key findings
(Buerkle et al., 2000)	RCT	60	Patients given **morphine** (1mg) and **clonidine** (150μg) intra-articularly in combination had lower VAS pain scores at 2 hours post-surgery and lower need for rescue analgesia compared to groups given either agent in isolation or saline placebo
(Calmet et al., 2004)	RCT	80	Following arthroscopic meniscectomy, patients receiving intra-articular **ketorolac** (60mg) had better post-operative pain control and less need for rescue analgesia compared to those receiving 10ml of 0.25% **bupivacaine**, 1mg of **morphine** or normal saline placebo.
(Cepeda et al., 1997)	RCT	112	Intra-articular and subcuticular **morphine** (10mg) and intraarticuular **bupivacaine** (20ml 0.5%) were compared with noraml saline placebo. Single dose morphine by either route provided superior pain conrol with lower pain scores at 6- and 3-hours post-surgery.
(Colbert et al., 1999)	RCT	88	Patients receiving intra-articular **tenoxicam** had lower pain scores at 30-180 minutes post-surgery and required less analgesia later than thos receiving the same drug intravenously.
(Convery et al., 1998)	RCT	60	Patients given 5mg **ketorolac** with 20ml of 0.25% **bupivacaine** into the joint after surgery provided similar analgesic control to 10mg ketorolac given intravenously with 20ml of 0.25% **bupivacaine** given into the joint.
(Cook et al., 1997)	RCT	63	Patients received either 40ml solution containing only normal saline, 0.25% **bupivacaine** or 20mg **tenoxicam** at the end of knee arthroscopy. Less analgesia was needed by the tenoxicam group but subjective pain reporting was similar in all groups.
(Dalsgaard et al., 1993)	RCT	52	Patients receiving 1mg of **morphine** intrarticularly at the end of surgery had lower pain scores at 8- and 24-hours after surgery and used less paracetamol compared to those receiving saline placebo.
(Drosos et al., 2002)	RCT	30	No significant difference seen in VAS pain scores between patients receiving intra-articular saline, 5mg **morphine** or 15mg **morphine** following diagnostic arthroscopy or arthroscopic meniscectomy.
(Elhakim et al., 1999)	RCT	60	Patients randomised to receive either saline placebo; 2% **lidocaine** and 10mg **pethidine**, or; 2% **lidocaine**, 10mg **pethidine** and 20mg **tenoxicam**. Combination of all three agents resulted in lower VAS pain scores for longer and less need for analgesic use.
(Elsharnouby et al., 2008)	RCT	108	Patients receiving 1g **magnesium sulfate** and 0.25% **bupivacaine** (20ml total) had significantly lower VAS pain scores and longer time to first analgesic use than thos receiving either agent in isolation or placebo.
(Eren et al., 2008)	RCT	90	Patients receving either 8mg **lornoxicam** or 50mg **bupivacaine** had less analgesic consumption after surgery than those receiving plcebo. Pain rating were lower for those receinving the lornoxicam than thos receiving the bupivacaine.
(Fagan et al., 2003)	RCT	40	Patients receiving pre-emptive injection of **bupivacaine with adrenaline** showed a trend toward needing less analgesia in the recovery room than those receiving the injection at completion of surgery.
(Farouk and Aly, 2009)	RCT	80	A combination of **magnesium** (150mg) and **morphine** (2mg) with 20 ml of 0.25% **bupivacaine** provided superior analgesic control (lower VAS scores and longer time to first analgesic) than either agent alone with bupivacaine or bupivacaine alone.

Author	Setting	Number	Key findings
(Franceschi et al., 2001)	RCT	90	**Ropivacaine** (75mg in 20ml saline) had quicker onset of effective analgesia post-opeatively than **morphine** (2mg in 20ml saline) with lower VAS pain scores in the first 4 hours and equivalent control in the first 24 hours.
(Goodwin et al., 2005, Goodwin and Parker, 2005)	RCT	50	**Bupivacaine with epinephrine** and **morphine** or **bupivacaine with epinephrine** alone given either pre- or post-operatively resulted in lower pain scores and narcotic onsumption than with epinephrine alone. There was a trend toward superior control in those receiving the injection pre-operatively.
(Goodwin and Parker, 2005)	RCT		Combinations of **bupivacaine, morphine** and **epinephrine** given pre- or post-surgery resulted in similar pain control.
(Grabowska-Gawel et al., 2003)		56	Patients received either 10ml 0.5% **bupivacaine** or 5mg **morphine** in normal saline. Mean time to rescue analgesia was shorter in the bupivacaine group but there was no difference in reported VAS pain scores.
(Graham et al., 2000)	RCT	36	Intra-articular analgesia given at completion of arthroscopy was equivalent to pre-operative intravenous regional analgesia with respect to post-opertive pain control
(Gupta et al., 1999)	RCT	100	Knee arthroscopy performed under LA (prilocaine (5mg/ml). **Morphine** (3mg), **ketorolac** (30mg) or a combination of the two was given at completion of surgery. A combination of morphine and ketorolac provided significantly superior analgesia than morphine alone or placebo.
(Hege-Scheuing et al., 1995)	RCT	59	**Morphine** (1mg) given either intra-articularly or intravenously at the end of arthroscopy had equivalent analgesic benefit.
(Izdes et al., 2003)	RCT	90	Patients receiving intra-articular **piroxicam** (20mg) and 25ml of 0.25% **bupivacaine** had longer analgesic duration in cases where synovial inflammation was confirmed present than when not present.
(Jacobson et al., 2006)	RCT	120	**Levobupivacaine** (5mg/ml) significantly reduced the need for analgesia in the first 24 hours post-surgery compared to **levobupivacaine** (2.5mg/ml) and **lidocaine** (10mg/ml) with **adrenaline**.
(Jaureguito et al., 1995)	RCT		Knee arthroscopy [performed under LA. Patients receiving intra-articular **morphine** (4mg) had lower VAS pain scores than those receiving 0.25% **bupivacaine** or saline placebo. Less supplemental pain medication was needed by the morphine group.
(Jawish et al., 1996)	RCT	33	Patients receiving a combination of 0.25% **bupivacaine** with 50µg of **fentanyl** had reduced post-operative pain for at least 9 hours post-surgery when compared to patients receiving 0.25% **bupivacaine** alone or saline placebo.
(Joshi et al., 1992)	RCT	20	Patients receiving intra-articular **morphine** (5mg) following knee arthroscopy had lower VAS pain scores and needed less rescue analgesia than those recevinign saline placebo. Low serum morphine metabolites suggested that the morphine was acting locally.
(Joshi et al., 1993)	RCT	40	Intra-articular **morphine** (5mg) either in isolation or incombination with 25ml of 0.25% **bupivacaine** resulted in significantly lower pain scores and need for supplementary analgesia than **bupivacaine** in isolation or saline placebo.

Author	Setting	Number	Key findings
(Juelsgaard et al., 1993)	RCT	47	There was no difference in reposrted VAS pain scores or acetaminophen use in the 48 hours after knee arthroscopy in patients receiving either 2 or 4mg of intra-articular **morphine** after surgery
(Kanbak et al., 1997)	RCT		Patients receiving 5mg **morphine** intra-articularly after arthroscopy had superior pain control in the 24 hours after surgery compared to those receiving 1mg **morphine** or saline placebo.
(Karaman et al., 2009)	RCT	40	No significant difference was found in control of post-operative pain and analgesic requirement between patients receiving 20ml of 0.5% **levobupivacaine** and 20ml of 0.5% **bupivacaine.**
(Kligman et al., 2002)	RCT	60	Infiltration of **morphine** (1mg) into the synovial tissue or outer third of meniscal tissue resulted in better pain control (lower VAS pain scores and less analgesic use) post-arthroscopy than if morphine (1mg) was given by the intra-articular route.
(Lundin et al., 1998)	RCT	50	Intra-articular **bupivacaine** 0.25% (40ml) with the addition of **morphine** 1mg compared to **bupivacaine** alone. Lower VAS pain scores noted with the addition of morphine in the 24 hours after surgery but no difference in supplementary analgesic use.
(Niemi et al., 1994)	RCT	80	Patients underwent knee arthroscopy under either spinal or LA (1% lidocaine with adrenaline) blockade. Intra-articular **morphine** (1mg) given at the end of the procedure resulted in reduced rescue analgesia requirement in the group that had LA block.
(Pooni et al., 1999)	RCT	107	Patients randomized to receive either intra-articular **bupivacaine** or **fantanyl** after knee arthroscopy reported similar pain scores except at 2-hours post-surgery when bupivacaine was superior
(Raj et al., 2004)	RCT	40	Patients receinving 10mg **morphine** intra-articularly repoted lower pain scores between 4- and 24-hours post-surgery and consumed less analgesia than patients receiving 10mg morphine via the intramuscular route.
(Rasmussen et al., 2002)	RCT	60	Patients randomized to receive either saline placebo; 150mg **bupivacaine** and 4mg **morphine,** or; 150mg **bupivacaine**, 4mg **morphine** and 40mg **methylprednisolone** intra-articulalry at the end of surgery.Bupivacaine with mprhine was effective at reducing pain and duration of immobilization, the addition of methylprednisolone futher reduce dpain and use of analgesics.
(Rautoma et al., 2000)	RCT	200	Pre-operative per oral diclofenac reduced post-operative pain scores compared to the intra-articular **ropivacaine** given at the time of surgery. Arthoscopy performed under spinal anaesthesia.
(Richardson et al., 1997)	RCT		Intra-articular morphine (1mg) was superior to bupivacaine (100mg) at reducing pain scores and need for supplementary anlgesia at 6- and 24-hours post-surgery. An intra-articular dose of 5mg morphine was more effective thatn 1mg intra-articular or 5mg intravenous at reducing VAS pain scores.
(Rosseland et al., 2004)	RCT	60	Intra-articular **saline** (1 or 10ml) was given following surgery via an intra-articular catheter in patients with at least moderate pain. Within 1 hour VAS pain scores reduced from 50 to 27 on a 100mm scale with both volumes.
(Rosseland et al., 2003)	RCT	40	Intra-articular **saline** (10ml) or **morphin**e (2mg in 10ml saline) was given following surgery via an intra-articular catheter in patients with at least moderate pain. Equivalent improvements in pain intesnity were found in both groups.

Author	Setting	Number	Key findings
(Rosseland et al., 1999)	RCT	90	Only patients with more intense pain after arthroscopy had beneift from intra-articular **morphine** (2mg) with regard reduced pain intensity and analgesia requirement. In most patients **morphine** (1 or 2mg) was equivalent to saline placebo.
(Samoladas et al., 2006)	RCT	60	Patientes received either 10 or 20ml of 7.5mg/ml **ropivacaine**. Both provided excellent pain control for two hours, however after that the lower dose group reported increased pain and need for supplementary analgesia.
(Santanen et al., 2001)	RCT	100	Knee arthroscopy performed under spinal anaesthesia. 20ml of 0.5% **ropivacaine** failed to reduce VAS pain scores or need for rescue analgesia when compared to saline control.
(Solheim et al., 2006)	RCT	40	Patients received intra-articular **morphine** (5mg) or saline placebo via intra-articular catheter 1 hour post-surgery if they developed at least moderate pain. Morphine was of no greater benefit than saline. Timing of catheter removal did not influence the outcome.
(Souza et al., 2002)	RCT	60	Patients receiving either saline placebo, 10ml 0.25% **bupivacaine**, 2mg **morphine** or 100µg **fentanyl** intra-articularly at the end of arthroscopy did not differ significantly in reported pain intensity.
(Tamosiunas et al., 2005)	RCT	48	Patients receiving 20ml of 0.5% **bupivacaine** with the addition of 1µg/kg of **clonidine** controlled post-operative pain more effectivley than **bupivacaine** in isolation or placebo.
(Townshend et al., 2009)	RCT	137	Patients receiving 20ml of 0.5% bupivacaine either intra-articulalry or infiltrated around the portals reported equivalent pain scores at 1-hour post-surgery.
(VanNess and Gittins, 1994)	RCT	81	Patients receiving intra-artticular **morphine** (2mg) reported significantly less pain and lower analgesic requirements in the 24-hours after surgery than those receiving 30ml of 0.25% **bupivacaine with epinephrine**..
(Varrassi et al., 1999)	RCT	48	Intra-articular **buprenorphine** (100µg) and intra-articular **bupivacaine** (50mg) resulted in lower VAS pain scores in the 6-hours after surgery than intra-articular saline or intra-muscular buprenorphine. Analgesic use was less in thoe treated with intra-articular **buprenorphine** or **bupivacaine.**
(Vranken et al., 2001)	RCT	60	**Sufentanil** (5 or 10µg) given intra-articulalry resulted in lower VAS pain scores than in control (intravenous sufentanil). Post-operative analgesic use was also lower in the treatment group.
(White et al., 1990)	RCT		Patients treated with **prilocaine with adenaline** reported prolonged time to first dose of oral analgesia but overall there was no difference in pain scores.
(Yang et al., 1998)	RCT	60	Patients receiving intra-articular **neostigmine** (500µg) had lower VAS pain scores 1-hour after surgery and had longer lasting duration of analgesia compared to those receiving intra-articular **morphine** (2mg) or saline placebo. No significant effects were seen with neostigmine 125 or 250µg.
(Zeidan et al., 2008)	RCT	90	Intra-articular administration of **tramadol** (100mg) and 0.25% **bupivacaine** to 20ml vloume had lower VAS scores, longer time to rescue analgesia and less analgesic use in the first 24-hours compared to when either agent was given in isolation.

Table 2. Studies assessing the benefit of intra-articular analgesic agents following knee arthroscopy. Treatments are in bold.

In summary a myriad of agents have been studied for their potential use in attenuating post-operative pain following knee arthroscopy. While the amide local anesthetic agents are the most widely studied their continuing benefit and use is questionable as portal infiltration has been shown to be as effective at providing pain control for a procedure that is generally very well tolerated. Knee arthroscopy performed under local anesthetic is a different entity although far less frequent.

Hip and ankle arthroscopy are far less studied and the ideal intra-articular agent is uncertain in these joints. A multi-model intra-articular analgesic bolus may be the best approach in these joints that require significant traction and subsequent injury to the capsule that can cause greater discomfort after surgery.

2.3 The potential for articular chondrocyte toxicity

The potential for deleterious effects of local anesthetic agents on articular chondrocytes was increasingly noted with the use of arthroscopic pain pumps following glenohumeral arthroscopy(Busfield and Romero, 2009, Hansen et al., 2007, Solomon et al., 2009). Increasingly however studies are alerting the practicing clinician to the potential for toxic effects secondary to amide local anesthetics given as a single bolus injection. Most of these are laboratory-based studies. Although some have questioned the relevance given the long use of intra-articular local anesthetic without seemingly any complication the serve as a caution.

The aim of this section is to provide an over view of the basic science evidence on the potential for local anesthetic agents to cause articular chondrocyte toxicity.

2.3.1 In vitro reports

A number of different laboratory modesl utilizing cell lines from a variety of animal species have been used in the study of local anaesthetic toxicity. A toxic effect in canine chondrocytes exposed to bupivacaine 0.5% using a proven in vitro model by Anz et al. They reported an almost 100% reduction in cell viability after two days exposure to bupivacaine. Bupivacaine conferred an anti-inflammatory effect in their study, evidenced by reduced nitric oxide and PGE rise in the presence of interleukin-1, but their conclusion maintained that continuous exposure to bupivacine resulted in a clear toxic effect toward the canine chondrocytes(Anz et al., 2009). Again using a canine osteochondral model the toxic effect of bupivacaine was again confirmed, with or without the addition of methylparaben(Hennig et al., 2010). Exposure to the local anaesthetic alone for 5 or 30 minutes caused significant cell death, although this was only significant statistically at the 30 minute exposure.

Miyazaki et al demonstrated a concentration dependent reduction in bovine chondrocyte viability after treatment with lidocaine (0.125, 0.25, 0.5 or 1%) (Miyazaki et al., 2011). Glycosaminoglycan (GAG)content of the cells was also noted to be reduced as the concentration of the local anaesthetic was increased. GAG and lactate production were higher in the cells treated with 0.5 and 1% lidocaine. The authors felt that this finding conferred a reparative response by the cells.

Using bovine articular chondrocytes in alginate bead cultures Karpie et al exposed these to 1 or 2% lidocaine for 15 to 60 minutes(Karpie and Chu, 2007). A dose and time dependent increase in cell toxicity was reported. An intact surface on the osteochondral core or variation in the pH of the treatments (pH 7.4, 7.0, 5.0) failed to confer any protective effect (this is in contrast to other studies - see below). Others have also reported time and concentration dependent reductions in cell viability using a bovine disc model(Lo et al., 2009). In this case osteochondral cores were harvested from the radiocarpal joint of cows and these were treated with either lidocaine (1%), bupivacaine (0.25%) or ropivacaine (0.5%).

The toxic effects of bupivacine (0.125, 0.25 and 0.5%) on the the articular chondrocyte from a bovine cell line were well demonstrated (Chu et al., 2008). Cells were cultured in a 3-dimensional alginate-bead culture. Specimens were exposed for 15, 30 or 60 minutes and analysis was performed at 1 and 24 hours and at 1 week. A clear time and concentration dependent respose to the local anaetshetic treatments was observed. Treatment with 0.125% bupivacaine for 15 minutes was not significantly different to the saline control. Almost complete loss of cell viability was noted with 0.5% bupivacaine. Analysis of osteochondral cores with an intact superficial cell layer suggested that an the superficial layer of the articular cartilage provided some protective benefit when intact. This may be significant in deciding during surgery whether or not intra-articular analgesic agents are safe to administer.

To test the respective toxic effects on chondrocytes of lidocaine, mepivacaine and bupivacaine Park et al used an equine model (Park et al., 2011). Bupivacaine (0.5%) was the most toxic of the agents used with cell viability reduced to 29 +/- 8% after 30 minutes. Cell viability after treatment with saline was 96%. Lidocaine and mepivacaine were both less toxic with mepivacine exerting the least toxic effect of the three.

A number of studies have used human cell lines which is arguably more useful for the extrapolation of results into clinical pratice. Dragoo et al used a custom made bioreactor to mimic the metabolism of synovial fluid to simulate the use of a pain pump following arthroscopic surgery(Dragoo et al., 2008). They found that both lignocaine (1%) and bupivacaine (0.25 or 0.5%) resulted in reduced cell viability but that the rates of necrosis were noted with the presence of epinephrine. Cell viability was similar at 24 and 48 hours in the bupivaine group, but there was a greater toxic effect seen at 72 hours. Further work using the same bioreactor model demonstrated that epineprhine, at levels of 1:100000-200000, conferred no significant increase in cell death compared to acidic media with a pH of 4.5-5.0 and local anaesthetics in combination with epinephrine (Dragoo et al., 2010). The authors suggest that local anaesthetic agents containing epinephrine should be used with caution as these are often titrated to a low pH.

Syed et al reported significant toxic effects of bupivacaine either alone or in combination with triamcinolone in a monlayer culture model using human articular chondrocytes (Syed et al., 2011). When the treatments were administered to the osteochondral plug with an intact surface however, the toxic effect of bupivacaine in isolation was no more than that of the control - again suggesting there is a benefit to an intact articular surface with regard exposure to potentially toxic agents.

Using chondrocytes harvested from osteoarthritic human knees it was demonstrated that exposure to lidocaine, bupivacaine or ropivacaine for 24 or 120 hours resulted in significant levels of cell death(Grishko et al., 2010). In the lignocaine 2% group massive necrosis was seen at 24 hours. After 120 hours exposure there were significant dereases in cell viability in all treatments groups with the exception of those cells treated with 0.2% ropivacaine. As viability decreased a concomitant rise in cell apoptosis was noted.

Jacobs et al harvested human articular chondrocytes from the knees of human tissue donors or patients undergoing total knee arthroplasty(Jacobs et al., 2011). They treated the articular chondrcytes with either 1% or 2% lidocaine with or without epinephrine and used saline as a control. Cell death between 91-99% was seen for each of the three treatments. A prolonged exposure time was also associated with higher rates of cell death.

Ropivacaine 0.5% was found to be significantly less toxic to human chondrocytes than bupivacaine 0.5% (Piper and Kim, 2008). Normal human articular cartilage was harvested from the femoral head or tibial plateau in in patients underoing surgical procedures. Full thickness explants and cultured chondrocytes were treated with either ropivacaine or bupivacaine for 30 minutes. Cell viability in the explant cultures fell to 95% and 78% after treatment with ropivacaine and bupivacaine respectively. Viability in the cell cultures fell to 64% and 37%. The viability of the cells in the explant cultures treated with ropivacaine did not differ significantly to that in the controls treated with saline. Ropivacaine may therefore confer a much more acceptable risk than bupivacaine - an important consideration if using it as an intra-articular agent following arthroscopy.

However, others failed to find a difference between these two agents using a simple monolayer culture model. Both ropivacaine and bupivacaine conferred simlar toxic effects to the articular chondrocytes either in isolation or if they were used in combination with magnesium sulfate(Baker et al., 2011b, Baker et al., 2011d). Lignocaine combined with magnesium sulfate was less toxic than either ropivacaine, bupivacaine or levobupivacaine combined with magnesium suflate after an exposure time of only 15 minutes(Baker et al., 2011b).

A useful finding for the practicing surgeon in the studies that have assessed human cells in in vitro settings is the recurrent finding that ropivacaine is less toxic than bupivacaine(Baker et al., 2011b, Baker et al., 2011d, Piper and Kim, 2008). If ropivacaine confers a less toxic effect, then as long as it provides equally efficacious analgesic control, then these studies support its use. Notably, Piper et al also found ropivacaine to be less toxic in the explant culture with cells embedded in an intact matrix, potentially a better representation of the in vivo state.

2.3.2 In vivo studies

In vivo models shoulde in theory provide the best simulation of what may happen in pratcice. However, consideration needs to be given to the culture model used and also the species studied. Arguably the ideal model is unknown to date and no human in vivo studies at the time of writing have been able to demonstrate a lasting deleterious effect of local anaesthetic on articular chondrocytes.

The effect of a single intra-articular injection of 0.5% bupivacaine into a stifle joint compared to 0.9% saline control was studied(Chu et al., 2010). Six months following injection gross and histological appearances showed that the chondral surfaces remained intact. They diod note howeevr, that there was a reduction in chondrocyte density of up to 50% in the joint treated with local anaesthetic compared to the saline control.

In an in vivo rabbit study three groups recieved continuous infusions of either saline, bupivacaine or bupivacaine with epinephrine over 48 hours(Gomoll et al., 2006). One week after treatment the animals were sacrificed and osteochondral and synovial samples analysed. Bupivacaine with or without epinephrine resulted in cell viability reduction by 20 to 32%. Histological analysis was worse in both treatment gourps compared to saline control.

A similar treatment regime did not result in long term changes in articular cartilage(Gomoll et al., 2009). When the rabbits were sacrificed three months after the infusion of the saline of local anaesthetic there was no significant difference found between treatment and control groups. An increase in cartilage metabolism in the treatment groups was noted suggesting that the cartilage was undergoing a reparative process. This study provides conflicting information to the earlier one noted by Chu et al creating more difficulty in ascertaining the true chronic effect of intra-articular local anaesthetic use.

In another, histological changes in rabbit knee joint articular cartilage have been reported (Dogan et al., 2004). Knees were injected with either 0.9% saline, bupivacaine or neostigmine. Histological analysis performed at 1, 2 and 10 days confirmed more toxic changes in both treatment groups compared to saline control.

2.3.3 The mechaisn of local anaesthetic mediated chondroctoxicity

Despite a number of studies reporting the potential toxic effects the mechanism by which these agents exert their effect is uncertain. Mitochondrial dysfunction is thought to be a key factor in articular chondrocyte death(Grishko et al., 2010). Grishko et al demonstrated mitochondrial DNA damage and a reduction in ATP and mitochondrial protein levels in response to treatment with a variety of local anaesthetics at varying concentrations.

In another study cells exposed to lidocaine or bupivacine in isolation had rates of cell death just over 10%(Bogatch et al., 2010). When the local anaesthetics were mixed with the cell culture medium this rate rose to over 96% in each instance. Crystal formation was seen when the bupivacine was mixed with culture medium. Acididc phosphate buffered saline resulted in increased cell death only when the acidity was increased to a pH less than 3.4. Based on these results the authors propose an incompatibility between the synovial fluid and the local anaesthetic is responsible for the majority of chondrocyte death rather than the local anaesthetic agent itself.

3. Summary

A number of different agents have been trialed as intra-articular analgesic agents following arthroscopy in the lower limb. Many of the reported trials have focussed on the use of amide local anaesthetic sgents as these are the most widely used in clinical practice. Depsite multiple studies there is no agent that appears clearly superior to the rest. Bupivacaine or ropivacaine appear the most likely to offer the greatest analgesic control by this route and a small number of studies are supportive of a multi-modal infiltration. Magnesium sulfate for one may be an ideal synergist.

Although Townsend et al have offered evidence that intra-articular local anaesthetc can be avoided in knee arthroscopy without compromising analgesic control, the ideal mode of analgesic control in hip and ankle arthroscopy is still uncertain. Recent reports of chondrolysis in shoulder arthroscopy prompted a number of investigations in the potential toxic effect that amide local anaesthetcis may have on articular chondrocytes.

Ropivacaine appears to less toxic than bupivacaine and a combination of ropivacaine and magnesium has also been suggested as a more acceptable alternative approach to intra-articular local anaesthesia(Baker et al., 2011b, Webb and Ghosh, 2009). The potential diffculties in applying laboratory findings to the clinical setting has been noted(Webb and Ghosh, 2009). In the arthroscopic setting, a number of variables including the articular surface disease state, the dilutional effect of the arthroscopic fluid and absorbance of injected agents into surrounding synovium and adjacent soft tissues could all modify the effect the local anaesthetic has on the articular chondrocyte. The potential for toxic effects on articular chondrocytes by local anaesthetic needs to be further investigated.

4. References

Aasbo, V., Raeder, J. C., Grogaard, B. & Roise, O. 1996. No additional analgesic effect of intra-articular morphine or bupivacaine compared with placebo after elective knee arthroscopy. *Acta Anaesthesiol Scand,* 40, 585-8.

Al-Metwalli, R. R., Mowafi, H. A., Ismail, S. A., Siddiqui, A. K., Al-Ghamdi, A. M., Shafi, M. A. & El-Saleh, A. R. 2008. Effect of intra-articular dexmedetomidine on postoperative analgesia after arthroscopic knee surgery. *Br J Anaesth,* 101, 395-9.

Alagol, A., Calpur, O. U., Kaya, G., Pamukcu, Z. & Turan, F. N. 2004. The use of intraarticular tramadol for postoperative analgesia after arthroscopic knee surgery: a comparison of different intraarticular and intravenous doses. *Knee Surg Sports Traumatol Arthrosc,* 12, 184-8.

Anz, A., Smith, M. J., Stoker, A., Linville, C., Markway, H., Branson, K. & Cook, J. L. 2009. The effect of bupivacaine and morphine in a coculture model of diarthrodial joints. *Arthroscopy,* 25, 225-31.

Baker, J. F., Byrne, D. P., Hunter, K. & Mulhall, K. J. 2011a. Post-operative opiate requirements after hip arthroscopy. *Knee Surg Sports Traumatol Arthrosc,* 19, 1399-402.

Baker, J. F., Byrne, D. P., Walsh, P. M. & Mulhall, K. J. 2011b. Human chondrocyte viability after treatment with local anesthetic and/or magnesium: results from an in vitro study. *Arthroscopy,* 27, 213-7.

Baker, J. F., McGuire, C. M., Byrne, D. P., Hunter, K., Eustace, N. & Mulhall, K. J. 2011c. Analgesic control after hip arthroscopy: a randomised, double-blinded trial comparing portal with intra-articular infiltration of bupivacaine. *Hip Int,* 21, 373-377.

Baker, J. F., Walsh, P. M., Byrne, D. P. & Mulhall, K. J. 2011d. In vitro assessment of human chondrocyte viability after treatment with local anaesthetic, magnesium sulphate or normal saline. *Knee Surg Sports Traumatol Arthrosc.*

Batra, Y. K., Mahajan, R., Kumar, S., Rajeev, S. & Singh Dhillon, M. 2008. A dose-ranging study of intraarticular midazolam for pain relief after knee arthroscopy. *Anesth Analg,* 107, 669-72.

Bogatch, M. T., Ferachi, D. G., Kyle, B., Popinchalk, S., Howell, M. H., Ge, D., You, Z. & Savoie, F. H. 2010. Is chemical incompatibility responsible for chondrocyte death induced by local anaesthetics? *Am J Sports Med,* 38, 520-6.

Buerkle, H., Huge, V., Wolfgart, M., Steinbeck, J., Mertes, N., Van Aken, H. & Prien, T. 2000. Intra-articular clonidine analgesia after knee arthroscopy. *Eur J Anaesthesiol,* 17, 295-9.

Busfield, B. T. & Romero, D. M. 2009. Pain pump use after shoulder arthroscopy as a cause of glenohumeral chondrolysis. *Arthroscopy,* 25, 647-52.

Calmet, J., Esteve, C., Boada, S. & Gine, J. 2004. Analgesic effect of intra-articular ketorolac in knee arthroscopy: comparison of morphine and bupivacaine. *Knee Surg Sports Traumatol Arthrosc,* 12, 552-5.

Cepeda, M. S., Uribe, C., Betancourt, J., Rugeles, J. & Carr, D. B. 1997. Pain relief after knee arthroscopy: intra-articular morphine, intra-articular bupivacaine, or subcutaneous morphine? *Reg Anesth,* 22, 233-8.

Chu, C. R., Coyle, C. H., Chu, C. T., Szczodry, M., Seshadri, V., Karpie, J. C., Cieslak, K. M. & Pringle, E. K. 2010. In vivo effects of single intra-articular injection of 0.5% bupivacaine on articular cartilage. *J Bone Joint Surg Am,* 92, 599-608.

Chu, C. R., Izzo, N. J., Coyle, C. H., Papas, N. E. & Logar, A. 2008. The in vitro effects of bupivacaine on articular chondrocytes. *J Bone Joint Surg Br,* 90, 814-20.

Colbert, S. T., Curran, E., O'Hanlon, D. M., Moran, R. & McCarroll, M. 1999. Intra-articular tenoxicam improves postoperative analgesia in knee arthroscopy. *Can J Anaesth,* 46, 653-7.

Convery, P. N., Milligan, K. R., Quinn, P., Scott, K. & Clarke, R. C. 1998. Low-dose intra-articular ketorolac for pain relief following arthroscopy of the knee joint. *Anaesthesia,* 53, 1125-9.

Cook, T. M., Tuckey, J. P. & Nolan, J. P. 1997. Analgesia after day-case knee arthroscopy: double-blind study of intra-articular tenoxicam, intra-articular bupivacaine and placebo. *Br J Anaesth*, 78, 163-8.

Dalsgaard, J., Felsby, S., Juelsgaard, P. & Frokjaer, J. 1993. [Analgesic effect of low-dose intra-articular morphine after ambulatory knee arthroscopy]. *Ugeskr Laeger*, 155, 4166-9.

Dogan, N., Erdem, A. F., Erman, Z. & Kizilkaya, M. 2004. The effects of bupivacaine and neostigmine on articular cartilage and synovium in the rabbit knee joint. *J Int Med Res*, 32, 513-9.

Dragoo, J. L., Korotkova, T., Kanwar, R. & Wood, B. 2008. The effect of local anesthetics administered via pain pump on chondrocyte viability. *Am J Sports Med*, 36, 1484-8.

Dragoo, J. L., Korotkova, T., Kim, H. J. & Jagadish, A. 2010. Chondrotoxicity of low pH, epinephrine, and preservatives found in local anesthetics containing epinephrine. *Am J Sports Med*, 38, 1154-9.

Drosos, G. I., Vlachonikolis, I. G., Papoutsidakis, A. N., Gavalas, N. S. & Anthopoulos, G. 2002. Intra-articular morphine and postoperative analgesia after knee arthroscopy. *Knee*, 9, 335-40.

Elhakim, M., Nafie, M., Eid, A. & Hassin, M. 1999. Combination of intra-articular tenoxicam, lidocaine, and pethidine for outpatient knee arthroscopy. *Acta Anaesthesiol Scand*, 43, 803-8.

Elsharnouby, N. M., Eid, H. E., Abou Elezz, N. F. & Moharram, A. N. 2008. Intraarticular injection of magnesium sulphate and/or bupivacaine for postoperative analgesia after arthroscopic knee surgery. *Anesth Analg*, 106, 1548-52, table of contents.

Eren, M., Koltka, K., Koknel Talu, G., Asik, M. & Ozyalcin, S. 2008. [Comparison of analgesic activity of intraarticular lornoxicam, bupivacaine and saline after knee arthroscopy]. *Agri*, 20, 17-22.

Fagan, D. J., Martin, W. & Smith, A. 2003. A randomized, double-blind trial of pre-emptive local anesthesia in day-case knee arthroscopy. *Arthroscopy*, 19, 50-3.

Farouk, S. & Aly, A. 2009. A comparison of intra-articular magnesium and/or morphine with bupivacaine for postoperative analgesia after arthroscopic knee surgery. *J Anesth*, 23, 508-12.

Franceschi, F., Rizzello, G., Cataldo, R. & Denaro, V. 2001. Comparison of morphine and ropivacaine following knee arthroscopy. *Arthroscopy*, 17, 477-80.

Gomoll, A. H., Kang, R. W., Williams, J. M., Bach, B. R. & Cole, B. J. 2006. Chondrolysis after continuous intra-articular bupivacaine infusion: an experimental model investigating chondrotoxicity in the rabbit shoulder. *Arthroscopy*, 22, 813-9.

Gomoll, A. H., Yanke, A. B., Kang, R. W., Chubinskaya, S., Williams, J. M., Bach, B. R. & Cole, B. J. 2009. Long-term effects of bupivacaine on cartilage in a rabbit shoulder model. *Am J Sports Med*, 37, 72-7.

Goodwin, R. C., Amjadi, F. & Parker, R. D. 2005. Short-term analgesic effects of intra-articular injections after knee arthroscopy. *Arthroscopy*, 21, 307-12.

Goodwin, R. C. & Parker, R. D. 2005. Comparison of the analgesic effects of intra-articular injections administered preoperatively and postoperatively in knee arthroscopy. *J Knee Surg*, 18, 17-24.

Grabowska-Gawel, A., Gawel, K., Hagner, W. & Bilinski, P. J. 2003. Morphine or bupivacaine in controlling postoperative pain in patients subjected to knee joint arthroscopy. *Ortop Traumatol Rehabil*, 5, 758-62.

Graham, N. M., Shanahan, M. D., Barry, P., Burgert, S. & Talkhani, I. 2000. Postoperative analgesia after arthroscopic knee surgery: a randomized, prospective, double-blind study of intravenous regional analgesia versus intra-articular analgesia. *Arthroscopy,* 16, 64-6.

Grishko, V., Xu, M., Wilson, G. & Pearsall, A. W. t. 2010. Apoptosis and mitochondrial dysfunction in human chondrocytes following exposure to lidocaine, bupivacaine, and ropivacaine. *J Bone Joint Surg Am,* 92, 609-18.

Gupta, A., Axelsson, K., Allvin, R., Liszka-Hackzell, J., Rawal, N., Althoff, B. & Augustini, B. G. 1999. Postoperative pain following knee arthroscopy: the effects of intra-articular ketorolac and/or morphine. *Reg Anesth Pain Med,* 24, 225-30.

Hansen, B. P., Beck, C. L., Beck, E. P. & Townsley, R. W. 2007. Postarthroscopic glenohumeral chondrolysis. *Am J Sports Med,* 35, 1628-34.

Hege-Scheuing, G., Michaelsen, K., Buhler, A., Kustermann, J. & Seeling, W. 1995. [Analgesia with intra-articular morphine following knee joint arthroscopy? A double-blind, randomized study with patient-controlled analgesia]. *Anaesthesist,* 44, 351-8.

Hennig, G. S., Hosgood, G., Bubenik-Angapen, L. J., Lauer, S. K. & Morgan, T. W. 2010. Evaluation of chondrocyte death in canine osteochondral explants exposed to a 0.5% solution of bupivacaine. *Am J Vet Res,* 71, 875-83.

Izdes, S., Orhun, S., Turanli, S., Erkilic, E. & Kanbak, O. 2003. The effects of preoperative inflammation on the analgesic efficacy of intraarticular piroxicam for outpatient knee arthroscopy. *Anesth Analg,* 97, 1016-9, table of contents.

Jacobs, T. F., Vansintjan, P. S., Roels, N., Herregods, S. S., Verbruggen, G., Herregods, L. L. & Almqvist, K. F. 2011. The effect of Lidocaine on the viability of cultivated mature human cartilage cells: an in vitro study. *Knee Surg Sports Traumatol Arthrosc.*

Jacobson, E., Assareh, H., Cannerfelt, R., Anderson, R. E. & Jakobsson, J. G. 2006. The postoperative analgesic effects of intra-articular levobupivacaine in elective day-case arthroscopy of the knee: a prospective, randomized, double-blind clinical study. *Knee Surg Sports Traumatol Arthrosc,* 14, 120-4.

Jaureguito, J. W., Wilcox, J. F., Cohn, S. J., Thisted, R. A. & Reider, B. 1995. A comparison of intraarticular morphine and bupivacaine for pain control after outpatient knee arthroscopy. A prospective, randomized, double-blinded study. *Am J Sports Med,* 23, 350-3.

Jawish, D., Antakly, M. C., Dagher, F., Nasser, E. & Geahchan, N. 1996. [Intra-articular analgesia after arthroscopy of the knee]. *Cah Anesthesiol,* 44, 415-7.

Joshi, G. P., McCarroll, S. M., Cooney, C. M., Blunnie, W. P., O'Brien, T. M. & Lawrence, A. J. 1992. Intra-articular morphine for pain relief after knee arthroscopy. *J Bone Joint Surg Br,* 74, 749-51.

Joshi, G. P., McCarroll, S. M., O'Brien, T. M. & Lenane, P. 1993. Intraarticular analgesia following knee arthroscopy. *Anesth Analg,* 76, 333-6.

Juelsgaard, P., Dalsgaard, J., Felsby, S. & Frokjaer, J. 1993. [Analgesic effect of 2 different doses of intra-articular morphine after ambulatory knee arthroscopy. A randomized, prospective, double-blind study]. *Ugeskr Laeger,* 155, 4169-72.

Kanbak, M., Akpolat, N., Ocal, T., Doral, M. N., Ercan, M. & Erdem, K. 1997. Intraarticular morphine administration provides pain relief after knee arthroscopy. *Eur J Anaesthesiol,* 14, 153-6.

Karaman, Y., Kayali, C., Ozturk, H., Kaya, A. & Bor, C. 2009. A comparison of analgesic effect of intra-articular levobupivacaine with bupivacaine following knee arthroscopy. *Saudi Med J,* 30, 629-32.

Karpie, J. C. & Chu, C. R. 2007. Lidocaine exhibits dose- and time-dependent cytotoxic effects on bovine articular chondrocytes in vitro. *Am J Sports Med,* 35, 1621-7.

Kligman, M., Bruskin, A., Sckliamser, J., Vered, R. & Roffman, M. 2002. Intra-synovial, compared to intra-articular morphine provides better pain relief following knee arthroscopy menisectomy. *Can J Anaesth,* 49, 380-3.

Lo, I. K., Sciore, P., Chung, M., Liang, S., Boorman, R. B., Thornton, G. M., Rattner, J. B. & Muldrew, K. 2009. Local anesthetics induce chondrocyte death in bovine articular cartilage disks in a dose- and duration-dependent manner. *Arthroscopy,* 25, 707-15.

Lundin, O., Rydgren, B., Sward, L. & Karlsson, J. 1998. Analgesic effects of intra-articular morphine during and after knee arthroscopy: a comparison of two methods. *Arthroscopy,* 14, 192-6.

Middleton, F., Coakes, J., Umarji, S., Palmer, S., Venn, R. & Panayiotou, S. 2006. The efficacy of intra-articular bupivacaine for relief of pain following arthroscopy of the ankle. *J Bone Joint Surg Br,* 88, 1603-5.

Miyazaki, T., Kobayashi, S., Takeno, K., Yayama, T., Meir, A. & Baba, H. 2011. Lidocaine cytotoxicity to the bovine articular chondrocytes in vitro: changes in cell viability and proteoglycan metabolism. *Knee Surg Sports Traumatol Arthrosc.*

Niemi, L., Pitkanen, M., Tuominen, M., Bjorkenheim, J. M. & Rosenberg, P. H. 1994. Intraarticular morphine for pain relief after knee arthroscopy performed under regional anaesthesia. *Acta Anaesthesiol Scand,* 38, 402-5.

Park, J., Sutradhar, B. C., Hong, G., Choi, S. H. & Kim, G. 2011. Comparison of the cytotoxic effects of bupivacaine, lidocaine, and mepivacaine in equine articular chondrocytes. *Vet Anaesth Analg,* 38, 127-33.

Piper, S. L. & Kim, H. T. 2008. Comparison of ropivacaine and bupivacaine toxicity in human articular chondrocytes. *J Bone Joint Surg Am,* 90, 986-91.

Pooni, J. S., Hickmott, K., Mercer, D., Myles, P. & Khan, Z. 1999. Comparison of intra-articular fentanyl and intra-articular bupivacaine for post-operative pain relief after knee arthroscopy. *Eur J Anaesthesiol,* 16, 708-11.

Raj, N., Sehgal, A., Hall, J. E., Sharma, A., Murrin, K. R. & Groves, N. D. 2004. Comparison of the analgesic efficacy and plasma concentrations of high-dose intra-articular and intramuscular morphine for knee arthroscopy. *Eur J Anaesthesiol,* 21, 932-7.

Rasmussen, S., Lorentzen, J. S., Larsen, A. S., Thomsen, S. T. & Kehlet, H. 2002. Combined intra-articular glucocorticoid, bupivacaine and morphine reduces pain and convalescence after diagnostic knee arthroscopy. *Acta Orthop Scand,* 73, 175-8.

Rautoma, P., Santanen, U., Avela, R., Luurila, H., Perhoniemi, V. & Erkola, O. 2000. Diclofenac premedication but not intra-articular ropivacaine alleviates pain following day-case knee arthroscopy. *Can J Anaesth,* 47, 220-4.

Richardson, M. D., Bjorksten, A. R., Hart, J. A. & McCullough, K. 1997. The efficacy of intra-articular morphine for postoperative knee arthroscopy analgesia. *Arthroscopy,* 13, 584-9.

Rosseland, L. A. 2005. No evidence for analgesic effect of intra-articular morphine after knee arthroscopy: a qualitative systematic review. *Reg Anesth Pain Med,* 30, 83-98.

Rosseland, L. A., Helgesen, K. G., Breivik, H. & Stubhaug, A. 2004. Moderate-to-severe pain after knee arthroscopy is relieved by intraarticular saline: a randomized controlled trial. *Anesth Analg,* 98, 1546-51, table of contents.

Rosseland, L. A., Stubhaug, A., Grevbo, F., Reikeras, O. & Breivik, H. 2003. Effective pain relief from intra-articular saline with or without morphine 2 mg in patients with moderate-to-severe pain after knee arthroscopy: a randomized, double-blind controlled clinical study. *Acta Anaesthesiol Scand,* 47, 732-8.

Rosseland, L. A., Stubhaug, A., Skoglund, A. & Breivik, H. 1999. Intra-articular morphine for pain relief after knee arthroscopy. *Acta Anaesthesiol Scand,* 43, 252-7.

Samoladas, E. P., Chalidis, B., Fotiadis, H., Terzidis, I., Ntobas, T. & Koimtzis, M. 2006. The intra-articular use of ropivacaine for the control of post knee arthroscopy pain. *J Orthop Surg Res,* 1, 17.

Santanen, U., Rautoma, P., Luurila, H. & Erkola, O. 2001. Intra-articular ropivacaine injection does not alleviate pain after day-case knee arthroscopy performed under spinal anaesthesia. *Ann Chir Gynaecol,* 90, 47-50.

Solheim, N., Rosseland, L. A. & Stubhaug, A. 2006. Intra-articular morphine 5 mg after knee arthroscopy does not produce significant pain relief when administered to patients with moderate to severe pain via an intra-articular catheter. *Reg Anesth Pain Med,* 31, 506-13.

Solomon, D. J., Navaie, M., Stedje-Larsen, E. T., Smith, J. C. & Provencher, M. T. 2009. Glenohumeral chondrolysis after arthroscopy: a systematic review of potential contributors and causal pathways. *Arthroscopy,* 25, 1329-42.

Souza, R. H., Issy, A. M. & Sakata, R. K. 2002. [Intra-articular analgesia with morphine, bupivacaine or fentanyl after knee video-arthroscopy surgery.]. *Rev Bras Anestesiol,* 52, 570-80.

Syed, H. M., Green, L., Bianski, B., Jobe, C. M. & Wongworawat, M. D. 2011. Bupivacaine and Triamcinolone May Be Toxic To Human Chondrocytes: A Pilot Study. *Clin Orthop Relat Res.*

Tamosiunas, R., Brazdzionyte, E., Tarnauskaite-Augutiene, A. & Tranauskaite-Keraitiene, G. 2005. [Postoperative analgesia with intraarticular local anesthetic bupivacaine and alpha2-agonist clonidine after arthroscopic knee surgery]. *Medicina (Kaunas),* 41, 547-52.

Townshend, D., Emmerson, K., Jones, S., Partington, P. & Muller, S. 2009. Intra-articular injection versus portal infiltration of 0.5% bupivacaine following arthroscopy of the knee: a prospective, randomised double-blinded trial. *J Bone Joint Surg Br,* 91, 601-3.

VanNess, S. A. & Gittins, M. E. 1994. Comparison of intra-articular morphine and bupivacaine following knee arthroscopy. *Orthop Rev,* 23, 743-7.

Varrassi, G., Marinangeli, F., Ciccozzi, A., Iovinelli, G., Facchetti, G. & Ciccone, A. 1999. Intra-articular buprenorphine after knee arthroscopy. A randomised, prospective, double-blind study. *Acta Anaesthesiol Scand,* 43, 51-5.

Vranken, J. H., Vissers, K. C., de Jongh, R. & Heylen, R. 2001. Intraarticular sufentanil administration facilitates recovery after day-case knee arthroscopy. *Anesth Analg,* 92, 625-8.

Webb, S. T. & Ghosh, S. 2009. Intra-articular bupivacaine: potentially chondrotoxic? *Br J Anaesth,* 102, 439-41.

White, A. P., Laurent, S. & Wilkinson, D. J. 1990. Intra-articular and subcutaneous prilocaine with adrenaline for pain relief in day case arthroscopy of the knee joint. *Ann R Coll Surg Engl,* 72, 350-2.

Yang, L. C., Chen, L. M., Wang, C. J. & Buerkle, H. 1998. Postoperative analgesia by intra-articular neostigmine in patients undergoing knee arthroscopy. *Anesthesiology,* 88, 334-9.

Zeidan, A., Kassem, R., Nahleh, N., Maaliki, H., El-Khatib, M., Struys, M. M. & Baraka, A. 2008. Intraarticular tramadol-bupivacaine combination prolongs the duration of postoperative analgesia after outpatient arthroscopic knee surgery. *Anesth Analg,* 107, 292-9.

9

Multimodal Analgesia for Postoperative Pain Management

G. Ulufer Sivrikaya
Sisli Etfal Training and Research Hospital, Department of 2nd Anesthesiology and Reanimation, Istanbul, Turkey

1. Introduction

The experience of pain is complex, multifaceted, and "an unpleasant sensory and emotional experience," as defined in part by the International Association for the Study of Pain. It is a personal, subjective experience that involves sensory, emotional and behavioral factors associated with actual or potential tissue injury (Rawal). The differential behavior response to surgical incision can be influenced by many variables including global (i.e., personality, gender, age, cultural background, pre-existing pain syndromes, genetic makeup, kind and type of surgical approach, cultural background) and specific (i.e., fear, anxiety, depression, anger, and coping) psychological factors (Eccleston, 2001). Only by considering all concomitant factors can physicians provide optimal treatment.

Millions of surgeries are performed on an annual basis, necessitating the frequent use of acute postoperative pain management. There are many types of surgery and, with few exceptions, all are painful. Fear of uncontrolled pain is among the primary concerns of many patients who are about to undergo surgery.

One of the most important factors in determining when a patient can be safely discharged from a surgical facility, and that also has a major influence on the patient's ability to resume his/her normal activities of daily living, is the adequacy of postoperative pain control. Pain is a predictable part of the postoperative experience. Unrelieved postoperative pain may result in clinical and psychological changes that increase morbidity and mortality as well as costs and that decrease quality of life (Carr& Goudas, 1999).

The guidelines for acute pain management in the perioperative setting published in 1992 and 1995 (Acute Pain, 1992; American Pain, 1995; Practice Guidelines, 1995) promoted aggressive treatment of acute pain and educate patients about the need to communicate unrelieved pain. Nonetheless these guidelines appear to have had little influence on practice patterns or on improved pain control for patients. In a study of Warfield and Kahn (Warfield&Kahn, 1995) they found three of four patients reported experiencing pain after surgery, and 80% of these patients rated pain after surgery as moderate to extreme. Since their study, newer drugs, techniques and protocols for postoperative pain management have been developed, and minimally invasive surgical techniques, such as endoscopic procedures, are used more frequently. These changes in practice patterns thought that they could affect the management of postoperative pain and patient attitudes about pain. But in a recent study (Apfelbaum, 2003) that assessed patients' postoperative pain experience and

the status of acute pain management in a random sample, approximately 80 percent of patients said (not very different the previous study mentioned above) they experienced acute pain after surgery. The authors concluded that; despite an increased focus on pain management programs and the development of new standards for pain management, many patients continue to experience intense pain after surgery.
Effective and appropriate pain management requires a proactive approach using a variety of treatment modalities to obtain an optimal outcome with respect to facilitating rapid recovery and returning to full function, allowing early discharge from hospital, improving quality of life for the patient and reducing morbidity (Rawal). Protocols for postoperative pain treatment should be made with considering patients' needs, surgical indications, and institutional resources. It is important to use effective state-of-the-art techniques combined with hospital protocols for early rehabilitation and recovery.
Many options are available for the treatment of postoperative pain, including systemic (i.e., opioid and nonopioid) analgesics and regional (i.e., neuraxial and peripheral) analgesic techniques. Multimodal analgesia is achieved by combining different analgesics that act by different mechanisms and at different sites in the nervous system, resulting in additive or synergistic analgesia with lowered adverse effects of sole administration of individual analgesics (Kehlet&Dahl, 1993). It also refers to concurrent application of analgesic pharmacotherapy in combination with regional analgesia (Elvir Lazo&White, 2010).
This chapter's aim is to overview on the topic of multimodal analgesia for postoperative pain management and to provide an update on the drugs and techniques used for this approach.

2. Consequences of postoperative pain

When an appropriate analgesic treatment is not given for postoperative pain, various adverse effects might occur in the respiratory, cardiovascular, gastrointestinal, urinary, endocrinological systems, as well as in patient's metabolisms and mentality. These changes were relievable with application of appropriate types of analgesic regimens.
Postoperative pain, especially when poorly controlled, may produce a range of detrimental acute (i.e., adverse physiologic responses) (Vadivelu et al, 2010) and chronic effects (i.e., delayed long-term recovery and chronic pain) (Perkins&Kehlet, 2000). Good pain control after surgery is important to prevent negative outcomes such as tachycardia, hypertension, myocardial ischemia, decrease in alveolar ventilation, immobility, deep venous thrombosis and poor wound healing (Vadivelu et al, 2010; Nett, 2010).
Pathophysiology of acute pain, includes of changes in neuroendocrine, respiratory and renal function, gastrointestinal activity, circulatory and autonomic nervous system activity.
Unsufficient pain management can cause acute and chronic effects:

2.1 Acute effects

- Emotional and physical suffering for the patient
- Sleep disturbance (with negative impact on mood and mobilisation)
- Respiratory system side effects (leading to atelectasis, retention of secretions and pneumonia)
  - Decreased respiratory motion
  - Inhibition of cough and sputum excretion
- Cardiovascular side effects (such as hypertension and arrhythmias)

- Increased oxygen consumption (with negative impact in the case of coronary artery disease, leading to coronary ischemia and myocardial infarction)
- Impaired gastrointestinal motility (while opioids induce constipation or nausea, untreated pain may also be an important cause of impaired bowel movement or postoperative nausea and vomiting-PONV)
- Delays mobilisation and promotes thromboembolism (postoperative pain is one of the major causes for delayed mobilisation)
- Increased sympathetic activity
  - increased release of catecholamines (resulting increase in systemic vascular resistance, cardiac work and myocardial oxygen consumption associated negative effects in patients with coronary artery diseases)
  - reduced blood flow in lower extremities (resulting a higher risk of deep vein thrombosis)

2.2 Chronic effects

- Severe acute pain is a risk factor for the development of chronic pain
- Sleep disturbance (with negative impact on mood and mobilisation)
- Risk of behavioural changes (frequently in children for a prolonged period after surgical pain)
- Poor wound healing
- Delay in long-term recovery

Chronic pain is a potential adverse outcome from surgery. It is costly to society in terms of suffering and disability. For humanitarian and economic reasons, the problem of chronic pain after surgery should be addressed. In a review of Perkins et al. (Perkins&Kehlet, 2000) they showed there was a significant variability in the incidence of chronic pain among surgical procedures (i.e. 3-56% for cholecystectomy, 0-37% for inguinal hernia surgery, 11-57% for breast surgery). They concluded that chronic pain after surgery was common as that has been confirmed with another review (Camann, 1998). Another conclusion of this study is; the intensity of acute postoperative pain was one of the most striking predictive factor for chronic pain, especially following breast surgery (Elia, 2005), thoracic surgery (Carli F,2002; Viscusi, 2004) and hernia repair (Birnbach, 1989).

3. Multimodal approach to postoperative pain

Advances in the knowledge of molecular mechanisms have led to the development of multimodal analgesia and new pharmaceutical products to treat postoperative pain.

Postoperative pain treatment may not be enough to provide major improvements in some outcomes because it is unlikely that a unimodal intervention can be effective in addressing a complex problem such as perioperative outcomes (Boisseau, 2001; Kehlet&Nolte, 2001). The analgesic benefits of controlling postoperative pain are generally maximized when a multimodal strategy to facilitate the patient's convalescence is implemented (Kehlet, 1997). Pain involves multiple mechanisms that ideally require treatment using a multimodal (or 'balanced') analgesic technique (White&Kehlet, 2010) Principles of a multimodal strategy include control of postoperative pain to allow early mobilization, early enteral nutrition, education, and attenuation of the perioperative stress response through the use of regional anesthetic techniques and a combination of analgesic agents (i.e., multimodal analgesia).

The concept of multimodal analgesia was introduced more than a decade ago as a technique to improve analgesia and reduce the incidence of opioid-related adverse events. Multimodal analgesia is achieved by combining different analgesics that act by different mechanisms at different sites in the nervous system, reducing the incidence of side effects owing to the lower doses of the individual drugs (Buvanendran&Kroin 2009). For example, epidural opioids can be administered in combination with epidural local anesthetics; intravenous opioids can be administered in combination with Nonsteroidal Antiinflammatory Drug (NSAID)s, which have a dose sparing effect for systemically administered opioids. It also refers to concurrent application of analgesic pharmacotherapy in combination with regional analgesia (Elvir Lazo&White, 2010; Rawal).
In the literature some different definitions of multimodal analgesia exists. In some contexts, multimodal analgesia refers to systemic administration of analgesic drugs with different mechanisms of action, whereas in other situations it refers to concurrent application of analgesic pharmacotherapy in combination with regional analgesia. Multimodal analgesia is based on to choice paracetamol and NSAIDs for low intensity pain with opioid analgesics and/or local analgesia techniques being used for moderate and high intensity pain as indicated. (Elvir Lazo&White, 2010; Rawal) (Table 1)

<table>
<tr><th>Mild intensity pain</th><th>Moderate intensity pain</th><th>Severe intensity pain</th></tr>
<tr><td rowspan="3">For example:
Inguinal hernia
Varices
Laparoscopy</td><td rowspan="2">For example:
Hip replacement
Hysterectomy
Jaw surgery</td><td>For example:
Thoracotomy
Upper abdominal surgery
Aortic surgery
Knee replacement</td></tr>
<tr><td>(i) Paracetamol and wound infiltration with local anesthetic
(ii) NSAIDs (unless contraindicated) and
(iii) Epidural local analgesia or major peripheral nerve or plexus block or opioid injection (IV PCA)</td></tr>
<tr><td colspan="2">(i) Paracetamol and wound infiltration with local anesthetic
(ii) NSAIDs (unless contraindicated) and
(iii) Peripheral nerve block
(single shot or continuous infusion) or opioid injection (IV PCA)</td></tr>
<tr><td colspan="3">(i) Paracetamol and wound infiltration with local anesthetic
(ii) NSAIDs (unless contraindicated) and
(iii) Regional block analgesia
Add weak opioid or rescue analgesia with small increments of intravenous strong opioid if necessary</td></tr>
</table>

Table 1. Treatment options in relation to magnitude of postoperative pain expected following different types of surgery (by permission from Publisher AstraZeneca)

A lower incidence of adverse effects and improved analgesia has been demonstrated with multimodal analgesia techniques, which may provide for shorter hospitalization times, improved recovery and function, and possibly decreased healthcare costs (Buvanendran & Kroin, 2009).

To achieve a maximum short-term and long-term benefits from multimodal analgesic therapies, the pain management would be initiated as a preventive in the preoperative period continued in the early postoperative period and extended into the postcharge period for 3-7 days (Bisgaard, 2006; White et al, 2007). A deficiency in the design of many of the published studies involving multimodal analgesic therapies is that the drug regimens were not continued into the postdischarge period (Ma, 2004). For example, only immediate pre- and postoperative administration of the cyclooxygenase 2 (COX-2) inhibitor rofecoxib as part of a multimodal analgesic regimen in outpatients undergoing inguinal hernia repair provided limited benefits beyond the early postoperative period (White&Kehlet, 2007). However, when the COX-2 inhibitors are administered for 3 to 5 days after ambulatory surgery, (Gan, 2004; Joshi, 2004) the greater benefits were achieved with respect to clinically relevant patient outcomes (eg, resumption of normal activities) and improvements in pain control. Bisgaard et al (Bisgaard, 2006) concluded that a multimodal analgesic regimen consisting of a preoperative single dose of dexamethasone, incisional local anesthetics (at the beginning and/or end of surgery), and continuous treatment with NSAIDs (or COX-2 inhibitors) during the first 3 to 4 days provided the best clinical outcome. Moreover, recent clinical studies suggest that when classical NSAIDs or more selective COX-2 inhibiting drugs were administered for 3–5 days after ambulatory surgery, a significant benefit was achieved with respect to clinically relevant patient outcomes (e.g., resumption of normal activities) and improvements in short-term pain control (Gan, 2004; White, 2007).

A multimodal analgesic regimen should be adjusted to meet the needs of the individual patient by taking into consideration their pre-existing medical conditions, types of surgery, and previous experiences related to both acute and chronic pain management. Critical multimodal protocols must be designed based on surgical procedures and structural organization to warrant improved outcome including having minimum side effects related to the treatment and rapid returning to social life and daily activities (Fanelli, 2008).

Several multimodal approaches have been advocated based on different combinations of anti-inflammatory drugs, and regional anesthesia (epidural, peripheral nerve blocks, paravertebral blocks, and local injection/infusion of local anesthetics) (Buvanendran, 2010; Mathiesen, 2009). Although each of these drugs and/or techniques has been demonstrated as being effective in reducing the need for postoperative intravenous opioids alone, the evidence supporting specific combinations of drugs and/or regional techniques is still limited.

3.1 Multidisciplinary approach

Faster recovery, reduced hospital stay, and decreased length of convalescence can occur if multimodal analgesia is combined with a rehabilitation program that is multidisciplinary and multimodal (Gajraj&Joshi, 2005).

Treatment of postoperative pain requires good multi-disciplinary and multi-professional co-operation. Multidisciplinary team consists of the anesthesiologist himself has overall responsibility, pain nurse and specialist surgeon, sometimes pharmacist. In the ward the patient's physician and nurse, physiotherapist when needed are responsible for all care, in partnership with the pain team. The nurse is responsible to report the patient's intensity of pain to the physician and to treat the pain within the defined rules of the local guidelines. Also should pay attention to the effects and side effects of the pain treatment. The pain team nurse is the first point of contact while the anesthesiologist and pharmacist are available to provide specialist advice (Rawal).

All staff involved in the treatment of postoperative pain require regularly updated training emphasising the importance of team-working and co-operation. In this training programme the main headings should be included as; a. Physiology and pathophysiology of pain, b. Pharmacology of analgesics, c. Locally available treatment methods d. Monitoring routines with regard to treatment of pain and e. Local document for treatment and assessment of pain (Rawal).

It is important to understand of the postoperative pain experience from a patient's perspective, if health care professionals are to identify ways to improve care. In Apfelbaum et al study (Apfelbaum et al, 2003); when asked about attitudes regarding pain and pain medications, 75% of patients believed that it was necessary to experience some pain after surgery, and 8% of patients had postponed surgery because they were worried about the possibility of experiencing pain. Although most patients claimed to receive preoperative education on postoperative pain management, that study's findings suggested that a patient's real concern is not adequately addressed.

The patient himself and family members are also to be undertaken as the members of the multidisciplinary team. Education is an important role in this point. Patients are unlikely to be aware of postoperative pain treatment techniques and as the success of pain relief is influenced by their knowledge and beliefs, it is helpful to give patients (and parents in case of cognitively impaired, severely emotionally disturbed, children) detailed information about postoperative pain and pain treatment. Adequate information gives the patient realistic expectations of the care that can be provided (pain relief, not a "pain free status"). Patients who do not speak the local language, and patients whose level of education or cultural background differs significantly from that of their health care team need special concern. A preoperative discussion with the patient and relatives can be helpful about an effective postoperative pain management (Rawal).

It is important to emphasize the need for collaboration between the various health care providers involved in the patient's perioperative care (eg, anesthesiologists, surgeons, nurses, and physiotherapists) to integrate improved perioperative pain management strategies with the recently described fast-track recovery paradigms (White, 2007). This type of multi-disciplinary approach has been documented to improve the quality of the recovery process and reduce the hospital stay and postoperative morbidity, leading to a shorter period of convalescence after surgery (White&Kehlet, 2010).

3.2 Pre-emptive – Preventive analgesia

The concept of pre-emptive analgesia has its origins in the idea that painful stimuli, if not prevented by administration of preoperative analgesic drugs, could lead to spinal sensitization and neuroplasticity processes, resulting in increased pain intensity and duration after surgery. Many authors have studied the effects of different timing of administration of single drugs (*e.g.*, pre-, intra- or postoperative) and have reported no differences in efficacy (Moiniche, 2002).

This approach does not seem to offer any clinically significant advantages over so-called preventative multimodal analgesic regimens when an effective pro-active approach to pain management is initiated in the early postoperative period and extended into the postdischarge period (Sun, 2008). Starting with intensive pain therapy at the beginning and analgesia must be continued, using step-down techniques that involve a change in drugs or route of administration (*i.e.,* from the epidural and intravenous routes to *per os* administration) (Fanelli, 2008).
The main goals of preventive analgesia are: to decrease pain after tissue injury, to prevent spinal sensitization and to reduce the incidence of inflammatory or chronic pain (Senturk, 2002).

4. Drugs in postoperative pain management

Multimodal (or balanced) analgesia represents an increasingly popular approach to preventing postoperative pain. The approach involves administering a combination of opioid and nonopioid analgesics (and adjuvant agents) that act at different sites within the central and peripheral nervous systems in an effort to improve pain control, with fewer opioid-related side effects mainly sedation, nausea, vomiting pruritis, constipation (Elvir Lazo&White, 2010; Vadivelu, 2010).
The development of newer agents available for postoperative pain control opens up possibilities for newer combinations in multimodal analgesia. Multi-pharmacological therapy based on synergistic effects of two or more drugs gives better results than a mono-pharmacologic approach (Vadivelu, 2010).

4.1 Opioids

Opioid analgesics continue to play an important role in the acute treatment of moderate-to-severe pain in the early postoperative period. The problem about these drugs is the variety of perioperative complications eg, drowsiness and sedation, PONV, pruritus, urinary retention, ileus, constipation, ventilatory depression of them. These opioid-related adverse effects inhibit rapid recovery and rehabilitation (Buvanendran&Kroin, 2009; Vadivelu, 2010).
Their effects can be summarized as hyperpolarization of first- and second-order sensory neurons, with inhibition of synaptic transmission. They act by binding to μ receptors, which initially results in increased G protein activity; this, in turn, leads to K+ efflux and inhibition of Ca2+ influx into the cell. Opioids also stimulate the supraspinal descending inhibitory system, which further increases the hyperpolarization of second-order neurons by releasing 5-HT and glycine. Opioid receptors have been demonstrated *in vitro* in peripheral nerve terminals, but they are unable to influence the inflammatory reaction, resulting lack of effectiveness on postoperative pain during movement (Christie, 2000).
Opioids can be used in different ways; i.e intravenous, intramuscular, subcutaneous, transmucosal, epidural, intrathecal, transdermal. The most common route of postoperative systemic opioid analgesic administration is intravenous. When the most important source of nociceptive stimuli is visceral pain, good results may be achieved by intrathecal administration of small doses of opioids (Rathmell, 2005).
Patient controlled analgesia (PCA) optimizes delivery of analgesic opioids and minimizes the effects of pharmacokinetic and pharmacodynamics variability in individual patients. It can be programmed for several variables: demand (bolus) dose, lockout interval, continuous or basal infusion, and 4 h limit (Table 2). PCA provides superior postoperative analgesia and improves patient satisfaction when compared with traditional PRN analgesic regimens.

Drug *- Concentration	Bolus dose	Lockout interval (min)	Basal-Continuous infusion **
Morphine (1 mg/ml)	0.5-2 mg	5-10	0-2 mg/h
Fentanyl (0.01 mg/ml)	10-20 μg	5-10	0-60 μg/h
Alfentanil (0.1 mg/ml)	0.1-0.2 mg	5-8	
Sufentanil (0.002 mg/ml)	2-5 μg	4-10	0-8 μg/h
Meperidine (10 mg/ml)	5-25 mg	5-10	0-20 mg/h
Tramadol (4-5 mg/ml)	10-20 mg	6-10	0-20 mg/ml

* Individual patient requirements vary widely. Titrated loading doses can be used if necessary to establish initial analgesia.
** Continuous infusions are not initially recommended for opioid-naive adult patients

Table 2. Intravenous PCA Regimens

Opioid analgesics will likely remain the primary treatment option for patients who require rescue analgesic therapy in the postoperative period until more potent and rapid-acting nonopioid analgesics become available for routine clinical use.

4.1.1 Controlled-release opiods

Controlled-release opioids are not traditionally considered useful in the immediate postoperative period, but some studies have demonstrated that controlled-release oxycodone may be used for postoperative pain control when remifentanil is used for maintenance of anesthesia. Its preoperative administration leads to adequate plasma concentrations for postoperative analgesia and hyperalgesia treatment following short surgery (1-2 h) (Nishimori, 2006). In addition, controlled-release opioids are an optimal choice for step-down analgesia in the late postoperative and rehabilitation periods following orthopedic surgical procedures (de Beer J de, 2005).

4.1.2 Tramadol

Tramadol enhances inhibitory effects on pain transmission at the spinal level blocking nociceptive signal transduction both by opioid and monoaminergic mechanisms. Its opioid and nonopioid modes of action appear to act synergistically. The drug is available in formulations suitable for oral, rectal and parenteral administration. Tramadol has been shown to provide effective analgesia after intravenous and oral (in a few of newer clinical studies) administration for postoperative pain management. The main advantage of tramadol in postoperative analgesia is a relative lack of respiratory depression. The potential of abuse is also negligible.

4.2 Nonopioids

Opioid analgesics, once considered the standard approach to preventing acute postoperative pain, are being replaced by a combination of nonopioid analgesic drugs with diverse modes of action as part of a multimodal approach to preventing pain after ambulatory surgery.
Nonopioid analgesics are increasingly being used before, during, and after surgery to facilitate the recovery process especially after ambulatory surgery because of their anesthetic-and analgesic-sparing effects and their ability to reduce postoperative pain (with movement), opioid analgesic requirement, and side effects, thereby shortening the duration of the hospital

stay. Nonopioid analgesics will likely assume a greater role as preventive analgesics in the future as the number of minimally invasive (keyhole) surgery cases continues to expand.
Recent studies have confirmed that a rational combination of different nonopioid analgesics when given as part of multimodal analgesia reduces postoperative pain. The use of traditional NSAIDs, COX-2 inhibitors, acetaminophen, ketamine, dexmedetomidine, dextromethorphan, alpha2-agonists, gabapentin, pregabalin, and glucocorticoid steroids can provide beneficial effects when administered in appropriate doses as part of a multimodal analgesic regimen in the perioperative setting (Elvir Lazo&White, 2010).
Nonopioid drugs used in postoperative pain management can be classified as:

1. NSAIDs and COX-2 inhibitors
2. Acetaminophen
3. Paracetamol
4. Adjuvants
   a. Alpha-2 adrenergic agonists
      i. Clonidine
      ii. Dexmedetomidine
   b. N-methyl-D-aspartate antagonists (Antihyperalgesic drugs)
      i. Ketamine
      ii. Dextramethorphan
      iii. Magnesium
   c. Gabapentin-type drugs
      i. Gabapentin
      ii. Pregabalin
   d. Glucocorticoids
      i. Dexamethasone
   e. Newer drugs
      i. Capsaicin
      ii. Glyceryl trinitrate
      iii. Cholinergic drugs
         Nicotine
5. Local Anesthetics

4.2.1 NSAIDs and cyclooxygenase-2-selective inhibitors

NSAIDs are known to achieve pain relief by their effect on COX-1 and 2 with the various NSAIDs differing in the proportion to which they inhibit COX-1 and COX-2. They are acid compounds with analgesic, antipyretic and anti-inflammatory properties via inhibition of prostaglandin (PG) synthesis. Prostaglandins, including PG-E2, are responsible for reducing the pain threshold at the site of injury, resulting in central sensitization and a lower pain threshold in the surrounding uninjured tissue. The primary site of action of NSAIDs is believed to be in the periphery though recent research indicates that central inhibition of COX-2 may also play an important role in modulating nociception. NSAIDs inhibit the synthesis of prostaglandins both in the spinal cord and at the periphery, thus diminishing the hyperalgesic state after surgical trauma (Buvanendran&Kroin, 2009; Fanelli, 2008; McClane, 2010).
NSAIDs are administered orally, parenterally or by the rectal route.
NSAIDs are useful as the sole analgesic after minor surgical procedures. They provide moderate postoperative analgesia and thereby have a significant opioid-sparing effect of 20-

30% after major surgery (Power, 1999). This may be of clinical importance as NSAIDs may reduce the incidence of opioid-related side-effects (respiratory depression, sedation, nausea and vomiting, ileus, urinary bladder dysfunction and possibly sleep disturbances). Since the COX-2 enzyme, the primary target of NSAIDs, is inducible, it is not found in damaged tissues until a few hours following the onset of a noxious stimulus. This could explain the lack of efficacy of preemptive administration of these drugs (Ness, 2001).

NSAID use is not appropriate in all patients because of their age or renal or hematological status or because of previous dyspeptic symptoms (McClane, 2010). COX-2-selective inhibitors (celecoxib, etoricoxib, rofecoxib- is no longer in use due to adverse cardiovascular events-) have the advantage over NSAIDs in the perioperative setting of not increasing the risk of bleeding (Buvanendran&Kroin, 2009).

Many patients now receive a NSAID as a routine part of their postoperative analgesic management. Recent practice guidelines for acute pain management in the perioperative setting specifically state 'unless contraindicated, all patients should receive around-the-clock regimen of NSAIDs, COX-2 inhibitors, or acetaminophen' (Ashburn, et al, 2004).

4.2.2 Acetaminophen

Acetaminophen is antipyretic and analgesic but has little, if any, anti-inflammatory action. Its analgesic efficacy is not more than that of traditional analgesics; however, it has fewer side effects. Preparation of intravenous acetaminophen recently has been released in Europe. A 100 ml solution is presented as 10 mg/ml for administration over a period of 15 minutes. The onset of action is within five to 10 minutes, with the peak at one to two hours. Optimal analgesia for moderate to severe postoperative pain cannot be achieved using a single agent alone, but a balanced approach in combination with non-steroidal agents can result in up to a 40 to 50 percent reduction in opioid requirements (Vadivelu, 2010).

4.2.3 Paracetamol

Paracetamol has antipyretic and analgesic properties, but it is devoid of anti-inflammatory effects. It has an inhibitory action on central COX-2 and COX-3 enzymes, which would explain its antipyretic activity. The analgesic effect seems to be due to activation of descending serotonergic inhibitory pathways as well as inhibition of central NO synthases (Graham&Scott, 2005). Similar to other analgesic drugs, paracetamol shows differential properties in terms of pain control. Paracetamol may be more effective in treating episiotomy or abdominal pain rather than pain following orthopedic surgery or tooth extraction (Gray, et al, 2005; macario&Lipman, 2001). The different relative roles of peripheral COX enzymes in postoperative pain may explain these differing efficacies.

When paracetamol and NSAIDs are administered by an intravenous route, they show sparing effects on opioid consumption (about 25% and 30%, respectively); this effect begins 4 h after their first administration and is synergistic (Elia et al, 2005; Mirande, 2006).

4.2.4 Adjuvants

Adjuvant drugs are defined as substances that may improve pain treatment and pain control, but they are not commonly defined as analgesics. Adjuvants are compounds, which by themselves have undesirable side effects or low potency but in combination with opioids allow a reduction of narcotic dosing for postoperative pain control. Thus they can provide beneficial effects when administered in appropriate doses as part of a multimodal analgesic regimen in the perioperative setting (Fanelli et al, 2008; Vadivelu et al, 2010).

Multimodal analgesia incorporates the use of analgesic adjuncts with different mechanisms of action to enhance postoperative pain management. Adjuvants are important in postoperative pain management due to side effects of opioid analgesics, which hinder recovery, especially in the increasingly utilized ambulatory surgical procedures (Buvanendran&Kroin, 2007). Multiple adjuvants recently have been developed for the control of pain.

4.2.4.1 Alpha-2 adrenergic agonists

Alpha-2 adrenergic activation represents an intrinsic pain control network of the central nervous system. The alpha-2 adrenergic receptor has high density in the substantia gelatinosa of the dorsal horn in humans and that is believed to be the primary site of action by which alpha-2 adrenergic agonists can reduce pain (Buvanendran&Kroin, 2007).

4.2.4.1.1 Clonidine

Clonidine is originally classified as an anti-hypertensive drug with negative chronotropic activity, but has antinociceptive properties as well. In the spinal cord, clonidine acts at alpha-2 adrenergic receptors to stimulate acetylcholine release, which acts at both muscarinic and nicotinic receptor subtypes with analgesic effects (Fanelli et al, 2008).
Clonidine can be administered orally, intravenously, neuraxially or perineurally in combination with local anesthetics. However, the side effects could be significant. The most important ones are hypotension, bradycardia and sedation (Rawal). Data about the systemic administration of clonidine could support the usefulness of low-dose IV administration. Nonetheless due to the many side effects of systemic clonidine administration, the spinal route is preferred.
Low doses of clonidine proved to be a useful adjunct analgesic when given neuraxially and in combination with peripheral nerve blocks (Habib et al, 2005). Significant results in terms of block duration were obtained when clonidine was added to local anesthetics for epidural or perineural analgesia. At low doses (2 µg/kg), it was shown to increase the duration of perineural blockade. Animal studies suggest that the mechanism of clonidine's potentiation of lidocaine nerve block is inhibition of the hyperpolarization-activated cation current, not via its binding to alpha-2 adrenergic receptors (Jurna, 1995).

4.2.4.1.2 Dexmedetomidine

Dexmedetomidine is a relatively new, highly selective central alpha-2 agonist. Dexmedetomidine, when used as an adjunct, can reduce postoperative morphine consumption in various surgical settings using various routes such as intravenous (Dholakia et al, 2007; Gurbet et al, 2006; Lin et al, 2009). In a recent study the authors found that; the addition of dexmedetomidine to intravenous PCA morphine resulted in superior analgesia, significant morphine sparing, and less morphine-induced nausea,while it was devoid of additional sedation and untoward hemodynamic changes (Dholakia et al, 2007).

4.2.4.2 N-methyl-D-aspartate antagonists (Antihyperalgesic drugs)

With the discovery of the N-methyl-D-aspartate (NMDA) receptor and its links to nociceptive pain transmission and central sensitization, there has been renewed interest in utilizing noncompetitive NMDA receptor antagonists, such as ketamine, dextromethorphan, magnesium ions as potential antihyperalgesic agents.

4.2.4.2.1 Ketamine

Ketamine has been a well known general anesthetic and analgesic for the past 3 decades. There is evidence that low-dose ketamine may play an important role in postoperative pain management when used as an adjunct to opioids, local anesthetics, and other analgesic agents.

Ketamine, is the most commonly used antihyperalgesic drug. There is a definite role of ketamine in preventing opioid-induced hyperalgesia in patients receiving high doses of opioid for their postoperative pain relief (Mitra, 2008). It acts as an antagonist of NMDA receptors and may reduce the intensity of hyperalgesia following rapid μ opioid receptor stimulation by short-acting agonists such as remifentanil and, to a lesser extent, sufentanil and fentanyl. Perioperative administration of 2-10 μg/kg/min following a loading dose of 0.5 mg/kg decreases hyperalgesia and allodynia after thoracic and abdominal surgery (Bilgin et al, 2005; Joly et al, 2005), although doses may vary depending on the overall duration and amount of exposure to short-acting opioids.

Routes of administration include oral, intravenous,intramuscular, subcutaneous, epidural, transdermal, and intra-articular.

Clinical use of ketamine can be limited due to psychotomimetic adverse effects such as hallucinations, excessive sedation and bad dreams. Other common adverse effects are dizziness, blurred vision, and nausea and vomiting (Bell et al, 2006). Although high doses of ketamine have been implicated in causing psychomimetic effects, subanesthetic or low doses of ketamine have demonstrated significant analgesic efficacy without these side effects (Buvanendran&Kroin, 2009). It can be used in sub-anesthetic doses as an adjunct to provide postoperative pain relief in opioid-dependent patients (Mitra et al, 2004).

4.2.4.2.2 Dextramethorphan

Dextromethorphan has a similar mechanism of action with a lower affinity for the NMDA receptor. Following oral administration, it is rapidly absorbed from the gut and crosses the blood-brain barrier. A systematic review of perioperative dextromethorphan treatment for acute post-surgical pain concluded that the drug was a safe potential adjunct to classical opioid-based analgesia, but the results were inconsistent (Duedahl et al, 2006).

4.2.4.2.3 Magnesium

The magnesium ion was the first agent discovered to be an NMDA channel blocker. Similarly to ketamine and dextromethorphan, magnesium ions act by blocking the NMDA receptor pore. Since magnesium crosses the blood-brain barrier with difficulty in humans, it is not clear whether its therapeutic effects are related to NMDA antagonism in the central nervous system.

Several clinical studies have shown that magnesium increases postoperative analgesia, but the best dosage regimen remains to be determined (Lysakowski et al, 2007). At very high doses, perioperative intravenous magnesium sulfate has been reported to reduce postoperative morphine consumption but not postoperative pain scores (Koinig et al, 1998; Tramer et al, 1996).

4.2.4.3 Gabapentin-type drugs

Pregabalin and gabapentin bind to voltage-gated calcium channels in the spinal cord and brain. Both drugs are used for seizures and neuropathic pain. One advantage of pregabalin in clinical use is that it has higher bioavailability than gabapentin and linear pharmacokinetics. The gabapentinoid compounds have been used as part of multimodal analgesic in the postoperative period. Earlier clinical trials with gabapentin for early postsurgical pain have recently been reviewed (Buvanendran&Kroin, 2009).

4.2.4.3.1 Gabapentin

Gabapentin, a third-generation anti-epileptic drug, is a structural analogue of Gaba Aminobutyric Acid (GABA), an important neurotransmitter in the central nervous system. Its main action, however, is to inhibit the alpha2δ subunit of Ca2+ channels with a resultant decrease in neuronal hyperexcitability. During the immediate postoperative period, however, its activation of descending inhibitory pathways may be more relevant and might explain its synergistic effect with opioids (Hurley et al, 2006).

Most of the reviews and meta-analyses concur that perioperative gabapentin helps to produce a significant opioid-sparing effect and probably also improves postoperative pain score relative to the control group (Hartrick et al, 2009; Tiipana et al, 2007).

4.2.4.3.2 Pregabalin

Pregabalin a structural analog of GABA and a derivative of gabapentin (S+ 3-isobutyl GABA). It is a novel drug with a heightened research interest in the analgesic, sedative, anxiolytic, and opioid-sparing effects, in various pain settings, including postoperative pain.

Its main advantages may be faster onset and reduced adverse side effects. Some studies suggest pregabalin to have effective sedative and opioid-sparing effects (Hartrick et al, 2009; Mathiesen et al, 2008), useful characteristics for the control of acute pain. Research on its established role as an analgesic adjuvant as a part of multimodal analgesia for acute pain control is ongoing.

4.2.4.4 Glucocorticoids

Glucocorticoids, including dexamethasone, have been used to reduce inflammation and postoperative pain in surgical procedures (Salerno et al, 2006). Glucocorticoid steroids can provide beneficial effects when administered in appropriate doses as part of a multimodal analgesic regimen in the perioperative setting (White, 2005, 2007).

4.2.4.4.1 Dexamethasone

Dexamethasone is a synthetic glucocorticoid with high potency and a long duration of action (half-life: 2 days), and has low mineralocorticoid activity. Although dexamethasone reduces PG synthesis, its possible analgesic effects have not yet been demonstrated.

In patients undergoing total hip arthroplasty under spinal anesthesia with propofol sedation a single preoperative intravenous dose of dexamethasone decreased the pain upon standing at 24 h compared to placebo (Kardash et al, 2008). In a recent study, it did not reduce postoperative pain scores and analgesic requirements after laparoscopic cholecystectomy. The main advantage of postoperative dexamethasone is its ability to reduce postoperative nausea and vomiting (Feo et al, 2006).

4.2.4.5 Newer drugs

4.2.4.5.1 Capcaisin

Capsaicin (8-methyl-N-vanillyl-6-nonenamide) is a non narcotic and acts peripherally. It can be used as a cream and also as an injectable analgesic.

Capsaicin cream is usually combined with narcotic analgesics and NSAIDs to relieve a variety of painful ailments such as back pain, arthritic joint pains, and strains and sprains. Injectable capsaicin is used for the control of post operative pain, such as after total knee replacement, total hip replacement, hernia repair, shoulder arthroscopy, and bunionectomy (Aasvang et al, 2008). Pre-administration of neural blockade before injection of capsaicin may greatly decrease the burning discomfort.

Capsaicin appears to be a relatively safe drug. In the elderly who are sensitive to respiratory depression that can occur with opioids, capsaicin can be particularly beneficial as an adjuvant. The only absolute contraindication being patient hypersensitivity. Relative contraindications include age less than 2 years, patients with elevated liver enzymes, patients on ACE inhibitors, and patients showing signs of septic arthritis and joint infections (Vadivelu et al, 2010).

4.2.4.5.2 Glyceryl trinitrate

The organic nitrates, such as glyceryl trinitrate (GTN), act as nitric oxide donors.

High dose nitroglyserin patches, such as 30 mg daily, are hyperalgesic, whereas doses less than 6 mg per day are analgesic under different circumstances. Previously it has been observed that patients with past histories of angina who had spinal block, in which the nitroglycerin transdermal patch was applied prophylactically, required fewer analgesic after operation (Lauretti et al, 1999).

4.2.4.5.3 Cholinergic drugs

Acetylcholine may cause analgesia through direct action on spinal cholinergic muscarinic receptors M1 and M3 and nicotinic receptors subtypes.

4.2.4.5.3.1 Nicotine

In a study in nonsmoker patients having radical retropubic prostatectomy under general anesthesia, the application of a 7 mg nicotine patch 30–60 min before surgery for postoperative 24 hrs, resulted with lower cumulative PCA morphine consumption versus placebo group. But the intensity of nausea was greater in the nicotine group (Habib et al, 2008).

Table 3 summarizes the doses and routes of administration of frequently used drugs.

	Administration	**Dosage**
OPIOIDS		
Morphine	(i) Intravenous. (ii) Subcutaneous by continuous infusion or intermittent boluses via indwelling cannula. (iii) Intramuscular (not recommended due to incidence of pain. 5-10 mg 3-4 hourly).	IV PCA Bolus: 1-2 mg, lockout: 5-15 min (usually 7-8 min), no background infusion. Subcutaneous 0.1-0.15 mg/kg 4-6 hourly, adapted in relation to pain score, sedation and respiratory rate.
Codeine	Oral	3 mg/kg/day combined with paracetamol. A minimum of 30 mg codeine/tablet is required

	Administration	Dosage
OPIOIDS		
Tramadol	(i) Intravenous: inject slowly (risk of high incidence of nausea and vomiting). (ii) Intramuscular. (iii) Oral administration as soon as possible.	0.75-1.0 mg/kg 50-100 mg 6 hourly.
NONOPIOIDS		
Paracetamol	Oral	4 x 1 g paracetamol/day (2 g propacetamol/day). Dose to be reduced (e.g. 3 x 1 g/day) in case of hepatic insufficiency.
Combination of paracetamol and codeine	Oral	Paracetamol 500 mg + codeine 30 mg. 4 x 1 g paracetamol/day.
NSAIDs	(i) Intravenous administration should start at least 30-60 min before end of surgery. (ii) Oral administration should start as soon as possible. Duration: 3-5 days. (iii) Rectal	Ketorolac: 3 x 30-40 mg/day (only IV form) Diclofenac: 2 x 75 mg/day Ketoprofen: 4 x 50 mg/day (ii) Selective NSAIDs include: Meloxicam 15 mg once daily Celecoxib: 200 mg/day.
Acetaminophen	Intravenous	100 ml solution (10 mg/ml) administration over a period of 15 minutes.
ADJUVANTS		
Clonidine	(i) Oral (ii) Intravenous (iii) Combined with local anesthetics-neuraxially or perineurally	3- 5 µg/kg (oral) 1 µg/kg (intravenous) 1-2 µg/kg (epidural) or 75-100 µg (intrathecal)
Ketamine	Intravenous	Loading dose of 0.5 mg/kg followed by 2-10 µg/kg/min

* The doses and routes of administration of drugs described above are general examples and each patient should be assessed individually before prescribing

Table 3. The doses and routes of administration of frequently used drugs * (modified table by permission from Publisher AstraZeneca)

4.2.5 Local anesthetics

Sodium channel blocking drugs are usually used in the management of both acute and chronic pain. When dealing with postoperative pain, local anesthetics such as lidocaine and bupivacaine mostly preferred (McCleane, 2010).

Local anesthetics block sodium channels, thereby, preventing transmission of nerve impulse along the axonal fibre. This is a local effect at the site of injection. Tissue anesthesia occurs after the injection of the local anesthetics into tissue at appropriate concentration, but it lasts after the duration of the drug ended. However, local anesthetics are also absorbed into the systemic circulation from the site of injection and, depending on the dose and rate of absorption, may have systemic analgesic effects (Gupta,2010; McCleane, 2010).

Local anesthetic solutions delivered through an epidural or perineural route are the most important treatments for decreasing incident pain, hormonal stress and sympathetic responses during and after surgery (Chelly, 2001; Liu, 2007). Generally, higher doses are used intraoperatively and then reduced to reach differential motor-sensory block in the postoperative period. The best results are achieved when local anesthetic solutions are infused neuraxially with lipophilic opioids, such as sufentanil and fentanyl at adequate concentrations (George, 2006; de-Leon-Casaola&Lema, 1996).

In some studies the effectiveness of the intravenous infusion of lidocaine in reducing postoperative pain and facilitating the recovery process have been demonstrated (Kaba et al, 2007; Lauwick et al, 2008). Yardeni and colleagues (Yardeni et al, 2009) suggested that, perioperative administration of intravenous lidocaine could improve early postoperative pain control and reduce surgery-induced immune alterations. The injection of local anesthetic around wound edges has been proven to reduce postoperative pain, but only for the duration of that local anesthetic (Moinichi et al, 1998). Several concerns about these drugs have been expressed in the literature including the risk of infection, chondrolysis and systemic local anesthetics toxicity when they used locally.

The maximum doses for local anesthetics are summarized in Table 4.

Local anesthetic	**Maximum total dosage**
Prokain	400 mg
Chlorprocaine	800 mg
Lidocaine	4 mg/kg (without epinephrine) 7 mg/kg(with epinephrine) **or** 300 mg
Prilocaine	6 mg/kg (without epinephrine) 9 mg/kg(with epinephrine) **or** 500 mg
Bupivacaine	2 mg/kg (without epinephrine) 2.5 mg/kg(with epinephrine) **or** 150 mg
Levobupivacaine	2.5-3 mg/kg (insufficient data) **or** 150 mg
Ropivacaine	3-4 mg/kg (without or with epinephrine)

Table 4. Maximum doses of frequently used local anesthetics

5. Techniques in postoperative pain management

One approach for multimodal analgesia is the use of regional anesthesia and analgesia to inhibit the neural conduction from the surgical site to the spinal cord and decrease spinal cord sensitization (Buvanendran&Kroin, 2009). A variety of neuraxial and peripheral regional analgesic techniques can provide analgesia superior to that with systemic opioids and may even result in improvement in various outcomes. However, there are some risks associated with the use of such techniques. The clinician should evaluate the risks and benefits of these techniques on an individual basis in determining the appropriateness of neuraxial or peripheral regional techniques for each patient, especially in light of some of the controversies about the use of these techniques in the presence of various anticoagulants.

Neuraxial (primarily epidural) and peripheral regional analgesic techniques (e.g., brachial plexus, lumbar plexus, femoral, sciatic-popliteal, and scalp nerve blocks), also a variety of wound infiltration techniques may be used for the effective treatment of postoperative pain. In general, the analgesia provided by epidural and peripheral techniques (particularly when local anesthetics are used) is superior to that with systemic opioids, (i.e., superior analgesia and decreased opioid-related side effects) and use of these techniques may even reduce morbidity and mortality (Wu&Fleisher 2000).

Techniques used in postopetaive pain management are:

1. Neuraxial Techniques
2. Peripheral Regional Analgesia Techniques
3. Infiltration Techniques
   a. Wound Infiltration
   b. Topical Application
   c. Local Infiltration Analgesia
4. Other - Nonpharmacological Techniques

5.1 Neuraxial techniques

Spinal or epidural analgesia techniques in single or continuous forms can be used in postoperative pain management. The use of epidural anesthesia and analgesia is an integral part of the multimodal approach because of the superior analgesia and physiologic benefits conferred by epidural analgesia.

Among the most commonly used pain-relieving techniques, there is evidence that the epidural local anesthetic or local anesthetic-opioid techniques are the most effective on providing dynamic pain relief after major surgical procedures (Kehlet et al, 1999). Epidural local anesthetic application comes in as the major component of multimodal analgesia.

Postoperative epidural analgesia is usually accomplished with a combination of a long-acting local anesthetic and an opioid, in dilute concentrations (Table 5). Long-acting local anesthetics are preferred because they are associated with less tachyphylaxis. Thoracic epidural analgesia with local anesthetics and opioids for abdominal, thoracic and vascular surgery improves bowel recovery times while decreasing the risks of cardiovascular adverse events and of developing persistent pain (Liu, 2004; Nishimori et al, 2006;). In an unpublished study of ours (Sivrikaya et al, 2000), preemptive analgesia with epidural tramadol has supressed the peroperative stress response and also reduced the pain intensity in the early postoperative period in patients had abdominal hysterectomy under general anesthesia.

Maintenance techniques in epidural analgesia include:

Continuous Infusion: An easy technique that requires little intervention. The cumulative dose of local anesthetic is likely to be higher and side effects are more likely than with the other two techniques.

Intermittent Top-up: Results in benefits due to frequent patient/staff contact but can produce a high staff workload and patients may have to wait for treatment.

Patient-Controlled Epidural Analgesia (PCEA): This technique produces high patient satisfaction and reduced dose requirements compared with continuous infusion. However, sophisticated pumps are required and accurate catheter position is important for optimal efficacy (Rawal).

Local anesthetics / opioids	Ropivacaine 2% (2 mg/ml) **or** Levobupivacaine **or** Bupivacaine 0.1-0.2% (1-2 mg/ml)	Sufentanil 0.5-1 μg/ml **or** Fentanyl 2-4 μg/ml **or** Morphine 0.05-0.1 mg/ml **or** Clonidine 5-20 μg/ml (clinical application is limited by its side effects) **or** Epinephrine 2- 5 μg/ml
Dosage for continuous infusion (thoracic or lumbar level)	6-12 ml/h	
Dosage for patient controlled infusion (thorasic or lumbar level) **	Background: 4-6 ml/h Bolus dose: 2 ml (2-4 ml) Minimum lockout interval 10 min (10-30 min) Recommended maximum hourly dose (bolus + background): 12 ml	

* The tip of the catheter should be placed as close as possible to the surgical dermatomes: T_6-T_{10} for major intra-abdominal surgery, and L_2-L_4 for lower limb surgery.

** There are many possible variations in local anesthetic/opioid concentration yielding good results, the examples given here should be taken as a guideline; higher concentrations than the ones mentioned here are sometimes required but cannot be recommended as a routine for postoperative pain relief.

Table 5. Examples of local anesthetics and opioids and doses in epidural analgesia *
(by permission from Publisher AstraZeneca)

Continuous central neuraxial blockade is one of the most effective forms of postoperative analgesia, but it is also one of the most invasive. However, this technique remains the first choice for a number of indications, such as abdominal, thoracic, and major orthopedic surgery, where adequate pain relief cannot be achieved with other analgesia techniques alone. Continuous central neuraxial blockade can be achieved via two routes: Continuous epidural analgesia - the recommended first choice and continuous spinal analgesia - should be limited to selected cases only, as there is less experience with this technique.

5.2 Peripheral regional analgesia techniques

It is clear that local anesthetic techniques, particularly peripheral nerve blockade, will be one of the cornerstones of postoperative pain management. A variety of peripheral regional analgesic techniques (e.g. brachial plexus, lumbar plexus, femoral, paravertebral nerve blocks) as a single injection or continuous infusion can be used to enhance postoperative analgesia. Peripheral regional techniques may have several advantages over systemic opioids (i.e., superior analgesia and decreased opioid-related side effects). Also

the side effects associated with central neuraxial blockade, such as hypotension and wide motor blockade with reduced mobility and proprioception, and complications such as epidural Hematoma, epidural abscess and paraparesis can be avoided (Liu&Salinas, 2003).
Continuous peripheral nerve blocks are being increasingly used since they may provide more selective but still excellent postoperative analgesia with reduced need for opioids over an extended period (Table 6). The vailability of disposable local anesthetic infusion systems and the encouraging results from these early studies have led to the increasing popularity of these techniques for pain control in the postdischarge period (Elvir Lazo&White, 2010). This technique has become increasingly popular due to its ability to control moderate to severe pain and accelerate recovery especially after orthopedic surgery procedures (Capdevila et al, 2005; Ilfeld&Enneking, 2005; White, 2003).
Patient controlled regional analgesia (PCRA) can also be used to maintain peripheral nerve block. A low basal infusion rate (e.g. 3-5 ml/h) associated with small PCA boluses (e.g. 2.5-5 ml - lockout: 30-60 min) is the preferred technique (Rawal).

Site of catheter	Local anesthetics and dosage*
	Ropivacaine 0.2%-0.375% Bupivacaine 0.1-0.125% Levobupivacaine 0.1-0.2%
Interscalene	5-9 ml/h
Infraclavicular	5-9 ml/h
Axillary	5-10 ml/h
Femoral	7-10 ml/h
Popliteal	3-7 ml/h
Patient controlled regional analgesia	Background: 3-5 ml/h Bolus dose: 2,5-5 ml Lockout interval: 30-60 min

*Sometimes, higher concentrations are required in individual patients. As a standard, starting with a low concentration/dose is recommended to avoid sensory loss or motor block.

Table 6. Examples of local anesthetics and doses in continuous peripheral nerve analgesia and PCA (modified table after using by permission from Publisher AstraZeneca)

5.2.1 Paravertebral blocks

The evidence suggests that the use of paravertebral blocks provide effective postoperative pain control following breast and thoracic surgery as well as for inguinal hernia repair (Greengrass et al, 1996; Karmakar, 2011; Pusch et al, 1999). On their own, paravertebral blocks have been demonstrated to provide effective postoperative analgesia lasting up to 24 hrs (Chelly et al, 2011).
Chelly et al showed in their study that; a multimodal approach, including paravertebral blocks (prior to surgery), celecoxib (pre and post surgey), and ketamine (immediately prior to surgery), provides better postoperative pain control than PCA morphine alone in patients

undergoing open radical retropubic prostatectomy. This approach also allows a reduction in the postoperative need for opioids, lessens the related side effects (e.g., PONV, constipation, and bladder spasm), and facilitates earlier patient recovery which can be connoted that it fascilitates the patient's early recovery (Chelly et al, 2011).

5.3 Infiltration techniques

Local anesthetics can be administered for perioperative pain management via different routes (Table 7). It is crucial for improving the perioperative outcomes especially after day-case surgery (White&Kehlet, 2010).

	Local anesthetic	Volume	Additives
Intraarticular instillation			
Knee arthroscopy	0.75% Ropivacaine	20 ml	Morphine 1-2 mg
	0.5% Bupivacaine	20 ml	Morphine 1-2 mg
Shoulder arthroscopy	0.75% Ropivacaine	10-20 ml	
Intraperitoneal instillation			
Gynecological	0.75% Ropivacaine	20 ml	
Cholecystectomy	0.25% Ropivacaine	40-60 ml	
Wound infiltration			
Inguinal hernia Perianal surgery	0.25-0.5% Ropivacaine	30-40 ml	
	0.25-0.5% Levobupivacaine	30-40 ml	
	0.25-0.5% Bupivacaine	Up to 30 ml	
Thyroid surgery	0.25-0.5% Ropivacaine	10-20 ml	
	0.25-0.5% Levobupivacaine	10-20 ml	
	0.25-0.5% Bupivacaine	Up to 20 ml	

Table 7. Local anesthetic infiltration (by permission from Publisher AstraZeneca)

There are a few techniques for the delivery of the drugs locally into the tissues: intermittent injection, continuous infusion or a combination of two: Intermittent injections (also sometimes referred to as patient-controlled regional analgesia) have the advantage that pain relief can be timed in order to achieve maximal effect during the painful periods such as during mobilization. However, the disadvantage is that sleep quality may be disturbed, as patients sometimes wake up at night due to severe pain, which may be annoying and can also be a cause of patient dissatisfaction. Continuous local anesthetic administration has its advantage in that the patient has adequate pain relief most of the time. However, during periods of activity, the pain could be more severe, which may hamper mobilization. Methods using pumps that have a dual function with low-dose continuous infusion combined with self-administered bolus doses during mobilization are ideal. Several such pumps are available in the market today, including mechanical (elastometric) and electronic (Gupta, 2010).

5.3.1 Wound infiltration

Infiltrating local anesthetics into the skin and subcutaneous tissue prior to making an incision may be the simplest approach to analgesia. It is a safe procedure with few side effects and low risk for toxicity. Particularly, local anesthetic toxicity, wound infection and healing do not appear to be major problems (Buvanendran&Kroin, 2009).

Although the benefit of local wound infiltration has been documented (Barr-Dayan et al, 2004; Legeby et al, 2009; Park et al, 2002), controversy exists as to the appropriate timing of administering local anesthesia for surgery. A single injection of local anesthetics into the wound is unlikely to have long-lasting effects. Therefore, new techniques for wound infiltration have evolved during the last 10 years and several of them are today used routinely during ambulatory surgery and even in the inpatient setting. One such technique is the use of catheters inserted into incision, fascia, intra-articularly and intraabdominally for the intermittent injection or continuous infusion of local anesthetics and adjuvants for pain management (Gupta, 2010).

Continuous wound infusion of local anesthetics, which is mainly used in general surgery and orthopedics, is an interesting technique in postoperative pain therapy. Continuous wound infusion of local anesthetics is able to reduce postoperative opioid requirements and results in decreased pain scores (Gupta et al, 2004; Rasmussen et al, 2004). Recent studies indicate that rehabilitation seems to be enhanced and postoperative hospital stay may be shorter. Continuous wound infusion is an effective analgesic technique, which is simple to perform. Comparisons with other analgesic techniques, such as peripheral nerve blocks, epidural analgesia and other multimodal analgesic concepts are still required.

Hollmann and Durieux (Hollmann&Durieux, 2000) found that there was a reduction in ileus and hospital stay when lidocaine was given intravenously following major abdominal surgery. Therefore, when administered in larger doses during wound infiltration analgesia, it is possible that some of the analgesic effect seen is via systemic absorption and anti-inflammation.

Wound infiltration with local anesthetics is a simple, effective and inexpensive way of regimen which can be used in a multimodal analgesic regime without major complications. Nonetheless this technique still open some questions to be answered as; to the site of catheter placement, catheter type to be placed, the drugs and concentrations recommended, the technique of administration and side-effects of the technique, including toxicity of local anesthetics. Also it remains unclear as to whether this technique is useful in all types of surgery or should preferably be used for specific operations (Gupta, 2000).

5.3.2 Topical application

5.3.2.1 Local anesthetics

Lidocaine patches were applied to the wound area in the next two studies, and the evidence shows that these are particularly effective for wound pain when the patient coughes and they reduce the postoperative pain score at discharge (Habib et al, 2009; Saber et al, 2009). To place lidocaine patches over or at least close to the wound is suggested as a safe and promising modality to consider in the management of postoperative pain control.

5.3.2.2 Clonidine

Clonidine is an alpha adrenoreceptor agonist and these receptors are known to be located centrally. In a volunteer study (Pratab et al, 2007) clonidine had a significant peripheral action in enhancing duration of local anesthesia on superficial co-infiltration with lidocaine. Hence an opportunity with this co-administration to prolong the duration of pain relief apparent after postoperative wound infiltration could be possible.

5.3.2.3 Nonsteroidal anti-inflammatory drugs

The topical application of NSAIDs could produce significant pain relief as the systemic levels achieved by transdermal application. Topically use of NSAIDs has become popular in the ophthalmic field, in which it has been shown that topically applied NSAIDs can reduce postoperative pain and inflammation (Cho, 2009; Jones&Francis, 2009). In a study, the use of a topical diclofenac patch resulted with reduced wound pain and analgesic requirement in patients who have undergone laparoscopic gynecologic surgery (Alessandri et al, 2006). As a result NSAID patch formulations, to be placed directly over the wound, would have a useful pain-relieving effect. But there is still some studies needed to compare this application with systemic administration of the same drug and what the side effect frequency might be with such application (McCleane, 2010).

5.3.2.4 Glyceryl trinitrate

Experimental data suggest that the production of endogenous nitric oxide is necessary for tonic cholinergic inhibition of spinal pain transmission. In a study; transdermal nitroglycerin and the central cholinergic agent neostigmine have enhanced each other's antinociceptive effects at the dose studied (Lauretti et al, 2010). In two recent more studies transdermal nitroglycerin enhanced the analgesic effect of intrathecal neostigmine following abdominal hysterectomy (Ahmed et al, 2010) and intrathecal fentanyl with bupivacaine following gynecological surgery (Gang et al, 2010).

5.3.3 Local infiltration analgesia

The administration of large volumes of local anesthetics with or without adjuvants into different tissue planes perioperatively is called local infiltration analgesia (LIA) (Gupta, 2010).

It is a multimodal technique developed by Kerr et al. (Kerr at al, 2008) for the control of pain following knee and hip surgery. In their study it was based on systematic infiltration of a mixture of a long acting local anesthetics (ropivacaine), a NSAID (ketorolac), and adrenaline into the tissues around the surgical field (periarticularly intraoperatively and via an intra-articular catheter postoperatively) to achieve satisfactory pain control with little physiological disturbance. The technique allows virtually immediate mobilization and earlier discharge from hospital. A recent study by Essving et al (Essving et al, 2009) on unicompartmental knee arthroplasty performed with minimal invasive technique, using the LIA technique found significantly shorter hospital stay, lower morphine consumption and pain intensity compared with placebo.

5.4 Other – Nonpharmacological techniques

A number of non-pharmacological methods of pain management may be used in conjunction with pharmacological methods in the postoperative setting. These nonpharmacologic techniques, such as transcutaneous electrical nerve stimulation, acupuncture, psychological approaches (cold) and relaxing therapy and distraction, can be used in an attempt to alleviate postoperative pain.

5.4.1 Transcutaneous electrical nerve stimulation (TENS)

The use of TENS at paravertebral dermatomes corresponding to the surgical incision and/or acupoints has also been reported to improve postoperative pain management (Chen et al, 1998). Because this technique cause few if any adverse effects, its use as an adjunct to conventional pharmaceutical approaches should be considered as part of multimodal analgesic regimens in the future, particularly for patients in whom conventional analgesic techniques fail and/or are accompanied by severe medication-related adverse events (Chen et al, 1998; Usichenko, 2007; Wang et al, 1997).

5.4.2 Acupuncture

The term acupuncture describes a family of procedures involving the stimulation of anatomical points on the body using a variety of techniques. Acupuncture theory is based on two conditions: "yin," which is considered feminine, passive, dark, and cold, and "yang," which is masculine, aggressive, bright, and hot, as well as "qi," which is considered the vital energy that flows and cycles throughout the body. The acupuncture theory is to harmonize any imbalance in yin-yang and qi in a human body to restore the body to a healthy condition. Acupuncture is thought to unblock any obstruction to the flow of qi and, thereby, relieves pain.

Usichenko et al. (Usichenko, 2008) focused on randomized controlled trials of only auricular acupuncture (a popular method in which needles are placed in various parts of the earlobe) for postoperative pain control. They identified nine studies of acceptable quality (though none of the best quality), and concluded that the evidence that auricular acupuncture controls postoperative pain is promising but not compelling. Sun et al. (Sun et al, 2008) conducted a systematic review to quantitatively evaluate the efficacy of acupuncture and related techniques as adjunct analgesics for acute postoperative pain management. The authors concluded that perioperative acupuncture might be a useful adjunct for acute postoperative pain management. However, there are issues with applicability and generalizability of the procedure (Lee&Chan, 2006).

5.4.3 Cold

Iced-water or continuous flow cold therapy is used in orthopedic surgery after knee-surgery (Barber et al, 2000). It can be used both at hospital and at home. There are commercial systems, which are easy to use. The use of iced-water in other kinds of surgery needs further investigation.

5.4.4 Relaxing therapy and distraction

Music, or imagery, or hypnosis may have a positive effect in individual cases. There are commercial music CDs available for relaxation (Rawal).

6 Special aspects

6.1 Ambulatory procedures

The percentage of surgical procedures being performed on an outpatient basis continues to rise. Many more complex and potentially painful procedures in comorbid conditions of the surgical outpatients are being routinely performed in the ambulatory setting (White & Kehlet, 2010).

Postoperative pain management have some disadvantages in this population; a. pain after minor surgery or in ambulatory patients is more difficult to treat because many of the aforementioned techniques are not available or are too risky. b. The increasing number and complexity of elective operations that are being performed on an ambulatory (or short-stay) basis in which the use of conventional opioid-based intravenous patient controlled analgesia and central neuraxial (spinal and epidural) analgesia techniques are simply not practical for acute pain management. c. The pressure to discharge patients after surgery could limit the pain medications health care professionals are willing to prescribe and it may explain the inadequate management of acute pain after surgery.

Most common medical causes of delayed discharge after ambulatory surgery are; pain, drowsiness and nausea/vomiting (Vadivelu et al, 2010). Although many factors, in addition to pain, must be carefully controlled to minimize postoperative morbidity and facilitate the recovery process after elective surgery, the adequacy of pain control should remain a major focus of health care providers, caring for patients undergoing ambulatory surgical procedures (Elvir Lazo&White, 2010). Many patients undergoing ambulatory surgery continue to experience unacceptably high levels of pain after their operation. A survey by McGrath et al. showed that 30% of patients suffer moderate-to-severe pain following minor surgical procedures (McGrath et al, 2004).

To have a qualified postoperative pain control after ambulatory surgery, it is required that patient discharge is not delayed and that pain control remains effective once the patient is at home. It is important to avoid to use of long acting analgesics and to use regional anesthesia techniques for the anesthesia. Regional analgesia techniques offer a number of advantages for day case surgery patients such as: flexible duration of analgesia (with single shot techniques and/or with catheter infusions), flexible intensity of blockade (according to the type, concentration and volume of local anesthetic) and reduced need for opioids. Wound infiltration, intraperitoneal instillation, peripheral nerve blocks e.g. brachial plexus, paravertebral, femoral nerve blocks can be used in ambulatory surgery patients.

The adaptation of multimodal (or balanced) analgesic techniques as the standard approach for the prevention of pain in the ambulatory setting is one of the keys to improving the recovery process after day-case surgery (McGrath et al, 2004; White, 2007). Early studies evaluating approaches to facilitating the recovery process have demonstrated that the use of multimodal analgesic techniques can improve early recovery as well as other clinically meaningful outcomes after ambulatory surgery. These benefits have been confirmed in more recent studies (Elvir Lazo&White, 2010).

An aggressive multimodal perioperative analgesic regimen that provides effective pain relief, has minimal side-effects, is intrinsically safe, and can be managed by the patient and their family members away from a hospital or surgical center is the ideal one. Current evidence suggests that these improvements in patient outcome related to pain control can best be achieved by using a combination of preventive analgesic techniques involving both centrally and peripherally acting analgesic drugs, as well as novel approaches to administering drugs in locations remote from the hospital setting (White&Kehlet, 2010).

Nonopioid analgesics are increasingly being used as adjuvant before, during, and after surgery to facilitate the recovery process after ambulatory surgery because of their anesthetic and analgesic-sparing effects, their ability to reduce postoperative pain (with movement), and their opioid related side-effects (e.g., gastrointestinal and bladder dysfunction), thereby shortening the duration of the hospital stay and the convalescence period (White&Kehlet, 2010).

Patient-controlled regional analgesia (PCRA) encompasses a variety of techniques that provide effective postoperative pain relief without systemic exposure to opioids. Using PCRA, patients control the application of pre-programmed doses of local anesthetics, most frequently ropivacaine or bupivacaine (occasionally in combination with an opioid), via an indwelling catheter, which can be placed in different regions of the body depending upon the type of surgery. It is important to use suitable local anesthetics in low concentration and to inform patient adequately to avoid the risk of local anesthetic toxicity (Rawal, Vadivelu et al, 2010).

6.2 Stress response

Many detrimental pathophysiologic effects occur in the perioperative period and are associated with activation of nociceptors and the stress response. Uncontrolled pain may result in activation of the sympathetic nervous system, which can cause a variety of potentially harmful physiologic responses that may adversely influence the extent of morbidity and mortality (Vadivelu et al, 2010).

As afferent neural stimuli and activation of the autonomic nervous system and other reflexes by pain may serve as a major release mechanism of the endocrine metabolic responses and thus contribute to various organ dysfunctions, pain relief may be a powerful technique to modify surgical stress responses.

Systemic opioids (PCA or intermittent), NSAID, epidural opiod, lumbar and thorasic epidural local anesthetics are analgesic techniques are mostly used to supress the postoperative surgical stress responces but there is a pronounced differential effect of these various techniques on surgical stress responses (Kehlet&Holte, 2001). Any treatment with opioids, being epidural or PCA opioids, has very little effect on surgical stress responses and organ dysfunctions. Same applies to clonidine and also NSAIDs. Epidural anesthesia has the most profound inhibitory effect on surgical stress responses.

Several studies investigating lower extremity surgery have shown continuous lumbar epidural local anesthetic techniques to be most effective, probably because of a more effective afferent blockade. In abdominal procedures, there is a somewhat smaller efficacy of thoracic epidural local anesthetic techniques in modulating endocrine-metabolic responses, probably due to insufficient afferent blockade as well as the presence of other release mechanisms in eliciting the surgical stress response.

The neuraxial application of local anesthetics and opioids combined to general anesthesia (especially in patients undergoing major abdominal or thoracic procedures) as a multimodal strategy can provide superior pain relief, reduced hormonal and metabolic stress, enhanced normalization of gastrointestinal function, and thus a shortened postoperative recovery time, facilitating mobilization and physiotherapy (Schug&Chong, 2009). In a study by Sivrikaya et al (Sivrikaya et al, 2008) general anesthesia combined lumbar epidural analgesia can only partially attenuate the peroperative stress response and has some limited effects on recovery of gastrointestinal functions, nevertheless provided a better postoperative analgesia compared to general anesthesia alone. Epidural opioid techniques are less effective on the stress response, and are comparable with systemic opioid techniques and the use of NSAIDs. More data on the use of multimodal analgesic techniques with combinations of different analgesics are needed on this issue.

7. Conclusion

Postoperative pain is a complication of surgery, which, in turn, complicates recovery with functional impairment and drug-related adverse effects. Despite an increased focus on pain management programs and the development of new standards for pain management, many patients continue to experience intense pain after surgery.

Many factors must be considered before deciding on the type of pain therapy to be provided to the surgical patient. These include the patients' co-morbid conditions, psychological status, exposure to analgesic therapies, and the type of surgical procedure.

The multimodal approach may potentially decrease perioperative morbidity, reduce the length of hospital stay, and improve patient satisfaction without compromising safety. However, widespread implementation of these programs requires multidisciplinary collaboration, change in the traditional principles of postoperative care, additional resources, and expansion of the traditional acute pain service. Although a multi-pharmacologic approach may be universally recommended, drugs and their route of administration must be changed according to the type of surgery and hospital resources, and of course to the patient needs.

8. References

Aasvang E, Hansen J, Malmstrøm J, Asmussen T, *et al* (2008). The effect of wound instillation of a novel purified capsaicin formulation on postherniotomy pain: a double-blind, randomized, placebo-controlled study. *AnesthAnalg*, Vol.107, No.1(Jul), pp.282-91, ISSN 0003-2999.

Acute pain management: operative or medical procedures and trauma, part 1 (1992). Agency for Health Care Policy and Research. *Clin Pharm* , Vol.11, No.4(Apr), pp.309-31. ISSN 0278-2677.

Ahmed F, Garg A, Chawla V, Khandelwal M (2010). Transdermal nitroglycerine enhances postoperative analgesia of intrathecal neostigmine following abdominal hysterectomies. *Indian J Anaesth*, Vol.54, No. 1(Jan), pp.24-8, ISSN 0019-5049.

Alessandri F, Lijoi D, Mistrangelo E, Nicoletti a, *et al* (2006). Topical diclofenac patch for postoperative wound pain in laparoscopic gynaecologic surgery: a randomized study. *J Minim Invasive Gynecol*, Vol.13, No.3(May-June), pp.195-200, ISSN 1553-4650.

American Pain Society Quality of Care Committee. Quality improvement guidelines for the treatment of acute pain and cancer pain (1995). *JAMA* , Vol.274, No.23(Dec), pp.1874-80, ISSN 0098-7484.

American Society of Anesthesiologists Task Force on Acute Pain Management (2004). Practice guidelines for acute pain management in the perioperative setting. An updated report by the American Society of Anesthesiologists task force on acute pain management. *Anesthesiology,* Vol.100, No.6(June), pp.1573-81, ISSN 0003-3022.

Apfelbaum J, Chen C,Mehta S, Gan T (2003). Postoperative pain experience: results from a national survey suggest postoperative pain continues to be undermanaged. *Anesth Analg,* Vol.97, No.2(Aug), pp.534-40, ISSN 0003-2999.

Barber FA. A comparison of crushed ice and continuous flow cold therapy (2000). *Am J Knee Surg,* Vol.13, No.2(Spring), pp.97-101, ISSN 0899-7403.

Bar-Dayan A, Natour M, Bar-Zakai B, Zmora O, *et al* (2004). Preperitoneal bupivacaine attenuates pain following laparoscopic inguinal hernia repair. *Surg Endosc,* Vol.18, No.7(Jul), pp.1079-81, ISSN 0930-2794.

Bell R, Dahl J, Moore R, Kalso E. Perioperative ketamine for acute postoperative pain (2006). *Cochrane Database Syst Rev,* Vol.25, No.1(Jan), CD004603, ISSN 1469-493X(Electronic).

Bilgin H, Ozcan B, Bilgin T, Kerimoglu B, *et al* (2005). The influence of timing of systemic ketamine administration on postoperative morphine consumption. *J Clin Anesth,* Vol.17, No.8(Dec), pp.592-7, ISSN 0952-8180.

Birnbach DJ, Johnson MD, Arcario T, Datta S, *et al* (1989). Effect of diluent volume on analgesia produced by epidural fentanyl. *Anesth Analg,* Vol.68, No.6(Jun), pp.808-10, ISSN 0003-2999.

Bisgaard T (2006). Analgesic treatment after laparoscopic cholecystectomy: a critical assessment of the evidence. *Anesthesiology,* Vol.104, No.4(Apr), pp.835-46, ISSN 0003-3022.

Boisseau N, Rabary O, Padovani B, Staccini P, *et al* (2001). Improvement of 'dynamic analgesia' does not decrease atelectasis after thoracotomy. *Br J Anaesth,* Vol.87, No.4(Oct), pp.564-9, ISSN 0007-0912.

Buvanendran A, Kroin J (2007). Useful adjuvants for postoperative pain management. *Best Pract Res Clin Anaesthesiol,* Vol.21, No.1(Mar), pp.31-49, ISSN 1521-6896.

Buvanendran A, Kroin JS (2009). Multimodal analgesia for controlling acute postoperative pain. *Curr Opin Anaesthesiol,* Vol.22, No.5(Oct), pp.588-93, Review, ISSN 0952-7907.

Buvanendran A, Kroin JS, Della Valle CJ, Kari M, *et al* (2010). Perioperative oral pregabalin reduces chronic pain after total knee arthroplasty: a prospective, randomized, controlled trial. *Anesth Analg,* Vol.110, No.1(Jan), pp.199-207, ISSN 0003-2999.

Camann W, Abouleish A, Eisenach J, Hood D, *et al* (1998). Intrathecal sufentanil and epidural bupivacaine for labor analgesia: dose-response of individual agents and in combination. *Reg Anesth Pain Med,* Vol.23, No.5(Sep-Oct), pp.457-62, ISSN 0952-7907.

Capdevila X, Pirat P, Bringuier S, Gaertner R, *et al* (2005). Continuous peripheral nerve blocks in hospital wards after orthopedic surgery: a multicenter prospective analysis of the quality of postoperative analgesia and complications in 1,416 patients. *Anesthesiology,* Vol.103, No.5(Nov), pp.1035-45, ISSN 0003-3022.

Carli F, Mayo N, Klubien K, Schricker T, *et al* (2002). Epidural analgesia enhances functional exercise capacity and health-related quality of life after colonic surgery: results of a randomized trial. *Anesthesiology,* Vol.97, No.3(Sep), pp.540-9, ISSN 0003-3022.

Carr DB, Goudas LC (1999). Acute pain. *Lancet,* Vol.353(9169), No.12(Jun), pp.2051-8, Review, ISSN 0140-6736.

Chelly JE (2001). General concepts and indications. In: Chelly JE, Casati A, Fanelli G, editors. Continuous peripheral nerve block techniques. London: Mosby, pp.11-21.

Chelly JE, Ploskanych T, Dai F, Nelson JB (2011). Multimodal analgesic approach incorporating paravertebral blocks for open radical retropubic prostatectomy: a randomized double-blind placebo-controlled study. *Can J Anaesth*, Vol.58, No.4(Apr), pp.371-8, ISSN 0832-610X.

Chen L, Tang J, White PF, Sloninsky A, *et al* (1998). The effect of location of transcutaneous electrical nerve stimulation on postoperative opioid analgesic requirement: acupoint versus nonacupoint stimulation. *Anesth Analg*, Vol.87, No.5(Nov), pp.1129-34, ISSN 0003-2999.

Cho H, Wolf KJ, Wolf EJ (2009). Management of ocular inflammation and pain following cataract surgery: focus on bromfenac ophthalmic solution. *Clin Ophthalmol*, Vol.3, pp.199-210, ISSN 1177-5467.

Christie MJ, Connor M, Vaughan CW, Ingram SL, *et al* (2000). Cellular actions of opioids and other analgesics: implications for synergism in pain relief. *Clin Exp Pharmacol Physiol*, Vol.27, No.7(Jul), pp.520-3, ISSN 0305-1870.

de Beer Jde V, Winemaker MJ, Donnelly GA, Miceli PC, *et al* (2005). Efficacy and safety of controlled release oxycodone and standard therapies for postoperative pain after knee or hip replacement. *Can J Surg*, Vol.48, No.4(Aug), pp.277-83, ISSN 0008-428X.

de Leon-Casasola OA, Lema MJ (1996). Postoperative epidural opioid analgesia: what are the choices? *Anesth Analg*, Vol.83, No.4(Oct), pp.867-75, ISSN 0003-2999.

Dholakia C, Beverstein G, Garren M, Nemergut C, *et al* (2007). The impact of perioperative dexmedetomidine infusion on postoperative narcotic use and duration of stay after laparoscopic bariatric surgery. *J Gastrointest Surg*, Vol.11, No.11(Nov), pp.1556-9, ISSN 1091-255X.

Dolin SJ, Cashman JN, Bland JM (2009). Effectiveness of acute postoperative pain management: I. Evidence from published data. *Br J Anaesth*, Vol.89, No.3(Sep), pp.409-23, ISSN 0007-0912.

Duedahl TH, Romsing J, Moiniche S, Dahl JB (2006). A qualitative systematic review of peri-operative dextromethorphan in post-operative pain. *Acta Anaesthesiol Scand*, Vol.50, No.1(Jan), pp.1-13, ISSN 0001-5172.

Eccleston C (2001). Role of psychology in pain management. *Br J Anaesth*, Vol.87, No.1(Jul), pp.144-52, Review, ISSN 0007-0912.

Elia N, Lysakowski C, Tramèr MR (2005). Does multimodal analgesia with acetaminophen, nonsteroidal antiinflammatory drugs, or selective cyclooxygenase-2 inhibitors and patient-controlled analgesia morphine offer advantages over morphine alone? Meta-analyses of randomized trials. *Anesthesiology*, Vol.103, No.6(Dec), pp.1296-304, ISSN 0003-3022.

Elvir-Lazo OL, White PF (2010). Postoperative pain management after ambulatory surgery: role of multimodal analgesia. *Anesthesiol Clin*, Vol.28, No.2(Jun), pp.217-24, ISSN 1932-2275.

Essving P, Axelsson K, Kjellberg J, Wallgren O, *et al* (2009). Reduced hospital stay, morphine consumption, and pain intensity with local infiltration analgesia after unicompartmental knee arthroplasty. *Acta Orthop*, Vol.80, No.2(Apr), pp.213-9, ISSN 1745-3674.

Fanelli G, Berti M, Baciarello M (2008). Updating postoperative pain management: from multimodal to context-sensitive treatment. *Minerva Anestesiol*, Vol.74, No.9, pp 489-500, ISSN 0375-9393.

Feo CV, Sortini D, Ragazzi R, De Palma M, *et al* (2006). Randomized clinical trial of the effect of preoperative dexamethasone on nausea and vomiting after laparoscopic cholecystectomy. *Br J Surg*, Vol.93, No.3(Mar), pp.295-9, ISSN 0007-1323.

Gajraj N, Joshi G (2005). Role of cyclooxygenase-2 inhibitors in postoperative pain management. *Anesthesiol Clin North America*, Vol.23, No.1(Mar), pp.49-72, ISSN 0889-8537.

Gan TJ, Joshi GP, Viscusi E, Cheung RY, *et al* (2004). Preoperative parenteral parecoxib and follow-up oral valdecoxib reduce length of stay and improve quality of patient recovery after laparoscopic cholecystectomy surgery. *Anesth Analg*, Vol.98, No.6(Jun), pp.1665-73, ISSN 0889-8537.

Garg A, Ahmed F, Khandelwal M, Chawla V, *et al* (2010). The effect of transdermal nitroglycerine on intrathecal fentanyl with bupivacaine for postoperative analgesia following gynaecological surgery. *Anaesth Intensive Care*, Vol.38, No.2(Mar), pp.285-90, ISSN 0310-057X.

George MJ (2006). The site of action of epidurally administered opioids and its relevance to postoperative pain management. *Anaesthesia*, Vol.61, No.1(Jul), pp.659-64, ISSN 0003-2409.

Graham GG, Scott KF (2005). Mechanism of action of paracetamol. *Am J Ther*, Vol.12, No.1(Jan-Feb), pp.46-55, ISSN 1075-2765.

Gray A, Kehlet H, Bonnet F, Rawal N (2005). Predicting postoperative analgesia outcomes: NNT league tables or procedure-specific evidence? *Br J Anaesth*, Vol.94, No.6(Jun), pp.710-4, ISSN 0007-0912.

Greengrass R, O'Brien F, Lyerly K, Hardman D, *et al* (1996). Paravertebral block for breast cancer surgery. *Can J Anaesth*, Vol.43, No.8(Aug), pp.858-61, ISSN 0832-610X.

Gupta A, Perniola A, Axelsson K, Thörn SE, *et al* (2004). Postoperative pain after abdominal hysterectomy: a double-blind comparison between placebo and local anesthetic infused intraperitoneally. *Anesth Analg*, Vol.99, No.4(Oct), pp.1173-9, ISSN 0003-2999.

Gupta A (2010). Wound infiltration with local anaesthetics in ambulatory surgery. *Curr Opin Anaesthesiol*, Vol.23, No.6(dec), pp.708-13, Review, ISSN 0952-7907.

Gurbet A, Basagan-Mogol E, Turker G, Ugun F, *et al* (2006). Intraoperative infusion of dexmedetomidine reduces perioperative analgesic requirements. *Can J Anaesth*, Vol.53, No.7(Jul), pp.646-52, ISSN 0832-610X.

Habib A, Gan T (2005). Role of analgesic adjuncts in postoperative pain management. *Anesthesiol Clin North America*, Vol.23, No.1(Mar), pp.85-107, ISSN 0889-8537.

Habib AS, White WD, El Gasim MA, Saleh G, *et al* (2008). Transdermal nicotine for analgesia after radical retropubic prostatectomy. *Anesth Analg*, Vol.107, No.3(Sep), pp.999-1004, ISSN 0003-2999.

Habib AS, Polascik TJ, Weizer AZ, White WD, *et al* (2009). Lidocaine patch for postoperative analgesia after radical retropubic prostatectomy. *Anesth Analg*, Vol.108, No.6(Jun), pp.1950-53, ISSN 0003-2999.

Hartrick C, Van Hove I, Stegmann J, Oh C, *et al* (2009). Efficacy and tolerability of tapentadol immediate release and oxycodone HCl immediate release in patients awaiting primary joint replacement surgery for end-stage joint disease: a 10-day, phase III, randomized, double-blind, active- and placebo-controlled study. *Clin Ther*, Vol.31, No.2(Feb), pp.260-71, ISSN 0149-2918.

Hollmann MW, Durieux ME (2000). Local anesthetics and the inflammatory response: a new therapeutic indication? *Anesthesiology*, Vol.93, No.3(Sep), pp.858-75, ISSN 0003-3022.

Hurley RW, Cohen SP, Williams KA, Rowlingson AJ, *et al* (2006). The analgesic effects of perioperative gabapentin on postoperative pain: a meta-analysis. *Reg Anesth Pain Med*, Vol.31, No.3(May-Jun), pp.237-47, ISSN 1098-7339.

Ilfeld BM, Enneking FK (2005). Continuous peripheral nerve blocks at home: a review. *Anesth Analg* , Vol.100, No.6(Jun), pp.1822-33, Review, ISSN 0003-2999.

Joly V, Richebe P, Guignard B, Fletcher D, *et al* (2005). Remifentanil-induced postoperative hyperalgesia and its prevention with small-dose ketamine. *Anesthesiology*, Vol.103, No.1(Jul), pp.147-55, ISSN 0003-3022.

Jones J, Francis P (2009). Ophthalmic utility of topical bromfenac, a twice-daily nonsteroidal anti-inflammatory agent. *Expert Opin Pharmacother*, Vol.10, No.14(Oct), pp.2379-85, ISSN 1465-6566.

Joshi GP, Viscusi ER, Gan TJ, Minkowitz H, *et al* (2004). Effective treatment of laparoscopic cholecystectomy pain with intravenous followed by oral COX-2 specific inhibitor. *Anesth Analg*, Vol.98, No.2(Feb), pp.336-42, ISSN 0003-2999.

Jurna I (1995). [Antinociceptive effects of alpha(2)-adrenoceptor agonists ("analgesic" actions in animal experiments)agonists ("analgesic" actions in animal experiments).]. *Schmerz*, Vol.9, No.6(Nov), pp.286-92, ISSN 0932-433X.

Kaba A, Laurent SR, Detroz BJ, Sessler DI, *et al* (2007). Intravenous lidocaine infusion facilitates acute rehabilitation after laparoscopic colectomy. *Anesthesiology*, Vol.106, No.1(Jan), pp.11-8, ISSN 0003-3022.

Kardash KJ, Sarrazin F, Tessler MJ, Velly AM (2008). Single-dose dexamethasone reduces dynamic pain after total hip arthroplasty. *Anesth Analg*, Vol.106, No.4(Apr), pp.1253-57, ISSN 0003-2999.

Karmakar MK (2001). Thoracic paravertebral block. *Anesthesiology*, Vol.95, No.3(Sep), pp.771-80, Review, ISSN 0003-3022.

Kehlet H, Dahl JB (1993). The value of multimodal or balanced analgesia in the postoperative pain treatment. *Anesth Analg*, Vol.77, No.5(Nov), pp. 1048-56, Review, ISSN 0003-2999.

Kehlet H (1997). Multimodal approach to control postoperative pathophysiology and rehabilitation. *Br J Anaesth*, Vol.78, No.5(May), pp.606-17, ISSN 0007-0912.

Kehlet H, Werner M, Perkins F (1999). Balanced analgesia: what is it and what are its advantages in postoperative pain? *Drugs*, Vol.58, No.5(Nov), pp.793-7, ISSN 0012-6667.

Kehlet H, Holte K (2001). Effect of postoperative analgesia on surgical outcome. *Br J Anaesth*, Vol.87, No.1(Jul), pp.62-72, Review, ISSN 0007-0912.

Kerr DR, Kohan L (2008). Local infiltration analgesia: a technique for the control of acute postoperative pain following knee and hip surgery: a case study of 325 patients. *Acta Orthop*, Vol.79, No.2(Apr), pp.174-83, ISSN 1745-3674.

Koinig H, Wallner T, Marhofer P, Andel H, *et al* (1998). Magnesium sulfate reduces intra- and postoperative analgesic requirements. *Anesth Analg,* Vol.87, No.1(Jul), pp.206-10, ISSN 0003-2999.

Lauretti GR, de Oliveira R, Reis MP, Mattos AL, *et al* (1999). Transdermal nitroglycerine enhances spinal sufentanil postoperative analgesia following orthopedic surgery. *Anesthesiology,* Vol.90, No.3(Mar), pp.734-9, ISSN 0003-3022.

Lauretti GR, Oliveira AP, Julião MC, Reis MP, *et al* (2000). Transdermal nitroglycerine enhances spinal neostigmine postoperative analgesia following gynecological surgery. *Anesthesiology,* Vol.93, No.4(Oct), pp.943-6, ISSN 0003-3022.

Lauwick S, Kim DJ, Michelagnoli G, Mistraletti G, *et al* (2008). Intraoperative infusion of lidocaine reduces postoperative fentanyl requirements in patients undergoing laparoscopic cholecystectomy. *Can J Anaesth,* Vol.55, No.11(Nov), pp.754-60, ISSN 0832-610X.

Lee A, Chan S (2006). Acupuncture and anaesthesia. *Best Pract Res Clin Anaesthesiol,* Vol.20, No.2(Jun), pp.303-14, ISSN 1521-6896.

Legeby M, Jurell G, Beausang-Linder M, Olofsson C (2009). Placebo-controlled trial of local anaesthesia for treatment of pain after breast reconstruction. *Scand J Plast Reconstr Surg Hand Surg* , Vol.43, No.6, pp.315-9. ISSN 0284-4311.

Lin TF, Yeh YC, Lin FS, Wang YP, *et al* (2009). Effect of combining dexmedetomidine and morphine for intravenous patient-controlled analgesia. *Br J Anaesth,* Vol.102, Vol.1(Jan), pp. 117-22, ISSN 0007-0912.

Liu SS, Salinas FV (2003). Continuous plexus and peripheral nerve blocks for postoperative analgesia. *Anesth Analg,* Vol.96, No.1(Jan), pp. 263-72, Review, ISSN 0003-2999.

Liu SS (2004). Anesthesia and analgesia for colon surgery. *Reg Anesth Pain Med,* Vol.29, No.1(Jan-Feb), pp.52-7, ISSN 1098-7339.

Liu SS, Wu CL (2007). Effect of postoperative analgesia on major postoperative complications: a systematic update of the evidence. *Anesth Analg,* Vol.104, No.3(Mar), pp.689-702, ISSN 0003-2999.

Lysakowski C, Dumont L, Czarnetzki C, Tramer MR (2007). Magnesium as an adjuvant to postoperative analgesia: a systematic review of randomized trials. *Anesth Analg,* Vol.104, No.6(Jun), pp.1532-9, ISSN 0003-2999.

Ma H, Tang J, White PF, Zaentz A, *et al* (2004). Perioperative rofecoxib improves early recovery after outpatient herniorrhaphy. *Anesth Analg,* Vol.98, No.4(Apr), pp.970-5, ISSN 0003-2999.

Macario A, Lipman AG (2001). Ketorolac in the era of cyclo-oxygenase-2 selective nonsteroidal anti-inflammatory drugs: a systematic review of efficacy, side effects, and regulatory issues. *Pain Med* , Vol.2, No.4(Dec), pp.336-51, ISSN 1526-2375.

Mathiesen O, Møiniche S, Dahl J (2007). Gabapentin and postoperative pain: a qualitative and quantitative systematic review, with focus on procedure. *BMC Anesthesiol,* Vol.7, No.7(Jul), pp.6, ISSN 1471-2253.

Mathiesen O, Jacobsen L, Holm H, Randall S, *et al* (2008). Pregabalin and dexamethasone for postoperative pain control: a randomized controlled study in hip arthroplasty. *Br J Anaesth,* Vol.101, No.4(Oct), pp.535-41, ISSN 0007-0912.

Mathiesen O, Rasmussen ML, Dierking G, Leck H, *et al* (2009). Pregabalin and dexamethasone in combination with paracetamol for postoperative pain control after abdominal hysterectomy. A randomized clinical trial. *Acta Anaesthesiol Scand*, Vol.53, No.2(Feb), pp.227-35, ISSN 0001-5172.

McCleane G (2010). Topical application of analgesics: a clinical option in day case anaesthesia? *Curr Opin Anaesthesiol*, Vol.23, No.6(Dec), pp.704-7, ISSN 0952-7907.

McGrath B, Elgendy H, Chung F, Kamming D, *et al* (2004). Thirty percent of patients have moderate to severe pain 24 hr after ambulatory surgery: a survey of 5,703 patients. *Can J Anaesth*, Vol.51, No.9(Nov), 886-91, ISSN 0832-610X.

Miranda HF, Puig MM, Prieto JC, Pinardi G (2006). Synergism between paracetamol and nonsteroidal anti-inflammatory drugs in experimental acute pain. *Pain*, Vol.121, No.1-2(Mar), pp.22-8, ISSN 0304-3959.

Mitra S, Sinatra R (2004). Perioperative management of acute pain in the opioid-dependent patient. *Anesthesiology*, Vol.101, No.1(Jul), pp.212-27, ISSN 0003-3022.

Mitra S (2008). Opioid-induced hyperalgesia: pathophysiology and clinical implications. *J Opioid Manag*, Vol.4, No.3(May-Jun), pp. 123-30, ISSN 1551-7489.

Møiniche S, Mikkelsen S, Wetterslev J, Dahl JB (1998). A qualitative systematic review of incisional local anaesthesia for postoperative pain relief after abdominal operations. *Br J Anaesth*, Vol. 81, No.3(Sep), pp.377-83, ISSN 0007-0912.

Moiniche S, Kehlet H, Dahl JB (2002). A qualitative and quantitative systematic review of preemptive analgesia for postoperative pain relief: the role of timing of analgesia. *Anesthesiology*, Vol.96, No.3(Mar), pp.725-41, ISSN 0003-3022.

Ness TJ (2001). Pharmacology of peripheral analgesia. *Pain Pract*, Vol.1, No.3(Sep), pp.243-54, ISSN 1530-7085.

Nett MP (2010). Postoperative pain management. *Orthopedics*, Vol.33, No.9 Suppl(Sep), pp.23-6, ISSN 0147-7447.

Nishimori M, Ballantyne JC, Low JH (2006). Epidural pain relief *versus* systemic opioid-based pain relief for abdominal aortic surgery. *Cochrane Database Syst Rev*, Vol.19, No.3(Jul), CD005059, ISSN 1469-493X(Electronic).

Park JY, Lee GW, Kim Y, Yoo MJ (2002). The efficacy of continuous intrabursal infusion with morphine and bupivacaine for postoperative analgesia after subacromial arthroscopy. *Reg Anesth Pain Med*, Vol.27, No.2(Mar-Apr), pp.145-9, ISSN 1098-7339.

Perkins FM, Kehlet H (2000). Chronic pain as an outcome of surgery. A review of predictive factors. *Anesthesiology*, Vol.93, No.4(Oct), pp.1123-33; ISSN 0003-3022.

Power I, Barratt S. Analgesic agents for the postoperative period. Nonopioids (1999). *Surg Clin N Am*, Vol.79, No.2(Apr), pp.275-95, ISSN 0039-6109.

Practice guidelines for acute pain management in the perioperative setting: a report by the American Society of Anesthesiologists Task Force on Pain Management, Acute Pain Section (1995). *Anesthesiology*, Vol.82, No.4(Apr), pp.1071-81, ISSN 0003-3022.

Pratap JN, Shankar RK, Goroszeniuk T (2007). Co-injection of clonidine prolongs the anesthetic effect of lidocaine skin infiltration by a peripheral action. *Anesth Analg*, Vol.104, No.4(Apr), pp.982-3, ISSN 0003-2999.

Pusch F, Freitag H, Weinstabl C, Obwegeser R, *et al* (1999). Single-injection paravertebral block compared to general anesthesia in breast surgery. *Acta Anaesthesiol Scand*, Vol.43, No.7(Aug), pp.770-4, ISSN 0001-5172.

Rasmussen S, Kramhøft MU, Sperling KP, Pedersen JH.(2004) Increased flexion and reduced hospital stay with continuous intraarticular morphine and ropivacaine after primary total knee replacement: open intervention study of efficacy and safety in 154 patients. *Acta Orthop Scand,* Vol.75, No.5(Oct), pp.606-9, ISSN 0001-6470.

Rathmell JP, Lair TR, Nauman B (2005). The role of intrathecal drugs in the treatment of acute pain. *Anesth Analg,* Vol.101, No.5 Suppl(Nov), pp.S30-43, ISSN 0003-2999.

Rawal N (Co-Ordinator) Postoperative Pain Management - Good Clinical Practice, General recommendations and principles for succesful pain management. http://www.esraeurope.org/PostoperativePain Management.pdf

Saber AA, Elgamal AH, Rao AJ, Itawi EA, *et al* (2009). Early experience with lidocaine patch for postoperative pain control after laparoscopic ventral hernia repair. *Int J Surg,* Vol.7, No.1(Feb), pp.36-8, ISSN 1743-9191.

Salerno A, Hermann R (2006). Efficacy and safety of steroid use for postoperative pain relief. Update and review of the medical literature. *J Bone Joint Surg Am,* Vol.88, No.6(June), pp.1361-72, ISSN 0021-9355.

Schug S, Chong C (2009). Pain management after ambulatory surgery. *Curr Opin Anaesthesiol,* Vol.22, No.6(Dec), pp.738-43, ISSN 0952-7907.

Senturk M, Ozcan PE, Talu GK, Kiyan E, *et al* (2002). The effects of three different analgesia techniques on long-term postthoracotomy pain. *Anesth Analg,* Vol.94, No.1(Jan), pp.11-5, ISSN 0003-2999.

Sivrikaya GU, Eksioglu B, Basgul A, Enhos H, *et al* (2000). The effects of preemptive epidural tramadol on peroperative stress response and postoperative analgesia (Oral communication), 19th Annual ESRA Congress, 20–23 November 2000, Rome, Italy. *The International Monitor (IMRAPT),* Vol.12, No.3, pp.65.

Sivrikaya GU, Koc Bekil EH, Hanci A, Kilinc LT, *et al* (2008). The effect of combined epidural-general anaesthesia on intraoperative stress response and postoperative analgesic consumption and gastrointestinal function in lower abdominal surgery. *J Turk Anaesth Int Care,* Vol.36, No.6(Nov-Dec), pp.358-65, ISSN 1304-0871.

Sun T, Sacan O, White PF, Coleman J, et al (2008). Perioperative vs postoperative celecoxib on patient outcome after major plastic surgery procedures. *Anesth Analg,* Vol.106, No.3(Mar), pp.950-8, ISSN 0003-2999.

Sun Y, Gan T, Dubose J, Habib A (2008). Acupuncture and related techniques for postoperative pain: a systematic review of randomized controlled trials. *Br J Anaesth*Vol.101, No.2(Aug), pp.151-60, ISSN 0007-0912.

Tiippana E, Hamunen K, Kontinen V, Kalso E (2007). Do surgical patients benefit from perioperative gabapentin/pregabalin? Asystematic review of efficacy and safety. *Anesth Analg,* Vol.104, No.6(Jun), pp.1545-56, ISSN 0003-2999.

Tramer MR, Schneider J, Marti R-A, Rifat K (1996). Role of magnesium sulfate in postoperative analgesia. *Anesthesiology* , Vol.84, No.2(Feb), pp.340-7, ISSN 0003-3022.

Usichenko TI, Kuchling S, Witstruck T, Pavlovic D, et al (2007). Auricular acupuncture for pain relief after ambulatory knee surgery: a randomized trial. *CMAJ,* Vol.176, No.2(Jan), pp.179-83, ISSN 1488-2329.

Usichenko T, Lehmann C, Ernst E (2008). Auricular acupuncture for postoperative pain control: a systematic review of randomised clinical trials. *Anaesthesia,* Vol.63, Vol.12(Dec), pp.1343-8, ISSN 0003-2409.

Vadivelu N, Mitra S, Narayan D (2010). Recent advances in postoperative pain management. *Yale J Biol Med*, Vol.83, No.1(Mar), pp.11-25, Review, ISSN 0044-0086.

Viscusi ER, Reynolds L, Chung F, Atkinson LE, et al (2004). Patient-controlled transdermal fentanyl hydrochloride vs intravenous morphine pump for postoperative pain: a randomized controlled trial. *JAMA*, Vol.17, No.11(Mar), pp.1333-41, ISSN 0098-7484.

Wang B, Tang J, White PF, Naruse R, et al (1997). Effect of the intensity of transcutaneous acupoint electrical stimulation on the postoperative analgesic requirement. *Anesth Analg*, Vol.85, No.2(Aug), pp.406-13, ISSN 0003-2999.

Warfield CA, Kahn CH (1995). Acute pain management: programs in U.S. hospitals and experiences and attitudes among U.S adults. *Anesthesiology*Vol.83, No.5(Nov), pp.1090-4, ISSN 0003-3022.

White PF, Issioui T, Skrivanek GD, Early JS, et al (2003). Use of a continuous popliteal sciatic nerve block for the management of pain after major podiatric surgery: does it improve quality of recovery? *Anesth Analg*, Vol.97, No.5(Nov), pp.1303-9, ISSN 0003-2999.

White PF (2005). The changing role of nonopioid analgesic techniques in the management of postoperative pain. *Anesth Analg*, Vol.101, No.5 Suppl(Nov), pp.S5-22, ISSN 0003-2999.

White PF (2007). Multimodal pain management: the future is now! *Curr Opin Investig Drugs*, Vol.8, No.7(Jul), pp.517-8, ISSN 1472-4472.

White PF, Sacan O, Tufanogullari B, Eng M, et al (2007). Effect of short-term postoperative celecoxib administration on patient outcome after outpatient laparoscopic surgery. *Can J Anaesth*, Vol.54, No.5(May), pp.342-8, ISSN 0832-610X.

White PF, Kehlet H (2007). Postoperative pain management and patient outcome: time to return to work! [editorial]. *Anesth Analg*, Vol.104, No.3(Mar), pp.487–90, ISSN 0003-2999.

White PF, Kehlet H, Neal JM, Schricker T, et al (2007). Role of the anesthesiologist in fast-track surgery: from multimodal analgesia to perioperative medical care. *Anesth Analg*, Vol.104, No.6(Jun), pp.1380-96, ISSN 0003-2999.

White PF, Kehlet H (2010). Improving postoperative pain management: what are the unresolved issues? *Anesthesiology*, Vol.112, No.1(Jan), pp.220-5, ISSN 0003-3022.

Wu CL, Fleisher LA (2000). Outcomes research in regional anesthesia and analgesia. *Anesth Analg*, Vol.91, No.5(Nov), pp.1232-42, ISSN 0003-2999.

Yardeni IZ, Beilin B, Mayburd E, Levinson Y, et al (2009). The effect of perioperative intravenous lidocaine on postoperative pain and immune function. *Anesth Analg*, Vol.109, No.5(Nov), 1464-9, ISSN 0003-2999.

10

The Effect of General Anesthesia and General Anesthesia Plus Epidural Levobupivacaine or Bupivacaine on Hemodynami Stress Response and Postoperative Pain

Semra Calimli, Ahmet Topal,
Atilla Erol, Aybars Tavlan and Seref Otelcioglu
Selcuk university Meram Medical Faculty,
Turkey

1. Introduction

Levobupivacaine, a new long-acting local anesthetic, is reported to achieve an effective and safe epidural anesthesia, similar to the anesthesia achieved by bupivacaine. Levobupivacaine with a pharmacological structure similar to that of bupivacaine was shown to have a wider confidence interval, and less neurotoxic and cardiotoxic effects.

A large number of trials have been conducted on determining the anesthetic methods that decrease the stress response of major surgery. These trials usually compared the effects of general, epidural and general + epidural anesthetic methods on the stress response occurring in major surgery with respect to mortality and morbidity. While some authors recommended general + epidural anesthesia, some only recommended the general anesthesia.

A combination of epidural and general anesthesia is reported to reduce the requirement for analgesic and anesthetic agents. Intraoperative hemodynamic stability can be better achieved and the metabolic, endocrine and immunologic responses better suppressed. Management of these responses is important in reducing postoperative morbidity and mortality. With the combination of epidural and general anesthesia, recovery is faster, a higher anesthetic quality can be achieved and patients can be mobilized earlier (1-4). There are no adequate trials on the novel agent, levobupivacaine.

This trial was designed to compare the epidural bupivacaine or levobupivacaine combined with general anesthesia and general anesthesia alone in patients who will undergo TAH-BSO, with respect to stress response to surgery, intraoperative hemodynamics, requirement for peroperative anesthetics and analgesic agents, the quality of the postoperative analgesia, recovery from anesthesia and postoperative side effects.

2. Methods

This trial included 54 ASA I-II group patients in the age range of 18-65 who were scheduled to undergo TAH-BSO and who gave written consent to participate in the trial. Those with severe cardiac, pulmonary, hepatic diseases, renal failure, hemorrhagic diathesis, fever, infection and those with known hypersensitivity to investigational drugs were excluded from the trial. Non-premedicated cases were randomly assigned to three groups: general anesthesia + epidural bupivacaine (Group I, n=18), general anesthesia + epidural levobupivacaine (Group II, n=18) and general anesthesia (Group III, n=18). All the patients were monitored for EKG, non-invasive blood pressure, peripheral oxygen saturation (SpO_2), end-tidal carbon dioxide pressure ($EtCO_2$) and body temperature.

In Groups I and II, the epidural space was entered by a 16-gauge Tuohy epidural needle before the surgery using the loss of resistance method through the L3-L4 space while the patient was in the sitting position and an 18-gauge epidural catheter was inserted (Perifix, Braun, Germany). As a test dose, 2 ml of 2% lidocaine (Aritmal Ampul® Osel) was administered; five minutes later, Group I and Group II were administered 5 ml of 0.25% bupivacaine (Marcaine flacon® Eczacıbaşı, Turkey) and 0.25% levobupivacaine (Chirocaine flacon® Abbott, USA) respectively via epidural catheter, followed by administration of 10 ml of 0.25% bupivacaine to Group I and 10 ml of 0.25% levobupivacaine to Group II via epidural catheter five minutes later. The sensory block upper level, time to achieve sensory block at T6 dermatome and the Bromage Scale values were assessed.

Anesthetic induction was achieved in all patients (when reached the sensorial block level dermatome of T6 in Group I and Group II) by 2 mg kg^{-1} propofol (Propofol ampul® Fresenius Kabi) and 1 µg kg^{-1} remifentanil (Ultiva® Glaxo Wellcome) administered in 60 seconds. 0.6 mg kg^{-1} rocuronium (Esmeron® Organon) was used for achieving neuromuscular block. For all three groups, the maintenance of anesthesia was achieved using 1% sevoflurane (Sevorane® Abbott, USA) in 50% O_2-air mixture and 0.1 µg kg^{-1} min^{-1} remifentanil infusion (Perfusor Compact-Braun). Regarding the patients who would require an anesthesia duration of more than two hours, Group I was scheduled to receive an additional 5 ml of 0.25% bupivacaine and Group II was scheduled to receive an additional 5 ml of 0.25% levobupivacaine from the epidural catheter.

When the heart beat rate (HBR) and the mean blood pressure (MBP) was reduced by 20% of the control value, the concentration of the inhalation agent was reduced by 50%. 250 ml of ringer lactate solution was rapidly administered. In case of absence of improvement, the dose of remifentanil was decreased by 50%. If the low level persisted, atropine or ephedrine was administered as required. When the HBR and MBP increased by more than 20% of the control value, the concentration of the inhalation agent was increased by 50%. In the case of persistence of the high level, the dose of remifentanil was increased by 50%. For maintenance of the neuromuscular blockage, 0.15 mg kg^{-1} rocuronium iv was administered, where necessary.

The hemodynamic parameters, systolic blood pressure (SBP), diastolic blood pressure (DBP), MBP, HBR, and SpO_2 were recorded 2 and 5 minutes after the intubation, 2, 5, 10, 15, 30, 45, 60, 90 and 120 minutes after the skin incision and after the extubation. For measuring the glucose, cortisol, insulin and CRP levels, preoperative venous access was achieved followed by blood sampling in the first and 24th hours of operation. The glucose, glucose oxidase, cortisol and insulin values were measured by chemiluminescent immunoassay, CRP, and the immunoturbidimetric methods.

The postoperative recovery was evaluated by the spontaneous breathing time, extubation time, eye opening time and the time to reach an Aldrete recovery score of ≥9. Data were recorded on the amount of sevoflurane used (ml) (Datex Ohmeda, S5. Sweden), the total dose of remifentanil (mg), whether muscle relaxant was added and whether atropine or

ephedrine were required. Pain intensity was evaluated by the visual analogue scale (VAS) and the motor block was assessed by the Bromage scale; the hemodynamic data and the side effects (hypotension, respiratory depression, motor block, nausea-vomiting, itching, tremor) were recorded at 0 and 30 minutes, and 2, 6, 12 and 24 hours after the operation.
To relieve the postoperative pain, Group III was administered iv morphine and PCA at a concentration of 1 mg ml^{-1} concentration with a loading dose of 1 mg and a lock-out period of 6 minutes. In Group I, 0.125% bupivacaine + 0.025 mg ml^{-1} morphine, in Group II, 0.125% levobupivacaine + 0.025 mg ml^{-1} morphine and 5 ml of h^{-1} basal infusion were prepared for PCA with a 1 ml loading and a lock-out period of 20 minutes and PCA administration was initiated in the recovery room. The total amount of anesthetics used and the administered and requested amounts were recorded.
Statistical analysis were performed using the SPSS 12.0 software. The data were summarized as mean ± standard deviation and percentage. Comparisons between the three groups were assessed by one way variance analysis (Anova) in cases where the parametric conditions could be met and by Kruskal Wallis variance analysis in non-parametric conditions. In the three-group comparisons, post-hoc Tukey-HSD test and Bonferroni correction Mann-Whitney U test were used for significantly differing parameters. The comparison between the two groups was made with a t test. The chi-square test was used for comparing categorical data. Variance analysis was used to analysis the parametric data and Wilcoxon Signed Ranks test Bonferroni correction was used to analyze the non-parametric data for the analysis of the repeated measurements. The level of significance was set at $p<0.05$.

3. Results

The groups showed similarity in the mean values for age, weight, height, the ASA score and the duration of surgery ($p>0.05$) (Table 1).

	GROUP I	GROUP II	GROUP III	P
Age (year)	46.55 ± 4.97	47.53 ± 6.87	48.44 ± 8.75	0.246
Weight (kg)	70.88 ± 8.58	75.50 ± 15.27	79.55 ± 8.05	0.075
Hight (cm)	160.55 ± 5.29	162.16 ± 5.95	160.27 ± 4.61	0.520
Surgery time (min)	74.88 ± 18.31	72.83 ± 20.47	80.94 ± 13.35	0.365
ASA I / II	11 / 7	13 / 5	10 / 8	0.574

Table 1. Patient characteristics (Mean ± SD)

Time to achieve sensory block at T6 dermatome was 18.72±4.41 and 21.27±4.48 in Group I and Group II, respectively; the sensory block upper levels were 5.66±0.68 and 5.88±0.32 dermatome, respectively ($p>0.05$). The pre-operative Bromage scores were 0 in Group I and II ($p>0.05$).
The total doses of the intra-operatively administered remifentanil and sevoflurane were similar between Group I and Group II, however, statistically higher in Group III ($p<0.000$) (Table 2). While there was no statistically significant difference between Group I and Group II in the postoperative recovery evaluated by spontaneous respiratory time, extubation time, eye opening time and the time to reach an Aldrete recovery score of ≥9, Group III had a significantly longer recovery time compared to Groups I and II ($p<0.000$) (Table 2).

	GROUP I	GROUP II	GROUP III	P
Remifentanil (mg)	0.78 ± 0.38	0.77 ± 0.27	1.24 ± 0.38 *	0.000
Sevoflurane (ml)	21.38 ± 7.63	21.94 ± 8.93	44.44 ± 14.84 *	0.000
Spontaneous breathing time (min)	4.58 ± 2.46	4.11 ± 1.17	7.58 ± 2.68 *	0.000
Extubation time (min)	5.19 ± 2.81	4.27 ± 1.14	8.36 ± 2.66 *	0.000
Eye opening time (min)	6.36 ± 3.27	5.16 ± 1.79	9.80 ± 3.79 *	0.000
Time to Aldrete Score ≥9 (min)	7.91 ± 3,19	7.75 ± 2.49	13.11 ± 3.67 *	0.000

* p< 0.05 Compared with Group I and Group II
(Mean ± SD)

Table 2. Mean doses of drugs used in the operation and recovery times.

There was no statistically significant difference between the groups with respect to requirement for atropine and ephedrine (p>0.05). One, two and nine patients received additional muscle relaxant administration in Group I, II and III respectively. There was a statistically significant difference between the groups with respect to the requirement of muscle relaxant (p=0.002), which was higher in Group III relative to Groups I and II.

Regarding the MBP values, Group III had the highest values at 5, 10, 15, 30, 45 and 60 minutes of incision and after extubation (p<0.05).

The intra-group MBP values showed significant reductions relative to the control values during induction, 2, 5 minutes after intubation and 2, 5, 10, 15, 30, 45, 60 and 90 minutes after the surgical incision in Group 1; during induction, five minutes after the intubation, and 2, 5, 10, 15, 30, 45 and 60 minutes after the surgical incision in Group II; and during induction, 2, 5 minutes after the intubation and 2, 30 and 45 minutes after the surgical incision in Group 3 (p<0.05). While there was no statistically significant difference between the post-extubation MBP values and the control MBP values in Groups I and II (p>0.05), Group III exhibited a significant increase relative to the control value in Group III (p<0.013).

The HBR values were lower in Group III compared to Groups I and II in the 2nd and 5th minutes of intubation (p<0.05).

The intra-group HBR values showed significant reductions relative to the control values during induction, and 2, 5, 10, 15, 30, 45 and 60 minutes after the surgical incision in Group I; during induction, and 10, 15, 30, 45 and 60 minutes after the surgical incision in Group II; and during induction, five minutes after intubation, and 2, 5, 10, 45 and 60 minutes after the surgical incision in Group III (p<0.05).

Since the duration of surgery was below 100 minutes in all patients, there was no requirement for additional epidural local anesthetic administration and the follow-ups at 120 minutes could not be conducted (Table 1).

The mean control values for the parameters used to assess the response to surgical stress including glucose, insulin, cortisol and the CRP values were statistically similar between the three groups (p>0.05).

While the postoperative glucose values in the first and 24th hours were not significantly different, they were higher in Group III relative to Groups I and II (p>0.05). Regarding the intra-group comparison, the glucose values exhibited a significant increase relative to the control values one hour after the operation in all groups, and 24 hours after the operation in Groups I and III (p<0.05) (Figure 1).

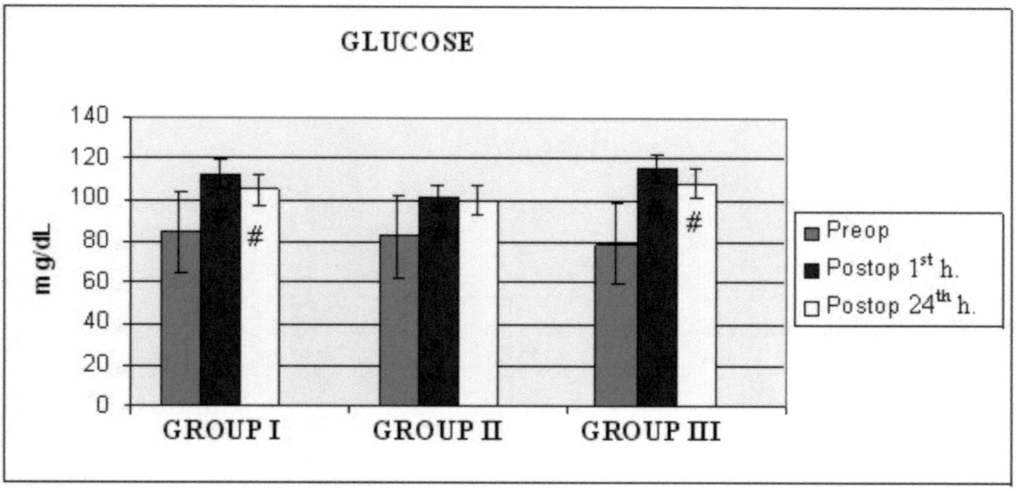

Compared with the control values ($p<0.05$)

Fig. 1. Changes in Glucose values when compared to Groups

There was no statistically significant difference between the groups in the 1st and 24th hour measurements of the insulin values ($p>0.05$). In Group I, the postoperative 1st and 24th hour values were different and the 24th hour values were higher ($p<0.05$). In Group III, the postoperative values in the first and 24th hours were higher than the control values ($p<0.05$) (Figure 2).

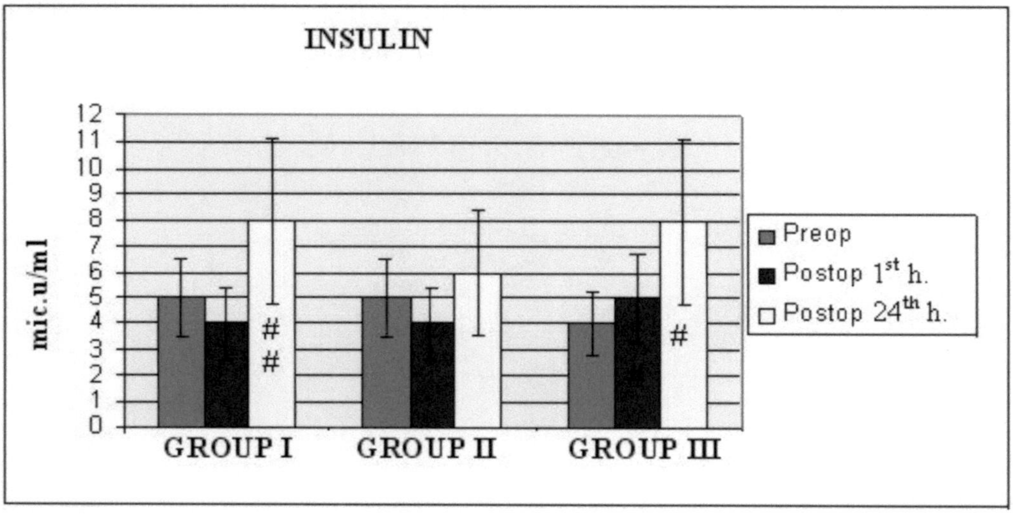

Compared with the control values ($p<0.05$)

Compared in Group I post op. 1th and 24th hours values ($p<0.05$).

Fig. 2. Changes in Insulin values when compared to Groups

The postoperative cortisol values at 1 hour differed between the groups and were highest in Group III ($p<0.05$). The intra-group comparison of the cortisol values revealed higher measurements one hour after the operation relative to the control values ($p<0.05$). The 24th hour postoperative cortisol values were higher than the control value only in Group III ($p<0.05$) (Figure 3).

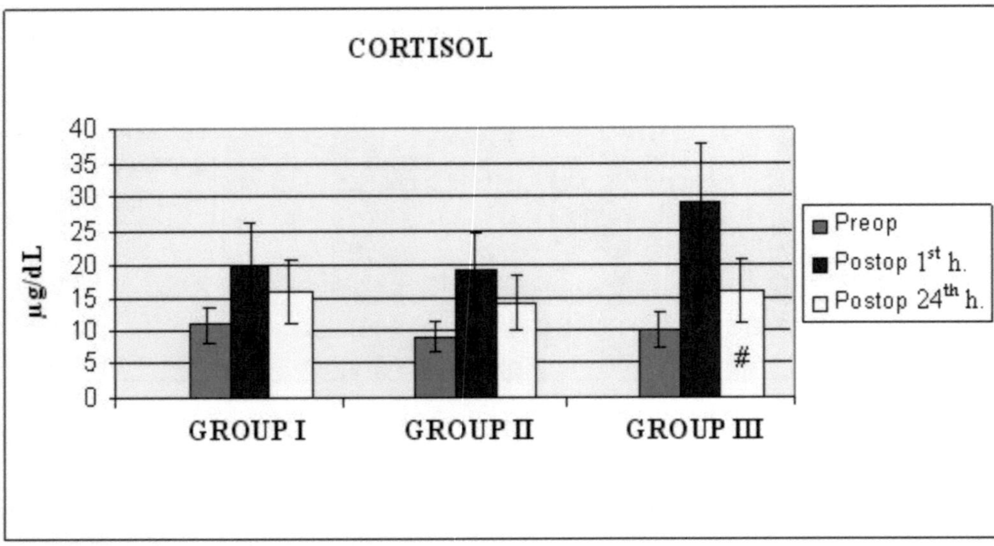

* Compared with the Groups ($p<0.05$)
# Compared with the control values ($p<0.05$).

Fig. 3. Changes in Cortisol values when compared to Groups

There was no difference between the groups in the CRP values. The intra-group comparison of the CRP values showed higher postoperative 24th hour values relative to the control values and the postoperative 1st hour values in all groups ($p<0.05$) (Figure 4).

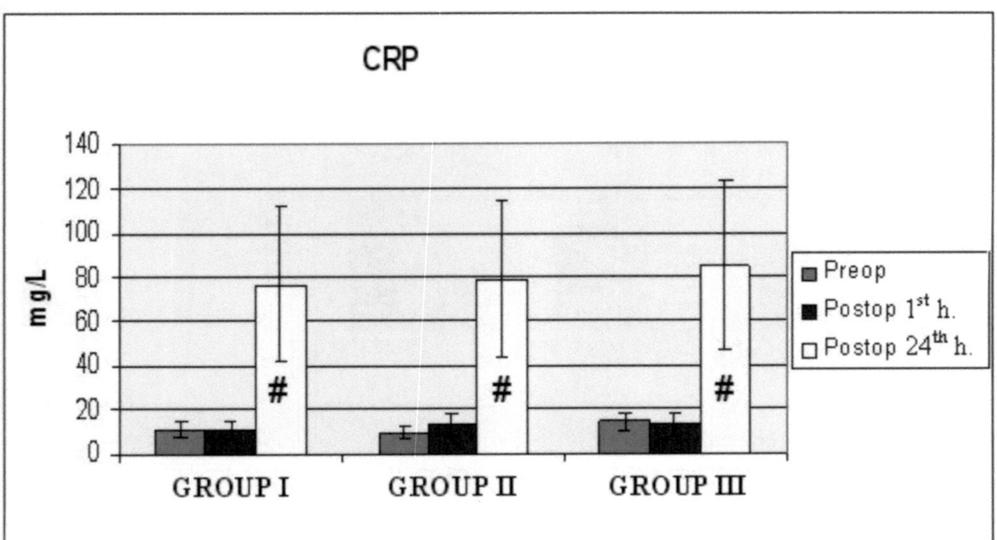

Compared with the control values ($p<0.05$)

Fig. 4. Changes in CRP values when compared to Groups

The comparison of the postoperative pain scores between the groups demonstrated the highest VAS value at minute 0 in Group III ($p<0.000$). Regarding the other measurement times, no significant difference was detected between the groups ($p>0.05$) (Table 3).

	GROUP I	GROUP II	GROUP III	P
Postop 0th min.	0.38 ± 1.14	1.33 ± 2.02	5.88 ± 1.99 *	0.000
Postop 30th min.	4.77 ± 1.95 #	4.50 ± 2.22 #	5.83 ± 1.75	0.172
Postop 2nd h	3.77 ± 2.21 #	3.22 ± 2.43	2.55 ± 1.72 #	0.388
Postop 6th h	2.11 ± 2.13	1.33 ± 1.74	1.33 ± 1.13 #	0.465
Postop 12th h	0.38 ± 0.69	0.50 ± 1.42	0.77 ± 1.16 #	0.325
Postop 24th h	0.25 ± 0.23	0.27 ± 0.75	0.33 ± 0.76 #	0.355
P	<0.05	<0.05	<0.05	

*Comparisons between-groups ($p<0.05$)
Comparison intra-groups ($p<0.05$).

Table 3. VAS values (Mean ± SD)

The comparison of the postoperative hemodynamic data revealed the highest MBP at minute 0 in Group III ($p<0.002$). None of the three groups exhibited postoperative hypotension or respiratory depression. Regarding the motor block, there was no significant difference between Groups I and II with respect to nausea-vomiting, itching, or tremor ($p>0.05$).

4. Discussion

In this trial investigating the extent of suppression of the stress response to surgery in patients undergoing general anesthesia + epidural anesthesia achieved with two different local anesthetics relative to the patients only receiving general anesthesia, the intraoperative hemodynamics, intraoperative anesthetic and analgesic agent requirement, the postoperative analgesia quality, the side effects and the recovery were also compared between the groups.

Bupivacaine is commonly used in epidural analgesia owing to its long-lasting effect and the sensory block it achieves that is more marked than the motor block. However, levobupivacaine was reported to be safer with respect to the central nervous system toxicity and cardiotoxicity in addition to exhibiting a local anesthetic effect similar to bupivacaine in the clinical trials. The tendency for sensory block is longer with levobupivacaine relative to bupivacaine. Following epidural administration of levobupivacaine, the duration of the motor block was observed to be shorter than that of the sensory block. Levobupivacaine was reported to be as effective as bupivacaine when combined with morphine or fentanyl in the treatment of postoperative pain. Some trials demonstrated that levobupivacaine exhibited small increases in the sensory block time relative to bupivacaine, in line with the results from this trial. This finding may be attributed to the relatively increased vasoconstrictor effect of levobupivacaine compared to bupivacaine (5-8).

In this trial, there was no difference between Group I and Group II in the time to achieve sensory block at T6. There was no difference between the two groups in the motor block levels measured until the time to achieve sensory block at T6 dermatome. The follow-ups conducted during the 24th postoperative hour revealed a smaller number of patients developing motor block in the group using levobupivacaine.

In the trial by Bader et al (9) where women undergoing cesarean section were administered 0.5% (150 mg) levobupivacaine or bupivacaine at the same dose via epidural anesthesia, the incidence of hypotension was detected to be lower in those receiving levobupivacaine (84.4% levobupivacaine, 100% bupivacaine).

Bardsley et al (10), upon administering 56.1 mg of levobupivacaine and 47.9 mg of bupivacaine via the iv route, and Kopacz and Allen (11), upon accidentally administering 17 ml of 0.75% of levobupivacaine intravenously to a patient, reported that levobupivacaine was safer for achieving direct depression of the myocardial contractility relative to bupivacaine.

In this trial, there was one patient in Group I and four patients in Group II who required intraoperative ephedrine for hypotension, although this was not statistically significant. In Group III, the arterial blood pressure values were higher at various measurement times and required higher anesthetic doses to achieve hemodynamic stability. None of the three groups exhibited EKG changes. The absence of EKG changes in Groups I and II may be attributed to the low concentration of the epidural local anesthetic used.

Luchetti M et al (12) compared epidural + general anesthesia and total intravenous anesthesia in patients undergoing laparoscopic cholecystectomy and reported that the epidural + general anesthesia group did not require intraoperative opioid use, did not exhibit an increase in side effects and had a faster recovery. In our trial, the amount of sevoflurane and remifentanil used was lower in the epidural + general anesthesia groups relative to the general anesthesia group and thus, recovery was faster in Groups I and II relative to Group III; this finding is in line with the literature.

In their trial where they compared general anesthesia combined with epidural anesthesia achieved by 2% lidocaine to general anesthesia alone, Lu CH et al (13) reported that the requirement for volatile anesthetics was lower in the epidural + general anesthesia group, in line with our results.

The stress response can be avoided and the mediator levels can be maintained at the preoperative values by epidural anesthesia administered before surgical stimulation (14). In addition, epidural analgesia achieved by local anesthetics or opioids should also be maintained in the postoperative period to be able to reduce the stress response at the maximum level (15). In this trial, Group I and Group II were administered local anesthetic solution from the epidural space approximately 20 minutes before the surgery. As the sensory block level reached the T6 dermatome, general anesthesia induction was performed and the surgery was initiated. Maintenance of analgesia was achieved by using postoperative epidural PCA. Postoperative iv morphine PCA was used in Group III. As such, suppression of the stress response was observed similarly to these trials (14, 15).

Latterman et al (16) demonstrated that the glucose response was more limited in the patients receiving epidural anesthesia relative to the group undergoing general anesthesia. In this trial, the plasma glucose value showed a limited increase relative to the control value at the 1st and 24th postoperative hours; this increase was slightly more in Group III. None of the groups exhibited an increase in the glucose level above 150 mg dL^{-1}.

The blood glucose level was detected to be lower with postoperative epidural fentanyl administration relative to iv fentanyl administration (17). Again after general anesthesia, the blood glucose level was observed to be better suppressed in association with general anesthesia + paravertebral anesthesia and analgesia versus postoperative iv morphine administration (18). In this trial, epidural morphine was combined with local anesthetic agents to achieve postoperative analgesia in Groups I and II. Iv morphine was used in Group III. Glucose level was better suppressed in Groups I and II relative to Group III.

The trials detected that the cortisol levels increased starting from the skin incision in cases undergoing general anesthesia + epidural analgesia; however, the blood cortisol levels were suppressed relative to the group receiving general anesthesia (19, 20). In another trial (21), epidural + general anesthesia and postoperative morphine administration were claimed to provide a better suppression of the blood cortisol level relative to the general anesthesia + postoperative iv morphine administration. In this trial, the postoperative 1st hour cortisol value was higher in Group III relative to Groups I and II. In all groups, the postoperative 1st hour cortisol value was higher than the control value; the postoperative cortisol value at 24 hours was significantly increased only in Group III. This shows that the cortisol response was better suppressed in the groups receiving epidural anesthesia and postoperative epidural analgesia relative to the group receiving general anesthesia and postoperative iv analgesia, even if partially.

Insulin, an anabolic and hypoglycemic hormone decreases following trauma as opposed to glucose and cortisol. This helps to maintain hyperglycemia and protect the metabolic status of the vital organs (22). In this trial, there was no difference between the groups in the insulin values measured preoperatively and in the first and 24th hours postoperatively. The increase in the insulin values in the 24th postoperative hour in Groups I and III may be related to the increase in glucose values.

Compared to general anesthesia, the increase in TNF-a and CRP levels was observed to be less with general + epidural anesthesia (1). In this trial, the 24th postoperative hour CRP values exhibited an increase compared to the control values in all groups. While there was no statistically significant difference between the groups, the values in Group III were higher relative to Groups I and II.

Chu CPW et al (2) compared general anesthesia followed by iv morphine, and combined spinal epidural anesthesia followed by epidural 1% bupivacaine and 2 $\mu g\ ml^{-1}$ fentanyl, and detected lower VAS scores in the first, 12th and 48th postoperative hours in the group receiving epidural anesthesia and postoperative epidural analgesia ($p<0.05$).

In this trial, morphine was combined with low-dose local anesthetic in patients using epidural PCA. Iv morphine PCA was used in the general anesthesia group. In the treatment of postoperative pain, the VAS scores were higher during the first hours in Group III relative to Groups I and II ($p<0.05$). This may result from the postoperative maintenance of analgesia in groups receiving preoperative epidural anesthesia. In the group receiving intravenous morphine PCA, the VAS scores gradually decreased and exhibited no significant difference compared to the other groups.

Enquist et al (3) demonstrated that epidural anesthesia blocking the neural afferent conduction whether combined with general anesthesia or alone resulted in suppression of the stress response to surgery in their trial on the effects of epidural anesthesia at various doses on surgical stress. The blood pressure values were higher during the first postoperative hours in the group of patients receiving epidural + general anesthesia relative to the general anesthesia group with no difference detected between the groups after three hours. In this trial, the MBP values were similarly higher in Group III during the first two hours relative to Groups I and II.

Nabil W. Doss et al (4) compared the thoracic epidural anesthesia and general anesthesia techniques in their trial performed using 0.2% ropivacaine in patients undergoing mastectomy and detected higher rates of nausea and vomiting in the general anesthesia group. Regarding hemodynamics, hypertension was more common in the general anesthesia group. The Aldrete recovery scores measured 1, 2 and 3 hours after the operation exhibited significant differences between the groups only in the first hour and were better in the thoracic epidural anesthesia group. In our trial, nausea-vomiting was less and the time of recovery from anesthesia was shorter in Groups I and II relative to Group III.

Morphine-related postoperative complications were most commonly in the form of nausea-vomiting, similar to the other trials. There was no significant difference between Groups I and II, and Group III with respect to nausea and vomiting. However, the number of patients with nausea and vomiting was higher in Group III. None of the patients had hypotension that required postoperative rapid fluid replacement or vasopressor agent use. Similarly, none of the patients developed respiratory depression. While there was no difference between the groups in itching, there were more patients with this compliant in Group III. There was no significant difference between the groups in tremor and only one patient in Group II had tremor.

In avoiding stress response, individual differences, the type and duration of surgery, tissue injury in major surgeries, the type of analgesia and the drugs used are also important as well as the method of anesthesia used.

As a result, we concluded that bupivacaine and levobupivacaine used in epidural anesthesia had similar effects, epidural + general anesthesia provided a better intraoperative hemodynamic stability relative to general anesthesia and reduced the requirement for anesthetic agents, provided a faster recovery, resulted in less side effects and achieved a better analgesia, particularly during the first postoperative hours. We believe that the stress response can be better suppressed by epidural + general anesthesia.

5. References

[1] Foster RH, Markham A. Levobupivacaine: A review of its pharmacology and use a local anesthetics. Drugs 2000; 59:531-79.

[2] McCellan KJ, Spencer CM. Levobupivacaine. Drugs 1998; 56:355-62.

[3] McLeod GA, Burke D. Review Article: Levobupivacaine. Anaesthesia 2001; 56:331-41.

[4] O' Sullivan EP. Comparison of 0.75 % levobupivacaine with 0.75 % racemic bupivacaine for peribulbar anaesthesia (letter). Anaesthesia 1999; 54:610.

[5] Bader AM, Tsen LC, Camann WR, Nephew E, Datta S. Clinical effects and maternal and fetal plasma concentrations of 0.5 % epidural levobupivacaine versus bupivacaine for cesarean delivery. Anesthesiology 1999; 90:1596-601.

[6] Bardsley H, Gristwood R, Baker H, Watson N, Nimmo W. A comparison of the cardiovascular effects levobupivacaine and rac-bupivacaine following intravenous administration to healty volunteers. Br J Clin Pharmacol 1998; 46(3):245-9.

[7] Kopacz DJ, Allen HW. Accidental intravascular injection of 0.75 % levobupivacaine during lumbar epidural anaesthesia. Anaesth Analg 1999; 89:1027-9.

[8] Luchetti M, Palamba R, Sica G, Massa G, Tufano R. Effectiveness and safety of combined epidural and general anesthesia for laparoscopic cholecystectomy. Reg Anesth 1996; 21(5):465-9.

[9] Lu CH, Borel CO, Wu CT, Yeh CC, Jao SW, Chao PC, Wong CS. Combined general-epidural anesthesia decreases the desflurane requirement for equivalent A-line ARX index in colorectal surgery.Acta Anaesthesiol Scand 2005; 49(8):1063-7.

[10] Chernow B, Alexander HR, Smallridge RC, Thompson WR, Cook D, Beardsley D, Fink MP, Lake CR, Fletcher JR. Hormanal responses to graded surgical stress. Arch Intern Med 1987; 147:1273-8.

[11] Moller IW, Dinesen K, Sondergard S, Knigge U, Kehlet H. Effect of patient-controlled analgesia on plasma catecholamine, cortisol and glucose concertrations after cholecystectomy. Br J Anaesth 1988; 61:160-4.

[12] Lattermann R, Carli F, Wykes L, Schricker T. Epidural Blockade Modifies Perioperative Glucose Production without Affecting Protein Catabolism. Anesthesiology 2002; 97:374-81.

[13] Salomaki TE, Leppahuoto J, Laitinen JO, Vuolteenaho O, Nuutinen DS. Epidural versus intravenous fentanyl for reducing hormonal, metabolic and physiologic responses after thoracotomy . Anesthesiology 1993; 79:672-9.

[14] Engquist A, Fog-Moller F, Christiansen C, Thode J, Vester-Andersen T, Madsen SN. Influence of epidural analgesia on the catecholamine and cyclic AMP responses to surgery. Acta Anaesthesiol Scand 1980; 24:17-21.

[15] Naito Y, Tamai S, Shingo K, Shindo K, Matsui T, Segawa H, Nakai Y, Mori K. Responses of plasma adrenocorticotropic hormone, cortizol and cytokines during and after upper abdominal surgery. Anesthesiology 1992; 77(3):426-31.

[16] Hase K, Meguro K. Perioperative stres response in elderly patients for elective gastrectomy the comparison between isoflurane anesthesia and sevoflurane anesthesia both combined with epidural anaesthesia. Masui 2000; 49:121-9.

[17] Qu DM, Jin YF, Ye TH, Cui YS, Li SQ, Zhang ZY. The effects of general anesthesia combined with epidural anesthesia on the stres response in thoracic surgery. Zhonghua Yi Xue Za Zhi 2003; 83(5):408-11.

[18] Christensen NJ, Hilsted J, Hegedus L, Madsbad S. Effects of surgical stress and insulin on cardiovascular function and norepinephrine kinetics. Am J Physiol. 1984; 247(1):29-34.

[19] Christopherson R, Beattie C, Frank SM, Norris EJ, Meinert CL, Gottlieb SO, Yates H, Rock P, Parker SD, Perler BA, et al. Perioperative morbidity in patients randomized to epidural or general anesthesia for lower extremity vascular surgery. Perioperative ischemia randomized anesthesia trial study group. Anesthesiology 1993; 79(3):422-34.

[20] CPW Chu, JCCM Yap, PP Chen, HH Hung. Postoperative outcome in Chinese patients having primary total knee artroplasty under general anaesthesia / intravenous patient-controlled analgesia compared to spinal-epidural anaesthesia / analgesia. Hong Kong Med J 2006; 12:442-7.

[21] Engquist A, Brant MR, Fernandez A. The blocking effect of epidural analgesia on the adrenocortical and hyperglisemic responses to surgery. Acta Anaesthesiol Scand 1977; 231:330-5.

[22] Doss NW, Ipe J, Crimi T, Rajpal S, Cohen S, Fogler RJ, Michael R, Gintautas J. Continuous thoracic epidural anesthesia with 0.2 % ropivacaine versus general anesthesia for perioperative management of modified radical mastectomy. Anesth Analg. 2001; 92(6):1552-7.

11

Propofol and Postoperative Pain: Systematic Review and Meta-Analysis

Antigona Hasani, Hysni Jashari, Valbon Gashi and Albion Dervishi
University Clinical Center of Kosova,
Department of Anesthesiology and Department of Pediatric Surgery, Prishtina,
Republic of Kosova

1. Introduction

If an intravenous or inhalator anesthetic, would include in itself all the components of general anesthesia, like hypnoses, analgesia, amnesia etc. it would represent a really ideal anesthetic.

Propofol is the drug of choice for induction and/or maintenance of anesthesia and sedation in the operating room and intensive care unit. It is a short-acting intravenous anaesthetic that features high blood-tissue solubility and allows a rapid induction and rapid emergence. Propofol has γ-aminobutyric acid agonist activity and produces dose dependent central nervous system depression resulting in sedation and hypnosis.

Analgesic properties of propofol are discussed in many studies, in recent years. However, evidence suggesting that the drug possesses analgesic activity still remains questionable (Fassoulaki, 2011).

The objective of this study is to systematically determine the effects of propofol in postoperative pain.

We have included double-blind, randomized, and controlled trials in humans, where postoperative analgesic effect of propofol was compared with another anesthetic or non-drug intervention.

The study was carried out according to the methods recommended by the Cochrane Collaboration (Higgins et al., 2009) and written in accordance with the PRISMA statement for reporting systematic reviews (Liberati et al., 2009, Moher et al., 2009).

Reports of randomized controlled trials were systemically sought using the Cochrane Library, PubMed, Embase, www.clinicaltrials.gov, and hand searching from the reference lists of identified papers.

Data were analyzed from 25 randomized controlled trials totaling 2033 adults and children. We developed standard data collection sheets to record details of trial design, interventions, and outcome measures for every trial. We extracted information about propofol and control group. Information about number of patients enrolled, type of surgical intervention and side effects, were also noted. Data on postoperative pain relief using pain scores time to first analgesic request and consumption of supplementary analgesics was taken from each report.

Qualitative analysis of postoperative effectiveness was evaluated by significant difference ($P < 0.05$ as reported in the original investigation) in pain relief using pain scores, time to

first analgesic request, and consumption of supplementary analgesics between the treatment groups, and by assessment of the clinical importance of observed differences.
Quantitative analyses of combined data were intended by calculation of the number of patients reporting any pain or no pain (pain response rate) between treatment groups.
Each trial was assessed for different measures of internal sensitivity. First, trials were checked for magnitude of pain intensity. Because it is difficult to detect an improvement with low or no pain, it was noted that pain scores were less than 30 mm on a visual analog scale (VAS) or less than moderate pain on a verbal rating scale or similar score. Second, it was noted that a power calculation of the statistical tests was performed. Trials with sample sizes less than 10 patients per treatment group were not considered in the study.
Meta-analyses were carried out by direct comparisons of intervention versus control and indirect comparisons between the networks of interventions shown to be significant individually.

2. Propofol

Propofol (2,6-diisopropyl phenol) is chemically inert phenolic compound with anesthetic properties. It has high lipid solubility, but is almost insoluble in water. The original preparation contained the solubilizing agent Ctenophore EL (polyethoxylated Castrol oil). Reformulation of the drug in an egg-oil-glycerol emulsion has eliminated hypersensitivity reactions that occurred with the original formulation (Sebel, 1989). The dose of propofol required to induce anesthesia measured by loss of eyelash reflex in 95% of healthy unpremedicated patients was 1.5-2.5 mg/kg. The range of induction times was 22-125 seconds. The rapid loss of consciousness was realized due to the immediate uptake of the lipid – soluble drug by the central nervous system (CNS).Within several minutes of intravenous administration, the plasma concentration of propofol decreases due to the distribution of the drug throughout the body and its uptake by peripheral tissues. As the plasma concentration falls, propofol diffuses from the CNS into the systemic circulation; when bolus doses of the anesthetic are used to induce anesthesia, there is a rapid recovery of full consciousness and awareness. These advantageous properties have contributed to the popularity of propofol as an induction agent for short procedures and day – case surgery (Short, 1999).
Propofol is also indicated for the maintenance of anesthesia computer-assisted continuous infusion and target-controlled infusion of propofol using a monitor of the hypnotic effects of propofol on the brain electroencephalographic Bispectral Index [BIS] monitor; it is possible to create a closed-loop delivery system for improving the titration of propofol during general anesthesia (Kwan, 1989, Singh, 1999).
Infusions of subanesthetic doses of propofol have been used to sedate patients for surgery under regional anesthesia, in diagnostic centers for sedation during gastroenterology and pulmonary medicine procedures, as well as in critical care areas for sedation of ventilator-dependent patients as an alternative to benzodiazepines and/or opioid analgesics (Mazurek, 2004).
Propofol is extensively bound to plasma proteins; approximately 97-98% is bound to albumin. After intravenous injection the plasma concentration of propofol decline. The initial fall is extremely rapid (half life 1-3 min), reflecting the distribution of the lipid - soluble drug from plasma to tissue.
Approximately 70% of a dose is excreted in the urine within 24 hours after administration, and 90% is excreted within 5 days. Clearance of propofol ranges from 1.6 to 3.4 liters per minute in

healthy 70 kg patients. As the age of the patient increases, total body clearance of propofol may decrease. Clearance rates ranging from 1.4 to 2.2 liters per minute in patients 18 to 35 years of age have been reported, in contrast to clearance rates of 1 to 1.8 liters per minute in patients 65 to 80 years of age. The propofol mean total body clearance rate was 2.09 +/- 0.65 1/min (mean SD), the volume of distribution at steady state was 159 +/- 57 I, and the elimination half-life was 116 +/- 34 min. Elderly patients (patients older than 60 yr) had significantly decreased clearance rates (1.58 +/- 0.42 vs. 2.19 +/- 0.64 1/min), whereas women (vs. men) had greater clearance rates (33 +/- 8 vs. 26 +/- 7 1 kg^{-1} min^{-1}) and volumes of distribution (2.50 +/- 0.81 vs. 2.05 +/- 0.65 1/kg). Patients undergoing major intraabdominal surgery had longer elimination half-life values (136 +/- 40 vs. 108 +/- 29 min). Patients required an average blood propofol concentration of 4.05 +/- 1.01 µg/ml for major surgery and 2.97 +/- 1.07 g/ml for nonmajor surgery. Blood propofol concentrations at which 50% of patients were awake and oriented after surgery were 1.07 and 0.95 µg/ml, respectively. The metabolic clearance of propofol exceeds hepatic blood flow, which has leaded to suggestion that propofol is also metabolized in extrahepatic sites. Approximately 70% of a dose is excreted in the urine within 24 hours after administration, and 90% is excreted within 5 days. Psychomotor performance returned to baseline at blood propofol concentrations of 0.38-0.43 g/ml (Shafer et al., 1988, White, 1989, Deegan, 1992; Zuppa et al., 2003).

Propofol causes a significant reduction in systemic blood pressure (more than 50% of preoperative level). This increase in blood pressure is a result of decrease in systemic vascular resistance. In addition to arterial vasodilatation, propofol produces venodilation (due both to a reduction in sympathetic activity and to a direct effect on the vascular smooth muscle), which contributes to its hypotensive effect. The fall in cardiac output is manifested with decrease in heart rate. (Machała & Szebla, 2008; Frolich, 2011).

Respiratory depression and apnea are more pronounced with propofol than thiopental. Propofol decreases tidal volume and increases respiratory rate. The ventilatory response to carbon dioxide and hypoxia is also significantly decreased, but propofol does not inhibit hypoxic pulmonary vasoconstriction. Propofol can produce bronchodilation in patients with chronic obstructive pulmonary disease and in patients with acute laryngospasm during emergence from anesthesia (Zeller et al., 2005).

Propofol decreases CMRO2 and CBF, as well as ICP.33 However, when larger doses are administered, the marked depressant effect on systemic arterial pressure can significantly decrease CPP. Cerebrovascular autoregulation in response to changes in systemic arterial pressure and reactivity of the cerebral blood flow to changes in carbon dioxide tension are not affected by propofol. Evidence for a possible neuroprotective effect has been reported in vitro preparations, and the use of propofol to produce EEG burst suppression has been proposed as a method for providing neuroprotection during aneurysm surgery. Its neuroprotective effect may at least partially be related to the antioxidant potential of propofol's phenol ring structure, which may act as a free-radical scavenger, decreasing free-radical induced lipid peroxidation. Recent studies reported that this antioxidant activity may offer many advantages in preventing the hypoperfusion/reperfusion phenomenon that can occur during surgery (Dagal & Lam, 2009; Girard et al., 2009; Ozturk et al., 2009; Menku et al., 2010).

Propofol produces cortical EEG changes that are similar to thiopental. However, sedative doses of propofol increase â-wave activity analogous to the benzodiazepines. Induction of anesthesia with propofol is occasionally accompanied by excitatory motor activity (so-called nonepileptic myoclonia). In a study involving patients without a history of seizure disorders, excitatory movements following propofol were not associated with EEG seizure activity.

Propofol appears to possess profound anticonvulsant properties. Propofol has been reported to decrease spike activity in patients with cortical electrodes implanted for resection of epileptogenic foci and has been used successfully to terminate status epilepticus. The duration of motor and EEG seizure activity following electroconvulsive therapy is significantly shorter with propofol than with other IV anesthetics. Propofol produces a decrease in the early components of somatosensory and motor evoked potentials but does not influence the early components of the auditory evoked potentials (Modica et al., 1990).

There is no evidence to suggest that propofol has any significant effects on renal or hepatic function.

Propofol is known to possess direct antiemetic effects. Its use for induction and maintenance of anesthesia has been shown to be associated with a lower incidence of postoperative nausea and vomiting (PONV) when compared to any other anesthetic drug or technique. The precise mechanism of propofol antiemetic effect of propofol has not been elucidated, several mechanisms have been proposed, including a direct depressant effect on the chemoreceptor trigger zone (CTZ), the vagal nuclei, and other centers implicated in PONV (Becker, 2010). A systematic review of PONV following maintenance of anesthesia with propofol or an inhalational anesthetic agent found that patients receiving propofol had a significantly lower frequency of PONV, regardless of induction agent, choice of inhalational agent, use of nitrous oxide, patient age, or use of an opioid (Soppitt et al., 2000). Another systematic review found that propofol may be effective in reducing PONV in the short term, but only when given as a continuous infusion for maintenance of anesthesia and when the PONV event rate is greater than 20% (Eberhart et al., 2006). There is evidence of a relationship between plasma propofol concentration and antiemetic efficacy. Gan et al., 1999, found that a median plasma propofol concentration of 343 ng/mL was associated with a reduction in PV in surgical patients. After a typical induction dose, plasma propofol levels remain above this antiemetic serum concentration threshold for approximately 30 minutes. Therefore, the common practice of selecting propofol for inducing anesthesia because of its antiemetic effects provides little benefit to a patient in terms of reducing the likelihood that the patient will develop PONV during the stay in the postanesthesia care unit and after discharge from the ambulatory surgery center.

Anticonvulsant effect of propofol is always described (Simpson et al., 1988). Theoretically, propofol should be strongly anticonvulsant, as it exhibits both GABAergic effects and persistent sodium current and calcium current blockade. However, a literature search of propofol associated tonic-clonic seizures retrieved more than 500 case reports, of which 81 were analyzed in more detail. The denominator is missing from these case reports, and hence the true incidence is unknown. Among the 172,592 anesthetics analyzed there were 53 generalized convulsions, of which 16 were thought to be primarily due to anesthesia. Fifteen of these cases were attributed to local anesthetic drug error, anti-epileptic drug withdrawal or cerebral anoxia/hypercarbia. This left a single case where the seizure was thought to be due to the anesthetic, propofol, an incidence of 1 per 172,592 anesthetics (Fredman et al, 1994).

Propofol has a remarkable safety profile (Sarani B, Gracias, 2008). Dose dependent hypotension is the commonest complication; particularly in volume depleted patients. Hypertriglyceridemia and pancreatitis are uncommon complications. Allergic complications, which may include bronchospasm, have been reported. High dose propofol infusions have been associated with the "propofol syndrome"; this is a potentially fatal complication characterized by severe metabolic acidosis and circulatory collapse (Murdoch &, Cohen, 1999). This is a rare complication first reported in pediatric patients and believed

to be due to decreased transmembrane electrical potential and alteration of electron transport across the inner mitochondrial membrane. And, of course pain during injection of propofol which could prevent in several ways (Jalota et al., 2011).
Finally, the favorable pharmacokinetic properties, like short half-life and high clearance rate, minimal side effects and other nonhypnotic positive effects make it safe and usefull in clinical practice.

3. Analgesic effects of propofol

General anesthetics and propofol modulate the function of the gama (γ)-aminobutyric acid $(GABA)_A$ receptors, the inhibitory neurotransmitter receptors in the central nervous system. GABA is the major inhibitory neurotransmitter in the central nervous system, with fast synaptic inhibition mediated by postsynaptic $GABA_A$ receptors. $GABA_A$ receptors are members of the superfamily of ligand-gated ion channels and are thought to consist of five subunits (α, β, and γ). The GABA-induced chloride current can be potentiated by some general anesthetics. The actions of propofol appear to be mediated by β3-containing $GABA_A$ receptors. Specific residue is located within the second transmembrane region of the β3 subunit of the $GABA_A$ receptor and has a influence in determining the action of propofol (Krasowski et. Al., 1998; Siegwart et al. 2002).
The hypnotic effect of propofol and probably analgesic effect is related to GABA accumulation and occupation of the GABA receptor. Occupation of receptors produced hyperpolarisation of the postsynaptic cell membrane and neuronal inhibition. Propofol at low concentration enhance the amplitude of response of GABA and prolong the duration of GABA mediated synaptic inhibition. At supraclinical concentrations propofol directly activate the receptors anion channel.
The analgesic effect of propofol may result as it acts at $GABA_A$ receptors (Dong & Xu, 2002). On the other hand, propofol induced potentiation of glycin receptors at the spinal level and might contribute to its antinociceptive actions and general anesthesia (Xu et al., 2004).
Spinal (NMDA) receptors were reported to be involved in the antinociceptive action of propofol. Prolonged firing of C-fiber nociceptors causes release of glutamate which acts on N-methyl-D-aspartate (NMDA) receptors in the spinal cord. Activation of NMDA receptors causes the spinal cord neuron to become more responsive to all of its inputs, resulting in central sensitization. NMDA-receptor antagonists can suppress central sensitization. NMDA-receptor activation not only increases the cell's response to pain stimuli, it also decreases neuronal sensitivity to opioid receptor agonists. In addition to preventing central sensitization, co-administration of NMDA-receptor antagonists with an opioid may prevent tolerance to opioid analgesia. Was reported that intrathecal administration of an NMDA receptor agonist inhibited the antinociceptive effect of propofol; in contrast, an NMDA receptor antagonist enhanced the antinociceptive action of propofol (Cheng et al., 2008). These studies demonstrated that propofol has a synergistic action with several nociceptive transmission cascades including amino acid and opioid systems in the spinal cord.
The above mentioned methods determined the probable way of analgesic action of propofol.

4. Methods

We followed the PRIZMA statement that recommends standards to improve the quality of reporting of meta-analyses.

Systematic search

The study was carried out according to the methods recommended by the Cochrane Collaboration and written in accordance with the PRISMA statement for reporting systematic reviews (Higgins et al., 2009 & Liberati et al., 2009).

This systematic review included studies published up to December 2010. We conducted a systemic search of the electronic databasas: PubMed, Cochrane Library, and Embase, www.clinicaltrials.gov, and hand searching from the reference lists of identified papers. We used the search terms "propofol" and ("postoperative analgesia" OR "analgesic effect"). Abstracts and unpublished studies were not considered. The search was limited to clinical trials and randomised controlled trials. Reference lists from identified studies and journals which appeared to be associated with the most retrieved citations were then hand-searched. The trials in languages other than English were not excluded. We prepared a flow diagram to summarize the study selection process according to PRISMA (Jaded et al., 1996) (Figure 1.).

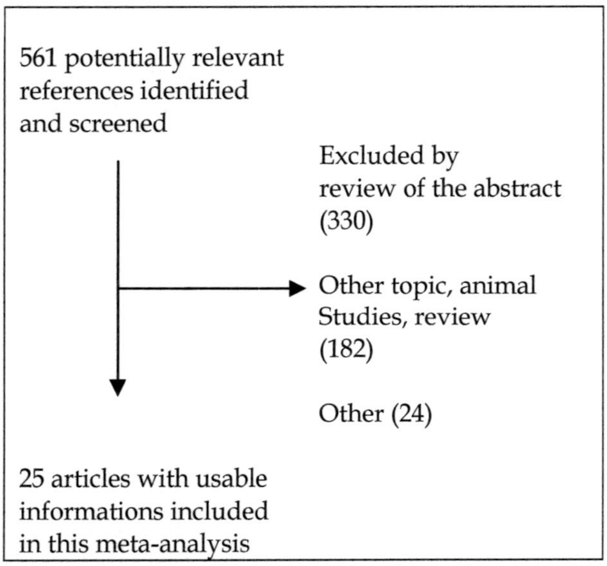

Fig. 1. Flow diagram of excluded and included studies according to PRIZMA statement

To minimize data duplication as a result of multiple reporting we compared papers from the same author. In addition, we searched www.clinicaltrials.gov for studies. Two authors (HJ and AD) screened and retrieved reports and excluded irrelevant studies. Relevant data were extracted by one author (VG) and checked by another (AH).

From each study we extracted details on patients' characteristics (adults and children, ASA status, age), type of surgery or no surgery and use of anesthetics in control group (Table 1.). Pain score, pain score method and use of postoperative analgesics, were also noted (Table 2). Side effects were noted in Table 3.

Study selection

To be considered for the review, the study was evaluated with regard to randomization method, allocation concealment, details of blinding measures, and withdrawals and dropouts using the modified 7-point 4-item Oxford scale (Figure 2) (Dong et al., 2002). This meant that adequate randomization was an absolute requirement for selection. However,

double-blinding was not a requirement, because adequate blinding was not felt to be possible in most studies. Each study was evaluated independently by authors and agreement was reached by consensus.
Selected studies included 25 randomised controlled trials that compared the use propofol during anesthesia and any drug or non-drug intervention, or a combination, with an active or inactive control, and reported the response rate and severity of pain after propofol anesthesia.

VALIDITY SCORE (0-7)	
Randomisation	*Double blinding*
0 None	0 None
1Mentioned	1 Mentioned
2Described and adequate	2 Described and adequate
Concealment of allocation	*Flow of patients*
0 None	0 None
1 Yes	1 Described but incomplete
	2 Described and adequate

Fig. 2. Modified Oxford Scale

Selected studies included 25 randomised controlled trials that compared the use propofol during anesthesia and any drug or non-drug intervention, or a combination, with an active or inactive control, and reported the response rate and severity of pain after propofol anesthesia.
The studies included in this review enrolled 1970, male and female patients, 1 to 80 year old, ASA I-III, who underwent surgical or non-surgical treatment resulting in the need for acute pain control. Relevant pain outcomes included number of patients who express pain, pain intensity, time to first analgesic request and supplemental analgesic demand were noted. All included studies had numerical data presented in the text or a table; if data were not presented as such, we extracted the information from the graphs if the scale allowed a sufficiently precise estimation.
We excluded trials including less than 10 patients and those reporting on chronic pain. Data from animal studies, abstracts, letters or reviews were not considered.
Information on number of patients, anesthetics and type of surgery was obtained from each report.
The data extracted from each of the included trials included: eligibility and exclusion criteria, study design, duration and degree of follow-up, randomization, allocation concealment, blinding, number and characteristics of participants, type of surgery, pain score, time to first analgesic request, and consumption of supplementary analgesics between the propofol and other treatment groups, and by assessment of the side effects (Table 1, 2 & 3).

Meta analyses

Qualitative analysis of postoperative effectiveness was evaluated by significant difference ($P < 0.05$ as reported in the original investigation) in pain relief using pain scores, time to first analgesic request, and consumption of supplementary analgesics between the treatment groups, and by assessment of the clinical importance of observed differences.

Reference	VS	Treatment	Control	No. of Patients	Type of Intervention
Briggs et al. 1982	3	Propofol	Thiopentone	40	Gynecologic procedures
Doze et al. 1988	4	Propofol	thiopental/isoflurane	120	Abdominal surgery
Borgeat et al. 1990	4	Propofol	thiopental/halothane	40	ENT surgery
Anker-Møller et al. 1991	4	Propofol	thiopental/saline	19	laser stimulation
V Hemelrijck et al. 1991	4	Propofol	desflurane	92	gynecological laparascopy
Hendolin et al. 1994	5	Propofol	thiopental/isoflurane	41	uvuloplasty
Jellish et al. 1995	5	Propofol	thiopental/isoflurane	102	middle ear surgery
Petersen-Felix et al. 1996	2	Propofol	alfentanyl	12	electric/laser/acoustical stimulation
Eriksson et al. 1996	5	desflurane	propofol	90	gynecological laparascopy
Zacny et al. 1966	3	propofol	fentanyl	12	ice-cold water
Davis et al. 1997	5	reifentanil	alfentanil/isofl/prop	129	strabismus surgery
Boccara et al. 1998	5	propofol	isoflurane	40	cosmetic abdominoplasty
Ozkose et al. 2001	6	Propofol,/fentanyl	sevoflurane/isofl & alfentanyl	60	laminectomy and discectomy operations
Hand et al. 2001	3	propofol	intralipids	48	tourniquet pain
Mukherjee et al. 2003	6	propofol,fentanyl, isoflurane	pr, remifentanil	100	middle ear surgery
Hofer et al. 2003	7	propofol	sevoflurane	305	gynaecologic or orthopedic procedures
Coolong et al 2003	4	propofol	thiopental	84	laparascopic procedures
Frölich et al. 2005	4	propofol	placebo	80	thermal pain
Cheng et al. 2008	7	propofol	isoflurane	80	open uterine surgery
Fassoulaki et al. 2008	7	sevofl/desfl	propofol	105	gynecological operations
Hasani et al. 2009	5	propofol	halothane	83	abdominal surgery
Bandschapp et al. 2010	7	propofol	intralipid/saline	14	electrical stimulation
Tan et al. 2010	6	propofol	sevoflurane	80	gynecological laparascopic
Pieters et al. 2010	7	propofol	sevoflurane	42	adenotonsillectomy
Shin et al. 2010	7	propofol & remifentanyl	sevoflurane and remifentanyl	214	brest cancer surgery

VS-Validity Score (Modified Oxford Scale)
NS - no significant difference between treatment groups or no significant difference in favor of the treatment; P< 0.05 - significant difference between treatment groups in favor of the treatment; NE - not evaluated.

Table 1. Details of study included.

References	Pain Score Method	Pain Score	Time to First Analgesic Request	Supplemental Analgesic Demand
Briggs et al. 1982	tibial pressure algesimetry	P<0.001	NE	NE
Doze et al. 1988	NE	NE	p>0.05	p>0.05
Borgeat et al. 1990	VAS	P<0.05	p>0.05	p>0.05
Anker-Møller et al. 1991	laser power meter	NS	NE	NE
Van Hemelrijck etal. 1991	VAS	NS	NS	NS
Hendolin et al. 1994	VAS	P<0.05	NS	NS
Jellish et al. 1995	VAS	NS	NS	NS
Petersen-Felix et al. 1996	VAS	NS	NE	NE
Eriksson et al. 1996	VAS	NS	NS	NS
Zacny et al. 1966	VAS	P<0.05	NE	NE
Davis et al. 1997	OPDS	NS	NS	NS
Boccara et al. 1998	VAS	P<0.05 for Iso	P<0.05 for Iso	P<0.05 for Iso
Ozkose et al. 2001	VAS	P<0.05	P<0.05	P<0.05
Hand et al. 2001	NRS	NE	P<0.05	P<0.05
Mukherjee et al. 2003	VAS	P<0.05	P<0.05	P<0.05
Hofer et al. 2003	VAS	NS	NS	NS
Coolong et al 2003	VNRS	NS	NS	NS
Frölich et al. 2005	VAS	P<0.05 more pain with propofol	NE	NE
Cheng et al. 2008	NAS	p<0.01	p<0.01	p<0.01
Fassoulaki et al. 2008	VAS	NS	NS	NS
Hasani et al. 2009	FPS	NS	NE	NE
Bandschapp et al. 2010	NRS	P<0.05	NE	NE
Tan et al. 2010	VAS	P=0.01	NS	NS
Pieters et al. 2010	CHEOPS	P<0.05	P<0.05	P<0.05
Shin et al. 2010	VAS	P> 0.001	P> 0.001	P> 0.001

NS - no significant difference between treatment groups or no significant difference in favor of the treatment; *P*<0.05 - significant difference between treatment groups in favor of the treatment; NE - not evaluated.

Table 2. Details of study included.

	Nauzea			Vomiting			Other side effects		
Study	**Propofol** n/N	**Control** n/N	***P***	**Propofol** n/N	**Control** n/N	***P***	**Propofol** n/N	**Control** n/N	***P***
Doze 1988	1/ 60	8 /60	P<0.05	3/ 60	16/60	P<0.05	10 në 60	34/60	P<0.05
Borgeat 1990	0/20	2/20	NS	0/20	2 në 20	NE	16/20	20/20	P<0.05
Vhemelrijck 1991			P<0.05			P<0.05	9/46	46/46	P<0.05
Hendolin 1994	0/20	2/21	NS	0/20	1/21		2 /21	2 /21	NS
Jellish 1995	3/34	20/68	P<0.05	5/34	15/68	NS			
Eriksson 1996			NS			NS			NS
Davis 1997				6/20	32/57	P<0.05	0/20	23/57	P<0.05
Boccara 1998	5/ 20	12/ 20	P<0.05						NS
Ozkose 2001				1 /20	22/40	P<0.05			
Mukherjee 2003			NS			NS			NS
Hofer 2003	50/155	75/146	P<0.001	34/155	50/146	P<0.01			
Coolong 2003			NS			NS			NS
Cheng 2008			NS			NS			NS
Hasani 2009			NS			NS			NS
Tan 2010			NS			NS			NS
Pieters 2010	1/19	7/19	P<0.05	1/19	7/19	P<0.05			NS
Shin 2010	29/96	40/90	P<0.005	29/ 96	40/90	P<0.005	50/96	42/90	NS

NS - no significant difference between treatment groups or no significant difference in favor of the treatment;
P<0.05 - significant difference between treatment groups in favor of the treatment; NE - not evaluated.

Table 3. Details of study included (side effects).

Quantitative analyses of combined data were intended by calculation of the number of patients reporting any pain or no pain (pain response rate) between treatment groups. For studies with multiple intervention groups, we partitioned the count of events and patients in the control group into two or more control groups within any meta-analysis to avoid a unit of analysis error. For the studies participating in the indirect comparisons, we partitioned the comparator group according to how many times it was used for indirect comparisons (across meta-analyses). The summary relative risks and 95% confidence intervals were estimated using a random effects Mantel-Haenszel method in RevMan 5.0 (Cochrane Collaboration). Statistical heterogeneity was assessed by the I^2 value.
The weight given to each study in this analysis (*i.e.*, how much influence each study had on the overall results) was determined by the precision of its estimate by taking into account study size and SDs of the pain in the individual trials. For the current use, a mean for each treatment group was calculated in every trial from all available recordings performed after anesthesia with propofol. Verbal rating pain scores and similar scores were converted to VAS pain scores (*e.g.*, a four-point verbal rating score including no, light, moderate, and severe pain was converted to 0, 25, 50, and 75 mm VAS, respectively).

5. Results

The systematic search in the databases identified 561 relevant articles. After screening, 25 studies potentially met the inclusion criteria. The full-text publications of these studies were examined in more detail. Four study was excluded, because it was reviews or editorial articles. In 90 studies the subject of investigation were animals and also were excluded. (Fig. 1).

The data of 25 randomized controlled studies were included in the present meta-analysis (Table 1,2 &3). A total of 1970 patients (909 with propofol), male and female were included. The patients were 1-85 year old. The 294 patients were children, aged 1-18 year (Borgeat et al.,1990, Pieters et al., 2010, Davis et al., 1997 & Hasani et al., 2009). The participans undergoing brest, ginecologic, orthopedic, ENT, abdominal, urogenital, spine, cosmetic or eye surgery. In 7 studies the participants were volunteer and have no surgery (total 163 volunteers) (Briggs et al., 1982, Anker-Møller et al., 1991, Zacny et al., 1996, Petersen-Felix et al., 1996, Hand et al., 2001, Frolich et al., 2005 & Bandschapp et al. ,2010).

The participants were randomly assigned to receive propofol and in control group: thiopental (Briggs et al.,1982 & Coolong et al.,2003); thiopental and saline (Anker-Møller et al., 1991); thiopental with halothane (Borgeat et al.,1990); or, thiopenthal with isoflurane (Doze et al., 1988 , Hendolin et al.,1994 & Jellish et al.,1995). In control grup the inhalation anesthetics used were halothane (Hasani et al., 2009), isoflurane (Boccara et al., 1998& Cheng et al.,2008), sevoflurane (Ozkose et al.,2001, Hofer et al., 2003, Tan et al., 2010, Pieters et al., 2010 & Shin et al., 2010) and desflurane (Van Hemelrijck et al.,1991&Fassoulaki et al., 2010). Also, the control groups contained opioids: fentanyl, remifentanil (Davis et al., 1997, Mukherjee et al., 2003 & Shin et al., 2010) and alfentanil (Petersen-Felix et al., 1996& Davis et al., 1997).

Intensity of pain scores was considered adequate (>30 mm VAS) in all trials. VAS (visual analogue score) pain score was not present in 9 studies. The pain scores used in studies was NRS-numeric rating scale (Hand et al., 2001&Bandschapp et al. ,2010), NAS-Numerical analogue score (Cheng et al., 2008), CHEOPS-Children's Hospital of Eastern Ontario Scale (Pieters et al., 2010), tibial pressure algesimetry (Briggs et al., 1982), VNSR-verbal numeric rating scale (Coolong et al., 2003), laser power meter (Anker-Møller et al., 1991), FPS- faces pain scale (Hasani et al., 2009) and OPDS-Objective Pain Discomfort Scale (Davis et al., 1997).

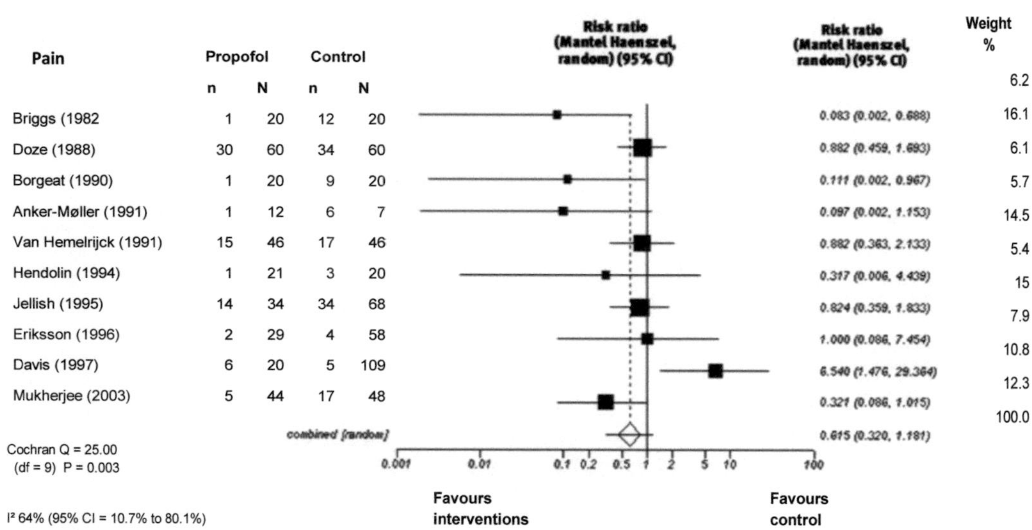

Fig. 3. Risk of postoperative pain after propofol anesthesia.

In selected 25 randomized controlled trials the postoperative pain was evaluated in patients treated with propofol. In 15 of them the degree of pain was given as the mean and, in our research to find risk ratio (Mantel Haenszel, random) we included 10 researches in which pain was expressed as present or absent.
Pain was rarely present in the groups treated with propofol 0.615 (95% CI 0.320-1.181) (Fig. 3).

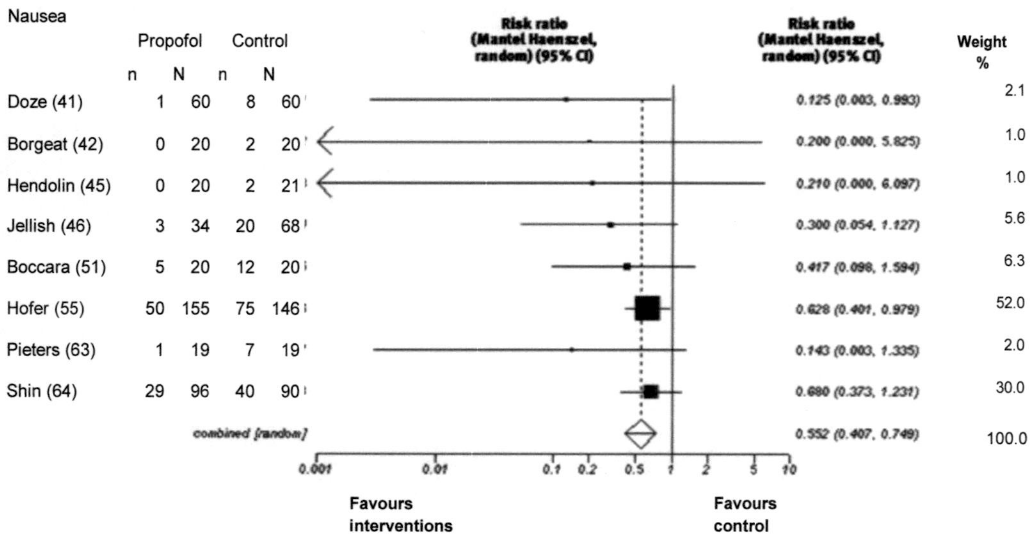

Fig. 4. Risk of postoperative nauzea after propofol anesthesia.

To study the presence of nausea we analyzed eight researches that have investigated this symptom in postoperative period. Nausea was the rare risk ratio 0.552 in intervention group (95% CI 0.407-0.749) (Fig. 4).

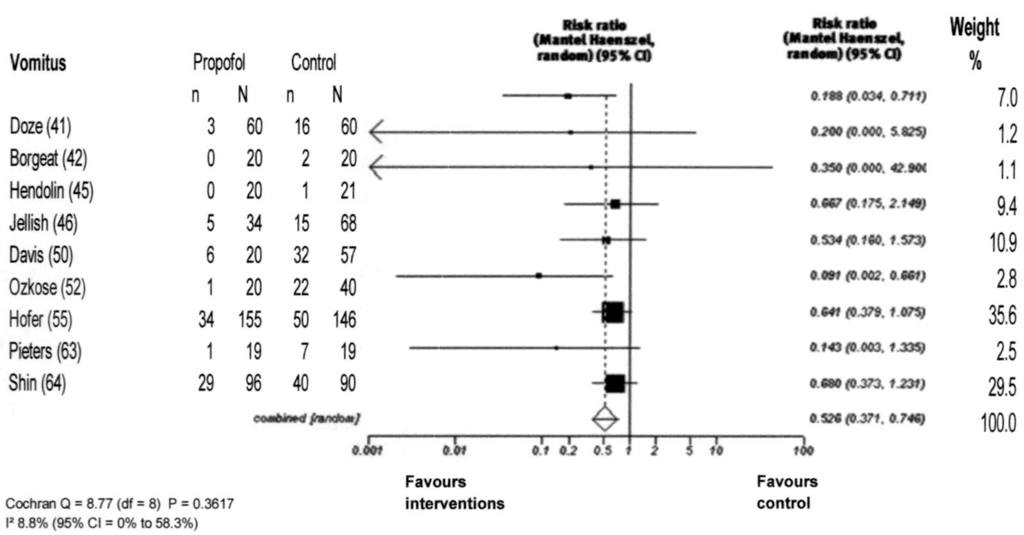

Fig. 5. Risk of postoperative vomiting after propofol anesthesia.

The presence of vomiting was analyzed in 9 researches. The risk ratio for vomiting was RR= 0.526 (95% CI 0.371-0.746) in intervention group with propofol (Fig. 5).

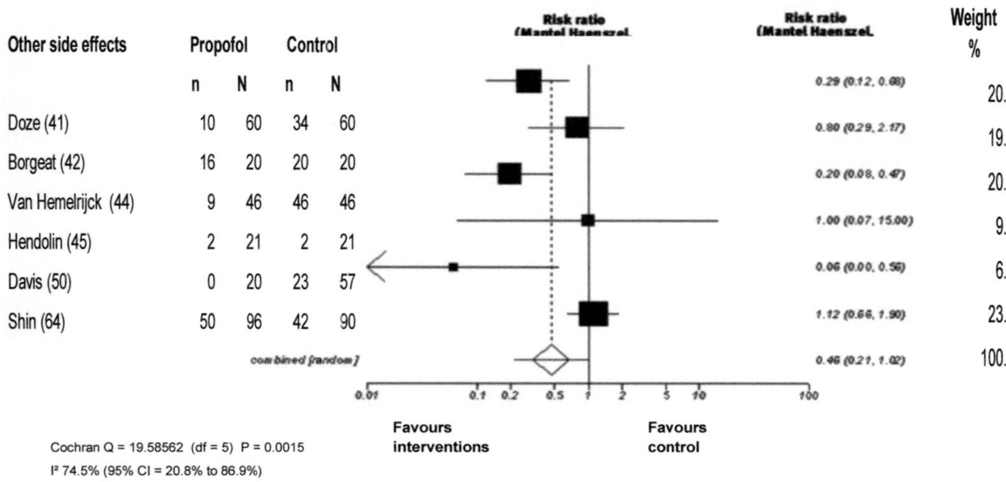

Fig. 6. Risk of the other side effects after propofol anesthesia during the postoperative period.

The other side effects which occurred in patients anesthetized with propofol were analyzed in 9 researches. In the term "the other side effects" was included: pain during propofol injection in induction period, bradycardia, hypotension, and spontaneous movements also described in perioperative period. Apnea, hypersalivation, laryngospasm and bronchospasm are also included in possible complications in postoperative period. The other side effects were also rare in the propofol anesthesia treated patients with the risk ratio 0.46 in intervention group (95% CI 0.21 to 1.02) (Fig. 6).

6. Discussion

Is propofol analgesic? ; still remain unclear. Experts held very different opinions on the value and clinical utility of an analgesic effect of propofol. The answers for this question were evaluated with pro *versus* con debates.

***PRO*: Propofol has analgesic effect**

Discussions about analgesic effect of propofol restarted with the study published in *Anesthesia & Analgesia* in January 2008 by Cheng et al. The trial was based in hypothesis that women scheduled for hysterectomy or myomectomy and anesthetized with volatile anesthesia, isoflurane induces a hyperalgesic state, and that patients anesthetized with propofol was neutral in its modulation of pain sensitivity. They found that patients anesthetized with isoflurane reported more postoperative pain than those anesthetized with propofol. The other finding was the difference in postoperative opioid use with more requirements in those anesthetized with isoflurane.

Two years later, in 2010 issue of *Anesthesia & Analgesia*, Tan et al. report on a trial that tests the hypothesis that patients undergoing day surgery anesthetized with propofol have less pain and a better quality of recovery compared with patients anesthetized with sevoflurane. In this prospective, double-blind, randomized trial, the authors used a study design in which one group had an induction with inhalation of sevoflurane followed by sevoflurane maintenance, whereas the other group had an IV induction with propofol followed by propofol maintenance. The subjects were treated during surgery with alfentanil, paracetamol, and diclofenac for pain and dexamethasone and ondansetron for nausea. Pain was treated after surgery using morphine until visual analog scale score was <4 and then oral oxycodone. The authors found that propofol provided a statistically significant ($P < 0.01$) difference, decrease in postoperative pain. Hendolin et al., 1994, found that propofol significantly reduced pain in the second hour compared with patients receiving isoflurane, corroborating the results of the present study.

The other study published in *Anesthesiology* August 2010 by Bandschapp et al., investigated the pain perception or central sensitization effects of propofol and its solvent (10% Intralipid) in healthy volunteers. They experienced decreased pain, hyperalgesia and allodynia elicited by intra-cutaneous electrical stimulation when they received a target-control infusion of propofol (2µg/ml) compared with controls (the solvent 10% Intralipid and saline). However, the results provide no evidence for a modulatory role of the solvent of propofol (10% Intralipid) in the analgesic and antihyperalgesic properties of propofol.

Propofol reduced pain by 40% and nearly abolished hypersensitivity which disappears on discontinuation of the drug. The EC_{50} for the analgesic effect of propofol was 3.2 µg/ml.

There is animal literature that addresses the modulatory effects of anesthetics in different nociceptive models.

In the 1990s, Ewen et al., found that in rats an IV infusion of propofol resulted in an initial decline followed by a rise in nociceptive threshold as the plasma concentration and degree of sedation increased. They suggest that smaller concentrations of propofol than sedative doses are responsible for hyperalgesia. However, the similar experiments in a postoperative pain models in mice were unable to detect any hyperalgesic phase at lower than sedative doses of propofol or on emergence (Udesky et al., 2005). Other groups have found an analgesic response to propofol, particularly in inflammatory pain models (Daniels&Roberts, 1998). A study in rodents by Guindon et al., 2007, demonstrated that in a test of inflammatory pain, locally injected propofol decreased pain behavior in a dose-dependent manner. The authors hypothesized that this antinociceptive activity was mediated, in part, by cannabinoid receptors 1 and 2 (CB1 and CB2). Gilron et al., 1999, however, showed that propofol suppressed hindpaw formalin-evoked expression of fos-like immunoreactivity (FLI) in spinal neurons, suggesting an important analgesic effect.

Clearly, most of the animal and human data on nociceptive effects mediated by propofol may provide advantages.

***CON:* Propofol has not analgesic effect**

On the other hand, many studies with propofol in both animals and humans have failed to demonstrate any evidence of analgesic-like activity.

In an animal study by Merrill et al., 2006, propofol produced anesthesia but failed to produce the experimental findings typically associated with nociception, suggesting that propofol lacks analgesic properties. Accurately, propofol sufficient to produce immobility did not prevent increased activation (c-fos expression) of spinal neurons by intraplantar formalin injection, a finding consistent with propofol lacking analgesic properties. Mice with a mutation of the gamma-aminobutyric acid type A receptor were resistant to propofol anesthesia, supporting the importance of this receptor for propofol's action. Another rodent study (Ng & Antognini, 2006) found that isoflurane and propofol both had similar effects on neuronal "windup" in the spinal cord, a factor associated with persistent pain. The study from Goto et al., 1994, reported that propofol, unlike pentobarbital, had no effect on second-phase nocifensive behavioral responses elicited by formalin injection in the hind paws of rats. Wilder-Smith et al. , 1995, also determined that propofol infusions did not affect thermal pain thresholds.

The human studies of interest, (Boccara et al., 1998) compared postoperative pain and analgesic requirements in patients receiving propofol or isoflurane for maintenance of anesthesia and reported that patients receiving propofol actually had increased pain and opioid requirements for the first 6 hours after surgery compared with patients receiving isoflurane. These findings were exactly the opposite of the findings of Cheng et al.

We conduct a more recent clinical study, published in *Anesthesia & Analgesia* in November 2008, by Fassoulaki et al., in patients undergoing abdominal hysterectomy or myomectomy under sevoflurane, desflurane or propofol anesthesia. Anesthesia was induced with propofol, morphine and cisatracrium; and maintained with sevoflurane or desflurane or propofol. Postoperative analgesia was maintained with morphine. They were unable to demonstrate any difference in postoperative pain scores or in the requirement for opioid analgesic medication among patients maintained with propofol, sevoflurane, or desflurane.

Presented data explained the inconsistency between the studies regarding the post-operative analgesic effect of propofol.

Our findings support the analgesic effect of propofol.

Postoperative nausea and vomiting (PONV) are unpleasant, often underestimated side effects of anesthesia and surgery, not devoid of medical complications. Prevention with antiemetics is only partially effective. Propofol has been shown recently to possess antiemetic properties in several situations.

The limitation of our analysis is mainly related to the methodological heterogeneity of several studies. The dose of propofol varied between the studies and my influenced the postoperative analgesic effect. The methods of postoperative pain assessment my bias the results of our meta-analyses. On the other hand, the number of analyzed clinical trials may also bias our results.

7. Conclusions

Our meta-analysis indicates that propofol provides a prolonged and improved postoperative analgesia with few adverse effects compared with an other inhalation and intravenous anaesthetics. However, propofol have improved antiemetic effect. The other side effects are minimal, with exception of pain during injection of propofol.

Propofol changed the practice of anesthesia, nevertheless postoperative analgesia with ordinary analgesics must be sustained.

Finally, we accomplished that propofol is not an analgesic, but many studies have certainly demonstrated analgesic properties of propofol.

8. References

Anker-Møller, E; Spangsberg, N; Arendt-Nielsen, L; Schultz, P; Kristensen, MS & Bjerring, P. (1991). Subhypnotic doses of thiopentone and propofol cause analgesia to experimentally induced acute pain. *Br J Anaesth* 66:185-8.

Bandschapp, O, Filitz, J, Ihmsen, H, Koppert, W & Ruppen W. (2010). Analgesic and antihyperalgesic properties of propofol in a human pain model. *Anesthesiology* 113:421–428.

Becker, DE. (2010) Nausea, vomiting, and hiccups: a review of mechanisms and treatment. Anesth Prog 57:150-6

Boccara, G, Mann, C, Pouzeratte, Y, Bellavoir, A, Rouvier, A & Colson, P. (1998). Improved postoperative analgesia with isoflurane than with propofol anaesthesia. *Can J Anaesth* 45:839–42.

Borgeat ,A, Popovic, V, Meier, D& Schwander, D. (1990). Comparison of propofol and thiopentone/halothane for short duration ENT surgical procedures in children. *Anesth Analg* 71:511–5.

Briggs, LP, Dundee, JW, Bahar, M & Clarke, RS.(1982). Comparison of the effect of diisopropyl phenol (ICI 35, 868) and thiopentone on response to somatic pain. *Br J Anaesth* 54:307–1.

Cheng, SS, Yeh, J& Flood, P. (2008). Anesthesia matters: patients anesthetized with propofol have less postoperative pain than those anesthetized with isoflurane. *Anesth Analg* 106:264-9.

Coolong, KJ, McGough, E, Vacchiano, C& Pellegrini, JE. (2003). Comparison of the effects of propofol versus thiopental induction on postoperative outcomes following surgical procedures longer than 2 hours. *AANA J* 71:215-22.

Dagal, A& Lam, AM. (2009). Cerebral autoregulation and anesthesia. *Curr Opin Anaesthesiol* 22:542-52.

Daniels, S& Roberts, RJ. (1998). Post-synaptic inhibitory mechanisms of anaesthesia; glycine receptors. *Toxicol Lett* 100–101:71–6.

Davis, PJ, Lerman, J, Suresh, S, McGowan, FX, Coté, CJ, Landsman, I & Henson LG. (1997). A randomized multicenter study of remifentanil compared with alfentanil, isoflurane, or propofol in anesthetized pediatric patients undergoing elective strabismus surgery. *Anesth Analg*. 84:982-9.

Deegan, RJ. (1992). Propofol: a review of the pharmacology and applications of an intravenous anesthetic agent. *Am J Med Sci* 304:45-9.

Dong, XP& Xu, TL. (2002). The actions of propofol on gamma-aminobutyric acid-A and glycine receptors in acutely dissociated spinal dorsal horn neurons of the rat. *Anesth Analg* 95:907-14.

Doze, VA, Shafer, A& White, PF. (1988). Propofol-nitrous versus thiopental-isoflurane-nitrous oxide for general anesthesia. *Anesthesiology* 69:63–71

Eberhart, LH; Frank, S; Lange, H; Morin, AM; Scherag, A; Wulf, H & Kranke, P. (2006). Systematic review on the recurrence of postoperative nausea and vomiting after a first episode in the recovery room - implications for the treatment of PONV and related clinical trials. *BMC Anesthesiol* 13;6:14

Ewen, A, Archer, DP, Samanani, N& Roth, SH. (1995). Hyperalgesia during sedation: effects of barbiturates and propofol in the rat. Can J Anaesth 42:532–40.

Fassoulaki, A. (2011). Is propofol an analgesic. *Eur J Anaesthesiol* 28:481-2.

Fassoulaki, A, Melemeni, A, Paraskeva, A, Siafaka, I& Sarantopoulos, C. (2008). Postoperative pain and analgesic requirements after anesthesia with sevoflurane, desflurane or propofol. *Anesth Analg* 107:1715–9.

Fredman, B; Husain, MM & White, PF. (1994). Anaesthesia for electroconvulsive therapy: use of propofol revisited. *Eur J Anaesthesiol* 11:423-5.

Frölich, MA; Arabshahi, A; Katholi, C; Prasain, J & Barnes S. (2011). Hemodynamic characteristics of midazolam, propofol, and dexmedetomidine in healthy volunteers. *J Clin Anesth* 23:218-23.

Gan, TJ; El-Molem, H; Ray, J & Glass, PS. (1999). Patient-controlled antiemesis: a randomized, double-blind comparison of two doses of propofol versus placebo. *Anesthesiology* 90:1564-70.

Gilron, I, Quirion, R& Coderre, TJ.(1999). Pre- versus postinjury effects of intravenous GABAergic anesthetics on formalin-induced Fos immunoreactivity in the rat spinal cord. *Anesth Analg* 88:414–20

Girard, F; Moumdjian, R; Boudreault, D; Chouinard, P; Bouthilier, A & Ruel, M. (2009). The effect of sedation on intracranial pressure in patients with an intracranial space-occupying lesion: remifentanil versus propofol. *Anesth Analg* 109:194-8.

Goto, T, Marota, JJ & Crosby, G. (1994). Pentobarbitone, but not propofol, produces pre-emptive analgesia in the rat formalin model. *Br J Anaesth* 72:662–7.

Guindon,J, LoVerme, J, Piomelli,D & Beaulieu,P. (2007). The antinociceptive effects of local injections of propofol in rats are mediated in part by cannabinoid CB1 and CB2 receptors. *Anesth Analg* 104:1563–9.

Hendolin, H, Kansanen, M, Kosk, E& Nuutinen, J. (1994).Propofol-nitrous oxide versus thiopentone-isoflurane-nitrous oxide anaesthesia for uvulopalatopharyngoplasty in patients with sleep apnea. *Acta Anaesthesiol Scand* 38:694–8.

Higgins, JPT & Green, S; eds. (2009). Cochrane handbook for the systematic reviews of interventions. Version 5.0.2. Cochrane Collaboration.

Jaded, AR, Moore, RA, Carroll, D, Jenkinson, C, Reynolds, DJ, Gavaghan, DJ & McQuay HJ.(1996). Assessing the quality of reports of randomized clinical trials: is blinding necessary? *Control Clin Trials* 17:1-12.

Jalota, L; Kalira, V; George, E; Shi, YY; Hornuss, C; Radke, O; Pace, NL & Apfel, CC. (2011). Prevention of pain on injection of propofol: systematic review and meta-analysis. Perioperative Clinical Research Core. *BMJ* 15;342:d1110.

Jewett, BA, Gibbs, LM, Tarasiuk, A& Kendig JJ. (1992). Propofol and barbiturate depression of spinal nociceptive neurotransmission.[see comment].*Anesthesiology* 77:1148–54

Krasowski, M. D., Koltchine, V. V., Rick, C. E., Ye, Q., Finn, S. E.& Harrison, N. L. (1998) Propofol and other intravenous anesthetics have sites of action on the γ-aminobutyric acid type A receptor distinct from that for isoflurane. *Mol. Pharmacol.* 53, 530-538.

Kwan, JW. (1989). High-technology i.v. infusion devices. Am *J Hosp Pharm* 46:320-35.

Liberati, A; Altman, DG; Tetzlaff, J; Mulrow, C; Gotzsche, PC; Ioannidis JP, et al. (2009). The PRISMA statement for reporting systematic reviews and meta-analyses of studies that evaluate healthcare interventions: explanation and elaboration. *BMJ* 339: b2700.

Machała, W & Szebla, R. (2008) . Effects of propofol induction on haemodynamics. *Anestezjol Intens Ter* 40:223-6.

Matsuki, A. (1991). A review of recent advances in total intravenous anesthesia. *Masui* 40:684-91.

Menku, A; Ogden, M & Saraymen, R.(2010). The protective effects of propofol and citicoline combination in experimental head injury in rats. *Turk Neurosurg* 20:57-62.

Merrill,AW, Barter,LS, Rudolph, U, Eger, EI II, Antognini, JF, Carstens,MI&Carstens,E. (2006). Propofol's effects on nociceptive behavior and spinal c-fos expression after intraplantar formalin injection in mice with a mutation in the gamma-aminobutyric acid-type (A) receptor beta3 subunit. *Anesth Analg* 103:478–83.

Modica, PA, Tempelhoff, R & White, PF. (1990). Pro- and anticonvulsant effects of anesthetics (Part I) *Anesth Analg* 70:303-15.

Modica, PA, Tempelhoff, R & White, PF (1990). Pro- and anticonvulsant effects of anesthetics (Part II) *Anesth Analg*. 70:433-44.

Moher, D; Liberati, A; Tetzlaff, J & Altman DG. (2009). PRISMA Group. Preferred reporting items for systematic reviews and meta-analyses: the PRISMA statement. *J Clin Epidemiol* 62:1006-12.

Murdoch, SD & Cohen, AT. (1999). Propofol-infusion syndrome in children. *Lancet* 12;353:2074-5.

Ng, KP& Antognini, JF.(2006). Isoflurane and propofol have similar effects on spinal neuronal windup at concentrations that block movement. Anesth Analg 103:1453–8.

Ozturk, E;l Demirbilek, S; Kadir But, A; Saricicek, V; Gulec, M; Akyol, O & Ozcan Ersoy, M. (2005). Antioxidant properties of propofol and erythropoietin after closed head injury in rats. Prog *Neuropsychopharmacol Biol Psychiatry* 29:922-7.

Sarani, B & Gracias, V. (2008). Safety and efficacy of propofol. *J Trauma* 64:242.

Siegwart, R., Jurd, R., Rudolph, U. (2002) Molecular determinants for the action of general anesthetics at recombinant $\alpha2\beta3\gamma2$ γ-aminobutyric acidA receptors. *J. Neurochem* 80, 140-148.

Simpson, KH; Halsall, PJ; Carr, CM & Stewart, KG. (1988). Propofol reduces seizure duration in patients having anaesthesia for electroconvulsive therapy. *Br J Anaesth* 61:343-4.

Singh, H. (1999). Bispectral index (BIS) monitoring during propofol-induced sedation and anaesthesia. *Eur J Anaesthesiol* 16:31-6.

Sebel, PS& Lowdon& JD. (1989) Propofol: a new intravenous anesthetic. Anesthesiology. 71:260-77.

Shafer, A; Doze, VA; Shafer, SL & White PF. (1988). Pharmacokinetics and pharmacodynamics of propofol infusions during general anesthesia. *Anesthesiology* 69:348-56.

Short, CE & Bufalari A. (1999). Propofol anesthesia.Vet *Clin North Am Small Anim Pract* 29:747-78.

Soppitt, AJ; Glass, PS; Howell, S; Weatherwax, K & Gan, TJ. (2000). The use of propofol for its antiemetic effect: a survey of clinical practice in the United States. *J Clin Anesth* 12:265-9.

Sun YY, Li KC, Chen J.(2005). Evidence for peripherally antinociceptive action of propofol in rats: behavioral and spinal neuronal responses to subcutaneous bee venom. *Brain Res* 1043:231–5

Tan, T, Bhinder, R, Carey, M & Briggs, L. (2010). Day-surgery patients anesthetized with propofol have less postoperative pain than those anesthetized with sevoflurane. *Anesth Analg* 111:83–5.

Trame`r, M; Moore, A & McQuay, H. (1997). Propofol anaesthesia and postoperative nausea and vomiting: quantitative systematic review of randomized controlled studies. *Br J Anaesth* 78:247–255.

Udesky, JO, Spence, NZ, Achiel,R, Lee, C& Flood, P. (2005). The role of nicotinic inhibition in ketamine-induced behavior. Anesth Analg 101:407–11.

Xu AJ, Duan SM & Zeng, YM. (2004). Effects of intrathecal NMDA and AMPA receptors agonists or antagonists on antinociception of propofol. *Acta Pharmacol Sin,* 25:9-14.

White, PF. (1989). Clinical uses of intravenous anesthetic and analgesic infusions. *Anesth Analg* 68:161-71.

White, PF. (2008). Propofol: its role in changing the practice of anesthesia. *Anesthesiology* 109:1132–1136.

Wilder-Smith, OH, Kolletzk, M & Wilder-Smith, CH.(1995). Sedation with intravenous infusions of propofol or thiopentone: effects on pain perception. *Anaesthesia;*50:218–22

Zeller, A; Arras, M; Lazaris, A; Jurd, R & Rudolph U. (2005). Distinct molecular targets for the central respiratory and cardiac actions of the general anesthetics etomidate and propofol. *FASEB* J 19:1677-9.

Zuppa, AF; Helfaer, MA & Adamson, PC. (2003). Propofol pharmacokinetics. *Pediatr Crit Care Med* 4:124-5.

Anker-Møller, E; Spangsberg, N; Arendt-Nielsen, L; Schultz, P; Kristensen, MS & Bjerring, P. (1991). Subhypnotic doses of thiopentone and propofol cause analgesia to experimentally induced acute pain. *Br J Anaesth* 66:185-8.

Bandschapp, O, Filitz, J, Ihmsen, H, Koppert, W & Ruppen W. (2010). Analgesic and antihyperalgesic properties of propofol in a human pain model. *Anesthesiology* 113:421–428.

Boccara, G, Mann, C, Pouzeratte, Y, Bellavoir, A, Rouvier, A & Colson, P. (1998). Improved postoperative analgesia with isoflurane than with propofol anaesthesia. *Can J Anaesth* 45:839–42.

Borgeat ,A, Popovic, V, Meier, D& Schwander, D. (1990). Comparison of propofol and thiopentone/halothane for short duration ENT surgical procedures in children. *Anesth Analg* 71:511–5.

Briggs, LP, Dundee, JW, Bahar, M & Clarke, RS.(1982). Comparison of the effect of diisopropyl phenol (ICI 35, 868) and thiopentone on response to somatic pain. *Br J Anaesth* 54:307–1.

Cheng, SS, Yeh, J& Flood, P. (2008). Anesthesia matters: patients anesthetized with propofol have less postoperative pain than those anesthetized with isoflurane. *Anesth Analg* 106:264-9.

Coolong, KJ, McGough, E, Vacchiano, C& Pellegrini, JE. (2003). Comparison of the effects of propofol versus thiopental induction on postoperative outcomes following surgical procedures longer than 2 hours. *AANA J* 71:215-22.

Davis, PJ, Lerman, J, Suresh, S, McGowan, FX, Coté, CJ, Landsman, I & Henson LG. (1997). A randomized multicenter study of remifentanil compared with alfentanil, isoflurane, or propofol in anesthetized pediatric patients undergoing elective strabismus surgery. *Anesth Analg*. 84:982-9.

Doze, VA, Shafer, A& White, PF. (1988). Propofol-nitrous versus thiopental-isoflurane-nitrous oxide for general anesthesia. *Anesthesiology* 69:63–71.

Eriksson, H & Korttila, K. (1996). Recovery profile after desflurane with or without ondansetron compared with propofol in patients undergoing outpatient gynecological laparoscopy. *Anesth Analg* 82:533–8.

Fassoulaki, A, Melemeni, A, Paraskeva, A, Siafaka, I& Sarantopoulos, C. (2008). Postoperative pain and analgesic requirements after anesthesia with sevoflurane, desflurane or propofol. *Anesth Analg* 107:1715–9.

Frölich, MA; Arabshahi, A; Katholi, C; Prasain, J & Barnes S. (2011). Hemodynamic characteristics of midazolam, propofol, and dexmedetomidine in healthy volunteers. *J Clin Anesth* 23:218-23.

Hand, R Jr, Riley, GP, Nick, ML, Shott, S & Faut-Callahan, M. (2001). The analgesic effects of subhypnotic doses of propofol in human volunteers with experimentally induced tourniquet pain. *AANA J* 69:466–70.

Hasani, A, Ozgen ,S & Baftiu, N. (2009). Emergence agitation in children after propofol versus halothane anesthesia. Med Sci Monit 2009; 15: CR302-CR306.

Hendolin, H, Kansanen, M, Kosk, E& Nuutinen, J. (1994).Propofol-nitrous oxide versus thiopentone-isoflurane-nitrous oxide anaesthesia for uvulopalatopharyngoplasty in patients with sleep apnea. *Acta Anaesthesiol Scand* 38:694–8.

Hofer, CK, Zollinger, A, Buchi,S, Klaghofer, R, Serafino, D, Buhlmann, S, Buddeberg, C, Pasch, T & Spahn, DR. (2003). Patient well-being after general anaesthesia: a prospective, randomized, controlled multi-centre trial comparing intravenous and inhalation anaesthesia. *Br J Anaesth* 91:631–7.

Jellish, WS, Leonetti, JP, Murdoch, JR & Fowles S. (1995). Propofol-based anesthesia as compared with standard anesthetic techniques for middle ear surgery. *J Clin Anesth* 7:292-6.

Mukherjee, K, Seavell, C, Rawlings, E & Weiss, A. (2003). A comparison of total intravenous with balanced anaesthesia for middle ear surgery: effects on postoperative nausea and vomiting, pain, and conditions of surgery. [see comment]. *Anaesthesia* 58:176–80.

Ozturk, E;l Demirbilek, S; Kadir But, A; Saricicek, V; Gulec, M; Akyol, O & Ozcan Ersoy, M. (2005). Antioxidant properties of propofol and erythropoietin after closed head injury in rats. Prog *Neuropsychopharmacol Biol Psychiatry* 29:922-7.

Petersen-Felix, S, Arendt-Nielsen, L, Bak, P, Fischer, M & Zbinden, AM. (1996). Psychophysical and electrophysiological responses to experimental pain may be influenced by sedation: comparison of the effects of a hypnotic (propofol) and an analgesic (alfentanil). *Br J Anaesth* 77:165-71.

Pieters, BJ, Penn, E, Nicklaus, P, Bruegger, D, Mehta, B &Weatherly, R. (2010). Emergence delirium and postoperative pain in children undergoing adenotonsillectomy: a comparison of propofol vs sevoflurane anesthesia. *Paediatr Anaesth* 20:944-50.

Shin, SW, Cho, AR, Lee, HJ, Kim, HJ, Byeon, GJ, Yoon, JW, Kim, KH & Kwon JY. (2010). Maintenance anaesthetics during remifentanil-based anaesthesia might affect postoperative pain control after breast cancer surgery. *Br J Anaesth* 105:661-7.

Tan, T, Bhinder, R, Carey, M & Briggs, L. (2010). Day-surgery patients anesthetized with propofol have less postoperative pain than those anesthetized with sevoflurane. *Anesth Analg* 111:83–5.

Van Hemelrijck, J, Smith, I & White, PF. (1991). Use of desflurane for outpatient anesthesia. A comparison with propofol and nitrous oxide. *Anesthesiology* 75:197-203.

Zacny, JP, Coalson, DW, Young, CJ, Klafta, JM, Lichtor, JL, Rupani, G, Thapar, P & Apfelbaum, JL. (1996). Propofol at conscious sedation doses produces mild analgesia to cold pressorinduced pain in healthy volunteers. *J Clin Anesth* 8:469–74.

12

Efficacy of Continuous Femoral Nerve Block with Stimulating Catheters Versus Nonstimulating Catheters - A Systematic-Narrative Review

Mario Dauri, Ludovica Celidonio, Sarit Nahmias,
Eleonora Fabbi, Filadelfo Coniglione and Maria Beatrice Silvi
Departement of Anesthesia and Intensive Care Unit, Tor Vergata University, Rome, Italy

1. Introduction

A femoral nerve block is simple to perform, has a high rate success, carries a low risk of complications, and it is widely used technique for surgical anesthesia and post-operative pain management of the lower extremity. It provides analgesia to the anterior thigh, including the flexor muscles of the hip and extensor muscles of the knee and therefore, it is well suited for surgeries that involve the hip, the knee or the anterior thigh zone. The femoral nerve block is often associated with sciatic nerve block in order to achieve a lower extremity analgesia.

The anterior approach to the femoral nerve block initially described as a 3-in-1 block by Winnie et al (Winnie et al., 1973), suggested that the femoral, lateral femoral cutaneous, and obturator nerves could be blocked from a single paravascular injection at a point inferior to the inguinal crease. Studies have since showed that the femoral can be reliably blocked by a single injection, the lateral femoral cutaneous nerves is blocked in 95%, but the obturator nerve is almost always spared (Parkinson et al., 1989). Therefore, a 3-in-1 block with the paravascular approach seems difficult to obtain, and, as a consequence, when all three nerves need to be anesthetized a posterior lumbar plexus block or a multitruncular block should be performed. The anterior approach to the femoral nerve is similar for "single shot" or continuous nerve blocks. A femoral nerve block can be obtained with single shot of local anesthetic or by using a continuous catheter technique. The localization of the femoral nerve can be obtained by the use of nerve stimulator or with ultrasound guidance. When using single shot technique, the local anesthetic agent is injected through the needle after location of the nerve with the nerve stimulator. When using continuous catheter techniques, the nerve can be stimulated via the needle through which the catheter is placed, or via both the needle and the catheter itself.

This narrative review summarizes the evidence derived from randomized controlled trials (RCTs) and retrospective analysis, in order to determine the efficacy of continuous femoral nerve block comparing the use of stimulating catheters with non-stimulating catheters for lower-extremity surgery. Furthermore, we explore the adjunctive use of ultrasonography for femoral nerve block.

1.1 Anatomy (Gray & Henry, 1918)

The Femoral Nerve, the largest branch of the lumbar plexus, arises from the dorsal divisions of the second, third, and fourth lumbar nerves. It descends through the fibers of the Psoas major, emerging from the muscle at the lower part of its lateral border, and passes down between it and the Iliacus, behind the iliac fascia; it then runs beneath the inguinal ligament, into the thigh, and splits into an anterior and a posterior division. At this level it is located lateral and posterior to the femoral artery.

The anterior division of the femoral nerve gives off (Table 1):

- Anterior cutaneous branches. The anterior cutaneous branches comprise the intermediate and medial cutaneous nerves
  - The intermediate cutaneous nerve pierces the fascia lata (and generally the Sartorius) and divides into two branches which supply the skin as low as the front of the knee. Here they communicate with the medial cutaneous nerve and the infrapatellar branch of the saphenous, to form the patellar plexus.
  - The medial cutaneous nerve passes obliquely across the upper part of the sheath of the femoral artery, and divides into two branches, an anterior and a posterior. Before dividing it gives off a few filaments, which supply the integument of the medial side of the thigh, accompanying the long saphenous vein. The anterior branch divides into two branches: one supplies the integument as low down as the medial side of the knee; the other crosses to the lateral side of the patella. The posterior branch descends along the medial border of the Sartorius muscle to the knee, where it pierces the fascia lata, communicates with the saphenous nerve, and gives off several cutaneous branches. It then passes down to supply the integument of the medial side of the leg.
- Muscular branches—The nerve to the Pectineus and the nerve to the Sartorius

The posterior division of the femoral nerve gives off (Table 1):

- The saphenous nerve - the largest cutaneous branch of the femoral nerve. It approaches the femoral artery where this vessel passes beneath the Sartorius, and lies in front of it, behind the aponeurotic covering of the adductor canal, as far as the opening in the lower part of the Adductor magnus. It descends vertically along the medial side of the knee behind the Sartorius, pierces the fascia lata, between the tendons of the Sartorius and Gracilis, and becomes subcutaneous. The nerve then passes along the tibial side of the leg, accompanied by the great saphenous vein, descends behind the medial border of the tibia, and, at the lower third of the leg, divides into two branches: one continues its course along the margin of the tibia, and ends at the ankle; the other passes in front of the ankle, and is distributed to the skin on the medial side of the foot, as far as the ball of the great toe. The saphenous nerve, about the middle of the thigh, gives off a branch which joins the subsartorial plexus. At the medial side of the knee it gives off a large infrapatellar branch, which pierces the Sartorius and fascia lata, and is distributed to the skin in front of the patella. Below the knee, the branches of the saphenous nerve are distributed to the skin of the front and medial side of the leg, communicating with the cutaneous branches of the femoral, or with filaments from the obturator nerve.
- Muscular branches supply the four parts of the Quadriceps femoris. The branch to the Rectus femoris enters the upper part of the muscle, and supplies a filament to the hip-joint. The branch to the Vastus lateralis enters the lower part of the muscle and gives off an articular filament to the knee-joint. The branch to the Vastus medialis enters the

muscle about its middle, and gives off a filament to the knee-joint. The branches to the Vastus intermedius, two or three in number, enter the muscle about the middle of the thigh and give off filament to the Articularis genu and the knee-joint.

- Articular branches
    - articular branch to the hip-joint is derived from the nerve to the Rectus femoris.
    - articular branches to the knee-joint are three in number. One is derived from the nerve to the Vastus lateralis, the second derived from the nerve to the Vastus medialis and the third branch is derived from the nerve to the Vastus intermedius.

Femoral Branches	
Anterior division provides sensory innervation to the skin of the anterior and medial thigh and motor innervation to the Sartorius and Pectineus muscles.	• Anterior cutaneous branches o intermediate cutaneous nerves o medial cutaneous nerves • Muscular branches o nerve to the Pectineus o nerve to the Sartorius
Posterior division provides sensory innervation to the medial part of the lower leg and motor innervation to the quadriceps muscle	• Saphenous nerve • Muscular branches (individual heads of the quadriceps muscle) • Articular branches o to the hip-joint o branches to the knee-joint

Table 1. Anatomy of femoral nerve

1.2 Indications

The femoral nerve block is mainly indicated for the pain control associated with unilateral anterior knee surgery (total knee arthroplasty, ACL). It is also ideal for surgery that involves the hip (femoral fracture repair) or anterior thigh. The block is often combined with a sciatic nerve block or with obturator nerve block if surgery is distal or posterior to the knee join.

1.3 Contraindications

- Infection or haematoma In the puncture site
- Local anesthetic allergy
- Lesion of the nerves to be stimulated distal to the puncture site
- Neurological deficit of the leg to be anaesthetised
- Refusal of the procedure by the patient

2. History of continuous nerve blocks

The first attempt to practice a continuous peripheral nerve blockade was done by Ansbro in 1946, who described a continuous block of the brachial plexus at a supraclavicular level (Ansbro, 1946). A continuous axillary block was performed in 1977 by Selander in patients who underwent hand surgery. (Selander, 1977).

The first use of an epidural catheter at the level of the lumbar plexus was reported by Brands and Callanan. Their conclusion was that continuous lumbar plexus blockade reduced administration of opioids and resulted in effective pain relief. (Brands E& Callanan VI, 1987 as cited in Navas et al., 2005). A continuous sciatic nerve block to relieve pain from ischaemic gangrene of the foot was described in 1984 by Smith et al. (Smith et al, 1984 as cited by Navas et al., 2005).

In order to provide reliable post-operative analgesia and prevent readmission due to failed catheter placement, it was necessary to develop methods to ensure accurate catheter positioning and to prevent catheter dislodgment.

Improvements in techniques and instruments have led to a painless, longer-lasting postoperative analgesia, with reduction of Opioids consumption, better functional recovery, increased patient satisfaction and reduced side-effects. New techniques and devices are increasingly appearing, and catheters are constantly being developed and improved (Navas et al., 2005)

3. Continuous femoral catheter placement technique (Fig 1- 2)

The patient should be in the supine position with legs spread slightly apart. After aseptic skin disinfection and sterile draping of the inguinal region, a local anesthetic is injected superficially. The stimulating needle insertion site is immediately below the inguinal crease, 1 to 2 cm lateral to the femoral artery pulsation. A 50-mm 18-gauge insulated stimulating needle is then connected to the peripheral nerve stimulator (PNS) with an initial current output of 1 mA (2 Hz, 0.1 ms). The stimulating needle has to be inserted with a 45° angle and advanced in a cephalad direction until quadriceps femoris muscle contractions were elicited (as evidenced by cephalad patellar movements). The needle position has to be adjusted until quadriceps femoris contractions are still elicited at a current of 0.5 mA or less. At this point, a 20-gauge catheter is introduced through the needle. The catheter is then advanced for 10 to 15 cm beyond the needle tip, needle is withdrawn and the catheter has to be secured in place. The local anesthetic of choice, has to be injected slowly through the catheter.

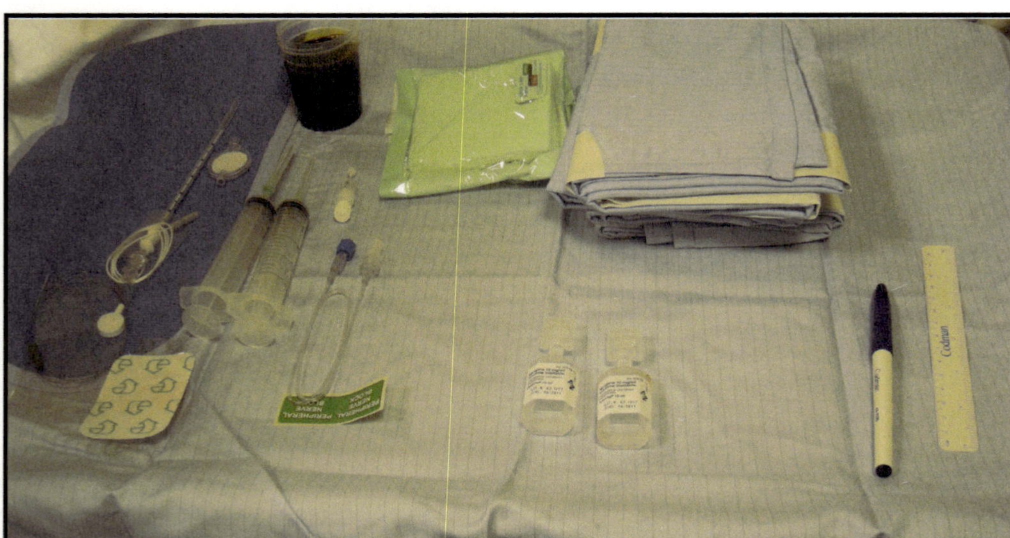

Fig. 1. Equipement

When stimulating catheter is being used, the catheter has to be connected to the PNS without changing the current output. The catheter is advanced 5 to 15 cm past the needle tip, and its position is adjusted until quadriceps femoris contractions are still elicited at a current output between 0.4 to 0.5 mA. At this point, the needle is withdrawn and quadriceps contractions are elicited via the catheter again to confirm the final perineural position of the catheter. (Dauri et al., 2007)

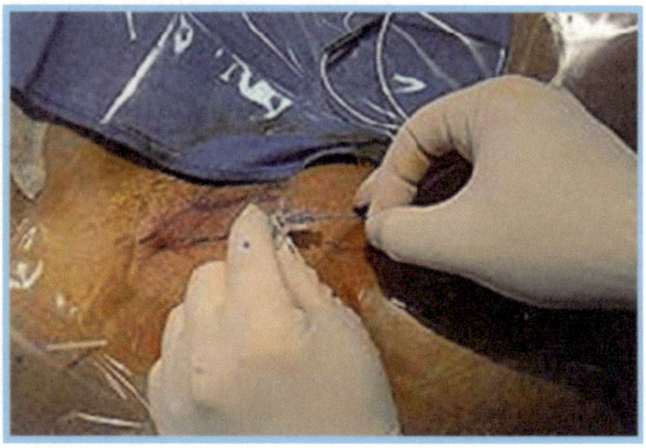

Fig. 2. Catheter placement

3.1 Local anesthetics

A number of local anesthetics may be used for femoral nerve blocks. In general, the volume of local anesthetic used to achieve a surgery anesthesia for a femoral nerve block will range from 15-20 ml. For 3-in-1 nerve block, the volume ranges from 25-30 ml. When postoperative analgesia is required, 0.5% of long acting anesthetic agents ropivacaine or levobupivacaine is often used. For postoperative analgesia, 1-2 mg/ml ropivacaine or 0.625-1.25 mg/ml levobupivacaine are used. The drugs are best administered by PCA pump with a basal rate infusion of 5-8 ml/h and bolus option.

3.2 Complications

- Vascular puncture
- Local infection
- Seizures (from systemic injection and local anesthetic toxicity)
- Neural ischemia and/or neural toxicity
- Local anesthetic toxicity:
    - CNS: tinnitus, confusion, metallic taste in the mouth
    - Cardiac: tachycardia, hypertension, arrhythmia
- Dislocation of the catheter
- Catheter breakage, formation of knots or loops
- Local anesthetic leakage (Gurnaney et al., 2011)

4. Continuous femoral block versus other techniques

Many studies were conducted in order to explore the benefits arising from continuous femoral nerve block compared with other analgesic techniques. Some of the studies conclusions are reported below:

- Continuous peripheral nerve blocks improve postoperative analgesia, patient satisfaction, and rehabilitation compared with IV narcotic therapy for lower extremity procedures (Capdevila et al., 1999; Singelyn et al., 1998; Ganapathy et al., 1999)
- Continuous femoral nerve blocks have been demonstrated to improve the outcome of total knee arthroplasty (capdevila et al., 1999; Chelly et al, 2001)
- Continuous femoral nerve block technique provides similar or better analgesia with fewer undesirable effects than intravenous PCA and the epidural technique during the first 48 h of postoperative management after total knee arthroplasty and after total hip arthroplasty (Singelyn et al., 1998; Singelyn et al., 1999).
- Outcome with continuous femoral nerve block has shown to be better than "single shot" femoral block and continuous epidural anesthesia. For analgesia after proximal lower limb orthopedic surgery, continuous three-in-one nerve blockade is as effective as epidural analgesia, with fewer side effects (urinary retention, nausea, and risk of spinal subarachnoid hemorrhage in anticoagulated patients) (Capdevila et al., 1999; Singelyn et al 1998)

5. Correlation between catheter position and the rate of effective sensory and motor blockades

Continuous femoral nerve block is commonly obtained with a peripheral nerve stimulator connected to a stimulating needle to localize the femoral nerve. The localization of the nerve is then followed by insertion of the catheter through the needle. Studies using blind advancement of femoral catheters indicate that catheter position in relation to the nerve is unpredictable. (Ganapathy et al., 1999; Capdevila et al., 2002) Therefore, even if the initial injection of local anesthetic through the needle produces adequate intraoperative anesthesia/analgesia, subsequent infusion through the catheter may not provide adequate postoperative analgesia. Furthermore, it is difficult to determine the correct catheter's position in order to obtain an effective postoperative analgesia; on the other side the proximity of the catheter to the femoral nerve could guarantee a better analgesia.
Few studies were conducted on the matter:

- Marhofer et al. used MRI scans in order to verify the distribution of local anesthetic. They showed that there is no evidence of cephalad spread of 30 ml of local anaesthetic when a 3-in-1 blockade is performed (Marhofer et al., 2000) .
- Ganapathy et al. used CT scans to verify the catheter position. They observed that only 40% of catheters are located in an 'ideal' position, defined as catheter-tip position at 2 cm of the cephalad extremity of the sacroiliac joint or between the sacral promontory and the lateral portion of the vertebral bodies of L4 and L5. (Ganapathy et al., 1999)
- Capdevila et al. used anteroposterior pelvic radiograph to determine the location of the distal tip of the catheter. They showed catheter location in a continuous 3-in-1 block to be unpredictable. Their conclusion was that during a continuous three-in-one block, the threaded catheter rarely reached the lumbar plexus and that the quality of sensory and motor blockade and initial pain relief depend on the location of the catheter tip under the fascia iliaca. (Capdevila et al., 2002) .

The reported results may highlight the theoretical advantages of using a stimulating catheter to ensure proper perineural catheter placement. The catheter's position could be fixed at a point where the desired motor response is observed at a stimulation intensity that guarantees its proximity to the femoral nerve.

6. Aim of the review

This narrative review summarizes the evidence derived from randomized controlled trials (RCTs) and retrospective analysis, in order to determine the benefits and harm comparing continuous femoral nerve block with stimulating catheters versus non-stimulating catheters for lower-extremity surgery; moreover we will explore the association with adjunctive ultrasonography (US) and stimulating perineural catheters for femoral nerve block.

7. Methods of searching literature

We searched PubMed, EMBASE, and the Cochrane Database using the following search terms: "ACL or anterior cruciate ligament" OR "knee arthroplasty" OR "knee surgery" AND "femoral nerve block" OR " peripheral nerve block" OR "regional anesthesia" AND "stimulating catheters" OR "non-stimulating catheters" AND "ultrasonography". Study were included in the review if they were randomized clinical trial (RCTs) and non randomized clinical trial comparing femoral nerve block with stimulating catheters versus non-stimulating catheters for elective knee surgery or RCTs comparing the insertion of stimulating catheters with or without ultrasonographic guidance; limits: English language, human adults. In addition to the systematic search of the bibliographic databases, the reference lists of all retrieved articles were screened for additional relevant trials.

8. Study description and results (Table 2)

An initial search yielded 8 potentially relevant clinical trial that were further examined. Two of these was subsequently excluded because it did not meet the inclusions criteria. A total of 733 patients were investigated: 311 patients with stimulating and 422 with nonstimulating catheters .

Salinas et Al. in 2004 (Salinas et al., 2004) published a prospective comparison of continuous femoral nerve block with nonstimulating catheter placement versus stimulating catheter-guided perineural placement, randomizing twenty volunteers; a stimulating catheter was placed on one side and an identical non-stimulating catheter on the contralateral side. Success of femoral block was defined as loss of sensation to cold and pinprick stimuli. Quality of successful block was determined by tolerance to transcutaneous electrical stimulation and force dynamometry of quadriceps strength. Despite the trial shown that block success was 100% via the stimulating catheters versus 85% via the nonstimulating catheters, they concluded that there was no statistically significant difference in block success between the two techniques.

Morin et Al. (Morin et al., 2005) in the following year published the results from the comparison between femoral nerve catheters inserted under continuous stimulation and catheters that were placed using the conventional technique of blind advancement in 81 patients undergoing major knee surgery. The aim of his randomized double blind trial was to determine whether accurate catheter positioning under continuous stimulation accelerates the onset of sensory and motor block, improves the quality of postoperative analgesia, and enhances functional recovery. He concluded that with continuous femoral nerve blocks, blind catheter advancement is as effective as the stimulating catheter technique with respect to onset time of sensory and motor block as well as for postoperative pain reduction and functional outcome.

A retrospective non randomized study of 419 patients was published in 2005 (Jack et al., 2005) comparing stimulating versus nonstimulating femoral catheter; it demonstrated no differences in term of visual analogue scale score and total morphine consumption with 3 days follow up. The conclusion was that the practical advantages of the stimulating catheter, as reported by previous investigators, were not obvious in this clinical situation.

In 2006 (Hayek et al., 2006) a randomized study was performed to evaluate whether a stimulating catheter allowed the use of lesser amounts of local anesthetics than a nonstimulating catheter concluding that the use of stimulating catheters in continuous femoral nerve blocks for TKA does not offer significant benefits over traditional nonstimulating catheters.

The experience from our department (Dauri et al., 2007) is about the evaluation of the efficacy of stimulating catheter to perform continuous femoral nerve block for anterior cruciate ligament reconstruction; data collection from 70 patient regarded pain scores, adverse effects, and need for supplemental anesthesia and analgesia other than a continuous postoperative infusion of ropivacaine 2 mg/mL through the continuous femoral nerve catheter set at 7 mL/h. Data collected shown that although the use of a stimulating catheter was associated with faster onset time for the femoral nerve block and lower additional analgesics postoperatively, the conclusions was that the clinical superiority (analgesia; lateral femoral cutaneous, and obturator nerve block) of stimulating catheters was not evident in this clinical setting.

	Study design	**Results**	**Conclusions**
Salinas et al., 2004	• Prospective , randomized double blind study in volounteers • SC= 20, NSC=20 Outcomes: • Block success • Overall tolerance to transcutaneous electrical stimulation • Overall depth of motor block	• Block success : • SC 100% , NSC 85%(p0.07) • Overall tolerance to transcutaneous electrical stimulation (p 0.009) and • overall depth of motor block(p 0.03) was significantly higher in the stimulating catheter-guided femoral nerve blocks	There was no statistically significant difference in block success between the two techniques. Stimulating catheter-guided placement provided an increased overall quality of continuous femoral perineural blockade.
Morin et al., 2005	• Randomized,controlled observer blinded trial in patients after major knee surgery • SC=38, NSC=43 Outcomes: • onset of sensory and motor block, • quality of postoperative analgesia • functional recovery	• onset time of sensory and motor block similar in both groups • no differences in the postoperative IV opioid consumption, and visual analog scale pain scores at rest and movement • No differences in maximal bending and stretching of the knee joint during the 5 days after surgery.	With continuous femoral nerve blocks, blind catheter advancement is as effective as the stimulating catheter technique with respect to onset time of sensory and motor block, for postoperative pain reduction and functional outcome.

	Study design	Results	Conclusions
Hayek et al., 2006	• randomized prospective study of patients undergoing TKA • SC=19, NSC=22 Outcomes: • amounts of local anesthetics • postoperative pain scores, • opioid use • side effects • acute functional orthopedic outcomes	• no statistically significant differences in the amount of ropivacaine administered (MD - 0.6, CI - 2.3 to 0.6. P=0.26) • No significant differences between groups for the amount of fentanyl dispensed by the IV patient-controlled anesthesia • No differences in numeric pain rating scale scores • No differences in acute functional orthopedic outcomes, side effects, or amounts of oral opioids consumed.	The use of stimulating catheters in continuous femoral nerve blocks for TKA does not offer significant benefits over traditional nonstimulating catheters.
Dauri et al., 2007	• prospective randomized controlled trial in patients undergoing anterior cruciate ligament reconstruction • SC=35, NSC=35 Outcomes: • pain score • adverse effects • need for supplemental anesthesia and analgesia other than a continuous • postoperative infusion of ropivacaine 2 mg/mL set at 7 mL/h.	• Onset time was faster in the SC group (SC: 6.4± 2.5, NSC: 8.3±2.9 min, *P* 0.006). • No differences in Visual analog scale. • The number of patient-controlled regional analgesia boluses (SC: 14.6 ± 12.6, NSC:23.2±13.6 mg ropivacaine 2 mg/mL, *P*_.008) as well as intravenous rescue ketorolac (SC: 34.3±35.7, NSC: 54±39.7 mg, *P* 0 .033) administered were higher in the NSC group.	Although the use of a stimulating catheter was associated with faster onset time for the femoral nerve block and lower additional analgesics postoperatively, the clinical superiority (analgesia; lateral femoral cutaneous, and obturator nerve block) of stimulating catheters was not evident in this clinical setting.
Barrington et al., 2008	• randomized, controlled, double-blind trial in patient undergoing TKA • SC=40, NSC=42 Outcomes: • Sensory blockade at 10 min, 20 min after injection of, lidocaine via femoral catheter and at postoperative days 1 (POD 1) and 2 (POD 2) • Morphine requirements • pain scores • markers of early recovery	• No differences on sensory blockade in the femoral nerve distribution • At 24 h, the 95% confidence interval for difference in morphine consumption between groups was -8 to 5 mg. • No difference between groups in visual analog scale scores at rest on POD 1 and POD 2, during active and passive physiotherapy • No differences in markers of early recovery after surgery.	In this study, blind catheter advancement was as reliable as a SC technique for establishing and maintaining CFNB for postoperative analgesia as a part of multimodal analgesia technique after TKA.

Table 2. Study included in analysis (SC= stimulating catheter, NSC= non stimulating catheter, TKA= Total knee arthroplasty, CFNB= continuous femoral nerve block)

Recently, a randomized clinical trial (Barrington et al., 2008) compared a stimulating catheter with a nonstimulating catheter technique for institution of continuous femoral nerve block and its effects on quality of analgesia after total knee arthroplasty performed under general anesthesia in 82 patients. Patients were randomized to have continuous femoral nerve block instituted using either a non-stimulating or a stimulating catheter technique. There were no differences in term of included morphine requirements, pain scores, and markers of early recovery. There was an increase in procedural time required for insertion of a SC compared with a NSC (10 and 6 min, respectively); however, this is of debatable clinical significance.

They concluded that blind catheter advancement was as reliable as a stimulating catheter technique for establishing and maintaining continuous femoral nerve block for postoperative analgesia as a part of multimodal analgesia technique after total knee arthroplasty.

In summary, although advantageous from a theoretical standpoint and in experimental designs (Salinas et al., 2004), randomized controlled trials in the clinical environment have yielded limited evidence to justify use of stimulating catheters for continuous femoral nerve block after knee surgery. The increased cost and need for additional catheter adjustments compared with nonstimulating catheter also make it hard to justify their use in this clinical setting.

9. Discussion: Focus on

Postoperative pain after major knee surgery is a major concern. It is severe in 60% of patients and moderate in another 30% (Singelyn et al., 1998; 2000). Pain has a major impact on patient satisfaction and postoperative well-being. In addition, pain impairs early intensive physical therapy and rehabilitation, probably the most influential factor for good postoperative knee rehabilitation (Singelyn & Gouverneur, 2000; Capdevila et al., 1999).

Continuous peripheral nerve blocks offer the potential benefits of extended postoperative analgesia, few side effects, improved patient satisfaction, and accelerated functional recovery after major knee surgery (Liu & Salinas, 2003); for this reason continuous femoral nerve block is often used to provide postoperative analgesia in this clinical setting (Singelyn et al.,1998; Capdevila et al., 1999)

9.1 Catheter tip

When performing a continuous femoral nerve block, efforts are made to place the catheter close to the nerve to achieve effective perioperative analgesia. Traditionally, catheter placement is performed through a stimulating needle, followed by injection of the local anesthetic and then blind advancement of the peripheral catheter beyond the needle tip. Secondary analgesic block failure rate (failure of a catheter to produce postoperative analgesia after having provided sufficient intraoperative analgesia with the bolus administration) with this technique ranges from 10% (Grant et al., 2001; Chelly & Casati, 2003) up to 40% (Salinas, 2003). This may be explained by the fact that the catheter can curl away from the needle during uncontrolled advancement (Salinas 2003). Correct catheter placement is confirmed by testing for a clinical effect of satisfactory analgesia or by sensory modality testing within the desired sensory distribution after injection of the local anesthetic. However, in case of insufficient block, the catheter cannot be further redirected.

The rational for using stimulating catheters, introduced in 1999 (Boezaart et al., 1999) is based on the assumption that catheter tips are directed close to nerves; in fact it provide the possibility to verify the position the catheter takes during advancement through the cannula. A study performed by Pham Dang et al (Pham Dang et al., 2003) concluded that the ability to electrostimulate nerves using an in situ catheter increases success rate in catheter placement for continuous peripheral nerve blocks. However, they were surprised to find that the amperage required to elicit motor responses is higher with the stimulating catheter than with the introducer needle. In a study performed by Morin et al (Morin et al., 2005), the authors did not find a relationship between the current that had to be applied via the stimulating catheter to evoke a motor response and any of the variables determined to judge the success of the catheter positioning. Viewing this works, doubts may arise regarding the reliability of stimulating catheter to elucidate motor contruction and to determine correct catheter positioning. Furthermore, A stimulation current 0.5mA or less is considered safe in order to avoid nerve injury and to deliver adequate stimulus to provoke a motor response. A stady performed by Bigeleisen et al (Bigeleisen et al., 2009) suggest that stimulation currents of more than 0.2 and no more than 0.5 mA could not rule out an intraneural position of the needle or catheter tip. Therefore, even with the use of low stimulation (0.2-0.5 mA) the tip of the stimulating catheters are not ascertained to be in the vicinity of the nerve of might be inside the nerve.
Placement of the catheter tip should ideally be as close as possible to the nerve to attain the minimal blocking concentration that will block the fibers responsible for transmission of painful stimuli. From a practical point, use of larger volumes may permit more successful blocks when nerves are less than ideally localized. This concept is expressed also by Pham Dang et al. (Pham Dang et al., 2009) affirming that interpretation of their data suggests that the failure of previous studies to show a superiority of stimulating catheters has perhaps been masked by methodological problems in previous investigations on the subject. In fact in their study, stimulating catheters seem to provide early analgesia within the femoral nerve distribution using low-dose initial bolus and subsequent low-volume infusion. Small doses of local anesthetics suffice if a catheter is correctly placed next the femoral nerve and that pain from unblocked obturator and sciatic nerves should be treated specifically (Pham Dang 2009).
Moreover, use of larger volumes of local anesthetics may potentially increase the risk of systemic toxicity and potentially increase motor block (Borgeat et al., 2001; Bergman et al., 2000).
More importantly, minimal motor weakness is desired for continuous femoral analgesia after total knee arthroplasty, because excessive quadriceps motor block may impair active knee extension required for rehabilitation protocols and potentially delay achievement of predetermined functional physical therapy goals. To better ascertain the difference between a well placed and a poorly placed catheter, one should use smaller amounts of local anesthetics. Hayek et al. (Hayek et al., 2006), analyzed data regarding the total amount of local anesthetic used in patient treated with stimulating catheter versus nonstimulating group founding no statistically significant differences in the amount of ropivacaine administered .
The question arises whether nerve proximity is really needed for the femoral nerve to be blocked effectively in routine clinical use. Several reasons argue against this necessity, particularly when larger volumes (40 ml) of local anaesthetic are used. Firstly, anatomical review suggests that, once the iliac fascia is penetrated, there are no relevant diffusion barriers for local anaesthetics. Secondly, catheters threaded 16–20 cm from the inguinal level radiographically deviated in 77% of cases but were as effective in motor blockade of the

femoral nerve, and only marginally less effective in sensory blockade of the femoral nerve, compared with radiographically well placed catheters (Capdevila et al., 2002). Thirdly, iliac fascia blocks performed without any nerve stimulation are as effective as femoral nerve blocks, in both children (Dalens et al.,1989) and adults (Capdevila et al., 1998), suggesting no clinically meaningful reason for placing catheter tips in close proximity to the femoral nerve. For these reasons, Birbaum affirmed that well designed studies should to be done to prove the superiority of stimulating catheters, but not for the femoral nerve (Birnbaum & Volk., 2006).
However , without direct visualization, catheter positions corresponding to the various stimulating tip-to-nerve distances could only be inferred on the basis of the neurostimulation recently developed by Johnson et al. (Jonson et al., 2007).
Another common problem to underling is the lack of control of the pain transmitted by the unblocked obturator nerve in all studies (Morin et al., 2005; Barrington et al., 2008) and the unblocked sciatic nerve in 2 studies (Morin et al., 2005; Hayek et al., 2006). These unblocked nerves constitute major confounding factors during assessment of the femoral block based on pain scores, given that the knee is innervated principally by the femoral, obturator, and sciatic nerves. In contrast to these studies, ours used a low dose of ropivacaine (0.2%) for initiation and maintenance of femoral nerve block and eliminated pain from obturator and sciatic nerves by blocking them.(Pham Dang et al., 2009).
It is conceivable that clinicians with less experience might find that the ability to verify accuracy of catheter placement with the stimulating catheter system improves their clinical outcomes. However the introduction of the stimulating catheter requires more expertise than introduction of the non-stimulating catheter. Placing the catheter to give good contractions often involves extra manipulation, reintroduction of the needle, or both. Thus, it would not (necessarily) expect the stimulating catheter to give better results in inexperienced hands.

9.2 Effect on neurostimulation of injectates used for perineural space expansion

A randomized clinical trial (Pham Dang et al., 2009) clinically assessed the electrophysiologic effect of dextrose 5% in water and of normal saline used for expansion of the perineural space before placing a stimulating catheter. They questioned if higher current was required with normal saline but not with dextrose 5% in water, as has been observed experimentally. This was a prospective randomized double-blind study of ASA I to II patients scheduled for total knee replacement. Patients were randomly assigned to receive unidentified injectate dextrose 5% in water (n = 25) or normal saline (n = 25). The primary outcome was the minimal intensity of stimulation (MIS) recorded before and after 2 and 5 mL of study injectates were flushed through the needle before placing a stimulating catheter for continuous femoral and sciatic nerve blocks. Secondary outcomes included, among other parameters, minimal intensity of stimulation recorded during placement of stimulating catheters.
Analysis of the primary outcome using a between-group comparison showed that minimal intensity of stimulation recorded during electrostimulation via the needle was significantly higher after normal saline than after dextrose 5% in water in all blocks and at each volume of injectate. This presumably reflects the electrophysiologic properties of normal saline versus dextrose 5% in water given the absence of difference between groups with all other parameters assessed in this study. To conclude, the use of normal saline for expanding the perineural space led to increased intensity for nerve electrostimulation, which may lead to potential errors when electrolocating the nerve. Dextrose 5% in water seemed to be a superior medium for perineural space expansion, which is in agreement with the animal and clinical studies of Tsui et al.(Tsui et al., 2005).

9.3 An alternative: Ultrasonographic guidance

Continuous femoral nerve blocks, have recently evolved towards being the gold standard for acute pain therapy after major reconstructive knee surgery, including total knee arthroplasty and certain techniques for anterior cruciate ligament reconstruction. As shown previously, accurate placement of femoral nerve catheters in close proximity to the femoral nerve, allows for a therapy with low infusion rates and minimal boluses, thus increasing its effectiveness and allowing for prolonged analgesia (48-72hours) with small portable disposable pumps in the outpatient setting. Neuro-stimulation and stimulating catheters, were the basis for perfecting continuous femoral blocks. While usually a simple technique, with minimal risks, occasionally, even in experienced hands, stimulating catheters present several shortcomings: lack of placement time consistency, increased costs, lack of direct visualization of local anesthetic spread, variability in stimulating catheter design and quality, uncertainty about nerve stimulation endpoints (Hayek, 2006; Jack et al., 2005; Morin et al., 2005; Salinas et al., 2004; Birnbaum et al., 2007).

An alternative for assisting with correct catheter placement is ultrasonographic guidance (Fig. 3- 4- 5).

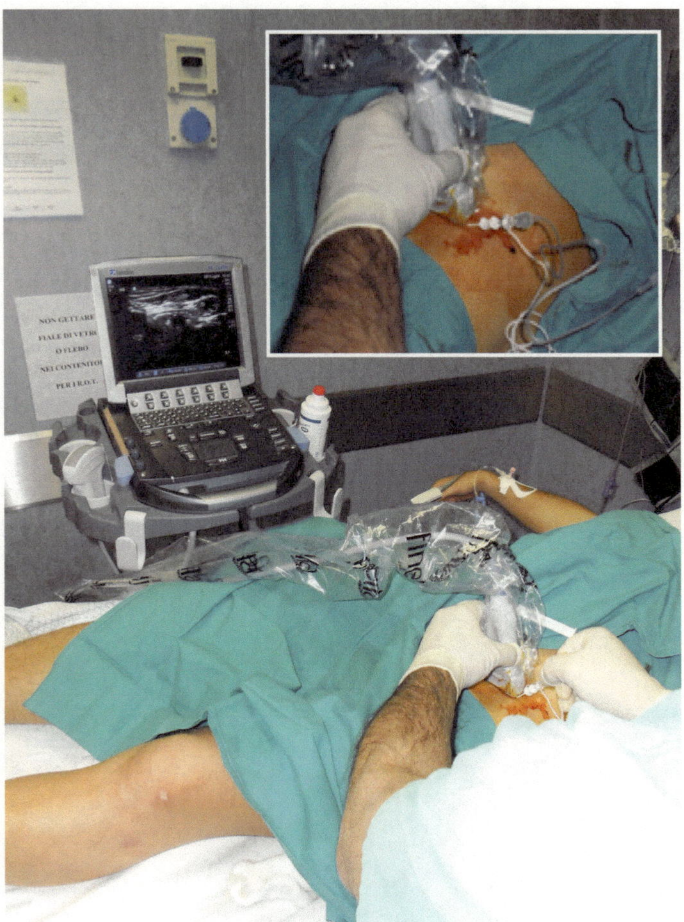

Fig. 3. Ultrasound-guided femoral nerve block: in plane approach

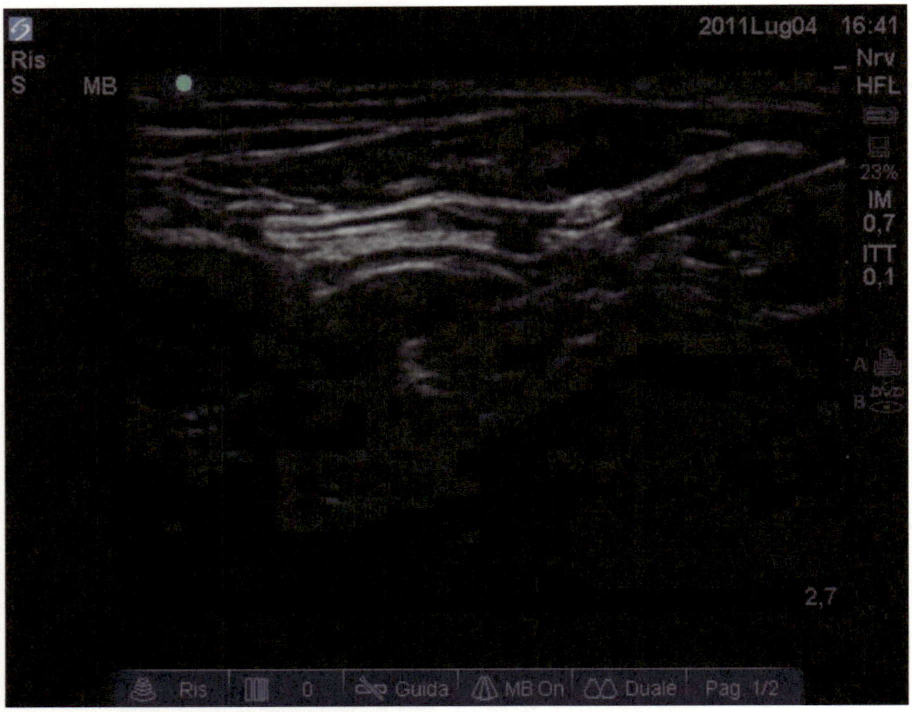

Fig. 4. Ultrasound guided femoral nerve block: needle insertion

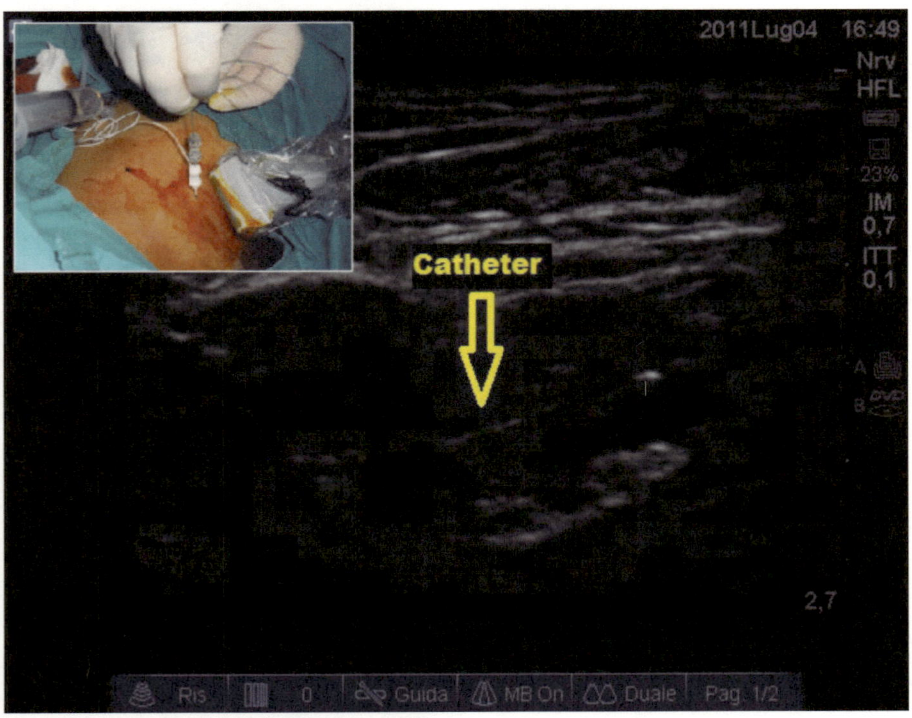

Fig. 5. Ultrasound guided femoral nerve block: catheter insertion

Ultrasound-guided regional anesthesia is an evolving field and its use has gained enormous popularity in the last 10 years. In one investigation, the onset of sensory blockade with ultrasound guidance was significantly shorter and the quality of sensory block significantly better compared with the nerve stimulator needle-assisted application of local anesthetic (Marhofer et al., 1997). Addition of ultrasound guidance to nerve stimulation could offer the benefits of rapid localization and visualization of local anesthetic spread, at the cost of several disadvantages: need for multiple assistants, increased time and cost; moreover the tip position can suggest proximity even though sufficient nerve stimulation is not achieved, injection of local anaesthetic usually produces a clinically effective block.

Other authors have reported both increased block density and lower anesthetic dose requirements with US-guided techniques when compared with conventional techniques using nerve stimulators (Marhofer, 1997-1998).

Mariano et al. (Mariano et al., 2009) performed a study were patients receiving a femoral perineural catheter for knee surgery were randomly assigned to either ultrasound guidance with a nonstimulating catheter or electrostimulation guidance with a stimulating catheter. The primary outcome was the catheter placement procedure time (minutes) starting when the ultrasound transducer (ultrasound group) or catheter insertion needle (electrostimulator group) first touched the patient and ending when the catheter insertion needle was removed after catheter insertion. He concluded that for femoral perineural catheter placement, an ultrasound-guided technique decreases the procedure time compared with nerve electro-stimulation alone while maintaining a similar success rate. Furthermore, patients in the ultrasound group reported less procedure-related pain during perineural catheter placement and had fewer inadvertent vascular punctures (20% less).

It is possible that using a combination of both approaches may offer additional benefits over either technique alone for brachial plexus perineural catheters (Mariano et al., 2009;Fredricksonet al., 2008). For continuous femoral nerve block the needle is inserted at the level of the inguinal crease along the long axis of the ultrasound probe. The needle shaft and needle tip are clearly visible with this approach during advancement of the needle toward the femoral nerve. Once the needle pierces the fascia iliaca lateral to the nerve, the needle tip is advanced 2 to 3 mm toward the nerve. This is contrary to the common method of placing the needle tip in close proximity to the nerve. At this point, 5 mL of dextrose 5% solution is injected to expand the perineural space, and electrical stimulation conforms a quadriceps or patellar twitch. The position of the needle in conjunction with the injected dextrose provides a path for catheter advancement toward the nerve and the catheter tip to lie in close approximation to the nerve. Had the needle tip initially been placed next to the femoral nerve, the catheter would have advanced medially past the nerve.

Another method to possibly improve catheter advancement is slight withdrawal of the catheter guide wire by 1 to 2 cm from the tip. This will provide more flexibility to the catheter tip but stiffness to the remainder of the catheter during advancement. This may further decrease the likelihood of catheter advancement away from the tract formed by the injected dextrose solution, thereby improving the ease of catheter insertion (Niazi et al., 2009). To date, however, the need for electro-stimulation in addition to ultrasound guidance remains controversial, especially for lower extremity perineural catheter placement (Chan et al., 2007; Walker & Roberts, 2007; Beach et al., 2006; Gürkan et al., 2008; Dingemans et al., 2007).

Moreover combining ultrasound with electro-stimulation does negate any cost advantages attributed to ultrasound guidance alone (Sandhu et al., 2004).

10. Conclusions

Randomized controlled trials in the clinical environment have yielded limited evidence to justify use of stimulating catheters for continuous femoral nerve block after knee surgery. It can be affirmed that failure of previous studies to show a superiority of stimulating catheters has perhaps been masked by methodological problems, above all regarding the dose and volume of local anesthetics used. However ultrasound guidance offer a safe and cost/effective technique for femoral catheter placement.

11. Future directions

It is important to design future trials in a consistent manner to make studies comparable and to enable a standard quantitative meta-analysis. Future study designs need to account for differences between the primary anesthetic block (bolus or a relatively large mass of concentrated local anesthetic via either the needle or catheter, typically with a long-acting agent) and the secondary analgesic block (infusion of a dilute local anesthetic). Injection of long-acting local anesthetic as the primary block renders interpretation of the secondary analgesic infusion difficult if not impossible for the first 12 to 24 hrs as the residual analgesic effects of the primary block may still be effective.

12. References

Ansbro P. A method of continuous brachial plexus block. *American Journal of Surgery* 1946; 121: 716 - 722

Barrington MJ, Olive DJ, McCutcheon CA, Scarff C, Said S, Kluger R, et al. Stimulating catheters for continuous femoral blockade after total knee arthroplasty: a randomized, controlled, double blind trial. *Anesth Analg*. 2008;106:1316Y1321.

Beach ML, Sites BD, Gallagher JD. Use of a nerve stimulator does not improve the efficacy of ultrasound-guided supraclavicular nerve blocks. *J Clin Anesth* 2006; 18:580–584.

Bergman BD, Hebl JR, Kent J, Horlocker TT. Neurologic complications of 405 consecutive continuous axillary catheters. *Anesth Analg* 2000;96:247-252.

Bigeleisen P.E, Moayeri N, Groen G.J. Extraneural versus Intraneural Stimulation Thresholds during Ultrasound-guided Supraclavicular Block. *Anesthesiology 2009; 110:1235–43*

Birnbaum J et al. "Electrical nerve stimualtion for plexus and nerve blocks" *Anaesthesist*. 2007 Nov; 56(11): 1156-62 .

Birnbaum J., Volk T. Use of a stimulating catheter for femoral nerve block. *British Journal of Anaesthesia* 96 (1): 139–42 (2006)

Boezaart AP, de Beer JF, duToit C, van Rooyen KA. New technique of continuous interscalene nerve block. *Can J Anaesth* 1999;46:275–81.

Borgeat A, Ekatodramis G, Kalberer F, Benz C. Acute and nonacute complications associated with interscalene block: A prospective study. *Anesthesiology* 2001;95:875-880.

Capdevila X, Barthelet Y, Biboulet P, et al. Effects of perioperative analgesic technique on the surgical outcome and duration of rehabilitation after major knee surgery. *Anesthesiology* 1999; 91:8–15.

Capdevila X, Biboulet P, Bouregba M, Barthelet Y, Rubenovitch J, d'Athis F. Comparison of the three-in-one and fascia iliaca compartment blocks in adults: clinical and radiographic analysis. *Anesth Analg* 1998; 86: 1039–44.

Capdevila X, Biboulet P, Morau D et al. Continuous three-inone block for postoperative pain after lower limb orthopedic surgery: where do the catheters go? *Anesth Analg* 2002; 94: 1001-6

Chan VW, Perlas A, McCartney CJ, Brull R, Xu D, Abbas S. Ultrasound guidance improves success rate of axillary brachial plexus block. *Can J Anaesth* 2007; 54:176-182..9,26-29.

Chelly JE, Casati A. Are nonstimulating catheters really inappropriate for continuous nerve block techniques? *Reg Anesth Pain Med* 2003;28:483-5.

Chelly JE, Greger J, Gebhard R et al. Continuous femoral blocks improve recovery and outcome of patients undergoing total knee arthroplasty. *J Arthroplasty* 2001; 16: 436—45.

Dalens B, Vanneuville G, Tanguy A. Comparison of the fascia iliaca compartment block with the 3-in-1 block in children. *Anesth Analg* 1989; 69: 705-13

Dauri M, Sidiropoulou T, Fabbi E, Giannelli M, Faria S, Mariani P, Sabato AF. Efficacy of continuous femoral nerve block with stimulating catheters versus nonstimulating catheters for anterior cruciate ligament reconstruction. *Reg Anesth Pain Med.* 2007 Jul-Aug;32(4):282-7.

Dingemans E, Williams SR, Arcand G, et al. Neurostimulation in ultrasound-guided infraclavicular block: a prospective randomized trial. *Anesth Analg* 2007; 104:1275-1280.

Fredrickson MJ, Ball CM, Dalgleish AJ. Successful continuous interscalene analgesia for ambulatory shoulder surgery in a private practice setting. *Reg Anesth Pain Med* 2008; 33:122-128.

Ganapathy S, Wasserman RA, Watson JT, et al. Modified continuous femoral three-in-one block for postoperative pain after total knee arthroplasty. *Anesth Analg* 1999;89:1197-202

Grant SA, Nielsen KC, Greengrass RA, et al. Continuous peripheral nerve block for ambulatory surgery. *Reg Anesth Pain Med* 2001;26:209-14.

Gray, Henry. Anatomy of the Human Body. Philadelphia: *Lea & Febiger*, 1918; Bartleby.com, 200.

Gürkan Y, Acar S, Solak M, Toker K. Comparison of nerve stimulation vs. ultrasound-guided lateral sagittal infraclavicular block. *Acta Anaesthesiol Scand* 2008; 52:851-855.

Gurnaney H, Kraemer FW, Ganesh A. Dermabond decreases pericatheter local anesthetic leakage after continuous perineural infusions. *Anesth Analg.* 2011 Jul;113(1):206.

Hayek SM, Ritchey RM, Sessler D, Helfand R, Samuel S, Xu M, Beven M, Bourdakos D, Barsoum W, Brooks P. Continuous femoral nerve analgesia after unilateral total knee arthroplasty: stimulating versus nonstimulating catheters. *Anesth Analg.* 2006 Dec;103(6):1565-70.

Jack NT, Liem EB, Vonhögen LH. Use of a stimulating catheter for total knee replacement surgery: preliminary results. *Br J Anaesth.*2005 Aug;95(2):250-4. Epub 2005 May 27.

Johnson CR, Barr RC, Klein SM. A computer model of electrical stimulation of peripheral nerves in regional anesthesia. *Anesthesiology.* 2007;106:323Y330.

Liu SS, Salinas FV. Continuous plexus and peripheral nerve blocks for postoperative analgesia. *Anesth Analg* 2003;96:263-72.

Marhofer P, Nael C, Sitwohl C et al. Magnetic resonance imaging of the distribution of local anesthetic during the three-in-one block. *Anesth Analg* 2000; 90: 119—24.

Marhofer P, Schrogendorfer K, Koinig H, et al. Ultrasonographic guidance improves sensory block and onset time of three-in-one blocks. *Anesth Analg* 1997;85:854-7.

Mariano ER, Afra R, Loland VJ, et al. Continuous interscalene brachial plexus block via an ultrasound-guided posterior approach: a randomized, triple-masked, placebo-controlled study. *Anesth Analg* 2009; 108:1688-1694.

Mariano ER, Loland VJ, Sandhu NS, Bellars RH, Bishop ML, Afra R, Ball ST, Meyer RS, Maldonado RC, Ilfeld BM. Ultrasound guidance versus electrical stimulation for femoral perineural catheter insertion. *J Ultrasound Med.* 2009 Nov;28(11):1453-60.

Morin AM, Eberhart LH, Behnke HK, Wagner S, Koch T, Wolf U, Nau W, Kill C, Geldner G, Wulf H. Does femoral nerve catheter placement with stimulating catheters improve effective placement? A randomized, controlled, and observer-blinded trial. *Anesth Analg.* 2005 May;100(5):1503-10.

Navas A.M, Gutieirrez T.V, Moreno M.E. Continuous peripheral nerve blockade in lower extremity surgery. *Acta Anaesthesiol Scand* 2005; 49: 1048 – 1055

Niazi AU, Prasad A, Ramlogan R, Chan VW. Methods to ease placement of stimulating catheters during in-plane ultrasound-guided femoral nerve block. *Reg Anesth Pain Med.* 2009 Jul-Aug;34(4):380-1.

Parkinson SK, Mueller JB, Little WL, Bailey SL. Extent of blockade with various approaches to the lumbar plexus. *Anesth Analg* 1989;68:243-248.

Pham-Dang C., Kick o, Collet T, et al. Continuous peripheral nerve blocks with stimulating catheters. *Reg Anesth Pain Med 2003;28:83-88.*

Pham Dang C, Difalco C, Guilley J, Venet G, Hauet P, Lejus C. Various possible positions of conventional catheters around the femoral nerve revealed by neurostimulation. *Reg Anesth Pain Med.* 2009 Jul-Aug;34(4):285-9.

Pham Dang C, Lelong A, Guilley J, Nguyen JM, Volteau C, Venet G, Perrier C, Lejus C, Blanloeil Y. Effect on neurostimulation of injectates used for perineural space expansion before placement of a stimulating catheter: normal saline versus dextrose 5% in water.*Reg Anesth Pain Med.* 2009 Sep-Oct;34(5):398-403.

Salinas FV, Neal JM, Sueda LA, Kopacz DJ, Liu SS. Prospective comparison of continuous femoral nerve block with nonstimulating catheter placement versus stimulating catheter-guided perineural placement in volunteers. *Reg Anesth Pain Med.* 2004 May-Jun;29(3):212-20

Salinas FV. Location, location, location: continuous peripheral nerve blocks and stimulating catheters. *Reg Anesth Pain Med* 2003;28:79–82.

Sandhu NS, Sidhu DS, Capan LM. The cost comparison of infraclavicular brachial plexus block by nerve stimulator and ultrasound guidance. *Anesth Analg* 2004; 98:267–268.

Selander D. Catheter technique in axillary block. *Acta Anaesth Scand* 1977;21:324–329.

Singelyn F, Deyaert M, Pendeville E et al. Effects of intravenous patient-controlled analgesia with morphine, continuous epidural analgesia and continuous three-in-one block on postoperative pain and knee rehabilitation after unilateraltotal knee arthroplasty. *Anesth Analg* 1998; 87: 88 – 92.

Singelyn F, Gouverneur JM. Postoperative analgesia after total hip arthroplasty: i.v. PCA with morphine, patientcontrolled epidural analgesia, or continuous '3-in-1' block?: a prospective evaluation by our acute pain service in more han 1,300 patients. *J Clin Anesth* 1999; 11: 550 – 4.

Singelyn FJ, Gouverneur JM. Extended "three-in-one" block after total knee arthroplasty: continuous versus patient-controlled techniques. *Anesth Analg* 2000;91:176–80.).

Tsui BC, Kropelin B, Ganapathy S, Finucane B. Dextrose 5% in water: fluid medium maintaining electrical stimulation of peripheral nerve during stimulating catheter placement. *Acta Anaesthesiol Scand.* 2005;49:1562Y1565.

Walker A, Roberts S. Stimulating catheters: a thing of the past? *Anesth Analg* 2007; 104:1001–1002.

Winnie AP, Ramamurthy S, Durrani Z. The inguinal paravascular technique of lumbar plexus anesthesia: The "3 in 1" block. *Anesth Analg* 1973;52:989-996.

13

Regional Anesthesia for the Trauma Patient

Stephen D. Lucas, Linda Le-Wendling and F. Kayser Enneking
Department of Anesthesiology,
University of Florida College of Medicine, Gainesville, Florida,
USA

1. Introduction

Trauma is the sixth most common cause of death globally [WHO, 2011]. In the United States, almost 30 million patients receive medical care for trauma every year [CDC, 2011], and trauma results in 30% of intensive care unit (ICU) admissions in the United States [Mackenzie et al., 2007]. In the Emergency Department, 91% of trauma patients are in pain [Berben et al., 2008], and two-thirds of those patients are discharged from the Emergency Department with moderate to severe pain [Berben et al., 2008]. Regional anesthesia (RA) can reduce pain in many of these patients. In this chapter, common problems with managing trauma patients that can be addressed with RA, and data suggesting that regional anesthesia can improve outcomes will be presented, as well as the different challenges to using RA in this patient population. We will also look into new and controversial areas of inquiry in this field.

2. Patients with traumatic injuries who can benefit from regional anesthesia

2.1 Thoracic trauma and rib fractures

Thoracic injury accounts for 25% of deaths among trauma patients. It is second only to head injury as a cause of trauma-related deaths in the United States [Trunkey & Lewis, 1980]. Rib fractures are common, and morbidity and mortality are directly correlated with the number of rib fractures [Flagel et al., 2005].Elderly patients have a particularly high incidence of rib fractures, with a higher rate of morbidity and mortality from these fractures than younger patients [Bulger et al., 2000; Shorr et al., 1989]. Improved analgesia, by various methods, has been shown to improve pulmonary function, including peak expiratory flow, maximum inspiratory force, tidal volume, and oxygen saturation [Luchette et al., 1994; Moon et al., 1999; Osinowo et al., 2004].

Thoracic epidural analgesia (TEA) has been shown to improve outcome after multiple rib fractures [Bulger et al., 2004;Flagel et al., 2005; Moon et al., 1999; Wisner, 1990].As early as 1990, a retrospective regression analysis of a trauma database revealed decreased pulmonary complications and decreased mortality in elderly patients with rib fractures that were treated with TEA as compared to parenteral opiates [Wisner, 1990].Moon et al showed improved pulmonary mechanics and decreased levels of the proinflammatory chemoattractant, interleukin 8, in a prospective, randomized trial that compared TEA with parenteral opioids in patients with thoracic trauma [Moon et al., 1999]. Another prospective study comparing TEA and parenteral opioid analgesia for patients with rib fractures showed decreased rates of nosocomial pneumonia and a shorter duration of mechanical ventilation in the TEA group [Bulger et al., 2004].However, one frequently cited meta-analysis is noteworthy to illustrate its limitations. Carrier et al reported that there was no significant difference when using epidural analgesia over other methods in terms of mortality, ICU length of stay, and duration of mechanical ventilation [Carrier et al., 2009]. Their analysis is of limited utility, however, because they included two studies using lumbar epidural catheters and three studies using only opiate medications with the epidural infusions; these are significant departures from recommended practices. Flagel et al performed a thorough analysis of a large, sophisticated trauma database [Flagel et al., 2005].They showed that TEA was associated with a reduction in mortality for all patients who sustained rib fractures, particularly those having more than four fractures. These findings have resulted in the recommendation that TEA be included in a widely proliferated pain management guideline for blunt thoracic trauma [Simon et al., 2005].

Despite all of the enthusiasm for epidural analgesia in patients with blunt thoracic trauma, there are considerable limitations to this approach. In the previously mentioned study by Bulger et al [Bulger et al., 2004], 282 patients of 408 admitted to the hospital had to be excluded for a variety of reasons. Thoracic epidural analgesia is contraindicated in patients on anticoagulants or those who have developed a coagulopathy [Horlocker et al., 2010].Brain or spinal injuries represent, at minimum, relative contraindications to the use of TEA, as most practitioners are uncomfortable placing epidurals in the face of elevated intracranial pressure. Possible spinal cord injury, even remote from the proposed insertion site, presents a dilemma, as an epidural may obscure or alter the neurologic examination. Spinal bone injuries may also make epidural placement more technically challenging. The hypotension caused by epidurals can frequently be a significant deterrent in critically ill patients who are already hemodynamically unstable from other causes.

Thoracic paravertebral catheterization (TPVC) has emerged as an enticing answer to some, if not all of the above mentioned concerns. A small pilot study showed comparable outcomes between TEA and TPVC when they were used in patients with unilateral rib fractures [Mohta et al., 2009].These findings are bolstered by similar results in the analogous case of analgesia after thoracotomy [Davies et al., 2006; Pintaric et al., 2011; Powell et al., 2011]. Davies et al presented a systematic review and meta-analysis of 10 randomized clinical trials comparing TPVC and TEA for thoracic surgery. They found no difference in pain scores, but did note a lower incidence of pulmonary complications, urinary retention, nausea and vomiting, and hypotension in the TPVC groups [Davies et al., 2006]. A large, prospective multicenter study of pneumonectomy in the United Kingdom found that TEA was associated with a higher incidence of major complications compared to TPVC [Powell et al., 2011]. A recent prospective randomized study comparing TEA and TPVC, with a primary endpoint of hemodynamic stability, found that TPVC was associated with similar analgesia levels to TEA, but with greater hemodynamic stability [Pintaric et al., 2011].

Should TPVC supplant TEA as the primary modality for providing analgesia for blunt thoracic trauma? A few caveats are in order. Epidural spread has been reported with thoracic paravertebral block [Purcell-Jones et al., 1989]. The authors have also experienced and reported the unintended placement of a catheter in the epidural space during TPVC placement [Lucas et al., 2011, Epub ahead of print]. Considerable controversy exists regarding the relative safety of paravertebral blocks vs. epidurals in the face of anticoagulation and coagulopathy, which will be discussed later in the chapter. Frequently, bilateral rib fractures or other injuries, such as an exploratory laparotomy incision, require bilateral blockade. Although studies on the use of TPVC are still quite undeveloped, findings by Richardson et al, in a literature review on bilateral paravertebral blocks, found a favorable side effect profile. The high local anesthetic load associated with bilateral TPVC is a worthwhile consideration for analgesia in thoracic trauma patients [Richardson et al., 2011].

The clinician is faced with a number of questions about how to proceed with regional analgesia techniques for blunt thoracic trauma. Does the patient need a catheter or not? The literature supports using either TEA or TPVC for more than three rib fractures, and in the elderly. The timing of catheter placement should be as early as *practicable*, although sometimes a short delay may be prudent to allow the anticoagulant effects to dissipate. Patients with very severe injuries may not benefit from early catheter placement, as the improvement in analgesia from RA may not likely alter the length of ventilator management. However, continuous and close monitoring in close consultation with Trauma Surgery and Critical Care Medicine can be used to determine when a patient will benefit from TPVC. Should TEA or bilateral TPVC be used? Extensive bilateral pathology is considered an indication for using thoracic epidural catheters over thoracic paravertebral catheters because of the extensive amount of local anesthetic required for multiple bilateral TPVC; however, there is scant literature to address this question. Another area of practical practice management in question is in regard to the number of catheters to place. Studies have shown loss of pinprick sensation in one to 13 dermatomes after a single-shot paravertebral block [Cheema et al., 1995; Saito et al., 2001]. Richardson et al measured somatosensory evoked potentials of the intercostal nerves and reliably ablated one, but only occasionally two or three nerve potentials [Richardson et al., 1998]. Most patients appear to reliably experience analgesia in approximately five dermatomes; therefore we recommend placing a second unilateral catheter for greater than four fractured ribs. This will provide some margin for error. As the process of adequately positioning and sedating these types of patients can be quite challenging, this seems to be a prudent approach. Figure 1 provides a simplified algorithm for managing these patients.

A number of different techniques have been reported for TPVC. When advancing a predetermined, fixed distance (1.0-1.5 cm) beyond the transverse process, loss of resistance, peripheral nerve stimulation(PNS), and various ultrasound-guided techniques have been described [Ben-Ari et al., 2009; Eason & Wyatt, 1979; Luyet et al., 2009; Naja et al., 2006]. Although any of these techniques can be used in different situations, it should be noted that ultrasound guidance and peripheral nerve stimulation can be technically limited in these patients, as they often have subcutaneous emphysema and hematomas. Measuring the depth of the transverse process and the parietal pleura on CT scan provides definitive information that can be used to guide the depth of needle insertion, thereby improving the safety margin and significantly expediting catheter placement. A CT scan also helps to determine the most severely injured ribs and flail segments.

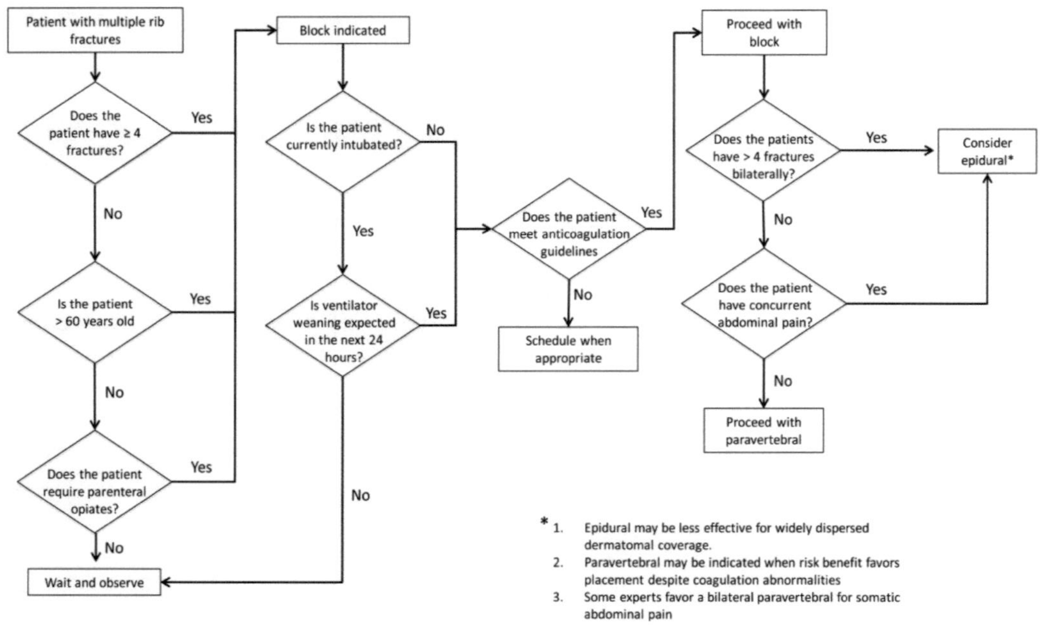

Fig. 1. Algorithm for managing analgesia in patients with multiple rib fractures.

2.2 Long bone fractures

Long bones are composed of a diaphysis, or hollow shaft, connected to the physis, or growth plate, at each end via the metaphysis. Long bones in the body include the humerus, radius, ulna, femur, tibia, fibula, and phalanges. Long bone fractures can result in significant pain, especially prior to stabilization, due to the significant number of nerve endings located in the periosteum and mineralized bone [Mach et al., 2002]. While sclerotome maps have been created to assist in the understanding of innervation to the bones, little evidence exists to confirm their accuracy. Classic studies, including those by Inman and Saunders in 1944 [Inman & Saunders, 1944], provide some evidence for the skeletal innervation [Ivanusic, 2007]. We will review anatomical considerations of the most common fractures and suggest strategies for analgesic management (Table 1).

Fracture	Innervation	Recommended Nerve Block for Analgesia	Considerations
Proximal femur	Femoral nerve Sciatic nerve Obturator nerve	-Single injection or continuous -Femoral nerve block, fascia iliaca block, or lumbar plexus block -Obturator nerve block	For surgical anesthesia, neuraxial anesthesia may decrease incidence of postoperative confusion

Midshaft and distal femur	Femoral nerve Sciatic nerve	-Single injection or continuous -Femoral nerve block -Sciatic nerve block	Greater predominance of sciatic nerve innervation
Proximal and midhumerus	-Brachial plexus, predominantly C5-C6 roots	-Single injection or continuous -Interscalene block, cervical paravertebral block, or supraclavicular block	Radial nerve injury may occur with midshaft humeral fractures
Distal humerus	-Brachial plexus, predominantly C6-C7-roots	-Single injection vs continuous -Interscalene block, cervical paravertebral, supraclavicular, or infraclavicular block	
Clavicle (distal)	Brachial plexus, predominantly C5-C6 roots	-Single injection vs continuous -Interscalene or cervical paravertebral	Possibility of brachial plexus injury due to surgical fixation
Clavicle (proximal)	Brachial plexus, predominantly C4, C5, C6 roots	-Single injection -Cervical paravertebral or deep cervical plexus	Skin overlying clavicle is innervated by supraclavicular nerves, which may be injured during surgery
Radius/Ulna	Brachial plexus, C5-T1	-Single injection -Supraclavicular block, infraclavicular block, or axillary block	
Tibia/Fibula	Sciatic nerve predominantly Possibly femoral nerve in proximal fractures such as tibial plateau	-Single injection or continuous -Sciatic nerve block (Labat or subgluteal or popliteal) -Femoral nerve block for more proximal fractures or to provide for skin sensation to medial lower extremity below knee	Compartment syndrome may occur, especially with young males in high-velocity accidents

Table 1. Regional Anesthesia Considerations for Common Long Bone Fractures

2.2.1 Femur fractures

Femur fractures represent a majority of the patients who suffer from long bone fractures, with one-third of these eventually undergoing surgical stabilization. Regional anesthesia for lower extremity fractures, including femur and hip fractures, has been extensively studied in the literature. Meta-analyses suggest that regional anesthesia, specifically neuraxial anesthesia, decreases the incidence of DVT and pulmonary embolism as well as the incidence of postoperative confusion, in addition to reducing the risk of postoperative pneumonia in patients who require surgical stabilization. Whether regional anesthesia affects mortality in the patient with a femur fracture has yet to be determined [Luger et al., 2010; Parker et al., 2004]. Evidence does suggest that analgesia is improved, and systemic analgesics are spared, when regional anesthesia techniques, such as perineural nerve blocks, are used to help manage pain in patients with hip fractures [Parker, 2002]. Femoral nerve blocks have also been shown to optimize patient positioning for performance of a neuraxial block [Sia et al., 2004; Yun, 2009].

Analgesia for proximal femur fractures may be obtained by blocking the femoral nerve, whether via a single injection or continuous block technique. Although the femur has innervations from multiple nerves, proximally, the femur is predominantly innervated by the femoral nerve, with contributions from the sciatic nerve and an articular branch of the obturator nerve [Locher et al., 2008].

There are a variety of methods available for performance of femoral nerve blocks. The femoral nerve can be anesthetized using stimulation, ultrasound [Beaudoin et al., 2010; Marhofer et al., 1998], or a fascial-pop technique [Candal-Couto et al., 2005; Dalens et al., 1989; Haddad et al., 1995]

Nerve stimulation approaches to the femoral nerve block are common but may cause significant discomfort in a patient with a fracture. The use of ultrasound has been popularized in the past decade for its various benefits. The femoral nerve can be easily visualized at the inguinal crease lateral to the femoral artery, below the fascia lata and iliaca, on the anteromedial aspect of the iliopsoas muscle as it attaches to the proximal femur. The needle can be readily identified since the femoral nerve is typically superficial in nature, and local anesthetic spread is obvious on ultrasound as it encircles the nerve.

In the absence of available ultrasound machines or nerve stimulators, the fascia iliaca compartment block can be easily performed using a simple blunt needle and local anesthetic. This technique has been successfully used in the emergency department setting [Foss et al., 2007; Monzon et al., 2007; Wathen et al., 2007]. The proceduralist draws a line connecting the pubic bone to the anterior superior iliac spine, and divides this line into thirds. At the marking between the distal third (near the anterior superior iliac spine) and middle third, a blunt needle is advanced one centimeter below this point until two pops are felt, the first as the needle punctures the fascia lata and the second as the needle punctures the fascia iliaca. Local anesthetic volumes similar to those used for stimulation-based approaches (20 mL) have been used successfully with the fascia iliaca block with good efficacy [Lopez et al., 2003]; however, weight-based dosing (0.3 mL/kg) [Monzon et al., 2007; Mouzopoulos et al., 2009] and higher doses may be considered to improve local anesthetic delivery [Candal-Couto et al., 2005]. As with any block performed with high volume, confirmation that no intravascular injection has occurred is necessary.

Sciatic nerve blocksbecome more important in more distal femur fractures and fractures of the leg and ankle. Various approaches to the sciatic nerve are utilized. For femur fractures, more proximal approaches, such as the classic Labat technique or the subgluteal approach [Di Benedetto et al, 2002; Franco et al., 2006], are appropriate. For leg and ankle fractures, a more distal approach, such as a popliteal catheter, may be more suitable, as sparing of the hamstring musculature is important for ambulation.

The subgluteal approach can be achieved with stimulation or ultrasound. Using the stimulation technique, the proceduralist elicits appropriate motor twitches, such as plantar/dorsiflexion and gastrocnemius twitches. When employing ultrasound [Danelli et al., 2009; Karmaker et al., 2007], a low frequency ultrasound probe allows visualization of the proximal femur and ischial tuberosity, as well as the sciatic nerve between these two bones. Confirmation of the nerve location on ultrasound can be done by tracing the nerve distally to the popliteal crease as the nerve divides into its two terminal branches: the common perineal and posterior tibial nerve [Bruhn et al., 2008].

2.2.2 Humerus and clavicle fractures

Proximal humerus fractures are the third, most common fracture in the elderly patient (4-5% of all fractures) after femur fractures and radial fractures [Court-Brown et al., 2001]. The most common mechanism of proximal humeral fractures in the elderly are falls [Chu et al., 2004]. Midhumeral fractures occur in 1-2% of patients, with the mechanism of this injury usually resulting from a direct blow to the arm or application of a bending force to the humeral shaft. This type of fracture typically occurs in the young, physically active patient [Ogawa et al., 1998]. Documentation of any radial nerve injury is important prior to proceeding with a regional anesthetic technique, especially with midhumeral shaft fractures in which the radial nerve may be injured from the trauma as it courses posteriorly alongside the humerus in the spiral groove [Ekholm et al., 2006]. Clavicle fractures also occur in the younger population and are usually related to direct or indirect trauma to the clavicle, commonly due to traffic accidents or a sports-related injury [Pecci et al., 2008; Postacchini et al., 2002; Robinson et al., 1998].

The humerus receives its innervation from the brachial plexus. Like the femur, multiple nerves are involved in providing sensation to the bone. Derivations of the C5 and C6 nerve root predominantly innervate the humerus. As the fracture becomes more distal, the innervation emanates from derivations of the C7 nerve root, and a regional anesthetic technique should be targeted accordingly.

Single injections may be performed using a cervical paravertebral, interscalene, or supraclavicular block. However, fractures of the humerus are painful, even after surgical stabilization, and a continuous approach is recommended for prolonged analgesia. Both stimulation and ultrasound-guided approaches have been utilized successfully. If using stimulation, biceps and deltoids are elicited as endpoints for a proximal humerus fracture and triceps stimulation for distal humeral fractures. As with femur fractures, use of stimulation may result in severe pain, and short but intense systemic analgesia may be needed for patient comfort. Ultrasound allows visualization of the brachial plexus from the root all the way to the terminal nerve, and can assist in minimizing needle attempts. By using ultrasound, nerves can be traced to their origin where they exit the intervertebral foramen as they convene in the interscalene groove, and

further down as they become situated posterolateral to the subclavian artery in the supraclavicular approach.
The clavicle is innervated from nerve roots that are more cephalad in origin [Choi et al., 2005]. While distal clavicle fractures can be anesthetized with a C5/C6 block, more medial fractures, which are more common, may be anesthetized as well by depositing local anesthetic near the C4 nerve root, which can be blocked and confirmed by ultrasound. The physician should be aware that numbness across the shoulder and upper chest wall may occur from surgical fixation due to injury to the supraclavicular nerve [Wang et al., 2010]. Furthermore, the brachial plexus lies between the first rib and clavicle as it courses to the upper extremity, and may be at risk for injury due to its proximity to a clavicle fracture.

2.2.3 Radial/ulnar fractures

Repair of radial and ulnar fractures are typically carried out in an outpatient setting, and analgesia prior to surgery is usually provided using oral systemic analgesics. Reduction of a dislocated fracture, however, is extremely painful and may be alleviated by either potent and short-acting anesthetics or a regional anesthetic technique [McManus et al., 2008]. Pain from the surgery itself is typically not severe beyond the initial perioperative phase [Chung et al., 2010], and single-injection brachial plexus blocks using a supraclavicular, infraclavicular [Chin et al., 2010], or axillary approach usually results in adequate intraoperative anesthesia and postoperative analgesia. Ultrasound guidance allows for minimal needle passes, sparing of volumes of local anesthetics, and faster onset [Liu et al., 2010; McCartney et al., 2010; Neal et al., 2010]. Because the radius and ulna are innervated by the entire brachial plexus, all branches of the brachial plexus should be considered when providing surgical anesthesia in the operating room; at the trunk level (supraclavicular), this includes the superior, middle and lower trunk, and at the cord level (infraclavicular), the lateral, posterior and medical cord should be covered. At the axillary level, all terminal nerves should be blocked, which includes the median, ulnar, radial, musculocutaneous, and medial cutaneous nerve of the forearm.

2.2.4 Tibia/fibula fractures

Fractures of the tibia and fibula may occur due to indirect (torsional injuries) or direct impact [Johner et al., 2000]. Open tibia and fibula fracture injuries occur due to high-velocity trauma, such as motor vehicle accidents [Ivarsson et al., 2008], while closed injuries occur due to falls or a sports-related injury. Isolated fibula fractures without concurrent tibial fractures are rare and usually require nonoperative treatment.
The tibia and fibula are predominantly innervated by the sciatic nerve. More proximally, the bones may receive innervation from the femoral nerve. For proximal tibia and fibula fractures, a combined femoral and sciatic nerve block is needed for more complete analgesia, especially if regional anesthesia is utilized for surgical repair Continuous blockade is the technique typically employed for proximal fractures, as many of these patients continue to have severe pain after surgical stabilization. Continuous blockade will also allow monitoring for severe pain out of proportion to what is deemed an appropriate analgesic regimen, as this may signify a developing compartment syndrome. It is important to be aware that patients with tibial fractures are at a particularly high risk of developing compartment syndrome [Park et al., 2009] (discussed in more detail below). Distal tibia and

fibula fractures, if uncomplicated, normally do not require more than a single-injection sciatic nerve block, with or without a saphenous nerve block depending on the medial cutaneous involvement of the injury or location of the surgical incision.

3. Challenges and opportunities

The anesthesiologist who performs RA for trauma patients has several challenges that must be addressed, and, thus, it is imperative to have a solid understanding of the complexities of compartment syndrome and coagulation issues in the trauma patient. Included in this chapter is a discussion on a number of technical challenges that frequently arise in trauma patients will be discussed, along with various solutions to these challenges. There are presently exciting opportunities in the field of RA for the trauma patient, one of which will be elucidated: the provision of RA in the prehospital or early hospital period.

3.1 Compartment syndrome

Compartment syndrome has been defined as a condition in which increased pressure within a closed compartment is compromising the circulation and function of the tissues within that space [Matsen, 1975].

In the setting of patients who have experienced trauma, we are primarily concerned with acute compartment syndrome (ACS). The most common sites of ACS are the forearm or leg, although it can occur in any closed compartment. Over 200,000 patients are diagnosed with ACS in the United States every year [Konstanantakos et al., 2007];fractures and various soft tissue injuries are the most common causes (Table 2) [McQueen et al., 2000] .Men are at a substantially greater risk than women, as are patients <35 years old [McQueen et al., 2000].

Tibial diaphyseal fracture
Soft tissue injury
Distal radius fracture
Crush syndrome
Diaphyseal fracture of the radius or ulna

Table 2. Most Common Causes of Acute Compartment Syndrome

The sine qua non of ACS management is early diagnosis and treatment, with extensive fasciotomy [Kashuk et al., 2009].Classically, the diagnosis of ACS is made by recognition of the 6 P's (Table 3) [Elliott & Johnstone, 2003].Of these, pulselessness and paralysis occur too late to effectively provide an intervention, and palpation abnormalities are difficult to discern in the traumatized patient. The other signs and symptoms all involve the need for the patient to sense the pain or parasthesia. For this reason, the use of RA in patients at risk for developing compartment syndrome is controversial [Davis et al., 2005; Thonse et al., 2004].

Pain out of proportion to injury
Parasthesia
Pain with forced dorsiflexion
Palpation (tense)
Paralysis
Pulselessness

Table 3. The 6 P's: Signs and Symptoms of Acute Compartment Syndrome

There are no randomized controlled trials comparing outcomes in patients at risk for ACS who had local anesthetic-based analgesia versus opioid-based analgesia. Clinical practice and recommendations have been founded on case reports and retrospective case series [Mar et al., 2009]; Clark's recent excellent editorial pointed out the usefulness of these case reports [Clark, 2011]. However, it is imperative that we carefully review these reports and not over-interpret their significance. It would seem an archaic practice to simply allow all patients at risk for ACS to suffer. Alternatives to RA, such as patient-controlled analgesia, have also been implicated as obscuring an ACS diagnosis [Richards et al., 2004].The literature on these topics will be briefly reviewed, and several recommendations for reasonable practices will be offered.

Recommendations against RA in patients at risk for ACS are based on the premise that any degree of sensory blockade will block the ischemic pain the patient is experiencing in a compromised compartment. Little distinction is made between a limb in which a patient has analgesia but still can sense a pinprick exam, and one that is completely insensate. A recent case report by Cometa illustrated a scenario of a patient with an initially good analgesic block who experienced increasing pain as he developed ACS [Cometa et al., 2011].Because of the prompt recognition of this increasing pain by the anesthesiologists involved, the patient underwent a timely and limb-saving fasciotomy. Although no clear-cut evidence exists to support it, most experts suspect that somewhere on a continuum of density of nerve blockade lies the "danger zone" of sensory blockade in which we are at risk of masking the symptoms of ACS. For this reason, prolonged duration of a dense blockade, such as with a long-acting, potent neuraxial block, are to be discouraged. Intraoperatively and immediately postoperatively, these patients will not be able to report the pain of ACS, so RA and general anesthesia (GA) represent a similar risk. If, however, a dense sensory block persists long after the operative period, then the choice of RA may place the patient at increased risk. For that reason, intraoperative RA - whether neuraxial, single shot peripheral nerve block, or dosing of a continuous perineural catheter - should be limited to short-acting local anesthetic regimens. A much more controversial question is whether a continuous regional anesthetic technique, aimed at providing analgesia but avoiding the "danger zone", should be offered to these patients. Epidural infusions have been implicated in delayed diagnosis of lower extremity ACS [Mar et al., 2009].Unfortunately, in this review of 35 cases, the infusion drugs and concentrations were not reported in the majority of the patients. Of those that were reported, some involved infusates that are much more concentrated than current practices. Eighteen of the 35 patients had symptoms of ACS while the epidural infusions were running. Interestingly, there is a paucity of reports of ACS diagnosis delay in peripheral nerve blockade (PNB), in either single-shot or continuous infusions. Upper limb nerve block has not been associated with delayed ACS diagnosis, but lower limb PNB has been reported in two cases, but the validity of that attribution is extremely doubtful [Mar et al., 2009].In one report, a femoral nerve block was cited for masking a lower leg ACS; as discussed previously, it is obvious that the femoral nerve supplies only cutaneous innervation of the medial lower leg via the saphenous nerve and a small portion of the proximal tibia anteriorly. It cannot block ischemic pain coming from lower leg muscles, all of which are innervated by the sciatic nerve. In the other case, an ankle block was presumed to mask an ACS in the foot, but although severe pain was reported, it was ignored.

There are no reported cases of delayed ACS diagnosis attributed to continuous perineural infusions. The absence of reports certainly does not imply that RA poses no risk to these patients, but may represent a number of factors, such as failure to report complications or avoidance of RA in these patients. Conversely, the literature certainly does not support a wholesale abandonment of RA in patients at risk. We would recommend avoiding long-lasting dense blockade, using minimally effective infusions, and promptly addressing insensate limbs by withholding infusions until pinprick sensation returns. Perhaps even more importantly is a high level of vigilance as was exhibited by Cometa et al [Cometa et al., 2011] and close cooperation between the orthopedic surgeons and anesthesiologists involved. Using RA in these patients should only be considered in centers with a willingness to dedicate resources to the close monitoring of these patients and with caregivers who are acutely aware of the risks involved.

Despite all the attention to the subjective symptoms of ACS, they have actually been found to be quite unreliable [Ulmer, 2002]. A reliable objective measure to diagnose ACS would drastically improve care. Most of the attention in the past has been centered on direct, invasive measurement of intracompartmental pressures [Al-Dadah et al., 2008; Harris, et al., 2006].These techniques have, to date, been somewhat limited by technical problems. The most promising use of this approach would appear to be the series reported by McQueen and Court-Brown, who suggest that maintaining a differential pressure between the diastolic blood pressure and an intracompartmental pressure greater than 30 mm Hg is protective [McQueen et al., 1996].Much more exciting is the prospect of a noninvasive modality, such as near-infrared spectroscopy or laser Doppler flowmetry capable of diagnosing ACS [Elliott & Johnstone, 2003]. Evidently, further research is needed in this area.

3.2 Regional anesthesia and anticoagulation

The trauma patient, depending on the injury, may be at risk for bleeding or clotting. Patients with a high volume blood loss and massive resuscitation can end up with a dilutional coagulopathy, while patients with lower extremity fractures, intracranial injuries, and immobility may be at risk for thromboembolic complications necessitating aggressive anticoagulation strategies. An increasing number of patients present with anticoagulants as part of their home medicine regimen (e.g. Plavix for patients with coronary stents). Close vigilance of the patient's coagulation status, whether hyper- or hypocoagulable, is important prior to initiation of a regional technique.

3.2.1 Venous thromboembolism risk in the trauma patient

Venous thromboembolism can lead to pulmonary embolism, the most common preventable cause of hospital death. In patients with major trauma who are not receiving thromboprophylaxis, rates of DVT can range anywhere between 40 and 80% [Geerts et al., 2008], with rates of pulmonary embolism between 1 and 2% depending on severity of the injury [Schuerer et al., 2005]. Pulmonary embolism is the 3rd leading cause of death for patients who survive beyond the first day [Geerts et al., 2008]. Independent predictors of DVT include spinal cord injury, lower extremity or pelvic fracture, surgery, increasing age, prolonged immobility, and delay in institution of thromboprophylaxis [Geerts et al., 2008].

The American College of Chest Physicians published their updated guidelines on antithrombotic and thrombolytic therapy in 2008 [Geerts et al., 2008]. Low-dose unfractionated heparin alone appears to be insufficient as thromboprophylaxis in trauma patients. The recommendation for patients with major trauma is the use of low molecular weight heparin (LMWH) thromboprophylaxis in the absence of major contraindications. If active bleeding or high risk for clinically significant bleeding is a contraindication for LMWH, mechanical thromboprophylaxis is appropriate. In the patient with hip fracture awaiting surgery, the recommendations include routine use of thromboprophylaxis with fondaparinux, LMWH, adjusted dose of a vitamin K antagonist, or low-dose unfractionated heparin if not at high risk for bleeding. Based on evidence and expert opinion, all these recommendations were grade 1 recommendations, indicating that the benefits of thromboprophylaxis outweigh the risks, burden, and costs of implementation. The panel did recognize that, for patients undergoing neuraxial procedures and deep peripheral blocks, the physician should exercise caution when selecting anticoagulant thromboprophylaxis [Geerts et al., 2008].

The EAST Practice Parameter Workgroup for DVT Prophylaxis also published guidelines on anticoagulation focusing on the trauma patient [Simon et al., EAST Practice Management Guidelines Work Group, 2005]. This group states that, while there is inadequate class I evidence for the general use of LMWH in venous thromboembolism prophylaxis, they do recommend that LMWH be standard for thromboprophylaxis in patients with complex pelvic, lower extremity, and spinal cord injuries who are not at risk for significant bleeding. These authors acknowledge that appropriate selection of the subset of patients to administer LMWH without increasing the risk of significant bleeding may be challenging.

3.2.2 American Society of Regional Anesthesia and Pain Medicine (ASRA) guidelines

The American Society of Regional Anesthesia and Pain Medicine (ASRA) convened a 3rd Consensus Conference on anticoagulation and published the guidelines in 2010 [Horlocker et al., 2010] .Recommendations were made with regard to optimal timing and placement of regional anesthetic techniques when patients have received anticoagulants. The guidelines focus on the appropriate timing of needle placement and catheter manipulation until the patient achieves a reasonable state of coagulation in order to avoid significant bleeding complications associated with needle and catheter placement (spinal hematomas, retroperitoneal hemorrhage). These recommendations were made for patients in the inpatient and outpatient setting, including patients in the intensive care unit who are to receive neuraxial, plexus, or deep peripheral blockade. Little mention is made of the trauma or ICU patient, and much of the literature presented was focused on the patient receiving a regional anesthetic technique in the perioperative setting.

The authors of the ASRA guidelines did acknowledge that fewer recommendations were being presented to allow for "flexibility and individuality in patient management", but stressed proper vigilance when managing a patient with a regional anesthetic and anticoagulation [Horlocker et al., 2010]. The guidelines represent a conservative but safe way to practice regional anesthesia in the anticoagulated patient, and are based on the pharmacologic activity of anticoagulants and large case series reported over a 20-year period. Recently, Chelly et al [Chelly & Schilling, 2008] described a series of orthopedic patients undergoing lumbar paravertebral and perineural blocks placed prior to the administration of thromboprophylaxis. The catheters were maintained during routine use of prophylactic dosing and withdrawn regardless of timing of the anticoagulant. The authors noted no significant hematomas.In another study, Buckenmeier described no bleeding complications in a series of 187 patients receiving continuous nerve blocks and LMWH [Buckenmaier et al., 2006]. These series might suggest that, with a high amount of vigilance and a great deal of technical skill, the ASRA guidelines (Table 4) [Horlocker et al., 2010] may represent too conservative an approach to the use of peripheral nerve blocks. However, neither series was powered to detect serious bleeding complications, and, thus, judgment about safety is not warranted.

Anticoagulant	Recommendations prior to block placement or catheter removal	Time from block placement to resuming anticoagulant	Time from catheter removal to resume anticoagulant
Subcutaneous unfractionated heparin (5000 U twice daily)	-Check platelet count for heparin-induced thrombocytopenia if patient on UFH for more than 4 days -No contraindication, may reduce bleeding by delaying dose until after block	No contraindication	No contraindication
Subcutaneous unfractionated heparin (>5000 U twice daily)	-Check platelet count for heparin-induced thrombocytopenia if patient on UFH for more than 4 days -No current recommendations	-Consider enhanced neurologic monitoring or -Consider switching to twice daily dosing	
Prophylactic LMWH	-12 hours -Anti-Xa level not predictive of bleeding	-If bloody catheter placement, consider postponement of dose for 24 hours -If not difficult placement, 6-8 hours	-2 hours
Therapeutic LMWH	-24 hours	Regardless of technique, postponement of LMWH for 24 hours -Contraindicated while catheter in situ	-2 hours

Warfarin	-Discontinue 4-5 d prior to procedure -INR < 1.5 Consider reversal agent to normalize INR	-INR < 1.5 ideal -Caution in INR 1.5-3 -Contraindicated INR >3	-INR < 1.5
Nonsteroidal antiinflammatory agents	No contraindication	No contraindication	No contraindication
Antiplatelet agents Plavix Ticlpidine	-7 days -if 5-7 days (for high risk patients) documentation of normalization of platelet function recommended -14 days	-Likely Contraindicated while continuous catheter in situ	No recommendation
Thrombolytic therapy	-No recommendation on length of time -Neuraxial techniques should be avoided if possible	Contraindicated	Avoidance for 10days after puncture of noncompressible vessels
Platelet GPIIb/IIIa inhibitors	-Abciximab 24-48 hours -Eptifibatide and tirofiban 4-8 hours -Document normal platelet function	Contraindicated	No recommendation
Fondiparinux (Arixtra)	Recommendations are to follow strict conditions in 2 studies	Contraindicated while continuous catheter in situ	-Follow strict conditions in 2 studies --or -Consider switching to alternative anticoagulant
Thrombin inhibitors	Contraindication	Contraindication	Contraindication
Herbals	No contraindication	No contraindication	No contraindication

*Note these recommendations are for single drug therapy and may not apply if patient receives concomitant anticoagulation with other agents

Table 4. ASRA guidelines for common anticoagulant management in the patient receiving a neuraxial, plexus or deep peripheral nerve block[Horlocker et al., 2010].*

3.2.3 Risks versus benefits

In the trauma patient, the risks of bleeding must be weighed against the benefits of regional anesthesia - for instance, the risk of bleeding from TPVC or thoracic epidural catheterization in a patient on LMWH versus the benefit of improved pulmonary function due to improved analgesia with minimal sedative effects, resulting in decreased incidence of hospital-acquired pneumonia [Bulger et al., 2004; Flagel et al., 2005; Karmakor et al, 2003].

When comparing a central neuraxial technique to a more peripheral technique (TEA versus TPVC or lumbar plexus block versus a lumbar epidural), one must always consider the closed nature of the spinal column. With a central neuraxial technique, compression of the epidural space may lead to devastating neurologic injury, including paraplegia, compared to a more peripheral technique in which bleeding into the paravertebral space may lead to extensive blood loss or compression neuropraxia but not paraplegia. The choice of a paravertebral block may be more appropriate in a patient on thromboprophylaxis therapy. Perineural blocks are usually performed at the terminal branches of the nerve (e.g. sciatic nerve block, popliteal nerve block, femoral nerve block, saphenous nerve block, axillary nerve block), and, while bleeding may result in neuropraxia and hematoma formation, the severity of the complications is less than that involving neuraxial or deep plexus blocks.

The decision to proceed should be based on a careful review of the patient's medical record. Informed consent for the patient and/or their family should include a review of the risks and benefits of the procedure, and their input into medical decision-making should be sought. While normal coagulation status would be preferable prior to the placement of a continuous catheter, this may not be possible or desirable. This decision requires astute clinical judgment on the part of the physician and a careful consideration of the risks versus benefits.

Even if the physician and patient both agree to maintain continuous epidural or paravertebral block with thromboprophylactic doses of anticoagulants, waiting until after the peak effect of a potent anticoagulant is prudent in order to avoid further bleeding complications in the already injured patient. Once a neuraxial technique or deep paraneuraxial or perineural technique is performed, maintenance on a prophylactic dose of a potent anticoagulant is reasonable to allow the patient to not only have improved analgesic but effective deep vein thrombosis prophylaxis as well. However, extreme vigilance is required, particularly during the high risk period that occurs when the catheter is removed.

4. Technical considerations

Anatomy can be distorted due to the patient's injuries. Swelling and subcutaneous emphysema may result in a difference in the standard sensations felt as the needle is advanced. If a loss of resistance approach is utilized, this may result in an indistinct or false sensation of loss. Even the use of ultrasound may not be helpful in the patient with subcutaneous emphysema, as the image is altered by the air underneath the skin. The use of CT scans to gauge the depth of the epidural space and paravertebral space is very important in allowing the physician to have an intelligent "guesstimate" of the depth of the targeted space.

Stimulating catheters may be utilized to guide catheters based on the motor response elicited via the catheter. While this provides an extra endpoint for confirmation of catheter placement, motor stimulation may result in further worsening of the patient's pain by stimulating muscle movement around a fractured bone. This, in turn, may produce increased analgesic requirements for block placement and an increase in time needed to thread a stimulating catheter.

In the patient placed in the lateral decubitus position on an ICU bed with an inflatable mattress, the spinal curvature may be altered and dependent on the patient's body habitus. Rotation of the spine or lateral displacement of the spine may lead to inaccurate placement of continuous blocks and difficulties in determining midline.

4.1 Confirmation of analgesic effects of the continuous block

In the nonobtunded and nonintubated patient, the efficacy of a continuous regional analgesic technique is simple to assess. Unfortunately, this is not the case in the intubated patient receiving sedatives. While there are many reasons for altered mental status and agitation in the intensive care unit, it is important to rule out severe pain as the cause.

In the patient who received an epidural catheter, accurate placement may be confirmed with a sympathectomy, which can be pronounced, and routinely requires management with fluids or pressors. While the sympathectomy confirms placement in the epidural space, it does not confirm which nerve roots are affected by the local anesthetic spreads, and analgesia may still be inadequate if the nerve roots to the fractured or injured site are spared.

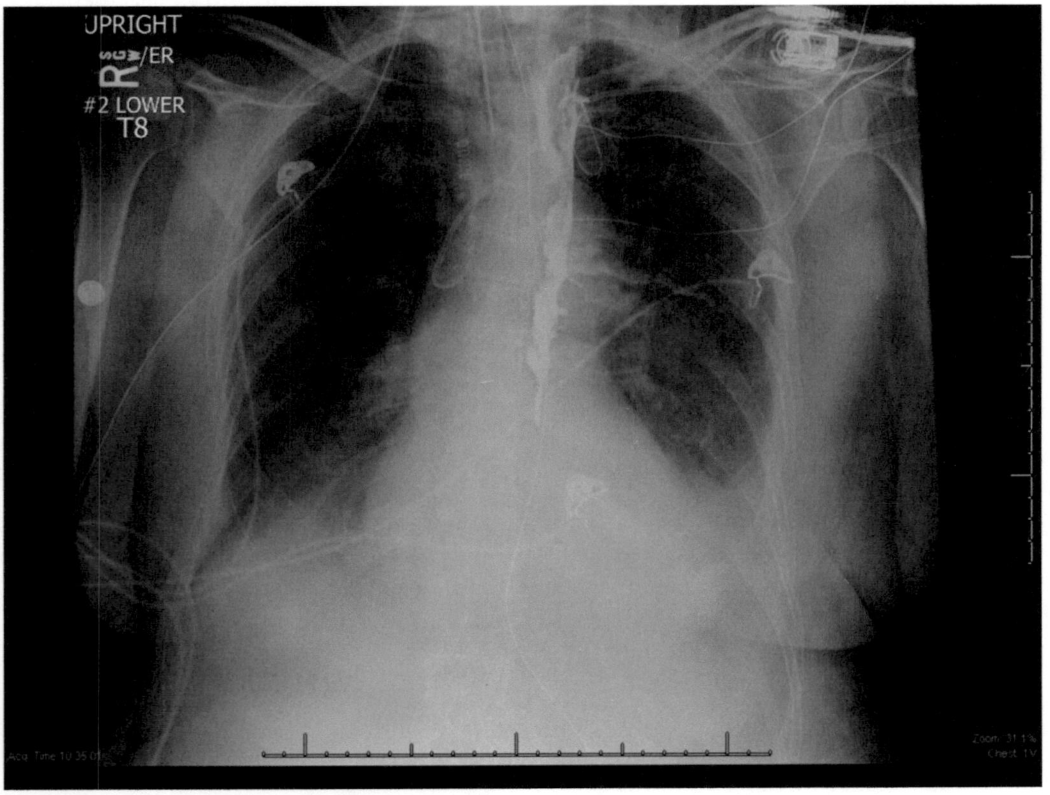

Fig. 2. Dye injection through paravertebral catheter and confirmation of spread of solution.

In the patient with perineural catheters, spread of local anesthetic, while not resulting in hemodynamic effects, can be visualized using ultrasound guidance, as these structures are superficial and can be visualized readily with this mode. In patients with paravertebral continuous blocks, the spread of local anesthetic is difficult to assess and may be inconsistent in its distribution. Therefore, dye injection through the catheter and visualization under fluoroscopy can be used as an alternative gauge of local anesthetic spread, assuming that the patient has no contraindications to contrast dye (Figure 2).
Nursing staff spend the most amount of time with these patients, and can provide important information concerning their perception of whether the patient demonstrates signs of improved or adequate comfort.

4.2 Early management with regional anesthesia

As previously noted, trauma patients often suffer moderate to severe pain in the Emergency Department [Berben et al., 2008]. In Europe, emergency response teams are frequently physician-based. Regional anesthesia performed in the field, prior to hospital admission, has been described for patients with femoral fractures [Lopez et al., 2003; Schiferer et al., 2007]. A simple fascia iliaca block and a nerve stimulator-guided femoral nerve block have been described. Both studies showed reasonably high success rates, with Schiferer reporting a 90% success rate in the RA group [Schiferer et al., 2007].Pain and anxiety scores were much lower in the RA group, as was heart rate. A mean treatment time of seven minutes in the RA group did delay transport time, which is of concern in this setting. While this paradigm will probably not take hold in the rest of the world, including the United States, it surely represents a call to action, to set up processes to provide earlier RA in the hospital setting.

5. Conclusion

Trauma patients represent a significant proportion of current surgical volume and of patients being cared for ICUs. Estimates suggest that this proportion will increase [Lopez et al., 2006]. These patients present many challenges and require extreme vigilance on the part of the health care team. An in-depth understanding of anatomy, physiology, and pharmacology is important when dealing with the trauma patient. Flexibility on the part of the physician to respond to the myriad challenges by adapting to different approaches and modalities is key. Clearly, RA can safely decrease suffering and improve outcomes in these patients when applied judiciously.

6. References

Al-Dadah, O.Q., Darrah, C., Cooper, A., Donell, S.T. & Patel, A.D. (2008). Continuous compartment pressure monitoring vs. clinical monitoring in tibial diaphysial fractures. *Injury* Oct; Vol. 39(No. 10): 1204-1209.

Beaudoin, F.L., Nagdev, A., Merchant, R.C. & Becker, B.M. (2010). Ultrasound-guided femoral nerve block in elderly patients with hip fractures. *American Journal of Emergency Medicine* Jan; Vol. 28(No. 1): 76-81.

Ben-Ari, A., Moreno, M., Chelly, J.E. & Bigeleisen, P.E. (2009). Ultrasound-guided paravertebral block using an intercostal approach. *Anesthesia & Analgesia* Nov; Vol. 109(No. 5): 1691-1694.

Berben, S.A., Meijs, T.H., van Dongen, R.T., van Vugt, A.B., Vloet, L.C., Mintjes-de Groot, J.J. & van Achterberg, T. (2008). Pain prevalence and pain relief in trauma patients in the Accident & Emergency department. *Injury* May; Vol. 39(No. 5): 578-85.

Bjurholm A., Kreicbergs, A., Brodin, E. & Schultzberg, M. (1988). Substance P - and CGRP-immunoreactive nerves in bone. *Peptides* Jan-Feb; Vol. 9(No. 1): 165-171.

Bruhn, J., Van Geffen, G.J., Gielen, M.J. & Scheffer, G.J. (2008). Visualization of the course of the sciatic nerve in adult volunteers by ultrasonography. *Acta Anaesthesiologica Scandinavica* Oct; Vol. 52(No. 9): 1298-1302.

Buckenmaier, C.C. 3rd, Shields, C.H., Auton, A.A., Evans, S.L., Croll, S.M., Bleckner, L.L., Brown, D.S. & Stojadinovic, A. (2006). Continuous peripheral nerve block in combat casualties receiving low-molecular weight heparin. *British Journal of Anaesthesia* Dec; Vol. 97(No. 6): 874-877.

Bulger, E.M., Arneson, M.A., Mock, C.N. & Jurkovich, G.J. (2000). Rib fractures in the elderly. *J Trauma* Feb; Vol. 48(No. 2): 1040-1046.

Bulger, E.M., Edwards, T., Klotz, P. & Jurkovich, G.J. (2004). Epidural analgesia improves outcome after multiple rib fractures. *Surgery* Aug; Vol. 136(No. 2): 426-430.

Candal-Couto, J.J., McVie, J.L., Haslam, N., Innes, A.R. & Rushmer, J. (2005). Pre-operative analgesia for patients with femoral neck fractures using a modified fascia iliaca block technique. *Injury* Apr; Vol. 36(No. 4): 505-510.

Carrier, F.M., Turgeon, A.F., Nicole, P.C., Trepanier, C.A., Fergusson, D.A., Thauvette, D. & Lessard, M.R. (2009). Effect of epidural analgesia in patients with traumatic rib fractures: a systematic review and meta-analysis of randomized controlled trials. *Can J Anesth* Mar; Vol. 56(No. 3): 230-242.

Centers for Disease Control and Prevention. (Last updated February 24, 2011). *Web-based injury statistics query and reporting system,* Accessed July 11, 2011, Available from:www.cdc.gov/injury/wisqars/index.html.

Cheema, S.P., Ilsley, D., Richardson, J. & Sabanathan, S. (1995). A thermographic study of paravertebral analgesia. *Anaesthesia* Feb; Vol. 50(No. 2): 118-1121.

Chelly, J.E. & Schilling, D. (2008). Thromboprophylaxis and peripheral nerve blocks in patients undergoing joint arthroplasty. *Journal of Arthroplasty* Apr; Vol. 23(No. 3): 350-354.

Chin, K.J., Singh, M., Velayutham, V. & Chee, V. (2010). Infraclavicular brachial plexus block for regional anaesthesia of the lower arm. *Cochrane Database of Systematic Reviews* Feb 17; (2): CD 005487.

Chu, S.P., Kelsey, J.L., Keegan, T.H., Sternfeld, B., Prill M., Quesenberry, C.P. & Sidney, S. Risk factors for proximal humerus fracture. (2004). *American Journal of Epidemiology* Aug; Vol. 160(No. 4): 360-367.

Chung, M.S., Roh, Y.H., Baek, G.H., Lee, Y.H., Rhee, S.H. & Gong, H.S. (2010). Evaluation of early postoperative pain and the effectiveness of perifracture site injections following volar plating for distal radius fractures. *Journal of Hand Surgery Am* Nov; Vol. 35(No. 11): 1787-1794.

Clark, L.L. (2011). The value of the case report in the age of evidence-based medicine. *Pain Med* May; Vol. 12(No. 5): 692-694.

Cometa, M.A., Esch, A.T. & Boezaart, A.P. (2011). Did continuous femoral and sciatic nerve block obscure the diagnosis or delay the treatment of acute lower leg compartment syndrome? A case report. *Pain Medicine* Vol. 12(No. 5): 823-828.

Court-Brown, C.M., Garg, A. & McQueen, M.M. (2001). The epidemiology of proximal humeral fractures. *Acta Orthopaedica Scandinavica* Aug; Vol. 72(No. 4): 365-371.

Choi DS, Atchabahian A, Brown AR. (2005). *Anesthesia and Analgesia* May; Vol. 100(No. 5): 1542-1543.

Dalens, B., Vanneuville, G. & Tanquy, A. (1989). Comparison of the fascia iliaca compartment block with the 3-in-1 block in children. *Anesthesia and Analgesia* Dec; Vol. 69(No. 6): 705-713.

Danelli, G., Ghisi, D., Fanelli, A., Ortu, A., Moschini, E., Berti, M., Ziegler, S. & Fanelli, G. (2009). The effects of ultrasound guidance and neurostimulation on the minimum effective anesthetic volume of mepivacaine 1.5% required to block the sciatic nerve using the subgluteal approach. *Anesthesia and Analgesia* Nov; Vol. 109(No. 5): 1674-1678.

Davies, R.G., Myles, P.S. & Graham, J.M. (2006). A comparison of the analgesic efficacy and side-effects of paravertebral vs. epidural blockade for thoracotomy - a systematic review and met-analysis of randomized controlled trials. *Br J Anaesth* Apr; Vol. 96(No. 4):418-426.

Davis, ET, Harris, A, Keene, D, Porter, K, Manji, M. (2005). The use of regional anaesthesia in patients at risk of acute compartment syndrome. Injury 2006; Vol. 37(No. 3): 128-133.

Di Benedetto, P., Casati, A., Bertini, L. & Fanelli, G. (2002). Posterior subgluteal approach to block the sciatic nerve: description of the technique and initial clinical experiences. *European Journal of Anaesthesiology* Sep; Vol. 19(No. 9): 682-686.

Eason, M.J. & Wyatt, R. (1979). Paravertebral thoracic block - a reappraisal. *Anaesthesia* Jul; Vol. 34(No. 7): 638-642.

Ekholm, R., Adami, J., Tidermark, J., Hansson, K., Tornkvis, H. & Ponzer, S. (2006). Fractures of the shaft of the humerus. An epidemiological study of 401 fractures. *Journal of Bone and Joint Surgery British* Nov; Vol. 88(No. 11): 1469-1473.

Elliott, K.G. & Johnstone, A.J. (2003). Diagnosing acute compartment syndrome. *Journal of Bone and Joint Surgery British* Jul; Vol. 85(No. 5): 625-632.

Flagel, B.T., Luchette, F.A., Reed, L., Esposito, T.J., Davis, K.A., Santaniello, J.M. & Gamelli, R.L. (2005). Half-a-dozen ribs: the breakpoint for mortality. *Surgery* Oct; Vol. 138(No. 4): 717-725.]

Foss, N.B., Kristensen, B.B., Bundgaard, M., Bak, M., Heiring, C., Virkelyst, C., Hougaard, S. & Kehlet, H. (2007). *Anesthesiology* Apr; Vol. 106(No. 4): 773-778.

Franco, C.D., Choksi, N., Rahman, A., Voronov, G. & Almachnouk, M.H. (2006). A subgluteal approach to the sciatic nerve in adults at 10 cm from the midline. *Regional Anesthesia and Pain Medicine* May-Jun; Vol. 31(No. 3): 215-220.

Geerts, W.H., Bergqvist, D., Pineo, G.F., Heit, J.A., Samama, C.M., Lassen, M.R. & Colwell, C.W.; American College of Chest Physicians. (2008). Prevention of venous thromboembolism: American College of Chest Physicians Evidence-Based Clinical Practice Guidelines (8th Edition). *Chest* Jun; Vol. 133(6 Suppl); 381S-453S.

Haddad, F.S. & Williams, R.L. (1995). Femoral nerve block in extracapsular femoral neck fractures. *Journal of Bone and Joint SurgeryBr* Nov; Vol. 77(No. 6): 922-923.

Harris, I.A., Kadir, A. & Donald, G. (2006). Continuous compartment pressure monitoring for tibia fractures: does it influence outcomes? *Journal of Trauma* Jun; Vol. 60(No. 6): 1330-1335.

Horlocker, T.T., Wedel, D.J., Rowlingson, J.C., Enneking, F.K., Kopp, S.L., Benzon, H.T., Brown, D.L., Heit, J.A., Mulroy, M.F., Rosenquist, R.W., Tryba, M., & Yuan, C.S. (2010). Regional anesthesia in the patient receiving antithrombotic or thrombolytic therapy: American Society of Regional Anesthesia and Pain Medicine Evidence-Based Guidelines (Third Edition). *Regional Anesthesia and Pain Medicine* Jan; Vol. 35(No. 1): 64-101.

Inman, V. & Saunders, J. Referred pain from skeletal structures. *Journal of Nervous and Mental Disease* 1944; 99: 660-667.

Ivanusic, J. The evidence for the spinal segmental innervation of bone. *Clinical Anatomy* 2007; Nov; Vol. 20(No. 8): 956-960.

Ivanusic, JJ. (2007). The evidence for the spinal segmental innervation of bone. *Clinical Anatomy* Nov; Vol. 20(No. 8): 956-960.

Ivarsson, B.J., Manaswi, A., Genovese, D., Crandall, J.R., Hurwitz, S.R., Burke, C. & Fakhry, S. (2008). Site, type, and local mechanism of tibial shaft fracture in drivers in frontal automobile crashes. *Forensic Science International* Mar; Vol. 175(No. 2-3): 186-192.

Johner, R., Staubli, H.U., Gunst, M. & Cordey, J. (2000). The point of view of the clinician: a prospective study of the mechanism of accidents and the morphology of tibial and fibular shaft structures. *Injury* Sep; Vol. 31 (Suppl 3): C45-49.

Karmakar, M.J., Critchley, L.A., Ho, A.M., Gin, T., Lee, T.W. & Yim, A.P. (2003). Continuous thoracic paravertebral infusion of bupivacaine for pain management in patients with multiple fractured ribs. *Chest* Feb; Vol. 123(No. 2): 424-431.

Karmakar, M.K., Kwok, W.H., Ho, A.M., Tsang, K., Chui, P.T. & Gin, T. (2007). Ultrasound-guided sciatic nerve block: description of a new approach at the subgluteal space. *British Journal of Anaesthesia* Mar; Vol. 98(No. 3): 390-395.

Kashuk, JL, Moore, EE, Pinski, S, Johnson, JL, Moore, JB, Morgan, S, Cothren, CC, Smith, W. (2009). Lower extremity compartment syndrome in the acute care surgery paradigm: safety lessons learned. Patient Safety in Surgery 2009; Vol. 3(No. 1): 11.

Konstantakos, E.K., Dalstrom, D.J., Nelles, M.E., Laughlin, R.T. & Prayson, M.J. (2007). Diagnosis and management of extremity compartment syndrome: an orthopedic perspective. *American Surgeon* Dec; Vol. 73(No. 12): 1199-1209.

Liu, S.S., Ngeow, J. & John, R.S.. (2010). Evidence basis for ultrasound-guided block characteristics: onset, quality, and duration. *Regional Anesthesia and Pain Medicine* Mar-Apr; Vol. 35(2 Suppl): S26-35.

Locher, S., Burmeister, H., Bohlen, T., Eichenberger, U., Stoupis, C., Moriggl, B., Siebenrock, K. & Curatolo, M. (2008). Radiological anatomy of the obturator nerve and its articular branches: basis to develop a method of radiofrequency denervation for hip joint pain. *Pain Medicine* Apr; Vol. 9(No. 3): 291-298.

Lopez, S., Gros, T., Bernard, N., Plasse, C. & Capdevila, X. (2003). Fascia iliaca compartment block for femoral bone fractures in prehospital care. *Regional Anesthesia and Pain Medicine* May-Jun; Vol. 28(No. 3): 203-207.

Lopez, A.D., Mathers, C.D., Ezzati, M., Jamison, D.T. & Murray, C.J.L. (Eds.). (2006). *Global Burden of Disease and Risk Factors.* Oxford University Press and the World Bank, New York, NY.

Lucas, S.D., Higdon, T.A. & Boezaart, A.P. (2011). Unintended epidural placement of a thoracic paravertebral catheter in a patient with severe chest trauma. *Pain Medicine* Jun 30; doi: 10.1111/j.1526-4637.2011.01180.x. [Epub ahead of print]

Luchette, F.A., Radafshar, S.M., Kaiser, R., Flynn, W. & Hassett, J.M. (1994). Prospective evaluation of epidural versus intrapleural catheters for analgesia in chest wall trauma. *Journal of Trauma* Jun; Vol. 36(No. 6): 865-869.

Luger, T.J., Kammerlander, C., Gosch, M., Luger, M.F., Kammerlander-Knauer, U., Roth, T. & Kreutziger, J. (2010). Neuroaxial versus general anaesthesia in geriatric patients for hip fracture surgery: does it matter? *Osteoporos International* Dec; Vol. 21(No. 4): S555-572.

Luyet, C., Eichenberger, U., Greif, R., Vogt, A., Szucs Farkas, Z. & Moriggl, B. (2009). Ultrasound-guided paravertebral puncture and placement of catheters in human cadavers: an imaging study. *British Journal of Anaesthesia* Apr; Vol. 102(No. 4): 534-539.

Mach, D.B., Rogers, S.D., Sabino, M.C., Luger, N.M., Schwei, M.J., Pomonis, J.D., Keyser, C.P., Clohisy, D.R., Adams, D.J., O'Leary, P. & Mantyh, P.W. (2002). Origins of skeletal pain: sensory and sympathetic innervation of the mouse femur. *Neuroscience* Vol. 113(No. 1): 155-156.

Mackenzie, E.J., Rivara, F.P., Jurkovich, G.J., Nathens, A.B., Frey, K.P., Egleston, B.L., Salkever, D.S., Weir, S. & Scharfstein, D.O. (2007). The National Study on Costs and Outcomes of Trauma. *J Trauma* Dec; Vol. 63(6 Suppl): S54-67.

Mar, G.J., Barrington, M.J. & McGuirk, B.R. (2009). Acute compartment syndrome of the lower limb and the effect of postoperative analgesia on diagnosis. *British Journal of Anaesthesia* Jan; Vol. 102(No. 1): 3-11.

Marhofer, P., Schrogendorfer, K., Wallner, T., Konig, H., Mayer, N. & Kapral, S. (1998). Ultrasonographic guidance reduces the amount of local anesthetic for 3-in-1 blocks. *Regional Anesthesia and Pain Medicine* Nov-Dec; Vol. 23(No. 6): 584-588.

Matsen, F.A. 3rd. (1975). Compartment syndrome. A unified concept. *Clinical Orthopaedics and Related Research* Nov-Dec; Vol. 113: 8-14.

McCartney, C.J., Lin, L. & Shastri, U. (2010). Evidence basis for the use of ultrasound for upper-extremity blocks. *Regional Anesthesia and Pain Medicine* Mar-Apr; Vol. 35(2 Suppl): S10-15.

McQueen, M.M. & Court-Brown, C.M. (1996). Compartment monitoring in tibial fractures. The pressure threshold for decompression. *Journal of Bone and Joint Surgery British* Jan; Vol. 78(No. 1): 99-104.

McQueen, M.M., Gaston, P. & Court-Brown, C.M. (2000). Acute compartment syndrome. Who is at risk? *Journal of Bone and Joint Surgery British* Mar; Vol. 82(No. 2): 200-203.

McManus, J.G., Morton, M.J., Crystal, C.S., McArthur, T.J., Helphenstine, J.S., Masneri, D.A., Young, S.E. & Miller, M.A. (2008). Use of ultrasound to assess acute fracture reduction in emergency care settings. *American Journal of Disaster Medicine* Jul-Aug; Vol. 3(No. 4): 241-247.

Mohta, M., Verma, P., Saxena, A.K., Sethi, A.K., Tyagi, A. & Girotra, G. (2009). Prospective, randomized comparison of continuous thoracic epidural and thoracic paravertebral infusion in patients with unilateral multiple fractured ribs-a pilot study. *Journal of Trauma* Apr; Vol. 66(No. 4): 1096-1101.

Monzon, D.G., Iserson, K.V. & Vazquez, J.A. (2007). Single fascia iliaca compartment block for post-hip fracture pain relief. *Journal of Emergency Medicine* Apr; Vol. 32(No. 3): 257-262.

Moon, M.R., Luchette, F.A., Gibson, S.W., Crews, J., Sudarshan, G., Hurst, J.M., Davis, K. Jr, Johannigman, J.A., Frame, S.B. & Fischer, J.E. (1999). Prospective, randomized comparison of epidural versus parenteral opioid analgesia in thoracic trauma. *Annals of Surgery* May; Vol. 229(No. 5): 684-691.

Mouzopoulos, G., Vasiliadis, G., Lasanianos, N., Nikolaras, G., Morakis, E. & Kaminaris, M. (2009). Fascia iliaca block prophylaxis for hip fracture patients at risk for delirium: a randomized placebo-controlled study. *Journal of Orthopaedics and Traumatology* Sep; Vol. 10(No. 3): 127-133.

Naja, Z.M., El-Rajab, M., Al-Tannir, M.A., Ziade, F.M., Tayara, K., Younes, F. & Lonnqvist, P.A. (2006). Thoracic paravertebral block: influence of the number of injections. *Regional Anesthesia and Pain Medicine* May-Jun; Vol. 31(No. 3): 196-201.

Neal, J.M., Brull, R., Chan, V.W., Grant, S.A., Horn, J.L., Liu, S.S., McCartney, C.J., Narouze, S.N., Perlas, A., Salinas, F.V., Sites, B.D. & Tsui, B.C. (2010). *Regional Anesthesia and Pain Medicine* Mar-Apr; Vol. 35(2 Suppl): S1-9.

Ogawa, K. & Yoshida, A. (1998). Throwing fracture of the humeral shaft. An analysis of 90 patients. *American Journal of Sports Medicine* Mar-Apr; Vol. 26(No. 2): 242-246.

Osinowo, O.A., Zahrani, M. & Softah, A. (2004). Effect of intercostal nerve block with 0.5% bupivacaine on peak expiratory flow rate and arterial oxygen saturation in rib fractures. *Journal of Trauma* ;Feb; Vol. 56(No. 2): 345-347.

Powell, E.S., Cook, D., Pearce, A.C., Davies, P., Bowler, G.M., Naidu, B. & Gao, F.; UKPOS Investigators. (2011). A prospective, multicentre, observational cohort study of analgesia and outcome after pneumonectomy. *Br J Anaesth* Mar; Vol. 106(No. 3): 364-370.

Park, S., Ahn, J., Gee, A.O., Kuntz, A.F. & Esterhai, J.L. (2009). Compartment syndrome in tibial fractures. *Journal of Orthopaedic Trauma* Aug; Vol. 23(No. 7): 514-518.

Parker, M.J., Griffiths, R. & Appadu, B.N. (2002). Nerve blocks (subcostal, lateral cutaneous, femoral, triple, psoas) for hip fractures. *Cochrane Database of Systematic Reviews* (1):CD001159.

Parker, M.J., Handoll, H.H. & Griffiths, R. (2004). Anaesthesia for hip fracture surgery in adults. *Cochrane Database of Systematic Reviews* Oct 18;(4):CD000521.

Pecci, M. & Kreher, J.B. Clavicle fractures. (2008). Clavicle fractures. *American Family Physician* Jan; Vol. 77(No. 1): 65-70.

Pintaric, T.S., Potocnik, I., Hadzic, A., Stupnik, T., Pintaric, M. & Jankovic, V.N. (2011). Comparison of continuous thoracic epidural with paravertebral block on perioperative analgesia and hemodynamic stability in patients having open lung surgery. *Regional Anesthesia and Pain Medicine* May-Jun; Vol. 36(No. 3): 256-260.

Postacchini, F., Gumina, S., De Santis, P. & Albo, F. (2002). Epidemiology of clavicle fractures. *Journal of Shoulder and Elbow Surgery* Oct; Vol. 11(No. 5): 452-456.

Purcell-Jones, G., Pither, C.E. & Justins, D.M. (1989). Paravertebral somatic nerve block: a clinical, radiographic and computed tomographic study in chronic pain patients. *Anesthesia and Analgesia* Jan; Vol. 68(No. 1): 32-39.

Richards, H., Langston, A., Kulkarni, R. & Downes, E.M. (2004). Does patient controlled analgesia delay the diagnosis of compartment syndrome following intramedullary nailing of the tibia? *Injury* Mar; Vol. 35(No. 3): 296-298.

Richardson, J., Jones, J. & Atkinson, R.. (1998). The effect of thoracic paravertebral blockade on intercostal somatosensory evoked potentials. *Anesthesia and Analgesia* Aug; Vol. 87(No. 2): 373-376.

Richardson, J., Lonnqvist, P.A. & Naja, Z. (2011). Bilateral thoracic paravertebral block: potential and practice. *British Journal of Anaesthesia* Feb; Vol. 106(No.2): 164-171.

Robinson, C.M. Fractures of the clavicle in the adult. (1998). Epidemiology and classification. *Journal of Bone and Joint Surgery British* May; Vol. 80(No. 3): 476-484.

Rogers, F.B., Cipolle, M.D., Velmahos, G .& Rozycki, G. Practice management guidelines for the management of venous thromboembolism in trauma patients, Accessed July 12, 2011, Available from: http://www.east.org/tpg/dvt.pdf.]

Saito, T., Den, S., Cheema, P.S., Tanuma, K., Carney, E., Carlsson, C. & Richardson, J. (2001). A single injection, multi-segmental paravertebral block- extension of somatosensory and sympathetic block in volunteers. *Acta Anaesthesiologica Scandinavica* Jan; Vol. 45(No. 1): 30-33.

Schiferer, A., Gore, C., Gorove, L., Lang, T., Steinlechner, B., Zimpfer, M. & Kober, A. (2007). A randomized controlled trial of femoral nerve blockade administered preclinically for pain relief in femoral trauma. *Anesthesia and Analgesia* Dec; Vol. 105(No. 6): 1852-1854.

Schuerer, D.J.E., Whinney, R.R., Freeman, B.D., Nash, J., Prasad, S., Krem, M.M., Mazuski, H.E. & Buchman, T.G. (2005). Evaluation of the applicability, efficacy, and safety of a thromboembolic event prophylaxis guideline designed for quality improvement of the traumatically injured patient. *Journal of Trauma* Apr; Vol. 58(No. 4): 731-739.

Shorr, R.M., Rodriguez, A., Indeck, M.C., Crittenden, M.D., Hartunian, S. & Cowley, R.A. (1989). Blunt chest trauma in the elderly. *Journal of Trauma* Feb; Vol. 29(No. 2): 234-237.]

Sia, S., Pelusio, F., Barbagli, R. & Rivituso, C. (2004). Analgesia before performing a spinal block in the sitting position in patients with femoral shaft fracture: a comparison between femoral nerve block and intravenous fentanyl. *Anesthesia and Analgesia* Oct; Vol. 99(No. 4): 1221-1224.

Simon, B.J., Cushman, J., Barraco, R., Lane, V. & Luchette, F.A., Miglietta, M., Roccaforte, D.J., Spector, R., EAST Practice Management Guidelines Work Group. (2005). Pain management guidelines for blunt thoracic trauma. *Journal of Trauma* Nov; Vol. 59(No. 5): 1256-1267.

Thonse, R, Ashford, RU, Williams, TI, Harrington, P. (2004). Differences in attitudes to analgesia in post-operative limb surgery put patients at risk of compartment syndrome. Injury 2004; Vol. 35 (No.3): 290-295.

Thurston, T.J. (1982). Distribution of nerves in long bones as shown by silver impregnation. *Journal of Anatomy* Jun; Vol. 134(Pt 4): 719-728.]

Trunkey, D.D., Lewis, F.R. (1980). Chest trauma. *Surgical Clinics of North America* Dec; Vol. 60(No.6): 1541-1549.

Ulmer, T. The clinical diagnosis of compartment syndrome of the lower leg: are clinical findings predictive of the disorder? Journal of Orthopaedic Trauma 2002; Vol. 16 (No. 8): 572-577.

Wang, K., Dowrick, A., Choi, J., Rahim, R. & Edwards, E. (2010). Post-operative numbness and patient satisfaction following plate fixation of clavicular fractures. *Injury* Oct; Vol. 41(No. 10): 1002-1005.

Wathen, J.E., Gao, D., Merritt, G., Georgopoulos, G. & Battan, F.K. (2007). A randomized controlled trial comparing a fascia iliaca compartment nerve block to a traditional systemic analgesic for femur fractures in a pediatric emergency department. *Annals of Emergency Medicine* Aug; Vol. 50(No. 2): 162-171.

Wisner, D.H. (1990). A stepwise logistic regression analysis of factors affecting morbidity and mortality after thoracic trauma: effect of epidural analgesia. *Journal of Trauma* Jul; Vol. 7(No. 7): 799-804.

World Health Organization. (2004). *Global Burden of Disease (GBD)*, Accessed July 11, 2011, Available from: www.who.int/healthinfo/global_burden_of_disease/en/.

Yun M.J., Kim, Y.H., Han, M.K., Kim, J.H., Hwang, J.W. & Do, S.H. (2009). Analgesia before a spinal block for femoral neck fracture: fascia iliaca compartment block. *Acta Anesthesiologica Scandinavica* Nov; Vol. 53(No. 10): 1282-1287.

Part 3

Opioids

14

Opioid Analgesics

Maree T. Smith[1,2] and Wei H. Goh[1]
[1]*Centre for Integrated Preclinical Drug Development, The University of Queensland, St Lucia Campus, Brisbane, Queensland*
[2]*School of Pharmacy, The University of Queensland, St Lucia Campus, Brisbane, Queensland*
Australia

1. Introduction

Intensive research on the neurobiology of pain over the past two decades has revealed many receptors, ion channels and enzymes with potential as novel targets for development of a new generation of analgesic agents. However, despite large investment in preclinical and clinical development of small molecules and biologics as potential novel pain therapeutics, very few have reached the clinic. Hence, drugs used in the clinical setting for the pharmacological management of pain continue to be those that were first recommended in 1986 by the World Health Organisation (WHO) for the management of chronic cancer pain (WHO, 1986). Twenty-five years on, the WHO 3-step Analgesic Ladder (Figure 1) is still used widely to guide the pharmacological management of pain and opioid analgesics are the mainstay for alleviation of moderate to severe nociceptive pain.

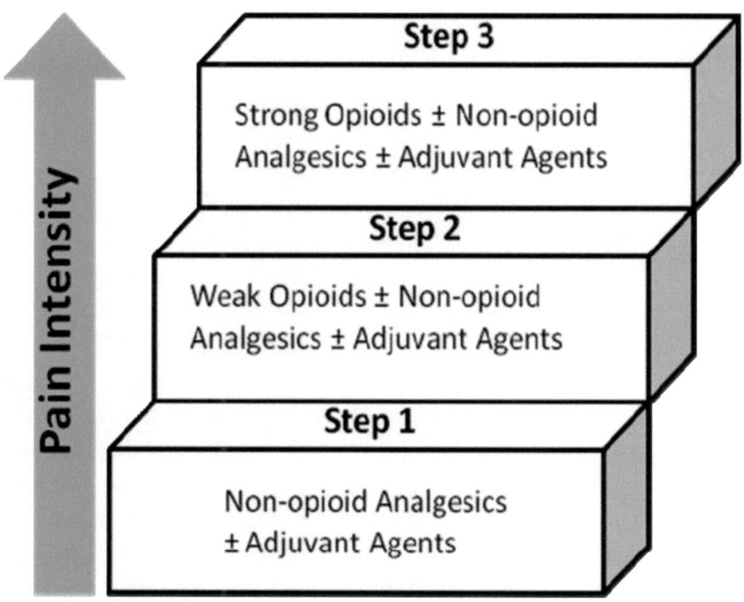

Fig. 1. World Health Organisation 3-Step Analgesic Ladder (WHO, 1986)

2. WHO Analgesic Ladder

The WHO Analgesic Ladder provides a succinct encapsulation of the guidelines for the management of chronic pain according to intensity (WHO, 1986). Specifically, for mild pain, non-opioid analgesics on Step 1 of the Analgesic Ladder including acetaminophen, aspirin and nonsteroidal anti-inflammatory drugs such as ibuprofen, are recommended. When the pain has a neuropathic component, addition of an adjuvant agent such as a tricyclic antidepressant, anticonvulsant or anti-arrhythmic agent, is recommended. Weak opioid analgesics such as codeine, tramadol and dextropropoxyphene are added to non-opioid analgesics when mild pain progresses to moderate pain (Step 2); adjuvants are again co-administered when the pain has a neuropathic component. Strong opioid analgesics are recommended for the management of moderate to severe nociceptive pain (Step 3) with morphine the strong opioid analgesic of choice due to its ready availability world-wide at low cost. Strong opioid analgesics are often co-administered with non-opioids, and adjuvants are added when pain has a neuropathic component (WHO, 1986).

According to the WHO guidelines, each patient should receive a period of individualized dose titration on a 'round the clock' rather than an 'as required' basis as this facilitates dosage optimization for the selected analgesic and/or adjuvant (WHO, 1986). Although many opioid analgesics have relatively short elimination half-lives (Table 1), most are available as sustained-release formulations that are administered once or twice-daily to optimize patient compliance as well as pain relief. For patients who experience break-through pain during ambulation or activities of daily living, additional bolus doses of immediate-release formulations are given on an "as required" basis. For most patients, the oral dosing route is preferred except where impaired gastrointestinal transit makes this impractical as in the immediate post-operative period or during labor.

3. Opioid analgesics

Opioid analgesics commonly used for the control of clinical pain include morphine, codeine, oxycodone, hydromorphone, buprenorphine, tramadol, fentanyl, remifentanil, pethidine and methadone. The potencies of these opioid analgesics differ markedly. Equi-analgesic doses and usual starting doses for the oral route derived from the acute pain setting are shown in Tables 2 and 3 respectively.

3.1 Opioid-related adverse effects

Apart from their desired analgesic action, clinically prescribed opioids also produce many undesired effects including respiratory depression, sedation, nausea, vomiting, constipation, pruritus, tolerance and dependence, to name but a few (Zollner & Stein, 2007). Although studies using μ-opioid (MOP) receptor knockout mice suggest that the analgesic and adverse effects of opioid analgesics are all produced by activation of the MOP receptor, clinical experience shows that there are marked between-opioid differences with respect to analgesic and tolerability profiles within the same patient (Smith, 2008). However, the precise mechanistic basis underpinning these observations is not well understood.

Opioid Analgesic	Elimination Half-life (h)	Duration of Action (h)
Codeine	3	4-6
Meperidine	3.5	4-6
Fentanyl	3.7	0.5-1 (IV); 72 (TD); 2-4 (TM)
Hydromorphone	2-3	4-5
Methadone	24#	4-6
Morphine	2.5	3-4
Oxycodone	3	8-12 (CR), 3-4 (IR)
Tramadol	5-7	4-6 (IR), 24 (ER)
Buprenorphine	3	6

#large inter-individual variability in range 12-150 h
IV = intravenous; TD = transdermal; TM = transmucosal
IR = immediate release; ER = extended release; CR = controlled release

Table 1. Typical Mean Elimination Half-lives and Durations of Action for Commonly Prescribed Opioid Analgesics (adapted from Mather & Smith 1998; Trescot et al., 2008; Argoff & Silvershein, 2009)

Opioid Analgesic	Dose × Conversion Factor
Codeine	x 0.16
Meperidine (IV)	× 0.4
Methadone	× 1.5
Oxycodone	× 1.5
Buprenorphine	× 50
Morphine (IV)	× 3
Morphine (oral)	× 1

IV = intravenous

Table 2. Opioid Analgesic Dose Conversion Table to Oral Morphine (adapted from Nissen et al., 2011)

Opioid Analgesic	Oral Administration	
	Dose	Inter-dosing Interval (h)
Codeine	15-60 mg	3-6
Fentanyl	100-200 μg (IV)	6[a]
Hydromorphone	2-4 mg	3-4
Methadone	5-10 mg	24
Morphine	15-30 mg (IR)	4 (IR)
Oxycodone	10 mg (CR), 5-10 mg (IR)	12 (CR), 4-6 (IR)
Tramadol	50-100 mg (IR), 100 mg (ER)	4-6 (IR), 24 (ER)

CR = controlled-release; ER = extended-release; IR = immediate-release; IV = intravenous;
[a]Not more than 4 doses per day.

Table 3. Common Starting Doses for Selected Opioid Analgesics (adapted from Mather & Smith; Argoff & Silvershein, 2009)

3.1.1 Respiratory depression

Opioid-related deaths continue to be reported in the acute pain setting underpinned by opioid-induced ventilatory impairment that often develops due to a combination of factors including opioid-induced central respiratory depression, sedation and/or upper airway obstruction (Macintyre et al., 2011). It is recommended that all patients be monitored for opioid-induced ventilatory impairment using sedation scores as a '6th vital sign' so that it can be detected early and appropriate intervention initiated (Macintyre et al., 2011).

3.2 Strategies for minimizing opioid-related adverse effects

It is essential to assess patients to ensure that adverse effects are genuinely opioid-related rather than being due to another medical problem. Strategies recommended (Swegle & Logemann, 2006) for minimizing opioid-related adverse effects are as follows:

1. Titrating opioid doses slowly
2. Dose reduction to assess if satisfactory analgesia can be obtained with tolerable side-effects
3. Symptom management including pro-active preventative treatment of nausea and constipation
4. Addition of, or increasing non-opioid or adjuvant analgesic doses for an opioid sparing effect
5. Opioid rotation
6. Changing the route of administration
7. Frequent re-assessment

3.3 Strategies for managing intolerable opioid-related adverse effects

For patients experiencing poor pain relief together with intolerable opioid-related side-effects such as severe vomiting, severe dysphagia or bowel obstruction, changing from the oral to the parenteral (e.g. intravenous, subcutaneous, intramuscular), rectal, buccal, sublingual, transdermal or spinal (epidural, intrathecal) route of administration, may reduce adverse effects to a tolerable level and restore satisfactory analgesia (Walsh, 2005). Another strategy for restoring satisfactory analgesia with tolerable side-effects in such patients is 'opioid rotation' that involves switching from one strong opioid analgesic to another (Smith, 2008; Knotkova et al., 2009; Vissers et al., 2010). Additional clinical strategies for restoring analgesia in patients experiencing inadequate pain relief and intolerable opioid-related side-effects include use of neurolytic blocks as an adjunct or alternative to pharmacotherapy (Eisenberg et al., 2005) or progression to use of anaesthetic intervention if 'opioid rotation' fails (Riley et al., 2007).

3.4 Tolerance to the analgesic effects of opioids

In the absence of disease progression, tolerance to the analgesic effects of an opioid manifests in patients with clinical pain as the need for progressively higher opioid doses in order to maintain the same level of pain relief (South & Smith, 2001). In rodent studies, analgesic tolerance is demonstrated by a rightward shift in the analgesia dose-response curve for a particular opioid administered after a period of chronic dosing relative to the dose-response curve determined for the same opioid in opioid-naïve animals (South & Smith, 2001).

3.5 Tolerance to opioid-related side-effects

As already noted, opioid-related adverse effects that may occur after the initation of opioid analgesic treatment in opioid-naïve patients include respiratory depression, somnolence, nausea, vomiting, miosis, pruritus, constipation, and euphoria/dysphoria. With chronic dosing, tolerance often develops to sedation, nausea and respiratory depression whereas tolerance to constipation and miosis is minimal (Chang et al., 2007).

3.6 Opioid analgesics and renal impairment

Several opioid analgesics including morphine, hydromorphone and meperidine are metabolized in the liver to pharmacologically active metabolites that may accumulate in patients with renal impairment. Hence, for patients with renal impairment, opioid analgesics including oxycodone and fentanyl that are devoid of active metabolites, are preferred (King et al., 2011).

4. Weak opioid analgesics

4.1 Codeine

Codeine (7,8-didehydro-4,5-epoxy-3-methoxy-17-methylmorphinan-6-ol) is an opioid alkaloid found in opium, the dried exudate of the unripe seed capsule of the opium poppy, *Papaver somniferum,* at 0.7 to 2.5% (Boerner, 1975). Due to its high consumption rates globally, codeine is generally synthesized by O-methylation of morphine, an abundant opium constituent at 10-15% (Lenz et al., 1986).

Codeine is a weak opioid analgesic that binds to the μ-opioid (MOP) receptor with low affinity (Ki = 0.7 μM) (Volpe et al., 2011). Its analgesic properties are generally thought to be derived from the fact that it is a prodrug for morphine as up to 10% of oral doses are O-demethylated to morphine by cytochrome P450 2D6 (CYP2D6), an enzyme subject to genetic polymorphism (Kadiev et al., 2008, Somogyi et al., 2007, Zollner & Stein, 2007). Supporting this notion, plasma morphine concentrations are virtually undetectable and codeine lacks efficacy in individuals with the poor metabolizer (PM) CYP2D6 phenotype (Poulsen et al., 1996). By contrast, codeine is extensively metabolized to morphine in those with the ultra-metabolizer (UM) phenotype who also have an increased risk of respiratory depression after regular doses of codeine (Kirchheiner et al., 2007).

Doses of codeine generally do not exceed 60 mg (Trescot et al., 2008). Codeine is available in a range of prescription and over-the-counter medicines, often in combination with paracetamol, aspirin or ibuprofen for pain relief (Moore et al., 1997; Moore et al., 2011). It is also the active ingredient in many cough suppressant mixtures and anti-diarrhoeal products (Schiller, 1995; Wee, 2008). Codeine is susceptible to metabolic drug-drug interactions with other commonly prescribed medications that are also metabolized by CYP2D6 including both CYP2D6 inhibitors (e.g. cimetidine) and CYP2D6 inducers (e.g. rifampicin) (Caraco et al., 1997; Zhou, 2009).

4.2 Meperidine (pethidine)

Meperidine (pethidine; ethyl-1-methyl-4-phenylpiperidine-4-carboxylate), is a synthetic MOP receptor agonist that binds with low affinity (Ki = 450 nM) at the MOP receptor (Volpe et al., 2011). Meperidine is a weak opioid analgesic with potency at ~10% that of morphine for the relief of acute post-operative pain (Latta et al., 2002). Meperidine is metabolized by hepatic esterases to pethidinic acid, an inactive metabolite, and by N-demethylation to a neurotoxic metabolite, normeperidine (Gilman et al., 1980, Armstrong et al., 2009). After multiple doses, normeperidine may accumulate in plasma and cerebrospinal fluid causing tremors, twitches, myoclonus and seizures as it has a longer plasma half-life than meperidine itself (Plummer et al., 1995; Simopoulos et al., 2002). Meperidine is contra-indicated in patients with impaired renal function as they are at increased risk of normeperidine neurotoxicity due to its faster accumulation (Marinella, 1997; Reutens & Stewart-Wynne, 1989). Generally, meperidine use is discouraged in favour of more efficacious and less toxic opioid analgesics (Latta et al., 2002).

4.3 Tramadol

Tramadol ((1RS,2RS)-2-[(dimethylamino)methyl]- 1 -(3-methoxyphenyl)-cyclo-hexanol hydrochloride) is a synthetic analgesic that is a racaemic mixture of two enantiomers that bind to the MOP receptor with low (10 μM) affinity (Volpe et al., 2011). After systemic administration, tramadol is metabolized in the liver by the enzyme CYP2D6, to its O-demethylated M1 metabolite, a potent μ-opioid agonist that contributes to its analgesic actions (Subrahmanyam et al., 2001). The (-)-enantiomer of tramadol mainly inhibits noradrenaline reuptake in the central nervous system (CNS) to augment descending inhibition of pain transmission in the spinal cord whereas the (+)-enantiomer preferentially inhibits serotonin reuptake (Reimann & Hennies, 1994). Thus, the pharmacology of tramadol is complex with its analgesic action being due to the combined effects of its two enantiomers and the M1 metabolite. For this reason, the US Food and Drug Administration (FDA) has classified tramadol as a nontraditional, centrally acting analgesic (Grond & Sablotzki, 2004).

For the relief of post-operative pain relief, tramadol is regarded as a "weak" opioid analgesic with potency at ~10% that of morphine but it does not produce significant constipation or respiratory depression and it has low abuse potential (Grond & Sablotzki, 2004). When tramadol is given in doses larger than the recommended doses, or if it is co-administered with medications that lower the seizure threshold such as selective serotonin reuptake inhibitors, tricyclic antidepressants and antipsychotic drugs, seizures may be induced (Gardner et al., 2000).

5. Strong opioid analgesics

5.1 Morphine

Morphine (7,8-didehydro-4,5,-epoxy-17-methyl-(5α,6α)-morphinan-3,6-diol) is extracted from opium due to its relatively high abundance at ~10-15% by weight (Boerner, 1975). Morphine was first isolated from opium in 1805 by Freidrich Sertűrner, a German pharmacist who named it "morphium" after Morpheus the Greek God of Dreams (Milne et al., 1996).

Morphine is the prototypic strong opioid analgesic that binds with high affinity (K_i = 1.2 nM) at the MOP receptor (Volpe et al., 2011). After oral administration in humans, morphine has low oral bioavailability at ~20% due to extensive first-pass metabolism in the liver to two major metabolites, viz morphine-6-glucuronide (M6G) and morphine-3-glucuronide (M3G) that account for ~10% and >50% of each dose, respectively (Milne et al., 1996). Morphine has a short elimination half-life at ~2 h consistent with its short duration of action at ~4 h (Mather & Smith, 1998).

M6G, like morphine, binds with high affinity at the MOP receptor and it is a more potent analgesic than morphine when given by central routes (Smith & South, 2001). By contrast, supraspinally administered M3G evokes dose-dependent neuro-excitatory effects and its actions generally oppose those of morphine in animal studies (Smith, 2000). The elimination half-lives of M3G and M6G are in the range 3-4 h (Mather & Smith, 1998).

After administration of single doses of morphine to patients with clinical pain, the plasma and CSF concentrations of M3G exceed those of morphine by several-fold (Hasselström & Säwe, 1993) and after chronic dosing, the plasma M3G concentrations exceed the corresponding morphine levels by as much as 10-20 fold (Smith et al., 1999). In patients with renal impairment, M6G and M3G may accumulate in the plasma and CSF, thereby increasing the risk of M6G-induced respiratory depression (Smith & South, 2001) and/or M3G-induced neuro-excitation (Smith, 2000).

Morphine is available in immediate-release and sustained-release oral tablet and capsule formulations as well as oral mixtures, rectal suppositories and sterile ampoules for parenteral administration by the intramuscular, intravenous, subcutaneous, epidural and intrathecal routes (Argoff & Silvershein, 2009). The duration of action for immediate-release oral morphine preparations is approximately 3-4 h whereas for oral sustained-released morphine tablets and capsules, the duration of action is 12-24 h (Mather & Smith, 1998). The convenience of once or twice daily dosing provided by sustained-release formulations improves patient compliance and pain relief outcomes (Argoff & Silvershein, 2009).

5.2 Oxycodone

Oxycodone ((5α-4,5-epoxy-14-hydroxy-3-methoxy-17-methylmorphinan-6-one) is a strong opioid analgesic that is a semi-synthetic derivative of the abundant opium alkaloid, thebaine (Lenz et al., 1986). After oral administration, the bioavailability of oxycodone is high at 60-87% (Leow et al., 1992; Lalovic et al., 2006). Oxycodone is extensively N-demethylated by the enzyme, CYP3A4, to the analgesically inactive metabolite, noroxycodone (Poyhia et al., 1992; Davis et al., 2003; Lalovic et al., 2004, 2006) with up to another 10% of each dose undergoing CYP2D6-catalyzed O-demethylation to the high affinity MOP receptor agonist oxymorphone (Lalovic et al., 2006). However, metabolically-derived oxymorphone does not contribute significantly to the analgesic actions of oxycodone for the relief of clinical pain because its circulating plasma concentrations are very low (~1 ng/mL) in both extensive metabolisers (EMs) and PMs (0.3 ng/mL) as it is rapidly further metabolized to its analgesically-inactive glucuronide conjugate (Lalovic et al., 2006; Zwisler et al., 2010). For patients with post-operative pain, there is no difference in analgesic outcomes between PMs and EMs (Zwisler et al., 2010), affirming earlier work by others showing that the analgesic effects of oxycodone are attributable to the parent opioid alone (Heiskanen et al., 1998; Lalovic et al., 1996).

Radioligand binding studies show that oxycodone has relatively low affinity (Ki = 26 nM) at the cloned MOP receptor (Volpe et al., 2011) and that it has a distinctly different binding profile from morphine in rat brain homogenate (Nielsen et al., 2007). This likely underpins the low extent of cross-tolerance between oxycodone and morphine in rodents (Nielsen et al., 2000) and the success of opioid rotation from morphine to oxycodone for the restoration of analgesia with tolerable opioid-related side-effects in humans (Narabayashi et al., 2008).

The potency of intravenous and oral oxycodone for the relief of both post-operative and chronic cancer pain is ~1.5 times that of morphine (Kalso et al., 1991; Heiskanen & Kalso, 1997; Bruera et al., 1998). However, when given by the epidural route for the relief of post-operative pain, the potency of oxycodone is much lower than that of morphine at ~11% (Backlund et al., 1997).

Oxycodone, like morphine, is available in immediate-release and sustained-release tablet formulations as well as in oral mixtures, rectal suppositories and ampoules for parenteral administration (Argoff & Silvershein, 2009).

5.3 Methadone

Methadone, 6-dimethylamino-4,4-diphenyl-heptan-3-one, is a synthetic, strong opioid analgesic that is a racaemic mixture of two enantiomers. The analgesic efficacy of methadone is multi-faceted as the R-enantiomer is a high affinity MOP receptor agonist (Ki = 3.4nM) whereas the S-enantiomer augments descending noradrenergic inhibition to block nociceptive signaling in the spinal cord, and both enantiomers have NMDA receptor antagonist activity (Davis and Walsh, 2001).

In humans, methadone has high but unpredictable oral bioavailability at ~80% (range 41-99%) with peak plasma concentrations observed at 2-4 h post-dosing (Trescot et al., 2008; Modesto-Lowe et al., 2010). There is a large degree of inter-individual variability in its long elimination half-life (12-150 h) (Trescot et al., 2008). These properties make it difficult to use for the relief of acute pain or for pain that is poorly controlled where rapid dose adjustments are needed (Davis & Walsh, 2001). Further adding to these difficulties, methadone is metabolized by CYP3A4-catalyzed N-demethylation to the analgesically inactive metabolite, normethadone, such that methadone is potentially subject to a large number of metabolic drug-drug interactions as many clinically used drugs are either CYP3A4 inhibitors or inducers (Fishman et al., 2002).

Apart from its use as a strong opioid analgesic for relief of moderate to severe pain, methadone is also widely used for opioid maintenance therapy in patients with heroin addiction (Fishman et al., 2002). Commercially available methadone formulations include oral tablets and mixtures, rectal suppositories and ampoules for parenteral administration (Manfredi et al., 2003). When converting patients from a strong opioid analgesic such as morphine to methadone, caution needs to be exercised. This is because morphine-methadone analgesic ratios vary significantly according to the previous morphine dosing regimen (Mancini et al., 2000).

For individuals receiving chronic methadone treatment for opioid dependence, cardiotoxicity characterized by prolonged QTc intervals are associated with methadone dose and concurrent stimulant use (Modesto-Lowe et al., 2010; Mayet et al., 2011). For individuals receiving methadone at doses exceeding 60 mg/day together with tricyclic antidepressants or other drugs that inhibit methadone metabolism, the QTc interval is lengthened thereby initiating Torsades de Pointes (Krantz et al., 2002, Ehret et al., 2007). QT prolongation with methadone is also influenced by other factors including hypokalaemia, hepatic failure and pre-existing heart disease (Ehret et al., 2007). Unfortunately, the general lack of awareness of the long and highly variable elimination half-life of methadone together with its many metabolic drug-drug interactions, has led to a dramatic increase in methadone-associated deaths (Trescot et al., 2008).

5.4 Hydromorphone

Hydromorphone, 4,5 alpha-epoxy-3-hydroxy-17-methyl morphinan-6-one, is a semi-synthetic opioid analgesic (Murray & Hagen, 2005) that binds with high affinity (Ki = 0.37 nM) at the MOP receptor (Volpe et al., 2011) and to a lesser extent at the δ-opioid (DOP) receptor but not at the κ-opioid (KOP) receptor (Murray & Hagen, 2005). Orally administered hydromorphone undergoes extensive first-pass metabolism in the liver to hydromorphone-3-glucuronide (H3G) that accounts for more than 50% of each dose. Although H3G, like M3G, is analgesically inactive, it produces dose-dependent neuro-excitatory effects after supraspinal administration in rodents with a potency ~2.5-fold higher than M3G (Wright et al., 2001). Chronic administration of hydromorphone in patients with renal impairment will result in H3G accumulation, raising the risk that neuro-excitatory side-effects will be produced (Smith, 2000; Mercadante & Arcuri, 2004).

The analgesic potency of parenteral hydromorphone is ~ 5-fold higher than that of morphine for the alleviation of moderate to severe acute pain (Bruera et al., 1996; Dunbar et al., 1996; Quigley, 2002; Horn & Nesbit, 2004) whereas for chronic cancer pain, the analgesic potency of hydromorphone is similar to that of morphine (Murray & Hagen, 2005).

Hydromorphone is available as immediate-release and controlled-release oral formulations (Guay, 2010) as well as ampoules for parenteral administration by either the epidural or intrathecal routes (Lee et al., 2011; Liu et al., 2011).

5.5 Buprenorphine

Buprenorphine, ((2S)-2-[(-)-(5R,6R,7R,14S)-9α-cyclopropylmethyl-4,5-epoxy-6,14-ethano-3-hydroxy-6-methoxymorphinan-7-yl]-3,3-dimethylbutan-2-ol), is also a semi-synthetic derivative of thebaine. Buprenorphine binds with high affinity (K_i = 0.2nM) at the MOP receptor (Volpe et al., 2011) and functionally it is a partial agonist (Pick et al., 1997). Buprenorphine also has antagonist actions at the κ-opioid (KOP) receptor and it interacts with the nociceptin (ORL-1) receptor (Pick et al., 1997). Buprenorphine produces dose-dependent analgesia with potency at ~25-50 times higher than morphine (Evans & Easthope, 2003). The slow onset and long duration of buprenorphine's pharmacodynamic actions are thought to be due to its slow binding to and dissociation from the MOP receptor (Evans & Easthope, 2003).

Consistent with its partial agonist activity at the MOP receptor, sublingual buprenorphine administered to healthy male volunteers in doses up to 70-fold higher than the recommended analgesic dose (0.3 mg) and 4-8 fold higher than doses (4-8 mg) used to treat opioid addiction, produced ceiling responses for subjective measures of drug liking in doses at 8 to 16 mg (Walsh et al., 1994). In the same subjects a ceiling effect for respiratory depression was observed at 16mg (Walsh et al., 1994). Because buprenorphine exhibited linear pharmacokinetics across the dose range tested, dose-limited sublingual absorption is not responsible for the ceiling effects (Walsh et al., 1994). The KOP antagonist activity of buprenorphine is thought to contribute to its good tolerability characterized by limited dysphoria or psychotomimetic effects (Johnson et al., 2005).

After oral administration, buprenorphine undergoes extensive first-pass metabolism in the liver catalyzed by the enzymes, CYP3A4 and CYP2C8 to produce the active N-dealkylated metabolite, norbuprenorphine (Picard et al., 2005). Consequently the oral bioavailability is low at ~14% and so buccal, sublingual, intranasal and transdermal formulations of buprenorphine have been developed that effectively by-pass first-pass metabolism and increase bioavailability to 30-60% (Evans & Easthope, 2003; Johnson et al., 2005; Davis, 2005). Due to its long half-life (~26 h) and ceiling pharmacodynamic effects, buprenorphine is used as an alternative to methadone for opioid maintenance therapy in opioid-dependent individuals (Robinson, 2002; Johnson et al., 2005). A combination product containing buprenorphine and naloxone in a 4:1 ratio respectively is available in some countries as a deterrent to illicit use of buprenorphine tablets for parenteral injection (Harris et al., 2004).

5.6 Fentanyl

Fentanyl, *N*-(1-(2-phenylethyl)-4-piperidinyl)-*N*-phenyl-propanamide, is a synthetic opioid analgesic (Horn & Nesbit, 2004) that binds with high affinity (Ki = 1.3 nM) at the MOP receptor (Volpe et al., 2011). Fentanyl is metabolized by CYP3A4 to its N-dealkylated metabolite, norfentanyl that is pharmacologically inactive (Horn & Nesbit, 2004).
After parenteral dosing, fentanyl is ~80-100 fold more potent than morphine with a rapid onset of action but only a short duration at < 60 min (Horn & Nesbit, 2004; Pasero, 2005; Stanley, 2005). For post-operative pain relief, fentanyl may be given by spinal routes whereas for breakthrough or procedural pain, the sublingual, transmucosal, intra-nasal, inhaled or parenteral routes are preferred (Lennernas et al., 2005; Hair et al., 2008; Peng & Sandler, 1999).
Fentanyl has high lipophilicity making it suitable for transdermal delivery. To this end, there are several transdermal patch formulations of fentanyl available for clinical use that effectively overcome fentanyl's short duration of action (Cachia & Ahmedzai, 2011). There is now a large body of evidence to support the use of fentanyl patches for the management of moderate to severe chronic cancer pain, with data suggesting improved pain relief and reduced opioid-related side-effects compared with sustained release oral morphine (Cachia & Ahmedzai, 2011).

5.7 Tapentadol

Tapentadol, [(-)-(1R,2R)-3-(3-dimethylamino-1-ethyl-2-methyl-propyl)-phenol], is a recently approved centrally acting analgesic with two complementary modes of action, viz moderate affinity activity at the MOP receptor (Ki = 0.1 μM) together with inhibitory effects on the NET transporter (Ki = 0.5 μM) to block the re-uptake of norepinephrine in the CNS and so augment descending inhibition to attenuate pain at the level of the spinal cord (Tzschentke et al., 2007; Hartrick, 2009; Wade & Spruill, 2009). After oral dosing, the oral bioavailability of tapentadol is relatively low at ~32% (Tzschentke et al., 2006) due to significant first-pass metabolism in the liver to the inactive glucuronide metabolite, tapentadol-O-glucuronide (Terlinden et al., 2010).
The immediate-release (IR) formulation of tapentadol was approved by the FDA in 2008 for the management of moderate-to-severe acute pain as the first new analgesic developed in over 25 years (Vadivelu et al., 2011). When compared with oxycodone in a head-to-head clinical trial for the relief of post-operative pain in patients following bunionectomy, tapentadol provided non-inferior analgesia to oxycodone with a superior gastrointestinal adverse effect profile characterized by significantly less nausea, vomiting, and constipation when compared with oxycodone (Hartrick, 2009; Vadivelu et al., 2011).
More recently, the FDA has approved an extended-release (ER) formulation of tapentadol for twice-daily oral administration for the management of moderate to severe chronic pain in adult patients (Vadivelu et al., 2011). In patients with end-stage joint disease administered IR tapentadol for two weeks followed by the ER formulation for a further 4-weeks, the superior gastrointestinal tolerability of tapentadol relative to oxycodone, was affirmed (Etropolski et al., 2011). Mechanistically, this may be due to an 'opioid-sparing' effect of the inhibitory actions of tapentadol at the NET transporter (Tzschentke et al., 2006).

5.8 Ultra-short acting opioid analgesics

For patients with cardiovascular instability, ultra-short acting structural analogues of fentanyl such as remifentanil, alfentanil and sufentanil are preferred for use as part of balanced analgesic regimens during anaesthesia (Horn & Nesbit, 2004).

5.8.1 Remifentanil

Remifentanil, 3-[4-methoxycarbonyl-4-[1-oxopropyl)phenylamino]-1-piperidine]propanoic acid, methyl ester) is a synthetic derivative of fentanyl with an ester function in its structure that makes it susceptible to hydrolysis by non-specific blood and tissue esterases (Egan et al., 1993). The very rapid metabolism of remifentanil to the inactive remifentanil acid metabolite by non-specific esterases underpins its activity as an ultra-short acting MOP agonist (Egan et al., 1993).

Parenteral remifentanil has a rapid onset of action (~1 min) and a rapid offset of action following discontinuation (~3–10 min) (Stroumpos et al., 2010) and it is indicated for the relief of pain associated with surgical procedures (Mesolella et al., 2004, Kucukemre et al., 2005).

Remifentanil's pharmacokinetics favour its use as an analgesic during labour (Leong et al., 2011), a notion supported by the findings of two recent clinical studies (Buehner et al., 2011; Ng et al., 2011). In the first study, 94% of 244 consecutive women in a small maternity unit who received remifentanil by patient-controlled analgesia (PCA) for relief of labour pain rated their analgesic outcomes as excellent, very good or good (Buehner et al., 2011). The safety profile of remifentanil was also good as the Apgar scores of neonates born to these women did not differ significantly from those for neonates born by normal vaginal delivery to women who received no analgesia (Buehner et al., 2011). In the second study, maternal satisfaction was higher in laboring women who received PCA remifentanil for analgesia compared with intramuscular pethidine (Ng et al., 2011) with no difference in the safety profile between these two opioid analgesics in the newborn infants (Ng et al., 2011).

6. Opioid rotation

For patients experiencing poor pain relief and intolerable opioid-related side-effects on one strong opioid analgesic, switching to a second strong opioid analgesic often results in restoration of satisfactory pain relief with tolerable opioid-related adverse effects (Knotkova et al., 2009; Vissers et al., 2010). The starting dose of the second opioid is selected to minimize potential risks whilst ideally restoring analgesic efficacy and must be informed by an estimate of its potency relative to the first opioid (Fine et al., 2009; Mercadante & Caraceni, 2011).

Both pharmacokinetic and pharmacodynamic factors may contribute to the clinical success of opioid rotation. For opioid analgesics such as morphine and hydromorphone that are avidly metabolized to the neuro-excitatory 'anti-analgesic' glucuronide metabolites, M3G and H3G respectively, opioid rotation facilitates clearance of these metabolites from the body enabling restoration of analgesia with the second opioid and resolution of neuro-excitatory side-effects (Smith, 2000). Additionally, opioid rotation exploits incomplete cross-tolerance between opioids possibly underpinned by subtle differences in their modulation of MOP receptor function (Smith, 2008; Slatkin, 2009).

7. Peripherally selective opioid antagonists for improving opioid-induced constipation

In patients receiving opioid analgesics for treatment of chronic pain, constipation is a very common side-effect that impairs quality of life and has a prevalence of >80% despite proactive laxative use (Clemens & Mikus, 2010; Diego et al., 2011). A recent approach to the treatment of opioid-induced constipation involves the recent development of quarternary ammonium opioid antagonists such as alvimopan and methylnaltrexone that have limited absorption across the gastrointestinal mucosa and do not cross the blood-brain-barrier, as well as products that incorporate low-dose oral naloxone that has very low oral bioavailability at 2% (Diego et al., 2011). These products selectively target opioid receptors in the gastrointestinal tract without affecting centrally-mediated analgesic mechanisms (Diego et al., 2011).

7.1 Alvimopan

Alvimopan, 2-([(2S)-2-([(3R,4R)-4-(3-hydroxyphenyl)-3,4-dimethylpiperidin-1-yl]methyl) -3-phenylpropanoyl]amino)acetic acid, is an orally active synthetic MOP receptor antagonist that is unable to cross the blood-brain-barrier due to the presence of a quaternary ammonium group in its chemical structure that is fully ionized at physiological pH (Foss et al., 2008; Diego et al., 2011). Thus after oral administration, its actions are confined to peripheral sites such as the gastrointestinal tract and it does not reverse centrally mediated analgesia (Foss et al., 2008; Karuppiah & Farrah, 2011). Alvimopan has been approved by the FDA for short-term use (maximum of 15 doses at twice-daily intervals) in hospitals to treat post-operative ileus that may be caused or exacerbated by opioid analgesics (Diego et al., 2011). Alvimopan accelerates the time to upper and lower gastrointestinal recovery following partial large or small bowel resection with primary anastomosis and decreases the time to hospital discharge by approximately one day (Diego et al., 2011; Karuppiah & Farrah, 2011).

The recommended dosing regimen for alvimopan is 12 mg at 0.5-5 h pre-surgery followed by 12 mg twice daily for a maximum of 15 doses (Karuppiah & Farrah, 2011). Alvimopan is generally well-tolerated when administered for seven days or less (Karuppiah & Farrah, 2011). However, with long-term use (e.g. 12 months) there is an increased risk of myocardial events (Bader et al., 2011; Karuppiah & Farrah, 2011).

7.2 Methylnaltrexone

Methylnaltrexone, (5α)-17-(cyclopropylmethyl)-3,14-dihydroxy-17-methyl-4,5-epoxymorphinanium-17-ium-6-one, is a quaternary ammonium derivative of the opioid receptor antagonist, naltrexone (Bader et al., 2011; Diego et al., 2011). Due to the quaternary ammonium group in its chemical structure that is ionized at physiological pH, methylnaltrexone does not cross the blood-brain-barrier and so centrally mediated analgesia is not reversed (Bader et al., Diego et al., 2011).

Methylnaltrexone has 8-fold and 120-fold higher binding affinity at the MOP receptor relative to the KOP and DOP receptors respectively (Bader et al., 2011). Following administration by the subcutaneous route at 0.15-5 mg/kg in humans, mean peak plasma concentrations of methylnaltrexone are observed at 0.5 h post-dosing and the elimination half-life is in the range 8-9 h (Rotshteyn et al., 2011). The mean bioavailability is high at 82% with minimal metabolism and so it has low potential for drug-drug interactions (Rotshteyn et al., 2011).

Methylnaltrexone is approved by the FDA and the European Medicines Agency (EMA) to treat opioid induced constipation in patients with advanced disease where other laxative regimens have failed (Iskedjian et al., 2010; Bader et al., 2011). Methylnaltrexone causes laxation in at least 50% of patients in less than 24 h over the first two weeks of treatment without impairing analgesia or causing serious adverse events (Bader et al., 2011).

7.3 Oral naloxone

Naloxone, (1*S*,5*R*,13*R*,17*S*)-10,17-dihydroxy- 4-(prop-2-en-1-yl)-12-oxa-4-azapentacyclo [9.6.1.$0^{1,13}$.$0^{5,17}$.$0^{7,18}$]octadeca-7(18),8,10-trien-14-one, is a non-selective opioid receptor antagonist (Lenz et al., 1986). In the clinical setting, parenteral naloxone is used to reverse life-threatening opioid agonist-induced respiratory depression (Diego et al., 2011). However, as naloxone crosses the blood-brain-barrier, it also reverses centrally mediated analgesia (Diego et al., 2011).
After oral administration, the bioavailability of naloxone is very low at 2% due to extensive first-pass metabolism which makes it possible to obtain a highly localized opioid antagonist action in the gastrointestinal tract whilst sparing the centrally mediated opioid analgesic effects of oral oxycodone (Leppert, 2010; Diego et al., 2011). The negligible oral bioavailability of naloxone is exploited in an oral prolonged-release tablet that contains oxycodone in combination with naloxone in a fixed 2:1 ratio resulting in less constipation and less laxative consumption relative treatment with oxycodone alone (Leppert, 2010).
The oxycodone plus naloxone oxycodone tablet is available in four tablet strengths; 5/2.5 mg, 10/5 mg, 20/10 mg and 40/20 mg oxycodone/naloxone respectively (Leppert, 2010).

8. Conclusion

Moderate to severe acute and chronic pain continues to be managed with opioid analgesics according to the principles succinctly summarized by Steps 2 and 3 of the WHO 3-step Analgesic Ladder. Weak opioid analgesics are added to non-opioid analgesics for the management of moderate pain with adjuvants added if pain has a neuropathic component. For moderate to severe pain, strong opioid analgesics are recommended with the addition of non-opioids and adjuvants, as required.

9. References

Argoff, C.E., Silvershein, D.I. (2009) A comparison of long- and short-acting opioids for the treatment of chronic noncancer pain: tailoring therapy to meet patient needs. *Mayo Clin Proc* 84: 602-12.

Armstrong, S.C., Wynn, G.H., Sandson, N.B. (2009) Pharmacokinetic drug interactions of synthetic opiate analgesics. *Psychosomatics* 50: 169-76.

Bader, S., Jaroslawski, K., Blum, H.E., Becker, G. (2011) Opioid-induced constipation in advanced illness: safety and efficacy of methylnaltrexone bromide. *Clin Med Insights Oncol* 5: 201-11.

Backlund, M., Lindgren, L., Kajimoto, Y., Rosenberg, P.H. (1997) Comparison of epidural morphine and oxycodone for pain after abdominal surgery. *J Clin Anesth* 9: 30-35.

Boerner, U. (1975) The metabolism of morphine and heroin and man. *Drug Metab Rev* 4: 39-73.

Bruera, E., Sloan, P., Mount, B., Scott, J., Suarez-Almazor, M. (1996) A randomized, double-blind, double-dummy, crossover trial comparing the safety and efficacy of oral sustained-release hydromorphone with immediate-release hydromorphone in patients with cancer pain. Canadian Palliative Care Clinical Trials Group. *J Clin Oncol* 14: 1713-1717.

Bruera, E., Belzile, M., Pituskin, E., Fainsinger, R., Darke, A., Harsanyi, Z., Babul, N., Ford, I. (1998) Randomized, double-blind, cross-over trial comparing safety and efficacy of oral controlled-release oxycodone with controlled-release morphine in patients with cancer pain. *J Clin Oncol* 16: 3222-3229.

Buehner, U., Broadbent, J.R., Chesterfield, B. (2011) Remifentanil patient-controlled analgesia for labour: a complete audit cycle. *Anaesth Intensive Care* 39: 666-70.

Cachia, E., Ahmedzai, S.H. (2011) Transdermal opioids for cancer pain. *Curr Opin Support Palliat Care* 5: 15-19.

Caraco, Y., Sheller, J., Wood, A.J. (1997) Pharmacogenetic determinants of codeine induction by rifampin: the impact on codeine's respiratory, psychomotor and miotic effects. *J Pharmacol Exp Ther* 281: 330-6.

Chang, G., Chen, L., Mao, J. (2007) Opioid tolerance and hyperalgesia. *Med Clin North Am* 91: 100-211.

Clemens, K.E., Mikus, G. (2010) Combined oral prolonged-release oxycodone and naloxone in opioid-induced bowel dysfunction: review of efficacy and safety data in the treatment of patients experiencing chronic pain. *Expert Opin Pharmacother* 11: 297-310.

Davis, M.P., Walsh, D. (2001) Methadone for relief of cancer pain: a review of pharmacokinetics, pharmacodynamics, drug interactions and protocols of administration. *Support Care Cancer* 9: 73-83.

Davis, M.P., Varga, J., Dickerson, D., Walsh, D., LeGrand, S.B., Lagman, R. (2003) Normal-release and controlled-release oxycodone: pharmacokinetics, pharmacodynamics and controversy. *Support Care Cancer* 11: 84-92.

Davis, M.P. (2005) Buprenorphine in cancer pain. *Support Care Cancer,* 13**,** 878-87.

Diego, L., Atayee, R., Helmons, P., Hsiao, G., von Gunten, C.F. (2011) Novel opioid antagonists for opioid-induced bowel dysfunction. *Expert Opin Investig Drugs* 20: 1047-56.

Dunbar, P.J., Chapman, C.R., Buckley, F.P., Gavrin, J.R. (1996) Clinical analgesic equivalence for morphine and hydromorphone with prolonged PCA. *Pain* 68: 265-270.

Egan, T.D., Lemmens, H.J., Fiset, P., Hermann, D.J., Muir, K.T., Stanski, D.R., Shafer, S.L. (1993) The pharmacokinetics of the new short-acting opioid remifentanil (G187084B) in healthy adult male volunteers. *Anesthesiology* 79: 881-92.

Ehret, G.B., Desmeules, J.A., Broers, B. (2007) Methadone-associated long QT syndrome: improving pharmacotherapy for dependence on illegal opioids and lessons learned for pharmacology. *Expert Opin Drug Saf* 6: 289-303.

Eisenberg, E., Marinangeli, F., Birkhahn, J., Paladini, A., Varrassi, G. (2005) Time to Modify the Analgesic Ladder. *Pain: Clinical Updates,* XIII.

Etropolski, M., Kelly, K., Okamoto, A., Rauschkolb, C. (2011) Comparable efficacy and superior gastrointestinal tolerability (nausea, vomiting, constipation) of tapentadol compared with oxycodone hydrochloride. *Adv Ther* 28: 401-17.

Evans, H.C., Easthope, S.E. (2003) Transdermal buprenorphine. *Drugs* 63: 1999-2001.

Fine, P.G., Portenoy, R.K. Ad hoc expert panel on evidence review and guidelines for opioid rotation (2009) Establishing "best practices" for opioid rotation: conclusions of an expert panel. *J Pain Symptom Manage* 38: 418-25.

Fishman, S.M., Wilsey, B., Mahajan, G., Molina, P. (2002) Methadone re-incarnated: novel clinical applications with related concerns. *Pain Med* **3**, 339-348.

Foss, J.F., Fisher, D.M., Schmith, V.D. (2008) Pharmacokinetics of alvimopan and its metabolite in healthy volunteers and patients in postoperative ileus trials. *Clin Pharmacol Ther* 83: 770-6.

Gardner, J.S., Blough, D., Drinkard, C.R., Shatin, D., Anderson, G., Graham, D., Alderfer, R. (2000) Tramadol and seizures: a surveillance study in a managed care population. *Pharmacotherapy* 20: 1423-1431.

Gilman, A.G., Goodman, L.S., Gilman, A. (1980) *Opioid Analgesics and Antagonists,* New York, Macmillan.

Grond, S., Sablotzki, A. (2004) Clinical pharmacology of tramadol. *Clin Pharmacokinet* 43: 879-923.

Guay, D.R. (2010) Oral hydromorphone extended-release. *Consult Pharm* 25: 816-28.

Hair, P.I., Keating, G.M., Mckeage, K. (2008) Transdermal matrix fentanyl membrane patch (matrifen): in severe cancer-related chronic pain. *Drugs* 68: 2001-9.

Harris, D.S., Mendelson, J.E., Lin, E.T., Upton, R.A., Jones, R.G. (2004) Pharmacokinetics and subjective effects of sublingual buprenorphine, alone or in combination with naloxone: lack of dose proportionality. *Clin Pharmacokinet* 43: 329-340.

Hartrick, C.T. (2009) Tapentadol immediate release for the relief of moderate-to-severe acute pain. *Expert Opin Pharmacother* 10: 2687-96.

Hasselstrom, J., Sawe, J. (1993) Morphine pharmacokinetics and metabolism in humans. Enterohepatic cycling and relative contribution of metabolites to active opioid concentrations. *Clin Pharmacokinet* 24: 344-54.

Heiskanen, T., Kalso, E. (1997) Controlled-release oxycodone and morphine in cancer related pain. *Pain* 73: 37-45.

Heiskanen, T., Olkkola, K.T., Kalso, E. (1998) Effects of blocking CYP2D6 on the pharmacokinetics and pharmacodynamics of oxycodone. *Clin Pharmacol Ther* 64: 603-611.

Horn, E., Nesbit, S.A. (2004) Pharmacology and pharmacokinetics of sedatives and analgesics. *Gastrointest Endosc Clin N Am* 14: 247-268.

Iskedjian, M., Iver, S, Lawrence Librach, S., Wang, M., Farah, B., Berbari, J. (2011) Methylnaltrexone in the treatment of opioid-induced constipation in cancer patients receiving palliative care: willingness-to-pay and cost-benefit analysis. *Pain Symptom Manage* 41: 104-115.

Johnson, R.E., Fudala, P.J., Payne, R. (2005) Buprenorphine: considerations for pain management. *J Pain Symptom Manage* 29: 297-326.

Kadiev, E., Patel, V., Rad, P., Thankachan, L., Tram, A., Weinlein, M., Woodfin, K., Raffa, R.B., Nagar, S. (2008) Role of pharmacogenetics in variable response to drugs: focus on opioids. *Expert Opin Drug Metab Toxicol* 4: 77-91.

Kalso, E., Poyhia, R., Onnela, P., Linko, K., Tigerstedt, I., Tammisto, T. (1991) Intravenous morphine and oxycodone for pain after abdominal surgery. *Acta Anaesthesiol Scand* 35: 642-646.

Karuppiah, S., Farrah, R. (2011) Alvimopan (entereg) for the treatment of postoperative ileus. *Am Fam Physician* 83: 978-9.

King, S., Forbes, K., Hanks, G.W., Ferro, C.J., Chambers, E.J. (2011) A systematic review of the use of opioid medication for those with moderate to severe cancer pain and renal impairment: a European Palliative Care Research Collaborative opioid guidelines project. *Palliat Med* 25: 525-52.

Kirchheiner, J., Schmidt, H., Tzvetkov, M., Keulen, J.T., Lotsch, J., Roots, I., Brockmoller, J. (2007) Pharmacokinetics of codeine and its metabolite morphine in ultra-rapid metabolizers due to CYP2D6 duplication. *Pharmacogenomics J* 7: 257-65.

Knotkova H, Fine PG, Portenoy RK (2009) Opioid rotation: the science and the limitations of the equianalgesic dose table. *J Pain Symptom Manage* 38: 426-39.

Krantz, M.J., Lewkowiez, L., Hays, H., Woodroffe. M.A., Robertson, A.D., Mehler, P.S. (2002) Torsade de pointes associated with very-high-dose methadone. *Ann Intern Med* 137: 501-4.

Kucukemre, F., Kunt, N., Kaygusuz, K., Kiliccioglu, F., Gurelik, B., Cetin, A. (2005) Remifentanil compared with morphine for postoperative patient-controlled analgesia after major abdominal surgery: a randomized controlled trial. *Eur J Anaesthesiol* 22: 378-85.

Lalovic, B., Phillips, B., Risler, L.L., Howald, W., Shen, D.D. (2004) Quantitative contribution of CYP2D6 and CYP3A to oxycodone metabolism in human liver and intestinal microsomes. *Drug Metab Dispos* 32: 447-454.

Lalovic, B., Kharasch, E., Hoffer, C., Risler, L., Liu-Chen, L.Y., Shen, D.D. (2006) Pharmacokinetics and pharmacodynamics of oral oxycodone in healthy human subjects: role of circulating active metabolites. *Clin Pharmacol Ther* 79: 461-79.

Latta, K.S., Ginsberg, B., Barkin, R.L. (2002) Meperidine: a critical review. *Am J Ther* 9: 53-68.

Lee, Y.S., Park, Y.C., Kim, J.H., Kim, W.Y., Yoon, S.Z., Moon, M.G., Min, T.J. (2011) Intrathecal hydromorphone added to hyperbaric bupivacaine for postoperative pain relief after knee arthroscopic surgery: a prospective, randomised, controlled trial. *Eur J Anaesthesiol* May 10; Epub ahead of print.

Lennernas, B., Hedner, T., Holmberg, M., Bredenberg, S., Nystrom, C., Lennernas, H. (2005) Pharmacokinetics and tolerability of different doses of fentanyl following sublingual administration of a rapidly dissolving tablet to cancer patients: a new approach to treatment of incident pain. *Br J Clin Pharmacol* 59: 249-53.

Lenz, G.R., Evans, S.M., Walters, D.E., Hopfinger, A.J. (1986) *Opiates*. Academic Press, Orlando, USA.

Leong, W.L., Sng, B.L., Sia, A.T. (2011) A comparison between remifentanil and meperidine for labor analgesia: a systematic review. *Anesth Analg* 113: 818-25.

Leow, K.P., Smith, M.T., Williams, B., Cramond, T. (1992) Single-dose and steady-state pharmacokinetics and pharmacodynamics of oxycodone in patients with cancer. *Clin Pharmacol Ther* 52: 487-495.

Leppert, W. (2010) The role of opioid receptor antagonists in the treatment of opioid-induced constipation: a review. *Adv Ther* 27: 714-30.

Liu, .SS., Bae, J.J., Bieltz, M., Wukovits, B., Ma, Y. (2011) A prospective survey of patient-controlled epidural analgesia with bupivacaine and clonidine after total hip replacement: A pre- and postchange comparison with bupivacaine and hydromorphone in 1,000 patients. *Anesth Analg* 2011 Aug 4 [Epub ahead of print].

Macintyre, P.E., Loadsman, J.A., Scott, D.A. (2011) Opioids, ventilation and acute pain management. *Anaesth Intensive Care* 39: 545-58.

Mancini, I., Lossignol, D.A., Body, J.J. (2000) Opioid switch to oral methadone in cancer pain. *Curr Opin Oncol* 12: 308-313.

Manfredi, P.L., Fole,y K.M., Payne, R., Houde, R., Inturrisi, C.E. (2003) Parenteral methadone: an essential medication for the treatment of pain. *J Pain Symptom Manage,* 26, 687-8.

Marinella, M.A. (1997) Meperidine-induced generalized seizures with normal renal function. *South Med J* 90: 556-8.

Mather. L.E., Smith, M.T. Opioid analgesics - clinical pharmacology and adverse effects. In: *Opioids in Pain Control – Basic and Clinical Aspects,* C. Stein (Ed.), Cambridge University Press, pp 188-211, 1999.

Mayet, S., Gossop, M., Lintzeris, N., Markides, V., Strang, J. (2011) Methadone maintenance, QTc and torsade de pointes: who needs an electrocardiogram and what is the prevalence of TQc prolongation? *Drug Alcohol Rev* 30: 388-96.

Mercadante, S., Arcuri, E. (2004) Opioids and renal function. *J Pain* 5: 2-19.

Mercadante, S., Caraceni, A. (2011) Conversion ratios for opioid switching in the treatment of cancer pain: a systematic review. *Palliat Med* 25: 504-15.

Mesolella, M., Lamarca, S., Galli, V., Ricciardiello, F., Cavaliere, M., Iengo, M. (2004) Use of Remifentanil for sedo-analgesia in stapedotomy: personal experience. *Acta Otorhinolaryngol Ital* 24: 315-20.

Michna, E., Blonsky, E.R., Schulman, S., Tzanis, E., Manley, A., Zhang, H., Iver, S., Randazzo, B. (2011) Subcutaneous methylnaltrexone for treatment of opioid-induced constipation in patients with chronic, nonmalignant pain: a randomized controlled study. *J Pain* 12: 554-62.

Milne, R.W., Nation, R.L., Somogyi, A.A. (1996) The disposition of morphine and its 3- and 6-glucuronide metabolites in humans and animals, and the importance of the metabolites to the pharmacological effects of morphine. *Drug Metab Rev* 28: 345-472.

Modesto-Lowe, V., Brooks, D., Petry, N. (2010) Methadone deaths: risk factors in pain and addicted populations. *J Gen Intern Med* 25: 305-9.

Moore, A., Collins, S., Carroll, D., McQuay, H. (1997) Paracetamol with and without codeine in acute pain: a quantitative systematic review. *Pain* 70: 193-201.

Moore, R.A., Derry, S., McQuay, J.H., Wiffen, P.J. (2011) Single dose oral analgesics for acute postoperative pain in adults. *Cochrane Database Syst Rev* Sep7;9:CD008659.

Murray, A., Hagen, N.A. (2005) Hydromorphone. *J Pain Symptom Manage* 29 (Suppl): S57-S66.

Narabayashi, M., Saijo, Y., Takenoshita, S., Chida, M., Shimoyama, N., Miura, T., Tani, K., Nishimura, K., Onozawa, Y., Hosokawa, T., Kamoto, T., Tsushima, T. (2008) Opioid rotation from oral morphine to oral oxycodone in cancer patients with intolerable adverse effects: an open-label trial. *Jpn J Clin Oncol* 38: 296-304.

Ng, T.K., Cheng, B.C., Chan, W.S., Lam, K.K., Chan, M.T. (2011) A double-blind randomised comparison of intravenous patient-controlled remifentanil with intramuscular pethidine for labour analgesia. *Anaesthesia* 66: 796-801.

Nielsen, C.K., Ross, F.B., Lotfipour, S., Saini, K.S., Edwards, S.R., Smith, M.T. (2007) Oxycodone and morphine have distinctly different pharmacological profiles: radioligand binding and behavioural studies in two rat models of neuropathic pain. *Pain* 132: 289-300.

Nielsen, C.K., Ross, F.B., Smith, M.T. (2000) Incomplete, asymmetric, and route-dependent cross-tolerance between oxycodone and morphine in the Dark Agouti rat. *J Pharmacol Exp Ther* 295: 91-9.

Nissen, L.M., Tett, S.E., Cramond, T., Williams, B., Smith, M.T. (2001) Opioid analgesic prescribing and use - an audit of analgesic prescribing by general practitioners and The Multidisciplinary Pain Centre at Royal Brisbane Hospital. *Br J Clin Pharmacol* 52: 693-8.

Pasero, C. (2005) Fentanyl for acute pain management. *J Perianesth Nurs* 20: 279-84.

Peng, P.W., Sandler, A.N. (1999) A review of the use of fentanyl analgesia in the management of acute pain in adults. *Anesthesiology* 90: 576-99.

Picard, N., Cresteil, T., Djebli, N., Marquet, P. (2005) In vitro metabolism study of buprenorphine: evidence for new metabolic pathways. *Drug Metab Dispos* 33: 689-95.

Pick, C.G., Peter, Y., Schreiber, S., Weizman, R. (1997) Pharmacological characterization of buprenorphine, a mixed agonist-antagonist with kappa 3 analgesia. *Brain Res* 744: 41-46.

Plummer, J.L., Gourlay, G.K., Cmielewski, P.L., Odontiadis, J., Harvey, I. (1995) Behavioural effects of norpethidine, a metabolite of pethidine, in rats. *Toxicology* 95: 37-44.

Poulsen, L., Brosen, K., Arendt-Nielsen, L., Gram, L.F., Elbaek, K., Sindrup, S.H. (1996) Codeine and morphine in extensive and poor metabolizers of sparteine: pharmacokinetics, analgesic effect and side effects. *Eur J Clin Pharmacol* 51: 289-95.

Poyhia, R., Seppala, T., Olkkola, K.T., Kalso, E. (1992) The pharmacokinetics and metabolism of oxycodone after intramuscular and oral administration to healthy subjects. *Br J Clin Pharmacol* 33: 617-621.

Quigley, C. (2002) Hydromorphone for acute and chronic pain. *Cochrane Database Syst Rev* CD003447.

Reimann, W., Hennies, H.H. (1994) Inhibition of spinal noradrenaline uptake in rats by the centrally acting analgesic tramadol. *Biochem Pharmacol* 47: 2289-93.

Reutens, D.C., Stewart-Wynne, E.G. (1989) Norpethidine induced myoclonus in a patient with renal failure. *J Neurol Neurosurg Psychiatry* 52: 1450-1.

Riley, J., Ross, J.R., Gretton, S..K, A'hern, R., Du Bois, R., Welsh, K., Thick, M.(2007) Proposed 5-step World Health Organization analgesic and side effect ladder. *European Journal of Pain Supplements* 1: 23-30.

Robinson, S.E. (2002) Buprenorphine: an analgesic with an expanding role in the treatment of opioid addiction. *CNS Drug Rev* 8: 377-90.

Rotshteyn, Y., Boyd, T.A., Yuan, C.S. (2011) Methylnaltrexone bromide: research update of pharmacokinetics following parenteral administration. *Expert Opin Drug Metab Toxicol* 7: 227-35.

Schiller, L.R. (1995) Review article: anti-diarrhoeal pharmacology and therapeutics. *Aliment Phrmacol Ther* 9: 87-106.

Simopoulos, T.T., Smith, H.S., Peeters-Asdourian, C., Stevens, D.S. (2002) Use of meperidine in patient-controlled analgesia and the development of a normeperidine toxic reaction. *Arch Surg* 137:84-8.

Slatkin, N.E. (2009) Opioid switching and rotation in primary care: implementation and clinical utility. *Curr Med Res Opin* 25: 2133-50.

Smith, M.T., Wright, A.W., Williams, B.E., Stuart, G., Cramond, T. (1999) Cerebrospinal fluid and plasma concentrations of morphine, morphine-3-glucuronide, and morphine-6-glucuronide in patients before and after initiation of intracerebroventricular morphine for cancer pain management. *Anesth Analg* 88: 109-16.

Smith, M.T. (2000) Neuroexcitatory effects of morphine and hydromorphone: evidence implicating the 3-glucuronide metabolites. *Clin Exp Pharmacol Physiol* 27: 524-8.

Smith, M.T. (2008) Differences between and combinations of opioids re-visited. Curr Opin *Anaesthesiol* 21: 596-601.

Somogyi, A.A., Barratt, D.T., Coller, J.K. (2007) Pharmacogenetics of opioids. *Clin Pharmacol Ther* 81: 429-44.

South, S.M., Smith, M.T (2001) Analgesic tolerance to opioids. *Pain – Clinical Updates* 9: 1-4.

Stanley, T.H. (2005) Fentanyl. *J Pain Symptom Manage* 29: S67-71.

Stroumpos, C., Manolaraki, M., Paspatis, G.A. (2010) Remifentanil, a different opioid: potential clinical applications and safety aspects. *Expert Opin Drug Saf* 9: 355-64.

Subrahmanyam, V., Renwick, A.B., Walters, D.G., Price, R.J., Tonelli, A.P., Lake, B.G. (2001) Identification of cytochrome P-450 isoforms responsible for cis-tramadol metabolism in human liver microsomes. *Drug Metab Dispos* 29: 1146-1155.

Swegle, J.M., Logemann, C. (2006) Management of common opioid-induced adverse effects. *Am Fam Physician* 74: 1347-54.

Terlinden, R., Kogel. B,Y., Englberger, W., Tzschentke, T.M. (2010) In vitro and in vivo characterization of tapentadol metabolites. *Methods Find Exp Clin Pharmacol* 32: 31-8.

Trescot, A.M., Datta, S., Lee, M., Hansen, H. (2008) Opioid pharmacology. *Pain Physician* 11: S133-53.

Tzschentke, T.M., De Vry, J., Terlinden, R., Hennies, H.H., Lange, C., Strassburger, W., Haurand, M., Kolb, J., Schneider, J., Buschmann, H., Finkam, M., Jahnel, U., Friedrichs, E. (2006) Tapentadol HCl. *Drugs Future* 31: 1053–61.

Tzschentke, T.M., Christoph, T., Kogel, B., Schiene, K., Hennies, H.H., Englberger, W., Haurand, M., Jahnel, U., Cremers, T.I., Friderichs, E., De Vry, J. (2007) (-)-(1R,2R)-3-(3-dimethylamino-1-ethyl2-methyl-propyl)-phenol hydrochloride (tapentadol HCl): a novel mu-opioid receptor agonist/norepinephrine reuptake inhibitor with broad-spectrum analgesic properties. *J Pharmacol Exp Ther* 323: 265-76.

Vadivelu, N., Timchenko, A., Huang, Y., Sinatra, R. (2011) Tapentadol extended-release for treatment of chronic pain: a review. *J Pain Res* 4: 211-8.

Vissers, K.C., Besse, K., Hans, G., Devulder, J., Morlion, B. (2010) Opioid rotation in the management of chronic pain: where is the evidence? *Pain Pract* 10: 85-93.

Volpe, D.A., McMahon Tobin, G.A., Mellon, R.D., Katki, A.G., Parker, R.J., Colatsky, T., Kropp, T.J., Verbois, S.L. (2011) Uniform assessment and raking of opioid mu receptor binding constants for selected opioid drugs. *Regul Toxicol Pharmacol* 59: 385-90.

Wade, W.E., Spruill, W.J. (2009) Tapentadol hydrochloride: a centrally acting oral analgesic. *Clin Ther* 31: 2804-18.

Walsh, S.L., Preston, K.L., Stitzer, M.L., Cone, E.J., Bigelow, G.E. (1994) Clinical pharmacology of buprenorphine: ceiling effects at high doses. *Clin Pharmacol Ther* 55: 569-80.

Walsh, D. (2005) Advances in opioid therapy and formulations. *Support Care Cancer* 13: 138-144.

Wee, B. (2008) Chronic cough. *Curr Opin Support Palliat Care* 2: 105-109.

World Health Organisation (1986) *Cancer Pain Relief*. Geneva: WHO.

Wright, A.W., Mather, L.E., Smith, M.T. (2001) Hydromorphone-3-glucuronide: a more potent neuro-excitant than its structural analogue, morphine-3-glucuronide. *Life Sci* 69: 409-420.

Zhou, S.F. (2009) Polymorphism of human cytochrome P450 2D6 and its clinical significance: part I. *Clin Pharmacokinet* 48: 689-723.

Zollner, C., Stein, C. (2007) Opioids. *Handb Exp Pharmacol* 177: 31-63.

Zwisler, S.T., Enggaard, T.P., Mikkelsen, S., Brosen, K., Sindrup, S.H. (2010) Impact of the CYP2D6 genotype on post-operative intravenous oxycodone analgesia. Acta Anaesthesiol Scand 54: 232-40.

15

Pain Management and Costs of a Combination of Oxycodone + Naloxone in Low Back Pain Patients

R. Rychlik, K. Viehmann, D. Daniel, P. Kiencke and J. Kresimon
Institute of Empirical Health Economics, Burscheid, Germany

1. Introduction

In industrial nations, low back pain (lbp) is one of the leading causes of physical limitation. It is also a main source of incapacitation, suffering and expense. According to the national institute of neurological disorders and stroke in the US, LBP accounts for more sick leave and disability than any other medical condition. In Germany, life time prevalence of LBP reaches up to 84 %, with the highest rate for people aged between 35 and 55. According to the German Health Report of the year 2002, the costs of rehabilitation and early retirement amounted to more than 15 billion € , and direct and indirect cost of illness up to 26 billion EURO. Thus the effective management of low back pain is a major health and economic concern.

In a minority of patients presenting for evaluation in a primary care setting, lbp can be reliably attributed to a specific underlying pathology, such as malignancy, vertebral compression fracture or inflammatory/infectious processes. The majority, 80-90%, of patients present primary or non-specific lbp. There is little documented knowledge of possible causes of non-specific lbp. Risk factors are probably related to genetic predisposition, lifestyle (e.g., overweight, lack of physical activity), physical strain and psychological distress.

Opioid analgesics are well established in the treatment of severe pain conditions and have internationally gained a strong position as a potent daily pain treatment option. Many physicians are still apprehensive about the administration of opioids within a continuous therapy, due to potential drug abuse and possible adverse effects, such as impaired gastrointestinal functioning.

To achieve a satisfactory balance between analgesia and side effects, the assessment and treatment of opioid side effects are fundamental aspects of the therapy. This may increase the likelihood of a favourable treatment outcome, potentially allow higher and more efficacious opioid doses, and improve quality of life by reducing other discomforting symptoms. Economic consequences of insufficiently treated chronic lbp and treatment of potential adverse drug effects also play a significant role from the society's point of view. Additional expenses may include costs that emerge from additional obligatory treatments, hospitalization and work incapacity.

2. Primary objective

The primary objective of this health services research study was to assess the health-related quality of life and the total costs (direct and indirect) of patients in Germany suffering from chronic back pain. Therapy with oxycodone + naloxone[1] was compared to therapy with other strong opioids (WHO-step III opioids).
Main aims are:

- Health related quality of life over a period of one year - patients on therapy with oxycodone + naloxone compared to therapy with other WHO-step III opioids.
- Costs for the pain therapy and therapy of AE/ADR in in- and out-patients.
- Patients' inability to work, days off work compared between both cohorts.
- The incidence of early retirement due to chronic back pain and the average age of these patients.

3. Secondary objective

The secondary objective of the study was to evaluate the data for effectiveness under daily routine conditions of the therapy with oxycodone + naloxone or other WHO-step III opioids (strong opioids).
Main issues were:

- The long-term effectiveness of treatment of chronic back pain under daily routine conditions with oxycodone + naloxone or other strong opioids (WHO-step III opioids).
- Frequency of the administration of rescue-medication (drugs additionally taken once only, as an emergency treatment of pain) under therapy with oxycodone + naloxone compared to other strong opioids (WHO-step III opioids).

4. Methods

In order to portray the actual costs ("true costs") incurred for patients suffering from chronic back pain, data had to be documented under daily routine conditions ("real-world-design"). Therefore, a cohort study design was chosen. Two cohorts were observed: Patients in the first cohort were treated with oxycodone + naloxone (cohort 1). Patients in the second cohort were treated with another WHO-step III opioid (cohort 2). In accordance with the statistical analysis plan, each participating physician was asked to document five patients per cohort. Because of the non-interventional study design, individual site-specific imbalances due to the cohort recruitment will be discussed from a statistical point of view.

4.1 Patient population

Opioid-naive and opioid-pretreated female and male adults (> 18 years) who suffered from chronic back pain below the costal arch and above the gluteal groove, who require a round-a-clock-treatment with WHO-step III opioids, were considered. Patients with cancer pain, herniated vertebral disks, or pain caused by an accident, were excluded. Patients who recently started therapy with oxycodone + naloxone or another WHO-step III opioid were also considered, as well as patients, who were switched from a WHO-step

[1] Targin®

II to a WHO-step III opioid or from one WHO-step III opiod to another WHO. The change of therapy was not allowed to be correlated to the study. Consequently, patients treated with oxycodone + naloxone or other WHO-step III opioids were eligible for the study.
For all patients, the summary of product characteristics (SPC) was considered with regard to patient's safety and need to perform daily activities.
Patients not treated according to the SPC were excluded from the study.

4.2 Inclusion and exclusion criteria

- Therapy with oxycodone + naloxone or another WHO-step III opioid was documented for all patients over an observation period of approximately twelve months, including prescription and administration of the medication (regular daily administration, period of administration).
- Patients were informed about the study and agreed to participate by signing and dating the informed consent form.
- Patients were able to comprehend the language as well as the contents of the study materials (patient information, informed consent form and patient questionnaires).
- Patients suffered from chronic back pain below the costal arch and above the gluteal groove.
- Patients with tumor pain, herniated vertebral disks, or pain caused by an accident, were excluded.
- Patients were more than 18 years old.
- oxycodone + naloxone or another WHO-step III opioids were not contraindicated.
- Female patients were neither pregnant nor breastfeeding.

Patients were excluded from the study if any of the following applied:

- A contraindication to the planned treatment regime occurred.
- The patient withdrew his/her consent to participate in the study.
- Newly diagnosed pregnancy.
- Administration of oxycodone + naloxone or another WHO-step III opioid was not in accordance with the specifications of the SPC.

4.3 Duration and conduct of the study

4.3.1 Study sites and number of patients

200 general practitioners and orthopedics, some of them specializing in pain therapy, should be achieved to participate at in this nation-wide, multi-center, non-interventional study. As stated in the observational plan, the enrolment of 2,000 patients (10 patients per physician, 5 patients per cohort) with chronic back pain was required to document patients at baseline (V1), after one week (V2), four weeks (V3), six months (V4) and after 12 months.

4.3.2 Time schedule

Screening and recruitment of the participating physicians were conducted by the Institute of Empirical Health Economics (IfEG) prior to the start of the study. IfEG CRAs started to visit the physicians´ medical centers in September 2008. Patients were enrolled by the physicians and observed for one year. Documentation started according to the project schedule after the patients had signed the informed consent form (ICF). An interim analysis was scheduled approximately six months after the beginning of the observation period. The study-report was due three months after last patient last visit (LPLV).

4.3.3 Patient information and informed consent form (ICF)

Prior to their participation, patients had to sign the ICF. The patient information describes the objectives, contents and risks of the study. Furthermore, the patients were informed that withdrawal from the observational study was possible at any point in time without further consequences. The patient obtained a copy of the patient information and the ICF. The physician is obligated to keep the signed ICF records at least for 15 years.

4.3.4 Documentation of treatment

Socio-demographic data, the clinical variables regarding progress of the disease, as well as the treatment costs incurred for the attending physician were documented on standardized case report forms (CRF). All consultations during the observation period due to chronic back pain were documented. The consultations took place as they would within the scope of the treatment of chronic back pain and no study-specific visits were indicated. Physicians sent the completed CRF by postal service to IfEG.

4.3.5 Documentation by patients

During the observation period, patients actively participated in the documentation by completing standardized health-related quality of life questionnaires (SF-36 v2 Health Survey) at four points in time. Visits took place every quarter and the quality of life questionnaires were completed during the visits.
Intensity of pain and stool consistency was recorded daily for the first four weeks, followed by recording every two weeks on patient diaries.
The patients also completed standardized questionnaires regarding constipation and the pain intensity of the last seven days during each consultation.

4.4 Variables

The variables considered for this report are described in the following sections.

4.4.1 Socio-demographic and administrative variables

The following data were collected regarding at the first visit (V1):

- gender
- date of birth (month/year)
- height
- weight
- ethnic group
- patient's ability to comprehend the patient information and informed consent
- family status
- educational school level and training level
- status of occupation
- status of ability to work (and correlation with chronic back pain)
- exemption from additional payments
- type of health insurance
- physicians' specialization and additional pain therapy qualifications

4.4.2 Clinical variables

The following clinical data were collected at V1:

- diagnosis of chronic back pain (back pain causing disease)
- concomitant diseases
- medical pre-treatment outside of pain therapy
- assessment of previous pain therapy prior to enrolment (by physician and patient)
- other disorders apart from pain indication experienced within the last week before the beginning of observational study (separately for opioid-naive patients and opioid-pretreated patients)
- previous and current drug therapy for chronic back pain treatment
- change/adjustment/withdrawal of therapy with oxycodone + naloxone or another opioid of WHO-step III
- dosage and application times of the therapy with oxycodone + naloxone or another opioid of WHO-step III
- concomitant medication
- rescue-medication
- assessment of pain, intensity of pain and general mobility of the patient (patient diary)
- average period of analgesia experienced by the patient

4.4.3 Variables of costs

The following variables of costs were included in the cost calculation. For all costs, a causal correlation to the underlying chronic back pain had to exist. Costs for the treatment of adverse events or adverse drug reactions were also included.

- ambulatory treatment costs (consultations including house calls, emergency treatments and medical specialist consultation) contributable to chronic back pain
- type (trade name and active ingredient) and amount (number of packages and package size) of prescribed and recommended drugs
- non-medicinal therapies
- inability to work within the last twelve months before the start and during the observation period
- early retirement
- reduction in earning capacity
- hospitalizations
- other medicinal interventions
- remedies and medical devices
- consultations at other physicians
- emergency treatments
- additional acquisitions or measures taken (e.g. conversion of an apartment)

4.5 Quality of life questionnaires

4.5.1 Quality of life questionnaires (SF-36 v2 Health Survey)

The SF-36 is a multi-purpose, short-form health survey with 36 questions. It provides an 8-scale profile of functional health and well-being scores, as well as a psychometrically-based physical and mental health summary and a preference-based health utility index. It is a

generic measure, as opposed to surveys that target a specific age, disease, or treatment group [16].
The taxonomy has three levels: (1) items; (2) eight scales with 2-10 items each; and (3) two summaries. All but one of the 36 items (self-reported health transition) are used to score the eight SF-36 scales. Each item is used in scoring only one scale.
The SF-36 has the following composition:

- Physical Functioning
- Role-Physical
- Physical Pain
- General Health
- Vitality
- Social Functioning
- Role-Emotional
- Mental Health

The calculations (pole reversal and recalibration of items, missing values, and transformation of scales) of the SF-36-subscales and the physical and mental summation scales are performed with the SSPS-program by Mogens Trab Damsgaard. The SSPS-program is described in the SF-36 manual. The totals from the 8 subscales are subsequently transformed to a percentage scale (co-domain 0-100). Norm-based scoring (NBS) algorithms are introduced for all eight scales and employ a linear T-score transformation with mean = 50 and standard deviation = 10. The weightings of subscales within summation scales are performed with the weight factor used in the American standard sample.
The SF-36 was completed for V1, V3 (after 4 weeks), V4 (after 6 months) and V5 (after 12 months).

4.5.2 Brief Pain Inventory Short Form (BPI-SF)

The Brief Pain Inventory is a standardized method applied for self assessment of pain and its outcomes in an abbreviated form. This inventory encompasses numeric rating scales for pain intensity and reduction in pain contributable to the treatment, as well as a graphic picture. Emphasise is placed on sensory pain components and the documentation of pain-related impairments.
The sum scale for pain intensity contains four questions: to most severe, minimum, and average pain severity experienced during the last 24 hours and at that moment (range 0-10 points per questions, total range 0-40 points). An increase in point score implies an increase in pain.
The sum scale for pain-related impairment consists of seven questions to self assessment of impairment in the daily routine (activity, mood, movement, occupation, relationships, sleep and vitality) within the last 24 hours (range 0-10 points per question, total range 0-70 points).
Cumulative values for pain intensity and pain-related impairment were calculated. An increase in cumulative values implies an increase in pain.
The third factor evaluated pain relief due to the analgesic therapy expressed as a percentage from the baseline value.
The BPI-SF was completed for V1 (beginning), V3 (after 4 weeks), V4 (after 6 months) and V5 (after 12 months).

4.6 Statistical analysis

4.6.1 Data entry

A data entry template for the complete documentation was designed by IfEG by using the program Oracle 11.1.06G. Data entry was conducted successively after CRFs were received.

4.6.2 Handling of dropouts

Patients were defined as dropouts if they were enrolled although the population criteria were not fulfilled, andif they did not receive any study-related medication. Dropouts were completely excluded from the effectiveness analysis.
Withdrawal patients were defined as patients who also include those patients who discontinued the therapy with oxycodone + naloxone or another WHO-step III opioid before the end of the observation period, withdrew their consent, or who became pregnant during the observation period. These patients are included in the effectiveness and efficacy analysis and are not considered to be dropouts, unless the therapy with oxycodone + naloxone or another WHO-step III opioid was administered for less than three months

4.6.3 Study population

The following populations were defined before data analysis:

- Safety-Population (SP): all patients who were included in the observational study and attended at least one follow-up visit
- Intent-to-Treat-Population (ITT-P): all patients for whom at least one examination regarding effectiveness (pain and bowel function) was conducted
- Per-Protocol-Population (PPP): all patients for whom all quarter and all BPI-SF assessment were completely documented

For the Per-Protocol-Population, only the CRFs completed for the whole observation period were considered, whereas for the Intent-To-Treat-Population, all available data were considered. Data in this paper refer to safety-population and intent-to-treat population only.

4.6.4 Statistical analysis

The data analyses are conducted with the software PASW 18.0 for Windows, as well as MS-Excel 2007 and MS-Access 2007. The evaluation is descriptive, based on the character of the documentation. An inferential statistic is performed for the comparison of the cohorts.

5. Analysis and results

5.1 Description of the study population

A total of 1.013 patients from 134 physicians were entered into the database (figure 1). 43 patients had to be excluded from the analysis: Of these, 24 patients did not receive any study-related medication and for 19 patients the physicians did not complete documentation to the end of the study. Therefore, 970 patients were included in the safety population (SP) comprising 583 patients from the cohort "oxycodone + naloxone" (cohort 1) and 371 from the cohort "other WHO-step III opioids" (cohort 2). No cohort classification was possible for 16 patients, because these patients did not take any strong opioid (oxycodone + naloxone or other WHO-step III opioids). 560 cohort 1 and 364 cohort 2 patients were feasible for the Intent-To-Treat-Population. For the Per-Protocol-Population, 569 patients were included: 345 of cohort 1 and 224 of cohort 2.

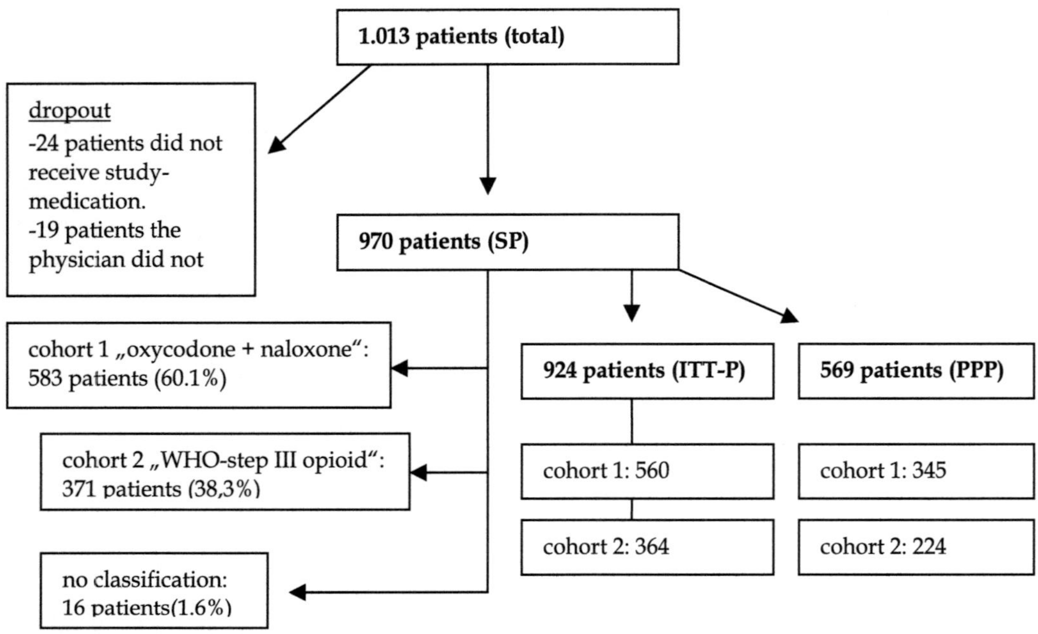

Fig. 1. Organigram of the study population

The majority of the patients were female (~60%) which refers to the epidemiological distribution in Germany within an aging population: the average age was around 64 years and by this most patients had been retired or were of least unable to work. Only 20% of the patients were employed (Table 1).

	cohort 1		cohort 2		
	N	rate	N	rate	p-value
female	350	62,5%	221	60,7%	P= 0,585
male	210	37,5%	143	39,3%	
age	560	63,4	364	64,9	p = 0,084
employed	121	21,6%	62	17,0%	p = 0,088
number of days off work 12 months before inclusion	81	75,0	40	95,4	p = 0,496

Table 1. Gender and age of the population

Almost all patients were classified as caucasians, more than half of the patients were married and app. 50% had an educational level above secondary general school. Less than 7% were ensured privately.
At visit 1 924 days off work in the last year were documented for both cohorts (560 in cohort 1). 17% of the included patients reported a reduction in earning capacity. 14,6% in cohort 1 and 16,8% in cohort 2 had been retired early due to chronic back pain.
Nearly 45% (!) of all patients reported a poor effectiveness of the applied pain therapies.
During the course of the study both physicians and patients assessed a higher effectiveness increase in cohort 1 compared to cohort 2. This refers also to tolerability.

5.2 Quality of life

5.2.1 SF-36

Figure 2 shows the results of the SF-36 evaluation for physical health.

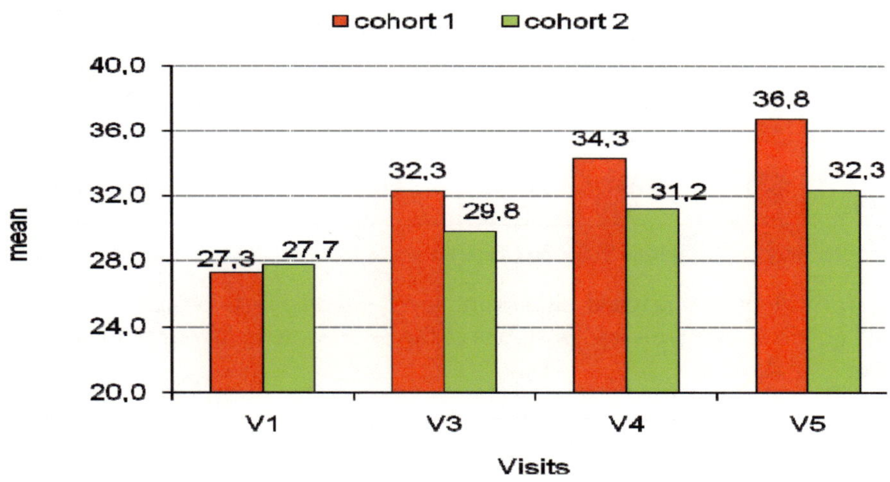

	cohort 1			cohort 2			
	number	mean	SD	number	mean	SD	p-value
Standardized physical health	356	9,65	10,29	244	4,55	8,90	p < 0,001

Fig. 2. Standardized physical health SF-36 (means)

The difference between the physical health of cohort 1 compared to cohort 2 were significant for the periods V5>V3, V3>V1, V4 >V1 and V4>V1 but not for V4>V3 and V5>V4. The results for both cohorts indicate a continuous improvement, which was more pronounced in cohort 1. This result is also mirrored by the data on standardized mental health (Figure 3).

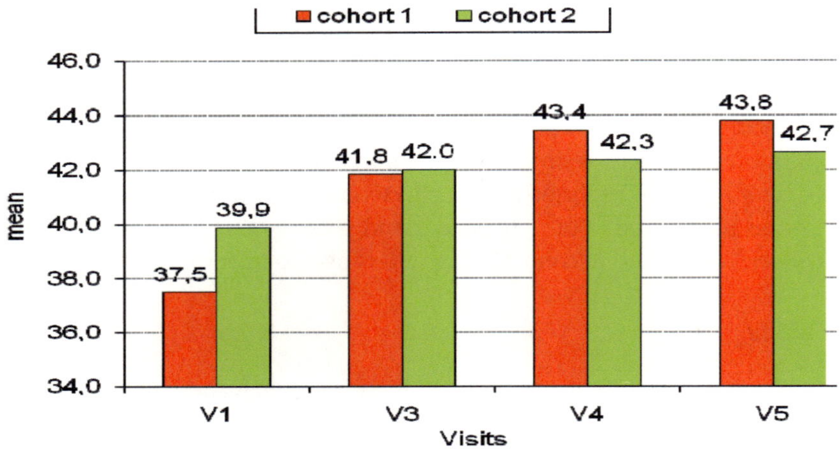

	cohort 1			cohort 2			
	number	mean	SD	number	mean	SD	p-value
Standardized mental health	356	6,34	12,82	244	2,58	12,33	p < 0,001

Fig. 3. Standardized mental health SF-36 (means)

In total statistical power reached significant level for all SF-36 positions except "Role-emotional" (Table 2). All items and positions of the SF-36 were in favour of the combination of oxycodone + naloxone.

SF-36 Positions	cohort 1			cohort 2			p-value
	number	mean	SD	number	mean	SD	
1 Physical function	392	23,09	29,79	272	8,52	26,36	< 0,001
2 Role-physical	370	31,28	44,62	261	16,44	41,15	< 0,001
3 Bodily Pain	379	25,66	25,97	263	11,97	19,10	< 0,001
4 General health	375	13,32	22,64	257	6,16	17,76	< 0,001
5 Vitality	376	16,21	22,64	261	5,77	18,69	< 0,001
6 Social functioning	377	19,46	28,50	263	6,65	25,91	< 0,001
7 Role-emotional	363	22,87	56,34	252	14,02	54,19	0,057
8 Mental health	376	15,13	22,88	261	6,27	19,75	< 0,001

Table 2. Summary of SF-36 positions

5.2.2 Brief Pain Inventory Short Form (BPI-SF)

The Brief Pain Inventory Short Form (BPI-SF) contains numeric rating scales for pain intensity and pain impairment as well as for pain relief. Fig. 4 shows the differences between the total scores of pain intensity. Significant differences were found between cohort 1 and cohort 2 at V5, V4 and V3 compared to V1. Significant differences were also determined for the time periods V3 to V5 and V3 to V4.

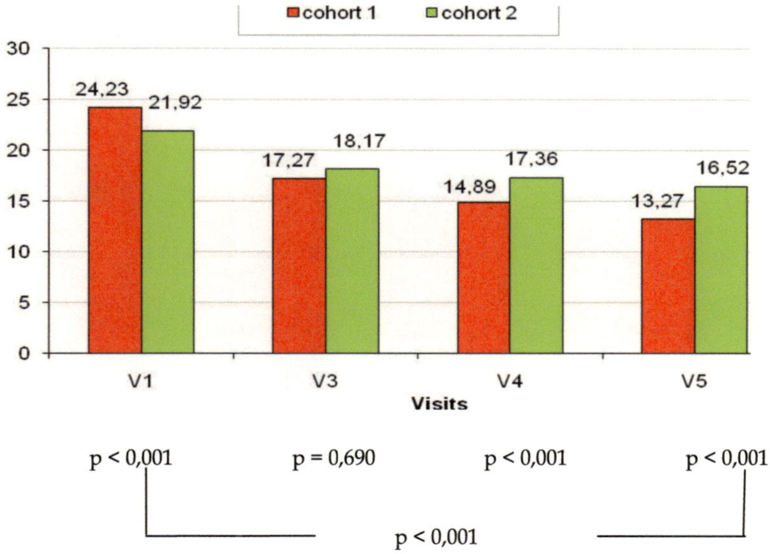

Fig. 4. Sum scale of pain intensity (means)
Brief Pain Inventory (BPI-Shortform)

Worst pain in the last 24 hours decreased in cohort 1 more over all periods than in cohort 2 although worst pain was significantly higher in cohort 1 at baseline (V1).
After 12 months (V5) both cohorts revealed highly significant differences (Fig. 5).

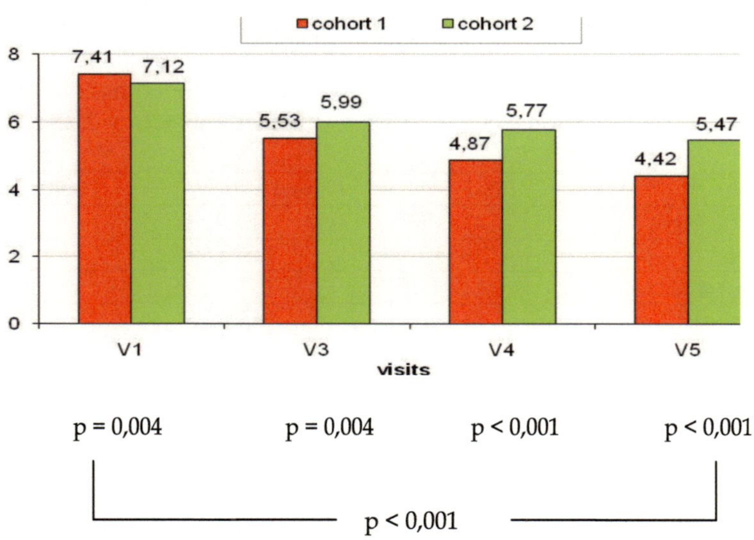

Fig. 5. Worst pain in the last 24 hours (means)
Brief Pain Inventory (BPI-Shortform)

Pain relief treatments or medications administered were also recorded. The patients had to mark the percentage that represents how much pain relief they have experienced (0%=no relief, 100%=complete relief). The pain relief of cohort 1 patients compared to cohort 2 was significant at V1 ($p < 0.001$) and at V5 ($p = 0.001$). At visit 1 the pain relief on average amounted to 39.2 % in cohort 1 and to 46.02 % in cohort 2. At the end of the study (V5) the averaged pain relief was 64.2 % in cohort 1 and 58.9 % in cohort 2 (Fig. 6).

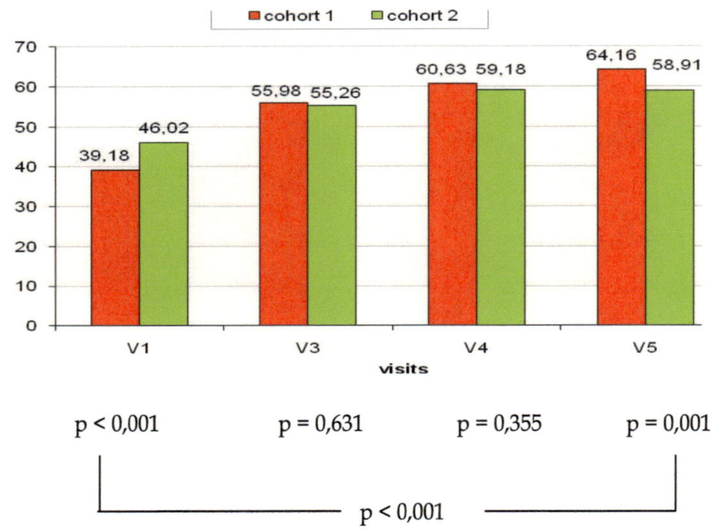

Fig. 6. Pain relief (means)
Brief Pain Inventory (BPI-Shortform)

6. Costs

Annual average direct costs of 2,403.45 € accumulated per patient in cohort 1 and 2,772.98 € per patient in cohort 2. The difference in annual average costs was not significant ($p = 0.195$). The approximately 13 % lower amount incurred in cohort 1 can be attributed to drug expenses, emergency treatment and hospitalisation/rehabilitation. The differences between both cohorts were significant for co-medication ($p < 0.001$) and rescue-medication ($p = 0.021$) (Tab. 3).

cost category	total	cohort 1	cohort 2
out-patient treatment	477,03 €	481,79 €	469,71 €
drug expenses	1.653,73 €	1.532,69 €	1.839,93 €
oxycodone + naloxone	812,17 €	1.270,16 €	107,57 €
opioid WHO-III	611,68 €	65,04 €	1.452,67 €
comedication	211,51 €	181,83 €	257,16 €
rescue medication	18,37 €	15,67 €	22,54 €
remedies	34,20 €	31,07 €	39,03 €
non-medical therapy	54,95 €	53,11 €	57,79 €
emergency treatments	64,76 €	52,57 €	83,52 €
hospitalization/rehabilitation	264,35 €	252,22 €	283,01 €
direct costs	2.549,02 €	2.403,45 €	2.772,98 €

Table 3. Direct costs categories

Fig. 7 shows the indirect costs for the cohorts. Higher averaged indirect costs per patient were calculated for cohort 2. The higher indirect costs resulted from higher costs due to reduction in earning capacity. Approximately 26 % less costs were documented for cohort 1 patients than for cohort 2 patients in this part of indirect costs.

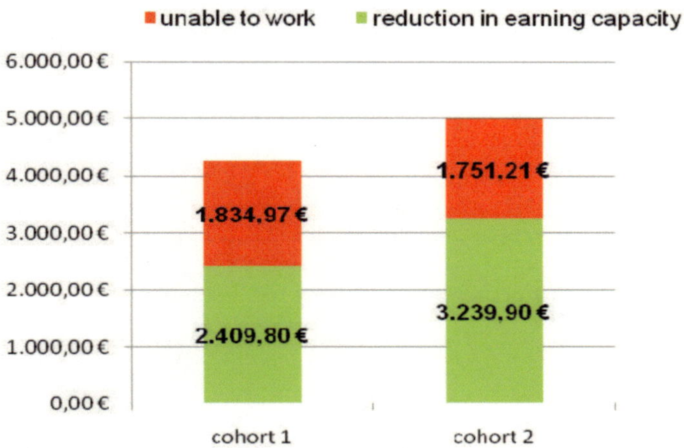

Fig. 7. Indirect cost categories for the cohorts

The incremental cost-effectiveness ratio (ICER) represents the ratio between the differences in treatment costs (ΔC) and treatment effects (ΔE) for cohort OXN and cohort "other strong opioids". It presents the cost of an additional effect unit. The ICER was tested against the main parameters (Tab. 4).

parameter	cohort 1		cohort 2		ICER	ΔC/ΔE
	ΔE	CER	ΔE	CER		
direct costs (C)	2,403 €		2,773 €		---	-370 €
SF-36 (physical health)	9.65	249 €	4.55	610 €	-72 €	-370 €/5.10
SF-36 (mental health)	6.34	379 €	2.58	1,074 €	-98 €	-370 €/3.76
BPI-SF (pain relief)	24.14	100 €	12.44	223 €	-32 €	-370 €/11.7
CER: Cost-Effectiveness Ratio; ICER: Incremental Cost-Effectiveness Ratio						

Table 4. Cost-effectiveness ratio

The following formula was used for the calculation of the incremental cost-effectiveness ratio:

$$ICER = \frac{\text{(costs of cohort OXN)-(costs of cohort "other strong opioids")}}{\text{(effect of cohort OXN)-(effect of cohort "other strong opioids")}} = \frac{\text{cost difference}}{\text{effect difference}}$$

$$ICER = \frac{\overline{C}_{\text{cohort OXN}} - \overline{C}_{\text{cohort "other strong opioids"}}}{\overline{E}_{\text{cohort OXN}} - \overline{E}_{\text{cohort "other strong opioids"}}} = \frac{\Delta\overline{C}}{\Delta\overline{E}}$$

Negative values were calculated for the ICER of the main parameters, which implies more effectiveness at a lower price for the alternative therapy with Oxycodone + Naloxone (Fig. 8).

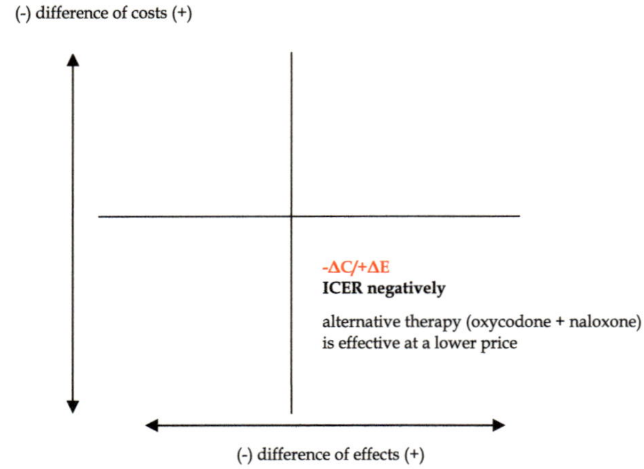

Fig. 8. Cost-effectiveness area

7. Conclusion

As a final conclusion it can be stated that patients of cohort 1 (oxycodone + naloxone) experienced a better quality of life and less back pain after twelve months compared to patients of cohort 2 (other WHO-step III opioids). According to the cost effectiveness-analysis therapy with oxycodone + naloxone is more effective and generates lower costs than cohort 2. These results and findings should be confirmed by a randomized, blinded controlled trial.

8. References

[1] http://www.ninds.nih.gov/disorders/backpain/detail-backpain.htm, stand 16.06.2008

[2] Arzneimittelkommission der deutschen Ärzteschaft: Therapieempfehlungen der Arzneimittelkommission der deutschen Ärzteschaft: Kreuzschmerzen. Arzneiverordnung in der Praxis; 3. Auflage 2007.

[3] Diemer W, Burchert H: Chronische Schmerzen - Kopf- und Rückenschmerzen, Tumorschmerzen. Gesundheitsberichterstattung. Heft 7 (2002)

[4] Roth SH, Fleischmann RM, Burch FX et al.: Around-the-clock, Controlled-Release Oxycodone Therapy for Osteoarthritis-Related Pain. Arch Intern Med. 160, 853-860 (2000)

[5] Furlan AD, Sandoval JA, Mailis-Gagnon A et al.: Opioids for Chronic Noncancer Pain: A Metaanalysis of Effectiveness and Side Effects. CMAJ. 174 (11), 1589-1594 (2006)

[6] Panchal SJ, Müller-Schwefe P, Wurzelmann JI: Opioid-Induced Bowel Dysfunction: Prevalence, Pathophysiology and Burden. Int J Clin Pract. 61 (7), 1181-1187 (2007)

[7] Rote Liste Win®, Ausgabe 2007/I, Version 3.3

[8] http://www.gelbe-liste.de (12/2007)

[9] http.//kbv.de/ebm2009/ebmgesamt.htm

[10] http://www.e-bis.de/ebm/; http://e-bis.de/goae/defaultFrame.htm

[11] http://drg.uni-muenster.de/de/webground/m.webground.php?menu=6

[12] Average of 2, 100 hospitals based on data oft he TK, stand 21.19.2009; http://www.tk-online.de

[13] Schulenburg JM et al. Deutsche Empfehlung zur gesundheitsökonomischen Evaluation - dritte und aktualisierte Fassung. Gesundh ökon Qual manag. 12, 285-290 (2007)

[14] RVaktuell. 11, 470 (2006)

16

The Role of Opioid Analgesics in the Treatment of Pain in Cancer Patients

Wojciech Leppert
Chair and Department of Palliative Medicine,
Poznan University of Medical Sciences, Poznan,
Poland

1. Introduction

Cancer pain treatment is based on the analgesic ladder, established in 1986 by the World Health Organization (WHO; see Fig. 1) (WHO, 1996). Cancer pain management guidelines in Europe are based on EAPC (European Association for Palliative Care) recommendations. Oral morphine is recommended by the Expert Working Group of the EAPC at the third step of the WHO analgesic ladder, which comprises additional opioids (i.e. oxycodone, fentanyl, buprenorphine, methadone, and hydromorphone) for the treatment of moderate-to-severe pain intensity (Hanks et al., 2001). The use of an analgesic ladder should be individualized with an appropriate application of supportive drugs (laxatives and antiemetics) for the prevention and treatment of opioid adverse effects (Leppert, 2009a) and nonpharmacological measures, such as radiotherapy and invasive procedures (nerve blockades and neurolytic blocks) (Eidelman et al., 2007).

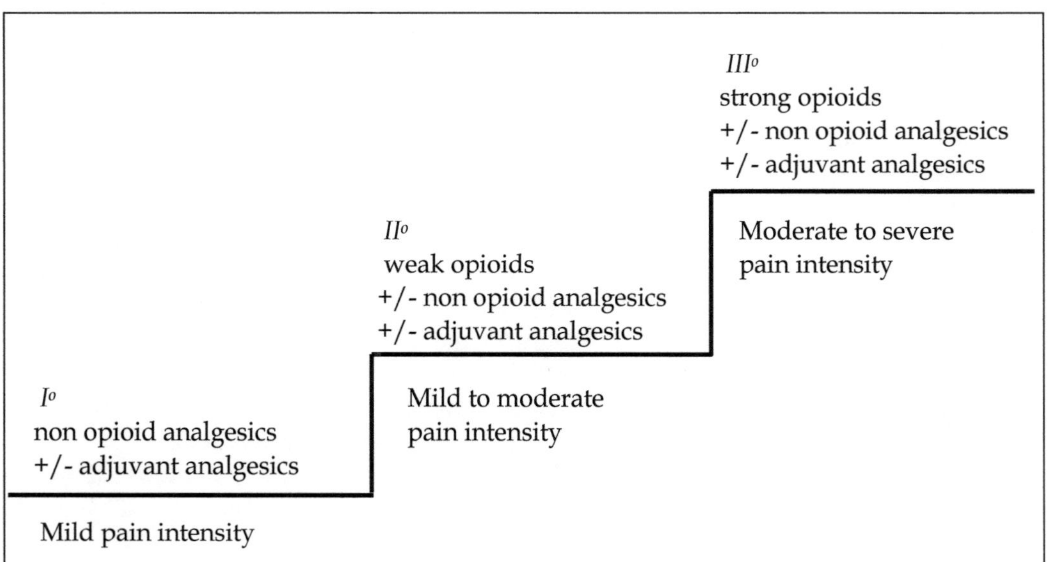

Fig. 1. World Health Organization three-step analgesic ladder

Each step of the WHO analgesic ladder: nonopioids (analgesics for mild pain, step 1 analgesics), weak opioids (analgesics for mild to moderate pain, step 2 opioid analgesics), and strong opioids (opioids for moderate-to-severe pain intensity, step 3 opioid analgesics) may be accompanied with adjuvant analgesics (coanalgesics), which can enhance opioid analgesia. In patients with bone pain, opioids may be combined with non-steroidal anti-inflammatory drugs (NSAIDs), glucocorticoids, and bisphosphonates along with local or systemic radiotherapy (Lussier et al., 2004). In patients with very severe neuropathic pain, a combination of opioids and NMDA (*N*-methyl D-aspartate)-receptor antagonists (e.g. ketamine) are recommended (Leppert, 2010a). Patients with neuropathic pain along with opioids may also receive anticonvulsants, and antidepressants (Bennett, 2011). Other drug groups used in patients with neuropathic pain component comprise local anesthetics and antiarrhytmics (Freynhagen & Bennett, 2009). Opioid analgesics should be supplemented with spasmolytics in patients with visceral colicky pain, especially in the course of bowel obstruction (Ripamonti et al., 2008).

2. Opioids for mild to moderate pain (weak opioids, step 2 opioid analgesics)

2.1 Tramadol

Tramadol displays opioid properties and acts on neurotransmission of noradrenalin and serotonin. Both enantiomers act synergistically and improve analgesia without increasing adverse effects. Tramadol is metabolized in the liver and excreted by the kidneys. The main metabolite is O-desmethyltramadol (M1), which displays analgesic activity with a higher affinity to μ-opioid receptors than the parent compound; (+)-M1 has 300 to 400 times greater affinity to μ-opioid receptors than tramadol and (-)-M1 mainly inhibits noradrenalin reuptake. Apart from O,N-didesmethyltramadol (M5, which has weak analgesic activity) and M1, other metabolites are inactive (Leppert and Mikolajczak, 2011). The elimination half-life of tramadol is 5 to 6 hours and that if M1 is 8 hours. During oral administration, 90% of tramadol is excreted by the kidneys and 10% in feces. Patients with renal impairment show a decreased excretion of tramadol and M1. In patients with advanced cirrhosis, there is a decrease in tramadol metabolism with decrease of hepatic clearance and increase in blood serum levels. In these patients, elimination half-life is increased 2.5-fold. The starting dose of immediate-release (IR) tramadol is 25 to 50 mg every 4 to 6 hour and that of controlled-release (CR) tablets or capsules is 50 to 100 mg twice daily; the daily dose should not exceed 400 mg (Dickman, 2007).

Patients devoid of CYP2D6 activity (poor metabolizers) need a tramadol dose higher by 30% than those with normal CYP2D6 activity (extensive metabolizers) (Stamer et al., 2003). Tramadol analgesia depends on CYP2D6 genotype, with less analgesia in poor metabolizers being associated with lack of (+)-M1 formation (Stamer et al., 2007). Genotyping is helpful in patients with duplication of CYP2D6 gene (ultrarapid metabolizers [UM]) who are at greater risk to develop tramadol adverse effects. Tramadol metabolism through CYP2D6 may cause interactions with drugs inhibiting this enzyme (eg, cimetidine and ranitidine).

Serotonin syndrome has been reported in patients taking selective serotonin reuptake inhibitors (SSRIs) in conjunction with tramadol or opioids (Gnanadesigan et al., 2005). SSRIs (eg, fluoxetine, paroxetine, and, to less extent, sertraline) used in conjunction with tramadol may cause serotonin syndrome because SSRIs inhibit tramadol metabolism and increase serotonin level; generally, they should not be coadministered with tramadol. Serotonin syndrome may appear with monoamine oxidase (MAO) inhibitors, olanzapine, risperidone, venlafaxine and mirtazapine (Davies and Glare, 2009).

The inhibition of tramadol metabolism to (+)M1 may attenuate tramadol analgesia. For example, coadministration of ondansetron (selective 5-HT_3 [hydroxytryptamine] receptor antagonist) blocks spinal 5-HT_3 receptors and competitively inhibits CYP2D6 although recent studies did not confirm such interaction (Rauers et al., 2010). Tramadol analgesia also may be impaired by coadministration of carbamazepine, which accelerates tramadol and M1 metabolism. Concomitant administration of tricyclic antidepressants increases the risk of seizures. Tramadol should be avoided in patients with history of epilepsy. In rats and mice, concomitant administration of tramadol and β-blocker and the 5-$HT_{1A/1B}$ antagonist pindolol enhances analgesia (Leppert, 2009b).

Respiratory depression is rare in the chronic use of tramadol. When it does occur, respiratory depression is connected with the opioid mode of tramadol action, so naloxone should be administered. For example, respiratory depression was reported in a cancer patient with renal impairment (creatinine clearance 30 mL/min) and with UM genotype after renal carcinoma resection. As respiratory symptoms appeared more than 10 hours after the first tramadol dose, the accumulation of M1 was the cause. The patient recovered after intravenous (IV) naloxone bolus administration (0.4 mg). This case highlights that tramadol should not be prescribed in patients with UM genotype and renal impairment (Stamer et al., 2008).

2.2 Codeine

Codeine is a methylated morphine derivative that is found naturally, along with morphine, in the poppy seed. Codeine displays analgesic and antitussive activity. Codeine is available as IR and CR formulations but also in the form of paracetamol combined preparations. IR codeine is administered every 4-6 h in chronic pain with a starting single dose of about 30 mg. The daily doses of dihydrocodeine and codeine usually do not exceed 240 mg and 300 mg, respectively; when these analgesics are ineffective, opioids for moderate-to-severe pain (strong opioids) are introduced.

Codeine is metabolized in the liver and its bioavailability is 30% to 40% after oral administration. After oral administration of codeine, maximal plasma concentration is attained within 1 to 2 hours with plasma half-life of 2.5 to 3.5 hours and analgesia maintained for 4 to 6 hours (IR formulations). Codeine is partially metabolized to morphine and its metabolites and to codeine metabolites norcodeine (NORC) and codeine-6-glucuronide (C-6-G) (Lötsch et al., 2006). The analgesic effect of codeine is about equal to 1/10th of morphine analgesia. Polymorphism of CYP2D6 is responsible for the formation of morphine, and its metabolites may affect codeine analgesia. Other codeine metabolites, C-6-G predominantly, also display analgesic activity and contribute to codeine analgesia (Vree et al., 2000). In healthy volunteers, codeine is metabolized to C-6-G (81.0% ± 9.3%), NORC (2.16% ± 1.44%), morphine (0.50% ± 0.39%), morphine-3-glucuronide (M-3-G; 2.10% ± 1.24%), morphine-6-glucuronide (M-6-G; 0.80% ± 0.63%), and normorphine (NORM; 2.44% ± 2.42%). The half-life of codeine is 1.47 hours ± 0.32 hours, and that of C-6-G is 2.75 hours ± 0.79 hours. The plasma AUC of C-6-G is about tenfold higher than that of codeine. Protein binding of codeine and C-6-G in vivo is 56.1% ± 2.5% and 34.0% ± 3.6%, respectively (Vree & Verwey-van Wissen, 1992).

Lötsch et al. explored the contributions from codeine and its metabolites to central nervous analgesic effects independent from O-demethylation of codeine to morphine. A pharmacokinetic/pharmacodynamic fit of the miotic effects by use of morphine as the only active compound was most significantly ($P < 0.0001$) improved when C-6-G as a second active moiety was added. CYP2D6-dependent formation of morphine does not explain exclusively the central nervous effects of codeine, and C-6-G is the most likely additional active moiety with possible contribution of NORC and the parent compound (Lötsch et al., 2006).

Gasche et al. depicted a patient who received oral codeine in a daily dose of 75 mg (25 mg three times a day) and who, after 4 days of treatment, experienced respiratory depression. The patient recovered after IV administration of naloxone (0.4 mg). The cause of the symptoms was CYP2D6 UM phenotype. The patient was concomitantly treated with clarithromycin and voriconazole, both known inhibitors of CYP3A4. This together with CYP2D6 gene duplication led to increased morphine formation. Blood concentrations of M-3-G and M-6-G were substantially elevated, also due to renal failure (Gasche et al., 2004). Recent reports (Kircheiner et al., 2007; Voronov et al., 2007) indicate that there is a significant risk of respiratory depression in infants whose mothers with CYP2D6 UM and UGT2B7•2/•2 genotypes taking codeine during breastfeeding (Madadi et al., 2009b). Guidelines for maternal codeine use during breastfeeding were issued in Canada (Madadi et al., 2009a) but it seems safer not to use codeine and substitute it with other analgesics in this patient group. Apart from morphine glucuronides, codeine and its metabolites (C-6-G and NORC) also contribute to codeine analgesic effects (Lötsch et al., 2006).

2.3 Dihydrocodeine

Dihydrocodeine (DHC) is a semi synthetic analogue of codeine. Apart from analgesic and antitussive activity, DHC also is used in the treatment of opioid addiction. After subcutaneous (sc) administration of DHC, 30 mg, analgesia is similar to that induced by 10 mg of morphine. After parenteral administration, DHC is twice as potent as codeine. Bioavailability of DHC after oral administration is 20%, which indicates that its analgesia after oral administration is slightly stronger than that of codeine (bioavailability after oral administration equals 30%–40%). After oral administration of DHC, the maximal serum concentration appears after 1.7 hours, plasma half-life varies 3.5 to 5.5 hours, and analgesia lasts 4-6 hours. DHC pharmacokinetics was assessed in 12 extensive metabolizers of CYP2D6 (Ammon et al., 1999). They received a single oral DHC dose of 60 mg, then after 60 hours, they were treated for 3 days with 60 mg dosed twice daily; for the next 3 days with 90 mg twice daily; and for 3 subsequent days 120 mg twice daily. In the 60 to 120 mg DHC dose range, pharmacokinetics of DHC and dihydromorphine (DHM) displayed linear characteristics: area under the curve (AUC), c_{max} (maximum serum concentration), and c_{ssmin} (minimum serum concentration at steady state) for both compounds increased depending on the drug dose (Rowell et al., 1983). Even though DHM displays higher affinity (about 100-fold) to the μ-opioid receptors and exhibits higher analgesic activity in comparison to the parent compound, the role of DHM and its glucuronides in DHC analgesia has not been unequivocally established. The starting dose of IR DHC is usually 30 mg every 4 to 6 hours, and that of CR tablets is 60 mg twice daily (Leppert, 2010b).

Renal clearance and the clearance to DHC metabolites, glucuronidation, and O-demethylation to dihydrocodeine-6-glucuronide (DHC-6-G) and DHM, respectively, are not dose dependent, which indicates that metabolism and excretion of DHC and its metabolites are also not dose dependent. Moreover, the ratio of DHC to DHM for AUC does not change depending on the dose, which suggests a lack of saturation effect of the O-demethylation process of DHC to DHM depending on CYP2D6 in patients normally metabolizing the substrates of this enzyme. Pharmacokinetic parameters were similar after single and multiple doses of 60 mg of DHC (Ammon et al., 1999). Single-dose and multiple-dose pharmacokinetics of IR and CR DHC formulations provide support for a twice-daily dosage schedule of CR DHC. DHC is metabolized in the liver to main metabolites: DHM, DHC-6-G, and nordihydrocodeine (NORDHC). NORDHC is further glucuronidated to NORDHC-6-glucuronide and O-demethylated to nordihydromorphine (NDHM). DHM undergoes glucuronidation to dihydromorphine-3-glucuronide (DHM-3-G) and dihydromorphine-6-glucuronide (DHM-6-G) and N-demethylation to NDHM. It may be concluded that DHC undergoes the first pass effect after oral administration, which is connected with the formation of significantly higher amount of metabolites after oral than after parenteral administration (Rowell et al., 1983). Studies performed to date (Schmidt et al., 2003; Webb et al., 2001) indicate that DHC analgesia is independent of CYP2D6 activity (Leppert and Majkowicz, 2010).

3. Opioids for moderate to severe pain (strong opioids, step 3 opioid analgesics)

3.1 Morphine

Morphine is the standard drug for the treatment of moderate to severe cancer pain and is a comparator for other strong opioids (Caraceni et al., 2011). This is predominantly due to large clinical experience and different routes of morphine administration (eg, oral, SC, IV, intrathecal, topical). Morphine is a hydrophilic opioid and a pure opioid agonist that acts predominantly through the activation of μ-opioid receptors (Flemming, 2010). Plasma half-life of IR formulations equals 2 to 3 hours and the bioavailability after oral morphine administration equals about 30% to 40%. Morphine undergoes glucuronidation; thus, there is little risk of pharmacokinetic interactions with other drugs.

The active metabolite responsible for analgesia is morphine-6-glucuronide (M-6-G). The accumulation of morphine and M-6-G may cause nausea and vomiting, sedation, and finally, respiratory depression. Morphine-3-glucuronide (M-3-G) is devoid of analgesic properties but may be responsible for neurotoxic effects and opioid hyperalgesia (paradoxical pain) (Gretton & Riley, 2008). The main drawback of morphine is the fact that M-3-G and M-6-G may accumulate especially in patients with renal impairment and renal failure, leading to possible intense adverse effects associated with accumulation of metabolites. In severe pain syndromes a change from oral to parenteral or intrathecal route of morphine administration may be beneficial. In case of renal problems, a switch from morphine to other opioids, such as fentanyl, methadone, or buprenorphine, is recommended. Similar to other opioids, morphine often causes constipation; therefore, the use of laxative prophylaxis is recommended. Common morphine adverse effects and possible management possibilities are showed in Table 1.

Numerous oral CR formulations of morphine, designed for 12-hour and 24-hour administration, were developed (Ridgway et al., 2010). Local administration of morphine prevents systemic adverse effects. The starting daily dose of oral morphine is usually 20 to 30 mg (for opioid-naïve patients) or 40 to 60 mg (for patients unsuccessfully treated with weak opioids) (Ripamonti et al., 2009). The dose of parenteral (SC or IV) morphine is one third of the morphine oral dose (Donnelly et al., 2002).

Adverse effect	Symptomatology	Treatment	Comments
Gastric stasis	Epigastric fullness, nausea	Metoclopramide 10 mg t.i.d.	If the symptom persists a switch to alternative opioid may be useful
Nausea/vomiting induced by vestibular stimulation	Symptoms appear on movement	Promethazine or cyclizine 25 mg t.i.d.	If intractable consider levomepromazine
Constipation	Flatulence, abdominal pain painful bowel movements,	Stool softener (macrogol or lactulose) plus stimulant (senna or bisacodyl). If no effect rectal measures or methylnaltrexone	If no effect consider switch to transdermal fentanyl or transdermal buprenorphine
Sedation	Drowsiness	Reduce dose of morphine, consider methylphedindate 5-10 mg o.d.-b.d.	May be caused by co-administered medications e.g. neuroleptics, benzodiazepines, antidepressants and co morbidities (hepatic/renal failure). Consider opioid switch
Neurotoxicity/ cognitive failure	Hyperalgesia, allodynia, myoclonic jerks/agitation, hallucinations	Reduce dose of morphine, haloperidol - 1 - 2 mg b.d. or risperidone 1 - 2 mg o.d.-b.d.	If no improvement consider opioid switch

Table 1. Common adverse effects of morphine and management possibilities

3.2 Oxycodone

Oral oxycodone is along with oral morphine recommended as a first choice opioid analgesic for the treatment of moderate to severe cancer-related pain (King et al., 2011). It is a semi synthetic thebaine derivative, a strong opioid that displays a significant affinity to κ-opioid receptors along with agonistic effect mediated by μ-opioid receptors. Limited cross-tolerance is observed between oxycodone and morphine in rats and in clinical studies (Maddocks et al, 1996). In comparison to morphine, oxycodone possesses lower affinity to μ-opioid receptors and similar lipid solubility. Oxycodone permeates the blood-brain barrier very quickly, which may explain its stronger analgesic effect in comparison to other opioids. Oxycodone does not display immunosuppressive effects in experimental studies. It has high oral bioavailability (60%–87%); the plasma half-life is 2 to 3 hours after IV administration, 3 hours after treatment with IR oral solution, and 8 hours after CR tablets. The bioavailability of rectal administration is similar to oral route (61%), but it displays greater variability.

Oxycodone is metabolized in the liver primarily to noroxycodone through CYP3A4 and, to a much less extent, to oxymorphone via CYP2D6. Noroxycodone is metabolized to noroxymorphone through CYP2D6, and oxymorphone is metabolized to noroxymorphone by CYP3A4. However, analgesia observed after oxycodone administration relies primarily on the parent compound. Noroxycodone has 17% of the potency of oxycodone. Oxymorphone, in spite of high affinity for μ-opioid receptors, is produced in very small amounts. Noroxymorphone is produced in a significant amount and displays significant affinity for opioid receptors. However, the blood–brain barrier is extremely impermeable to noroxymorphone; thus, its role in analgesia is negligible. Low blood–brain barrier permeability is also characteristic of noroxycodone and oxymorphone (Leppert, 2010c).

In patients with liver cirrhosis and hepatic diseases, the oxycodone dose should be reduced by half. Oxycodone is excreted through the kidneys. In patients with renal insufficiency, the oxycodone dose also should be reduced. In patients with renal failure, the oxycodone half-life is prolonged and ranges from 1.8 to 26 hours. The elimination of noroxycodone and oxymorphone also is impaired in patients with renal failure. CYP2D6 polymorphism probably does not influence oxycodone analgesia and adverse effects. Sertraline minimally inhibits CYP2D6 and intensifies adverse effects of oxycodone (eg, hallucinations, tremors), whereas fluoxetine and quinidine (significant CYP2D6 inhibitors) do not intensify oxycodone adverse effects. Oxycodone reduces oral bioavailability of cyclosporine by half. In healthy patients, rifampin, a CYP3A4 inducer, greatly decreased oral and IV oxycodone AUC by 86% and 53%, respectively ($P < 0.001$), and modestly reduced analgesia and increased plasma metabolite-to-parent compound ratios for noroxycodone and noroxymorphone ($P < 0.001$) (Nieminen et al., 2009). A pharmacodynamic interaction of oxycodone with other drugs acting on the central nervous system, such as benzodiazepines, neuroleptics, and antidepressants, may intensify oxycodone adverse effects, especially sedation, and respiratory depression may be intensified in the case of patients who are more sensitive to opioids.

3.3 Hydromorphone

Oral hydromorphone is an alternative to oral morphine and oral oxycodone as a first choice opioid analgesic for the treatment of moderate to severe cancer pain (Pigni et al, 2011). Hydromorphone has about 5 to 10 times more potent analgesic effect than morphine and similar pharmacodynamic properties. Hydromorphone analgesia is mainly due to μ-opioid-receptor agonist effects; it also features some affinity for δ- but not for κ-opioid receptors (Murray & Hagen, 1995). After hydromorphone administration, analgesia lasts for about 4 to 6 hours and the plasma half-life is about 2.5 hours; sustained-release oral preparations provide analgesia for 12-24 hours (Gardner-Nix & Mercadante, 2010).

The drug is metabolized mainly to hydromorphone-3-glucuronide that is devoid of analgesic activity and may accumulate in patients with renal failure; it may induce neurotoxic adverse effects to larger extent than the respective morphine metabolite (morphine-3-glucuronide) (Wright et al., 2001). Hydromorphone in small amount is also metabolized to 6-hydroxy-hydromorphone, but its role is unknown. Due to glucuronidation, the risk of hydromorphone pharmacokinetic interactions with other drugs seems to be low (Sarhill et al., 2001). Adverse effects are similar to those of morphine; however, hydromorphone less frequently induces nausea and vomiting, constipation, itching, and probably more slowly develops tolerance to analgesia (Wirz et al., 2008). In comparative studies conducted in cancer patients with pain hydromorphone displays similar analgesic efficacy to morphine (Miller et al., 1999) and oxycodone (Hagen and Babul, 1997).

Hydromorphone is especially useful for patients requiring high opioid doses via parenteral route due to strong analgesic effects and increased solubility that enables the possibility administering small volumes of the drug in SC injections.

3.4 Fentanyl

Fentanyl is a lipophilic opioid, μ-opioid–receptor agonist, with analgesic effect about 100 times more potent than that of morphine. In chronic pain treatment, transdermal fentanyl (TF) patches are applied, usually on the upper trunk. There are five types of patches that release 12, 25, 50, 75, and 100 μg/h equal to approximately 0.3, 0.6, 1.2, 1.8, and 2.4 mg fentanyl dose per day, respectively. Patches are changed every 72 hours. Patients need access to short-acting opioid preparations (i.e. oral or parenteral morphine, buccal fentanyl tablets, oral transmucosal fentanyl citrate [OTFC] or fentanyl spray) during TF therapy to effectively manage breakthrough pain episodes. Fentanyl is metabolized mainly to inactive norfentanyl; thus, it may be used in patients with renal impairment. Because the fentanyl metabolic pathway is through CYP3A4, the drugs inhibiting or inducing this enzyme should be avoided. Caution is recommended when using drugs metabolized via CYP3A4. In comparison to morphine, the advantages of TF include milder constipation, nausea, and drowsiness (Ahmedzai & Brooks, 1997).

When starting TF in opioid-naive or strong opioid–naïve patients, one patch at a dose of 12 and 25 μg/h is recommended, respectively. TF also may be used in opioid switch, especially in patients treated with morphine who suffer from intractable constipation. In an open-label study of 16 patients with cancer pain unable to take oral opioids, TF was effective and well tolerated (Leppert et al., 2000). A good analgesic effect was achieved in 11 patients, with a partial effect in an additional 2 patients. TF was effective and well-tolerated in patients formerly treated with weak opioids that did not provide satisfactory analgesia (Vielvoye-Kerkmeer et al., 2000). The indications for TF include patients' preferences, intense constipation during morphine treatment, morphine intolerance, nausea, and vomiting. TF should not be used in patients with unstable pain syndromes, especially with neuropathic pain component due to the long plasma half-life (20 h) of the drug, which hinders quick and effective dose titration. Fentanyl may be successfully used by other routes (e.g. SC, IV, intranasal inhaled, buccal) in the treatment of breakthrough pain (Slatkin et al., 2008).

3.5 Buprenorphine

Buprenorphine is a partial μ-opioid–receptor agonist and κ-receptor antagonist. A ceiling analgesic effect may be obtained at high doses (ie, 15 mg); however, such high doses are not used in clinical practice. The analgesic potency of buprenorphine is about 100 times greater than oral morphine (Likar et al., 2008). Buprenorphine may be administered sublingually due to low oral bioavailability at doses 0.2 to 0.8 mg, usually 3 times daily. It also may be administered by parenteral route (SC or IV).

Buprenorphine is metabolized to the active metabolite norbuprenorphine via CYP3A4. The parent compound and norbuprenorphine undergo glucuronidation; thus, the risk of pharmacokinetic interactions with other drugs is low. Compared with morphine, buprenorphine less frequently induces constipation, nausea, and vomiting, which is probably associated with higher lipophilicity. Buprenorphine is mainly excreted with feces (2/3) and 1/3 of the drug is excreted with urine therefore, it may be used in patients with renal failure. Respiratory depression is rare; however, when the symptom appears, naloxone injection should be administered at a dose of 2 mg, followed by continuous infusion (4 mg/h). Buprenorphine displays antihyperalgesic activity and may be successfully used in the treatment of neuropathic pain (Mercadante et al., 2007).

Buprenorphine is administered in transdermal patches (TB) releasing 35, 52.5, and 70 μg/h, which corresponds to 0.8, 1.2, and 1.6 mg/d, respectively. The patches are changed every 84 to 96 hours. In some countries, patches releasing 5 and 10 μg/h, changed weekly, are available. The starting dose for strong opioid-naïve patients is usually one patch of 35 μg/h. However, opioid-naive patients and those with renal or hepatic impairment may start with a dose of 17.5 μg/h. The treatment is usually well-tolerated. At doses up to 140 μg/h, TB does not display ceiling analgesia (Kress, 2009). Breakthrough pain may be treated with sublingual buprenorphine tablets or with IR morphine administered by oral or parenteral route (Mercadante et al., 2006).

3.6 Methadone

Methadone is a synthetic opioid and a racemate of dextrorotatory (S-methadone) and levorotatory (D-methadone) isomers. Methadone activates μ, κ, and Δ receptors (D-methadone); it displays moderate antagonistic effect to NMDA receptors (both enantiomers) and strongly inhibits the reuptake of serotonin and noradrenalin in the central nervous system (S-methadone). In high doses, methadone blocks potassium channels required for rapid cardiac muscle repolarization, which may explain the risk of developing ventricular arrhythmia.

Methadone is administered mostly to patients with cancer pain who undergo opioid switch; usually methadone is given every 8 hours. In comparison to morphine, 10 times less demand for laxatives and 2 times less nausea and vomiting were observed. Methadone may be administered as the first strong opioid to patients who have been treated with opioids for moderate pain or to opioid-naïve patients (the starting dose is usually 3–5 mg every 8 h) (Ripamonti et al., 1998) although EAPC recommends methadone as the second or the third-line opioid. Methadone can be administered to patients with renal impairment. It has weak immunosuppressive effect and does not suppress the functioning of natural killer cells. Methadone is tenfold less expensive than the CR morphine and 25-fold cheaper than TF.

Methadone is a highly lipophilic and basic drug with a high distribution volume (4.1 ± 0.65 L/kg) and a high affinity to tissues, where it cumulates after multiple administrations (in brain, lung, liver, gut, kidney, and muscles). The high affinity to tissues together with a gradual, retarded release to plasma is the cause of a prolonged half-life. The bioavailability of the drug after oral administration oscillates between 70% and 90%. The half-life is about 24 hours, but it occurs in the range of 8 to 120 hours. Analgesia lasts for 6 to 12 hours. A stable level is reached within 2 to 4 days. Methadone is metabolized mostly via liver enzymes, but also in the intestine wall via N-demethylation to inactive metabolites. The main enzyme responsible for methadone N-demethylation is CYP3A4 with a lesser CYP1A2 and CYP2D6 involvement and a significant CYP2B6 role. The drug is excreted mainly via the alimentary tract, but also through kidneys (depending on the urine pH). In chronic renal disease, methadone does not accumulate; in severe renal failure, a dose reduction may be considered. Methadone is not eliminated in the process of hemodialysis. Methadone is more difficult to use than other opioids due to complicated pharmacokinetics, numerous drug interactions, and possible QT prolongation; therefore, it should be used by physicians experienced in chronic pain management (Leppert, 2009c).

3.7 Tapentadol

Tapentadol chloride ([-]-[1*R*,2*R*]-3-[3-Dimethylamino-1-ethyl-2-methyl-propyl]-phenol hydrochloride) is an opioid with two analgesic mechanisms: agonist of μ-opioid receptors with 50 times less affinity than morphine, and inhibition of norepinephrine reuptake (Tzschentke et al., 2007). Bioavailability after oral administration is over 30%, the drug is metabolized to inactive metabolites through glucuronidation and excreted via kidneys (Kneip et al., 2008). In experimental studies tapentadol is effective in the treatment of neuropathic pain and in inflammatory pain. In clinical studies conducted in patients with low back pain, those with postoperative pain, and those with osteoarthritis, IR tapentadol at doses 50, 75, and 100 mg had more favorable adverse-effects profiles with less intense gastrointestinal adverse effects (ie, nausea, vomiting, constipation) in comparison to IR oxycodone at doses 10 and 15 mg. Clinical studies on tapentadol use in patients with cancer pain are ongoing.

4. Conclusions

Opioids are usually effective when administered alone or with adjuvant analgesics. The traditional WHO step-by-step approach should be used individually, based on the clinical assessment of pain type and intensity. Patients with severe pain intensity should use strong opioids (opioids for moderate-to-severe pain) without climbing up the analgesic ladder. Opioids may be combined with nonopioid analgesics and adjuvant analgesics appropriate for a given pain type. Understanding important attributes of commonly used opioids can help assist selection.

In case of lack of efficacy of orally or transdermally administered opioids, it may be beneficial to change the route of administration to parenteral or intrathecal (Enting et al., 2002). Another possibility is opioid switch that may improve analgesia and reduce adverse effects (Mercadante & Bruera, 2006). A good example may be patients suffering from severe constipation who may benefit when switching from morphine to TF (Ahmedzai & Brooks, 1997) and from codeine or DHC to tramadol (Leppert & Majkowicz, 2010). A newer approach is the concomitant use of two opioids, although little evidence supports such procedure (Fallon & Laird, 2011). Future studies may address genetic disposition responsible for individual patients' response to opioid analgesics (Lötsch et al., 2009).

5. References

Ahmedzai S, Brooks D. Transdermal Fentanyl versus Sustained-Release Oral Morphine in Cancer Pain: Preference, Efficacy and Quality of Life. J Pain Symptom Manage1997; 13: 254 - 261.

Ammon S, Hofmann U, Griese EU, Gugeler N, Mikus G. Pharmacokinetics of dihydrocodeine and its active metabolite after single and multiple oral dosing. Br J Clin Pharmacol 1999; 48: 317-322.

Benett MI. Effectiveness of antiepileptic or antidepressant drugs when added to opioids for cancer pain: a systematic review. Palliat Med 2011; 25: 553-559.

Caraceni A, Pigni A, Brunelli C. Is oral morphine still the first choice opioid for moderate to severe cancer pain? A systematic review within the European Palliative Care Research Collaborative guidelines project. Palliat Med 2011; 25: 402-409.

Davies MP, Glare P. Tramadol. In: Opioids in cancer pain. Second Edition; Davies MP, Glare P, Quigley C, Hardy JR. Eds. Oxford, Oxford University Press 2009, pp. 99-118.
Dickman A. Tramadol: a review of this atypical opioid. Eur J Palliat Care 2007; 14: 181-185.
Donnelly S, Davis MP, Walsh D, Naughton M. Morphine in cancer pain management: a practical guide. Support Care Cancer 2002; 10: 13 - 25.
Eidelman A, White T, Swarm RA: Interventional therapies for cancer pain management: important adjuvants to systemic analgesics. J Natl Compr Canc Netw 2007; 5: 753-760
Enting RH, Oldenmenger WH, van der Rijt CCD, Wilms EB, Elfrink EJ, Elswijk I, Sillevis Smitt PAE. A Prospective Study Evaluating the Response of Patients with Unrelieved Cancer Pain to Parenteral Opioids. Cancer 2002; 94: 3049 - 3056.
Fallon MT, Laird BJA. A systematic review of combination step III opioid therapy in cancer pain: An EPCRC opioid guideline project. Palliat Med 2011; 25: 597-603.
Flemming K. The Use of Morphine to Treat Cancer-Related Pain: A Synthesis of Quantitative and Qualitative Research. J Pain Symptom Manage 2010; 39: 139 - 154.
Freynhagen RJ, Benett MI. Diagnosis and management of neuropathic pain. BMJ 2009; 339: 391-395.
Gardner-Nix J, Mercadante S. The Role of OROS® Hydromorphone in the Management of Cancer Pain. Pain Pract 2010; 10: 72-77.
Gasche Y, Daali Y, Fathi M. et al. Codeine Intoxication Associated with Ultrarapid CYP2D6 Metabolism. N Engl J Med 2004; 351: 2827-2831.
Gnanadesigan N, Espinoza RT, Smith R, Israel M, Reuben DB. Interaction of serotonergic antidepressants and opioid analgesics: is serotonin syndrome going undetected? J Am Med Dir Assoc 2005; 6: 265-269
Gretton S, Riley J. Morphine metabolites: a review of their clinical effects. Eur J Palliat Care 2008; 15: 110 - 114.
Hagen NA, Babul N. Comparative clinical efficacy and safety of a novel controlled-release oxycodone formulation and controlled-release hydromorphone in the treatment of cancer pain. Cancer 1997; 79: 1428–1437.
Hanks GW, de Conno F, Cherny N, Hanna M, Kalso E, McQuay HJ, Mercadante S, et al. Expert Working Group of the Research Network of the European Association for Palliative Care: Morphine and alternative opioids in cancer pain: the EAPC recommendations. Br J Cancer 2001; 84: 587-593.
King SJ, Reid C, Forbes K, Hanks G. A systematic review of oxycodone in the management of cancer pain. Palliat Med 2011; 25: 454-470.
Kirchheiner J, Schmidt H, Tzetkov M, Keulen J-T, Lötsch J, Roots I, Brockmöller J. Pharmacokinetics of codeine and its metabolite morphine in ultra-rapid metabolizers due to CYP2D6 duplication. Pharmacogenomics J 2007; 7: 257-265.
Kneip C, Terlinden R, Beier H, Chen G. Investigations Into the Drug-Drug Interaction potential of tapentadol in Human Liver Microsomes and fresh Human Hepatocytes. Drug Metabol Lett 2008; 2: 67-75.
Kress HG. Clinical update on the pharmacology, efficacy and safety of transdermal buprenorphine. Eur J Pain 2009; 13: 219 - 230.
Leppert W, Luczak J, Gorzelinska L, Kozikowska J. Research from the Palliative Care Department in Poznan on treatment of neoplasm pain with Durogesic (transdermal fentanyl) (Polish). Przegl Lek 2000; 57: 59 - 64.

Leppert W, Majkowicz M. The impact of tramadol and dihydrocodeine treatment on quality of life of patients with cancer pain. Int J Clin Pract 2010; 64: 1681 - 1687.

Leppert W, Mikolajczak P. Analgesic Effects and Assays of Controlled-Release Tramadol and O-desmethyltramadol in Cancer Patients with Pain. Curr Pharmaceut Biotechnol 2011; 12: 306 - 312.

Leppert W. Dihydrocodeine as an analgesic for the treatment of moderate to severe chronic pain. Curr Drug Metab 2010; 11: 494-506.

Leppert W. Progress in pharmacological pain treatment with opioid analgesics (Polish). Wspolcz Onkol 2009; 13: 66-73.

Leppert W. Role of oxycodone and oxycodone/naloxone in cancer pain management. Pharmacol Rep 2010; 62: 578 - 591.

Leppert W. The role of ketamine in the management of neuropathic cancer pain - a Polish experience. Proceedings of the 3rd International Congress on Neuropathic pain, NeuPSIG, Athens (Greece), May 27 - 30, 2010, Ed. Christopher D. Wells. Medimond International Proceedings 2010, pp. 199 - 203.

Leppert W. The role of methadone in cancer pain treatment - a review. Int J Clin Pract 2009; 63: 1095 - 1109.

Leppert W. Tramadol as an analgesic for mild to moderate cancer pain. Pharmacol Rep 2009; 61: 978-992.

Likar R, Krainer B, Sittl R. Challenging the equipotency calculation for transdermal buprenorphine: four case studies. Int J Clin Pract 2008; 62: 152 - 156.

Lötsch J, Geisslinger G, Tegeder I. Genetic modulation of the pharmacological treatment of pain. Pharmacol Ther 2009; 124: 168-184.

Lötsch J, Skarke C, Schmidt H, Rohrbacher M, Hofmann U, Schwab M, Geisslinger G. Evidence for morphine-independent central nervous opioid effects after administration of codeine: Contribution of other codeine metabolites. Clin Pharmacol Ther 2006; 79: 35-48.

Lussier D, Huskey AG, Portenoy RK. Adjuvant Analgesics in Cancer Pain Management. Oncologist 2004; 9: 571-591.

Madadi P, Moretti M, Djokanovic N, Bozzo P, Nulman I, Ito S, Koren G. Guidelines for maternal codeine use during breastfeeding. Can Fam Phys 2009; 55: 1077-1078.

Madadi P, Ross CJD, Hayden MR, Carleton BC, Gaedigk A, Leeder JS, Koren G. Pharmacogenetics of Neonatal Opioid Toxicity Following Maternal Use of Codeine During Breastfeeding: A Case-Control Study. Clin Pharmacol Ther 2009; 85: 31-35.

Maddocks I, Somogyi A, Abbott F, Hayball P, Parker D. Attenuation of morphine-induced delirium in palliative care by substitution with infusion of oxycodone. J Pain Symptom Manage1996; 12: 182–189.

Mercadante S, Bruera E. Opioid switching: a systematic and critical review. Cancer Treat Rev 2006; 32: 304 - 315.

Mercadante S, Ferrera P, Villari P. Is there a ceiling effect of transdermal buprenorphine? Preliminary data in cancer patients. Support Care Cancer 2007; 15: 441 - 444.

Mercadante S, Villari P. Ferrera P. et al. Safety and effectiveness of intravenous morphine for episodic breakthrough pain in patients receiving transdermal buprenorphine. J Pain Symptom Manage 2006; 32: 175 - 179.

Miller MG, McCarthy N, O'Boyle CA et al. Continuous subcutaneous infusion of morphine vs. hydromorphone: a controlled trial. J Pain Symptom Manage 1999; 18: 9 - 16.

Murray A, Hagen NA. Hydromorphone. J Pain Symptom Manage 1995; 29 (Suppl): S57 - S66.

Nieminen TH, Hagelberg NM, Saari TI, Pertovaara A, Neuvonen M, Laine K, Neuvonen PJ, Olkkola KT. Rifampin Greatly Reduces the Plasma Concentrations of Intravenous and Oral Oxycodone. Anesthesiology 2009; 110: 1371-1378.

Pigni A, Brunelli C, Caraceni A. The role of hydromorphone in cancer pain treatment: a systematic review. Palliat Med 2011; 25: 471-477.

Rauers NI, Stuber F, Lee E.-H. et al. Antagonistic Effects of Ondansetron and Tramadol? A Randomized Placebo and Active Drug Controlled Study. J Pain 2010; 11: 1274-1281.

Ridgway D, Sopata M, Burneckis A, Jespersen L, Andersen C. Clinical Efficacy and Safety of Once-Daily Dosing of a Novel, Prolonged-Release Oral Morphine Tablet Compared With Twice-Daily Dosing of a Standard Controlled-Release Morphine Tablet in Patients With Cancer Pain: A Randomized, Double-Blind, Exploratory Crossover Study. J Pain Symptom Manage 2010; 39: 712 - 720.

Ripamonti C, Groff L, Brunelli C, Polastri D, Stavrakis A, De Conno F. Switching From Morphine to Oral Methadone in treating Cancer Pain: What Is the Equianalgesic Dose Ratio? J Clin Oncol 1998; 16: 3216 - 3221.

Ripamonti CI, Campa T, Fagnoni E, Brunelli C, Luzzani M, Maltoni M, De Conno F. on behalf of MERITO Study Group. Normal-release Oral Morphine Starting Dose in Cancer Patients With Pain. Clin J Pain 2009; 25: 386-390.

Ripamonti CI, Easson AM, Gerdes H. Management of malignant bowel obstruction. Eur J Cancer 2008; 44: 1105 - 1115.

Rowell FJ, Seymour RA, Rawlins MD. Pharmacokinetics of Intravenous and Oral Dihydrocodeine and its Acid Metabolites. Eur J Clin Pharmacol 1983; 25: 419-424. Sarhill N, Walsh D, Nelson KA. Hydromorphone: pharmacology and clinical applications in cancer patients. Support Care Cancer 2001; 9: 84 - 96.

Schmidt H, Vormfelde SV, Walchner-Bonjean M. et al. The role of active metabolites in dihydrocodeine effects. Int J Clin Pharmacol Ther 2003; 41: 95-106.

Slatkin NE, Xie F, Messina J, Segal TJ. Fentanyl Buccal Tablet for Relief of Breakthrough Pain in Opioid-Tolerant Patients With Cancer-Related Chronic Pain. J Support Oncol 2008; 5: 327 - 334.

Stamer U, Musshoff F, Kobilay M, Madea B, Hoeft A, Stuber F. Concentrations of Tramadol and O-desmethyltramadol Enantiomers in Different CY2D6 Genotypes. Clin Pharmacol Ther 2007; 82: 41-47.

Stamer U, Stuber F, Muders T, Musshoff F. Respiratory Depression with Tramadol in a Patient with Renal Impairment and CYP2D6 Gene Duplication. Anesth Analg 2008; 107: 926–929.

Stamer UM, Lehnen K, Höthker F, Bayerer B, Wolf S, Hoeft A, Stuber F. Impact of CYP2D6 genotype on postoperative tramadol analgesia. Pain 2003; 105: 231-238.

Tzschentke TM, Christoph T, Kögel B. et al. (-)-(1R,2R)-3-(3-Dimethylamino-1-ethyl-2-methyl-propyl)-phenol Hydrochloride (Tapentadol HCl): a Novel μ-Opioid Receptor Agonist/Norepinephrine Reuptake Inhibitor with Broad-Spectrum Analgesic Properties. J Pharmacol Exp Ther 2007; 323: 265 - 276.

Vielvoye-Kerkmeer APE, Mattern C, Uitendaal MP. Transdermal Fentanyl in Opioid-Naive Cancer Pain Patients: An Open Trial Using Transdermal Fentanyl for the Treatment of Chronic Cancer Pain in Opioid-Naive Patients and a Group Using Codeine. J Pain Symptom Manage 2000; 19: 185 - 192.

Voronov P, Przybylo HJ, Jagannathan N. Apnea in a child after oral codeine: a genetic variant - an ultra-rapid metabolizer. Pediatric Anesthesia 2007; 17: 684-687.

Vree TB, van Dongen RTM, Koopman-Kimenai PM. Codeine analgesia is due to codeine-6-glucuronide, not morphine. Int J Clin Pract 2000; 54: 395-398.

Vree TB, Verwey-van Wissen CP. Pharmacokinetics and metabolism of codeine in humans. Biopharm Drug Disp 1992; 13: 445-460.

Webb JA, Rostami-Hodjegan A, Abdul-Manap R, Hofmann U, Mikus G, Kamali F. Contribution of dihydrocodeine and dihydromorphine to analgesia following dihydrocodeine administration in man: a PK-PD modelling analysis. Br J Clin Pharmacol 2001; 52: 35-43.

Wirz S, Wartenberg HC, Nadstawek J. Less nausea, emesis, and constipation comparing hydromorphone and morphine? A prospective open-labeled investigation on cancer pain. Support Care Cancer 2008; 16: 999 – 1009.

World Health Organization: Cancer Pain Relief and Palliative Care. Geneva: World Health Organization, 1996.

Wright AW, Mather LE, Smith MT. Hydromorphone-3-glucuronide: a more potent neuro-excitant than its structural analogue, morphine-3-glucuronide. Life Sci 2001; 69: 409-420

Part 4

Chronic Pain

17

Epidural Lysis of Adhesions and Percutaneous Neuroplasty

Gabor B. Racz[1], Miles R. Day[1], James E. Heavner[1], Jeffrey P. Smith[1], Jared Scott[2], Carl E. Noe[3], Laslo Nagy[4] and Hana Ilner[1]
[1]*Texas Tech University Health Sciences Center, Lubbock, Texas*
[2]*Advanced Pain Medicine Associates, Wichita, Kansas*
[3]*University of Texas Southwestern Medical Center, Dallas, Texas*
[4]*Texas Tech University Health Sciences Center and Covenant Medical Center, Department of Pediatric Neurosurgery*
USA

1. Introduction

Chances are relatively high that each of us will experience low back pain at some point in our lives. The usual course is rapid improvement with 5% to 10% developing persistent symptoms.[1] In the 1990s the estimated cost of low back pain to the health industry was in the billions of dollars, and with a larger proportion of our population now reported to be older, this number can only be expected to increase. [2, 3] Treatment typically begins with conservative measures such as medication and physical therapy and may even include minimally and highly invasive pain management interventions. Surgery is sometimes required in patients who have progressive neurologic deficits or those who do not respond to conservative treatment sometimes chose surgery. A quandary sometimes arises, following a primary surgery, as to whether repeat surgery should be attempted or another alternative technique should be tried. This is the exact problem that the epidural adhesiolysis procedure was designed to address. Failed back surgery or postlaminectomy syndrome led to the development of the epidural adhesiolysis procedure.

It was shown to be effective in many patients with chronic pain after back surgery presumably by freeing up nerves and breaking down scar formation, delivering site-specific corticosteroids and local anesthetics, and reducing edema with the use of hyaluronidase and hypertonic saline. Epidural adhesiolysis has afforded patients a reduction in pain and neurologic symptoms without the expense and occasional long recovery period associated with repeat surgery, and often prevents the need for surgical intervention. Epidural adhesiolysis was given an evidence rating of strong correlating to a 1B or 1C evidence level for post–lumbar surgery syndrome in the most recent American Society of Interventional Pain Physicians evidence-based guidelines. The therapy is supported by observational studies and case series along with randomized-control trials. The recommendation was also made that this therapy could apply to most patients with post laminectomy syndrome or failed back syndrome in many circumstances with informed consent.[4] Additionally, current procedural terminology (CPT) codes have been assigned to the two different kinds of adhesiolysis: CPT 62263 for the three-times injections over 2 to 3 days, usually done in an inpatient hospital setting, and CPT 62264 for the one-time injection series surgery-center model that may need to be repeated 3 to 3.5 times in a 12-month period.

2. Pathophysiology of epidural fibrosis (scar tissue) as a cause of low back pain with radiculopathy

The etiology of chronic low back pain with radiculopathy after appropriate surgery is not well understood. Kuslich et al[5] addressed this issue when they studied 193 patients who had undergone lumbar spine operations given local anesthesic int the epidural space. It was postulated that sciatica could only be produced by stimulation of a swollen, stretched, restricted (i.e., scarred) or compressed nerve root.[5] Back pain could be produced by stimulation of several tissues, but the most common tissue of origin was the outer layer of the annulus fibrosus and the posterior longitudinal ligament. Stimulation for pain generation of the facet joint capsule rarely generated low back pain, and facet synovium and cartilage surfaces of the facet or muscles were never tender.[6]

The contribution of fibrosis to the etiology of low back pain has been debated.[7-9] There are many possible etiologies of epidural fibrosis, including surgical trauma, an annular tear, infection, hematoma, or intrathecal contrast material.[10] These etiologies have been well documented in the literature. LaRocca and Macnab[11] demonstrated the invasion of fibrous connective tissue into postoperative hematoma as a cause of epidural fibrosis, and Cooper et al[12] reported periradicular fibrosis and vascular abnormalities occurring with herniated intervertebral disks. McCarron et al[13] investigated the irritative effect of nucleus pulposus on the dural sac, adjacent nerve roots, and nerve root sleeves independent of the influence of direct compression on these structures. Evidence of an inflammatory reaction was identified by gross inspection and microscopic analysis of spinal cord sections after homogenized autogenous nucleus pulposus was injected into the lumbar epidural space of four dogs. In the control group consisting of four dogs injected with normal saline, the spinal cord sections were grossly normal. Parke and Watanabe[14] showed significant evidence of adhesions in cadavers with lumbar disk herniation.

It is widely accepted that postoperative scar renders the nerve susceptible to injury by a compressive phenomena.[9] It is natural for connective tissue or any kind of scar tissue to form fibrous layers (scar tissue) as a part of the process that transpires after disruption of the intact milieu.[15] Scar tissue is generally found in three components of the epidural space. Dorsal epidural scar tissue is formed by reabsorption of surgical hematoma and may be involved in pain generation.[16] In the ventral epidural space, dense scar tissue is formed by ventral defects in the disk, which may persist despite surgical treatment and continue to produce low back pain and radiculopathy past the surgical healing phase.[17] The lateral epidural space includes the epiradicular structures outside the root canals, known as the lateral recesses or "sleeves," which are susceptible to lateral disk defects, facet hypertrophy, and neuroforaminal stenosis.[18]

Although scar tissue itself is not tender, an entrapped nerve root is. Kuslich et al[5] surmised that the presence of scar tissue compounded the pain associated with the nerve root by fixing it in one position and thus increasing the susceptibility of the nerve root to tension or compression. They also concluded that no other tissues in the spine are capable of producing leg pain. In a study of the relationship between peridural scar evaluated by magnetic resonance imaging (MRI) and radicular pain after lumbar diskectomy, Ross et al[19] demonstrated that subjects with extensive peridural scarring were 3.2 times more likely to experience recurrent radicular pain.

This evidence also parallels a new study by Gilbert et al[20] in which lumbosacral nerve roots were identified as undergoing less strain than previously published during straight leg raise and in which hip motion greater than 60 degrees was determined to cause displacement of the nerve root in the lateral recess.

3. Fluid foraminotomy: Foraminal adhesiolysis or disentrapment

Relative or functional foraminal root entrapment syndrome secondary to epidural fibrosis with corresponding nerve root entrapment is frequently evident after an epidurogram and signified by lack of epidural contrast flow into epidural finger projections at those levels. The lysis procedure effectively serves as a fluid foraminotomy reducing foraminal stenosis caused by epidural fibrosis. In addition to increasing foraminal cross-sectional area, adhesiolysis serves to decompress distended epidural venous structures that may exert compression at nearby spinal levels (Fig. 1) and inevitably cause needle stick related epidural hematomas. Adhesiolysis has led to the development of flexible epiduroscopy that is being pioneered by, primarily initiated, pursued and to this day supported by Dr. James Heavner.[21,22]

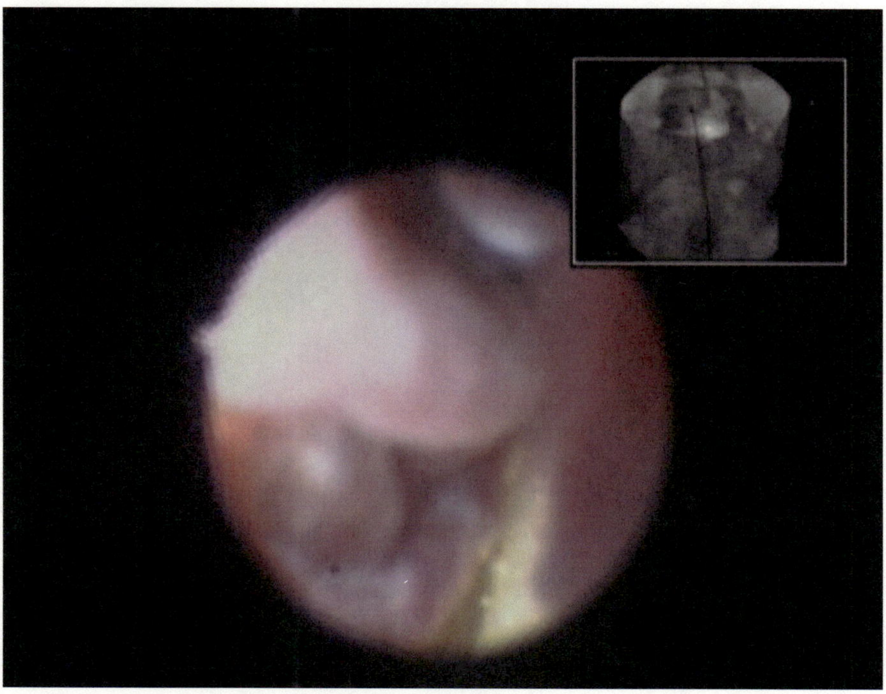

Fig. 1. Engorged blood vessels in the epidural cavity as observed during epiduroscopy. Insert in upper right corner is fluoroscopy showing location for epiduroscopy tip (left anterior border of L5)

4. Diagnosis and radiologic diagnosis of epidural fibrosis

As with any patient, a thorough musculoskeletal and neurologic examination should be performed. In addition to standard dural tension provocative tests, we recommend a provocative test called 'dural tug'. To perform the test, the patient should be instructed to sit up with a straight leg, bend forward flexing the lumbar spine until their back pain starts to become evident, and the head and neck flexed rapidly forward. During this maneuver, the dura is stretched cephalad and if adhered to structures such as the posterior longitudinal ligament, the most heavily innervated spinal canal structure, the movement of the dura will elicit back pain that is localized to the pain generator. A positive dural tug maneuver has been observed to resolve after percutaneous neuroplasty. (Fig 2 A-E)

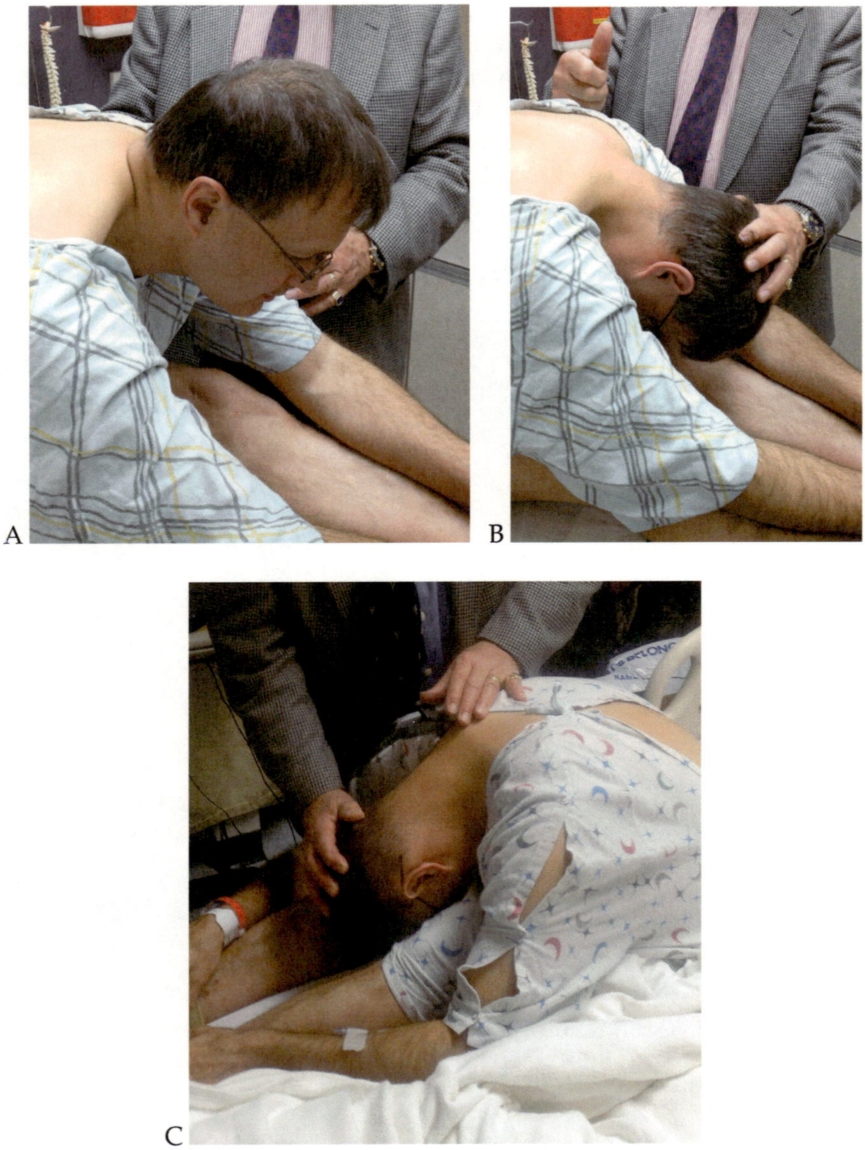

Fig. 2. A-C. A) The 'dural tug' maneuver being performed prior to percutaneous neuroplasty. B) Note pain reproduction prior to full neck flexion secondary to dural adhesions. C) Patient after percutaneous neuroplasty with pain free neck and back flexion due to treatment of dural adhesions.

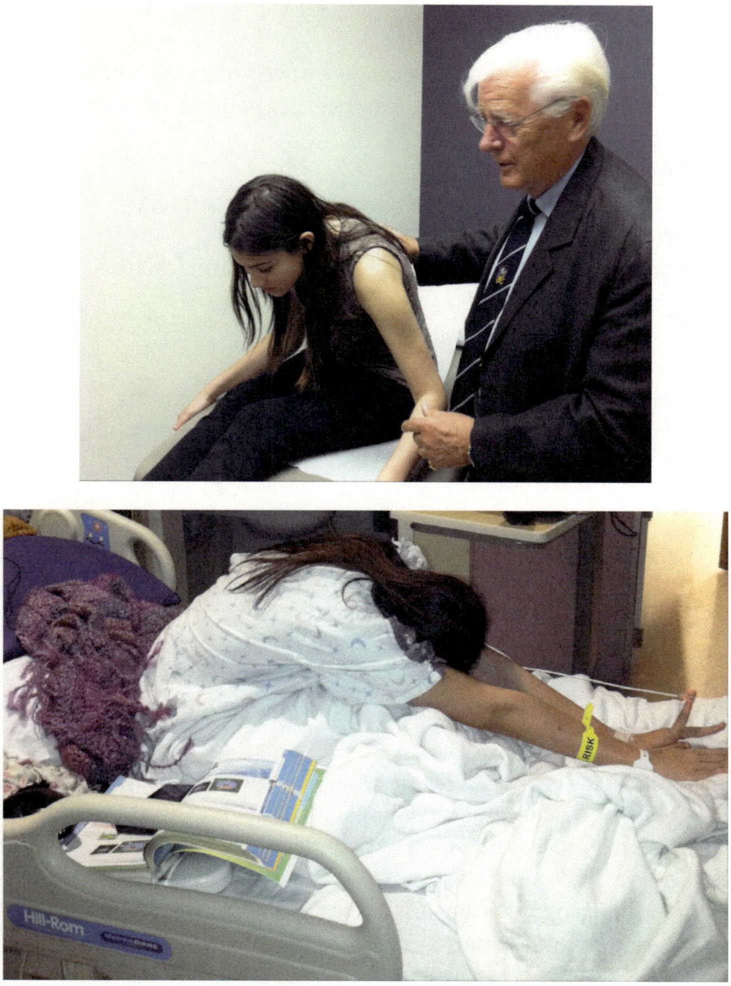

Fig. 2. D-E. D) There is decreased spine flexion prior to treatment secondary to dural adhesions. E) After treatment, the same patient demonstrates increased painless flexion of the spine.

MRI and computed tomography (CT) are diagnostic tools; sensitivity and specificity are 50% and 70%, respectively.[15] CT myelography may also be helpful, although none of the aforementioned modalities can identify epidural fibrosis with 100% reliability. In contrast, epidurography is a technique used with considerable success and it is believed that epidural fibrosis is best diagnosed by performing an epidurogram.[23-26] It can detect filling defects in good correlation with a patient's symptoms in real time.[26] A combination of several of these techniques would undoubtedly increase the ability to identify epidural fibrosis.

5. Current Procedural Terminology or CPT codes

The American Medical Association has developed Current Procedural Terminology codes for epidural adhesiolysis, which include 62264 for a single infusion and 62263 for a staged three-series infusion.

6. Indications for epidural adhesiolysis

Although originally designed to treat radiculopathy secondary to epidural fibrosis following surgery, the use of epidural adhesiolysis has been expanded to treat a multitude of pain etiologies. These include the following[27]:

1. Failed back surgery syndrome
2. Postlaminectomy syndrome of the neck and back after surgery
3. Disk disruption
4. Metastatic carcinoma of the spine leading to compression fracture
5. Multilevel degenerative arthritis
6. Facet pain
7. Spinal stenosis
8. Pain unresponsive to spinal cord stimulation and spinal opioids
9. Thoracic disk related chest wall and abdominal pain (after mapping)

7. Contraindications

The following are absolute contraindications for performing epidural adhesiolysis:

1. Sepsis
2. Chronic infection
3. Coagulopathy
4. Local infection at the procedure site
5. Patient refusal
6. Syrinx formation

A relative contraindication is the presence of arachnoiditis. With arachnoiditis, the tissue planes may be adherent to one another, increasing the chance of loculation of contrast or medication. It may also increase the chance of spread of the medications to the subdural or subarachnoid space, which can increase the chance of complications. Practitioners with limited experience with epidural adhesiolysis should consider referring these patients to a clinician with more training and experience.

8. Patient preparation

When epidural adhesiolysis has been deemed an appropriate treatment modality, the risks and benefits of the procedure should be discussed with the patient and informed consent obtained. The benefits are pain relief, improved physical function, and possible reversal of neurologic symptoms. Risks include, but are not limited to, bruising, bleeding, infection, reaction to medications used (i.e., hyaluronidase, local anesthetic, corticosteroids, hypertonic saline), damage to nerves or blood vessels, no or little pain relief, bowel/bladder incontinence, worsening of pain, and paralysis. Patients with a history of urinary incontinence should have a urodynamic evaluation by a urologist before the procedure to document the preexisting urodynamic etiology and pathology.

9. Anticoagulant medication

Medications that prolong bleeding and clotting parameters should be withheld before performing epidural adhesiolysis. The length of time varies depending on the medication taken. A consultation with the patient's primary physician should be obtained before stopping any of these medications, particularly in patients who require chronic anticoagulation such as those with drug-eluting heart stents or prosthetic heart valves. Nonsteroidal anti-inflammatory drugs and aspirin, respectively, should be withheld 4 days and 7 to 10 days before the procedure. Although there is much debate regarding these medications and neuraxial procedures, we tend to be on the conservative side. Clopidogrel (Plavix) should be stopped 7 days before, whereas ticlopidine (Ticlid) is withheld 10 to 14 days before the adhesiolysis.[28] Warfarin (Coumadin) stoppage is variable but 5 days is usually adequate.[27] Patients on subcutaneous heparin should have it withheld a minimum of 12 hours before the procedure, whereas those on low-molecular-weight heparin require a minimum of 24 hours.[28] Over-the-counter homeopathic medications that prolong bleeding parameters should also be withheld. These include fish oil, vitamin E, gingko biloba, garlic, ginseng, and St. John's Wort. Adequate coagulation status can be confirmed by the history, INR, prothrombin time, partial thromboplastin time, and a platelet function assay or bleeding time. The tests should be performed as close to the day of the procedure as possible. Tests performed only a few days after stopping the anticoagulant medication may come back elevated because not enough time has elapsed to allow the anticoagulant effects of the medication to resolve. The benefits of the procedure must be weighed against the potential sequelae of stopping the anticoagulant medication and this should be discussed thoroughly with the patient.

10. Preoperative laboratory

Before the procedure, a complete blood count and a clean-catch urinalysis are obtained to check for any undiagnosed infections. An elevated white count and/or a positive urinalysis should prompt the physician to postpone the procedure and refer the patient to the primary care physician for further workup and treatment. In addition, history of bleeding, abnormalities a prothrombin time, partial thromboplastin time, and platelet function assay or bleeding time, are obtained to check for coagulation abnormalities. Any elevated value warrants further investigation and postponement of the procedure until those studies are complete.

11. Technique

This procedure can be performed in the cervical, thoracic, lumbar, and caudal regions of the spine. The caudal and transforaminal placement of catheters will be described in detail, whereas highlights and slight changes in protocol will be provided for cervical and thoracic catheters. Our policy is to perform this procedure under strict sterile conditions in the operating room. Prophylactic antibiotics with broad neuraxial coverage are given before the procedure. Patients will receive either ceftriaxone 1 g intravenously or Levaquin 500 mg orally in those allergic to penicillin. The same dose is also given on day 2. An anesthesiologist or nurse anesthetist provides monitored anesthesia care.

12. Caudal approach

The patient is placed in the prone position with a pillow placed under the abdomen to correct the lumbar lordosis and a pillow under the ankles for patient comfort. The patient is asked to put his or her toes together and heels apart. This relaxes the gluteal muscles and facilitates identification of the sacral hiatus. After sterile preparation and draping, the sacral hiatus is identified via palpation just caudal to the sacral cornu or with fluoroscopic guidance. A skin wheal is raised with local anesthetic 1-inch lateral and 2 inches caudal to the sacral hiatus on the side opposite the documented radiculopathy. A distal subcutaneous approach theoretically provides some protection from meningitis, as a local skin infection would be much preferred over infection closer to the caudal epidural space. The skin is nicked with an 18-gauge cutting needle, and a 15- or 16-gauge RX Coudé (Epimed International) epidural needle is inserted through the nick at a 45-degree angle and guided fluoroscopically or by palpation to the sacral hiatus (Figs. 3 and 4).

When the needle is through the hiatus, the angle of the needle is dropped to approximately 30 degrees and advanced. The advantages of the RX Coudé needle over other needles are the angled tip, which enables easier direction of the catheter, and the tip of the needle is less sharp. The back edge of the distal opening of the needle is designed to be a noncutting surface that allows manipulation of the catheter in and out of the needle. A Touhy needle has the back edge of the distal opening, which is a cutting surface and can more easily shear a catheter. A properly placed needle will be inside the caudal canal below the level of the S3 foramen on anteroposterior (AP) and later fluoroscopic images. A needle placed above the level of the S3 foramen could potentially puncture a low-lying dura. The needle tip should cross the midline of the sacrum toward the side of the radiculopathy.

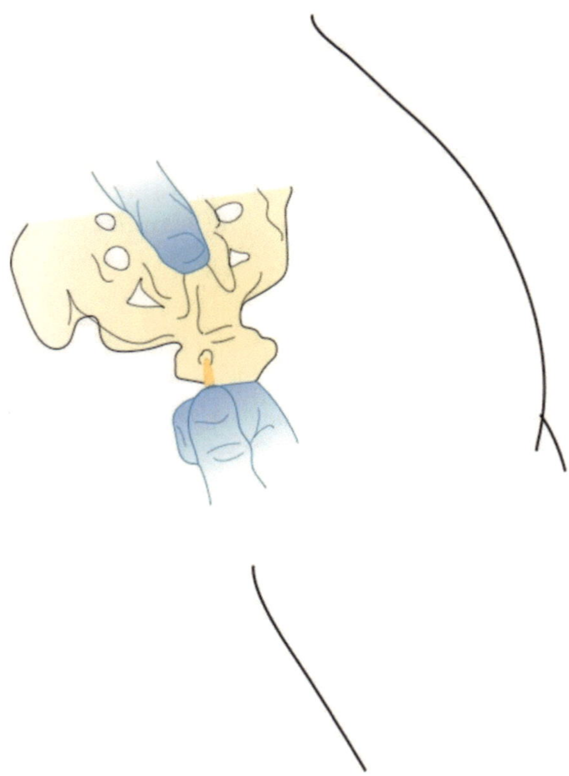

Fig. 3. Caudal lysis sequence – first find sacral hiatus and tip of coccyx.

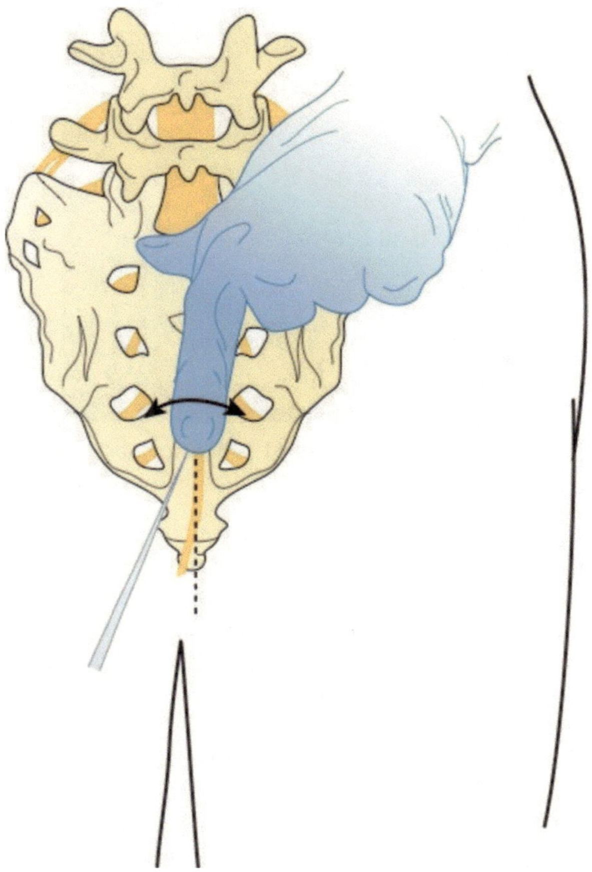

Fig. 4. Roll palpating index finger to identify the sacral cornu and thus the target sacral hiatus.

An epidurogram is performed using 10 mL of a non-ionic, water-soluble contrast agent. Confirm a negative aspiration for blood or cerebrospinal fluid before any injection of the contrast or medication. Omnipaque and Isovue are the two agents most frequently used and are suitable for myelography.[29, 30] Do not use ionic, water-insoluble agents such as Hypopaque or Renografin or ionic, water-soluble agents such as Conray. [31,32] These agents are not indicated for myelography. Accidental subarachnoid injections can lead to serious untoward events such as seizure and possibly death. Slowly inject the contrast agent and observe for filling defects. A normal epidurogram will have a "Christmas tree" pattern with the central canal being the trunk and the outline of the nerve roots making up the branches. An abnormal epidurogram will have areas where the contrast does not fill (Fig. 5). These are the areas of presumed scarring and typically correspond to the patient's radicular complaints. If vascular uptake is observed, the needle needs to be redirected.

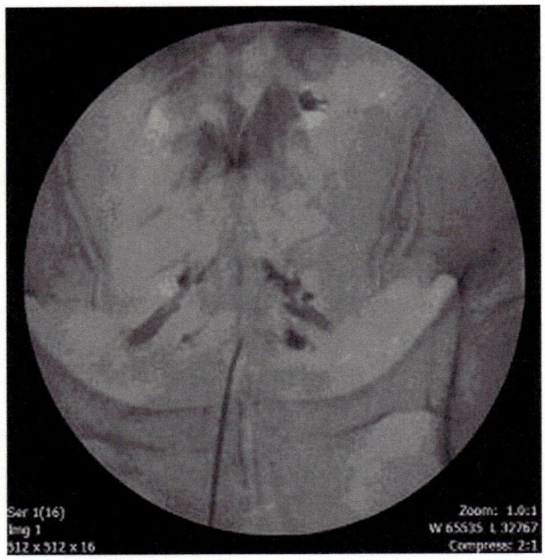

Fig. 5. Initial dye injection Omnipaque 240 (10 mL) showing sacral S3 runoff and filling defects at S2, S1, and right L5

After turning the distal opening of the needle ventral lateral, insert a TunL Kath or TunL-XL (stiffer) catheter (Epimed International) with a bend on the distal tip through the needle (Figs. 6 and 7). The bend should be 2.5 cm from the tip of the catheter and at a 30-degree angle. The bend will enable the catheter to be steered to the target level (Fig 8). Under continuous AP fluoroscopic guidance, advance the tip of the catheter toward the ventral-lateral epidural space of the desired level. The catheter can be steered by gently twisting the catheter in a clockwise or counterclockwise direction. Avoid "propellering" the tip (i.e., twisting the tip in circles) because this makes it more difficult to direct the catheter. Do not advance the catheter up the middle of the sacrum because this makes guiding the catheter to the ventral-lateral epidural space more difficult. Ideal location of the tip of the catheter in the AP projection is in the foramen just below the midportion of the pedicle shadow (Figs 9 and 10). Check a lateral projection to confirm that the catheter tip is in the ventral epidural space.

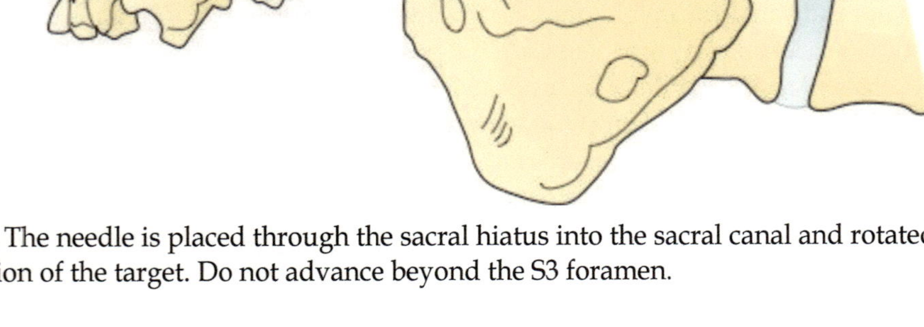

Fig. 6. The needle is placed through the sacral hiatus into the sacral canal and rotated in the direction of the target. Do not advance beyond the S3 foramen.

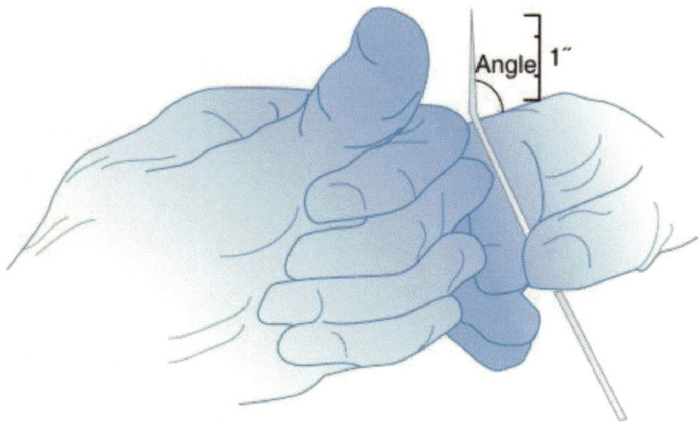

Fig. 7. The Epimed Racz catheter is marked for the location of the bend, or use the thumb as reference for the 15-degree angle bend

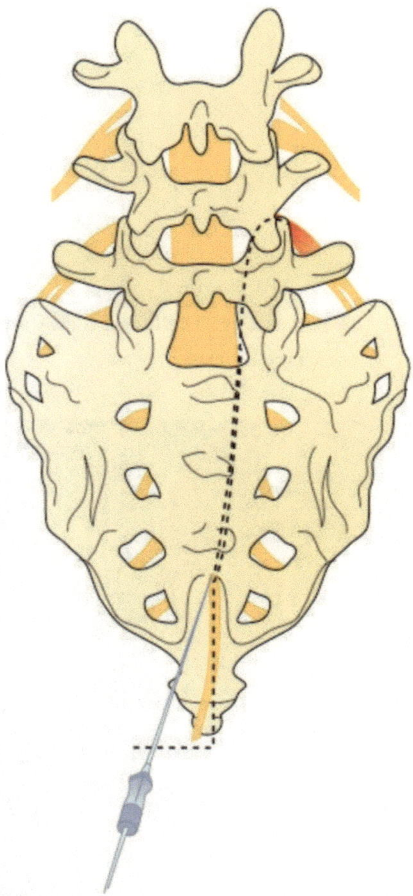

Fig. 8. The direction of the catheter is just near the midline; direct the curve under continuous fluoroscopic guidance to the ventral lateral target site. The needle rotation, as well as the catheter navigation, may need to be used to reach the target

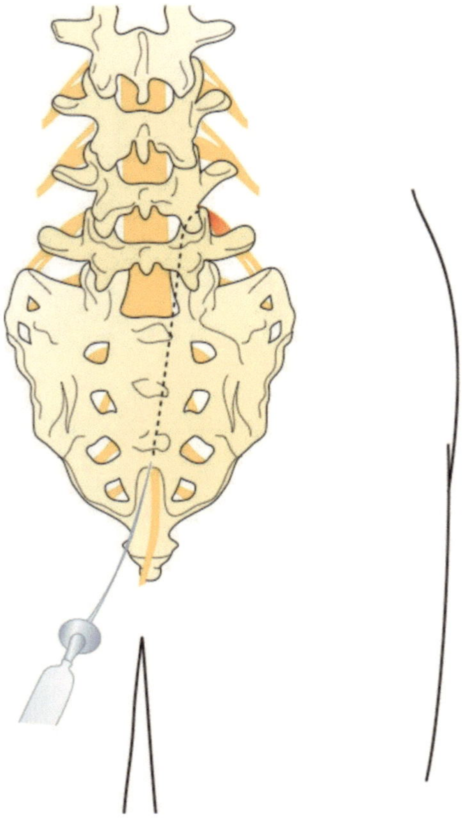

Fig. 9. The needle is removed, and the catheter is placed in the ventral lateral epidural space ventral to the nerve root

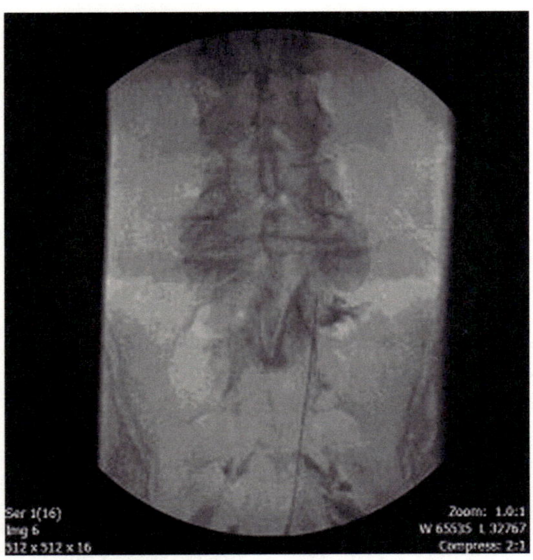

Fig. 10. Catheter (24xL) is threaded to lateral L5 neural foramen

Under real-time fluoroscopy, inject 2 to 3 mL of additional contrast through the catheter in an attempt to outline the "scarred in" nerve root (Fig 11). If vascular uptake is noted, reposition the catheter and reinject contrast. Preferably there should not be vascular runoff, but infrequently secondary to venous congestion, an epidural pattern is seen with a small amount of vascular spread. This is acceptable as long as the vascular uptake is venous in nature and not arterial. Extra caution should be taken when injecting the local anesthetic to prevent local anesthetic toxicity. Toxicity is volume and dose related and so far there has not been any reported complications from small volume venous spread. Any arterial spread of contrast always warrants repositioning of the catheter. We have never observed intra-arterial placement in 25 years of placing soft, spring-tipped catheters.

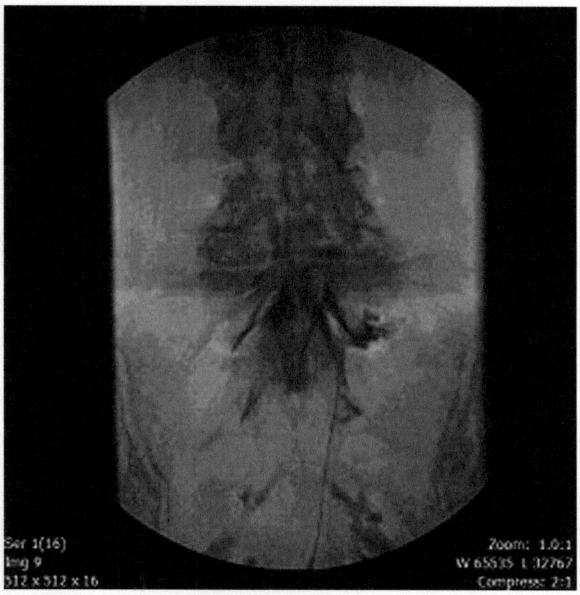

Fig. 11. Contrast injection Omnipaque 240, additional 5 mL opening right L5, S1, S2, and S3 perineural spaces; also left L5, S1, S2, and S3 in addition to right L4 spread in cephalad direction

Inject 1500 U of hyaluronidase dissolved in 10 mL of preservative-free normal saline. A newer development is the use of Hylenex or human-recombinant hyaluronidase, which carries the advantage of a reportedly increased effectiveness at the body's normal pH compared to bovine-recombinant hyaluronidase.[33] This injection may cause some discomfort, so a slow injection is preferable. Observe for "opening up"(i.e. visualization) of the "scarred in" nerve root (Figs 12 and 13 ; see also Fig. 11). A 3 mL test dose of a 10 mL local anesthetic/steroid (LA/S) solution is then given. Our institution used 4 mg of dexamethasone mixed with 9 mL of 0.2% ropivacaine. Ropivacaine is used instead of bupivacaine for two reasons: the former produces a preferential sensory versus a motor block, and it is less cardiotoxic than a racemic bupivacaine. Doses for other corticosteroids commonly used are 40 to 80 mg of methylprednisolone (Depo-Medrol), 25 to 50 mg of triamcinolone diacetate (Aristocort), 40 to 80 mg of triamcinolone acetonide (Kenalog), and 6 to 12 mg of betamethasone (Celestone Solu span). If, after 5 minutes, there is no evidence of intrathecal or intravascular injection of medication, inject the remaining 7 mL of the LA/S solution.

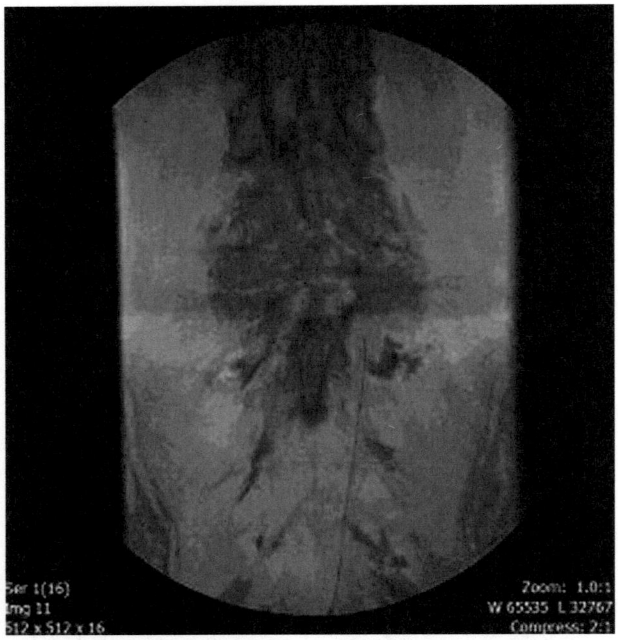

Fig. 12. Additional contrast and hyaluronidase injection opens up bilaterally formerly scarred areas. The Christmas tree appearance is obvious.

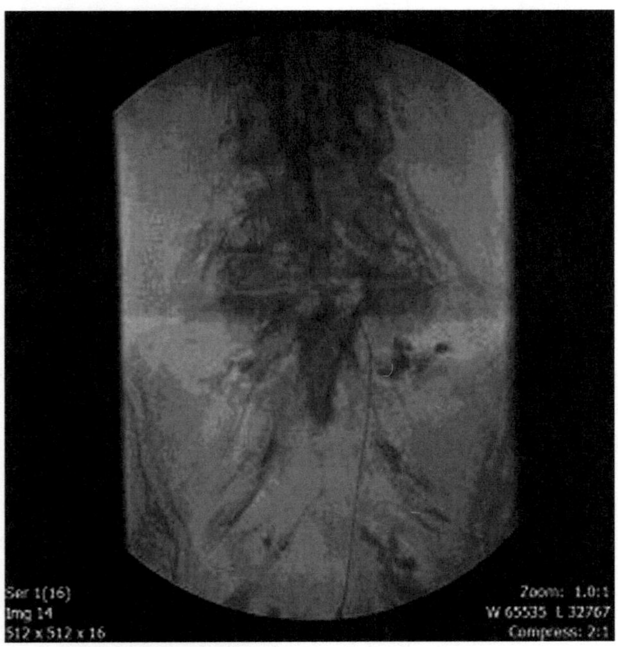

Fig. 13. Catheter advances to the desired symptomatic level of right L5 in the ventral lateral epidural space. Injection of contrast followed by 10 mL hyaluronidase 1,500 units opens up bilaterally L3-5, S1, S2, and S3 neural foramina.

Remove the needle under continuous fluoroscopic guidance to ensure the catheter remains at the target level (Fig 14). Secure the catheter to the skin using nonabsorbable suture and coat the skin puncture site with antimicrobial ointment. Apply a sterile dressing and attach a 0.2 μ m filter to the end of the catheter. Affix the exposed portion of the catheter to the patient with tape and transport the patient to the recovery area.

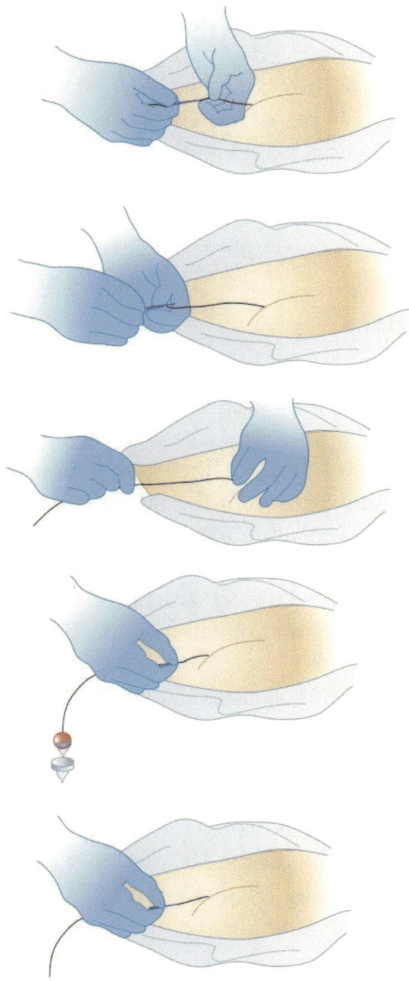

Fig. 14. Five picture sequence of removal of the needle to prevent dislodging the catheter from target site before suturing and application of dressing.

A 20- to 30-minute period should elapse between the last injection of the LA/S solution and the start of the hypertonic saline (10%) infusion. This is necessary to ensure that a subdural injection of the LA/S solution has not occurred. A subdural block mimics a subarachnoid block but it takes longer to establish, usually 16 to 18 minutes. Evidence for subdural or subarachnoid spread is the development of motor block. If the patient develops a subarachnoid or subdural block at any point during the procedure, the catheter should be removed and the remainder of the adhesiolysis canceled. The patient needs to be observed to document the resolution of the motor and sensory block and to document that 10 mL of the hypertonic saline is then infused through the catheter over 15 to 30 minutes. If the patient complains of discomfort, the infusion is stopped and an additional 2 to 3 mL of 0.2% ropivacaine is injected and the infusion is restarted. Alternatively, 50 to 75 μ g of fentanyl can be injected epidurally in lieu of the local anesthetic. After completion of the hypertonic saline infusion, the catheter is slowly flushed with 2 mL of preservative-free normal saline and the catheter is capped.

Our policy is to admit the patient for 24-hour observation status and do a second and a third hypertonic saline infusion the following day. On post–catheter insertion day 2, the catheter is twice injected (separated by 4- to 6-hour increments) with 10 mL of 0.2% ropivacaine without steroid and infused with 10 mL of hypertonic saline (10%) using the same technique and precautions as the day 1 infusion. At the end of the third infusion, the catheter is removed and a sterile dressing applied. The patient is discharged home with 5 days of oral cephalexin at 500 mg twice a day or oral levofloxacin (Levaquin) at 500 mg once a day for penicillin-allergic patients. Clinic follow-up is in 30 days.

13. Transforaminal catheters

Patients with an additional level of radiculopathy or those in whom the target level cannot be reached by the caudal approach may require placement of a second catheter. The second catheter is placed into the ventral epidural space via a transforaminal approach.

After the target level is identified with an AP fluoroscopic image, the superior endplate of the vertebra that comprises the caudal portion of the foramina is "squared," that is, the anterior and posterior shadows of the vertebral endplate are superimposed. The angle is typically 15 to 20 degrees in a caudocephalad direction. The fluoroscope is then oblique approximately 15 degrees to the side of the radiculopathy and adjusted until the spinous process is rotated to the opposite side. This fluoroscope positioning allows the best visualization of the superior articular process (SAP) that forms the inferoposterior portion of the targeted foramen. The image of the SAP should be superimposed on the shadow of the disk space on the oblique view. The tip of the SAP is the target for the needle placement (Fig 15). Raise a skin wheal slightly lateral to the shadow of the tip of the SAP. Pierce the skin with an 18-gauge needle and then insert a 15- or 16-gauge RX Coudé needle and advance using gun-barrel technique toward the tip of the SAP. Continue to advance the needle medially toward the SAP until the tip contacts bone. Rotate the tip of the needle 180 degrees laterally and advance about 5 mm (Fig 16). Rotate the needle back medially 180 degrees (Fig 17).

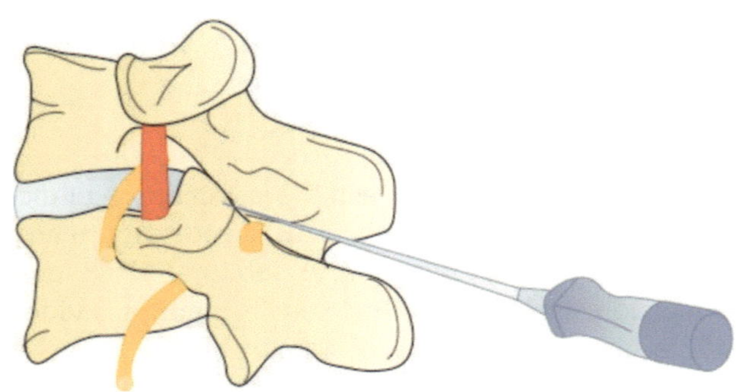

Fig. 15. Transforaminal lateral-oblique view. Target the SAP with the advancing RX Coude needle.

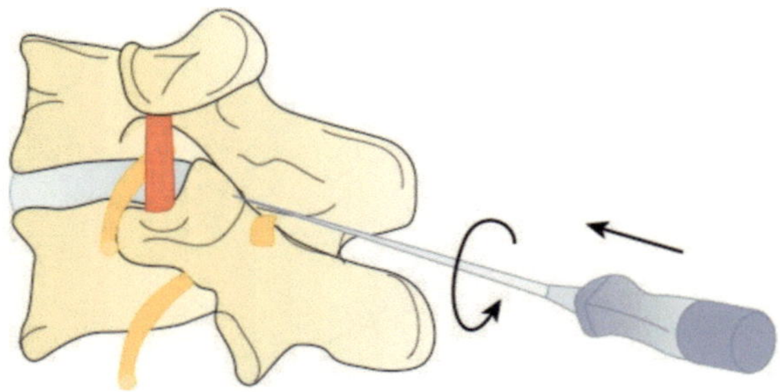

Fig. 16. Following bony contact with SAP. Lateral rotation of 180 degrees to allow passage toward the target.

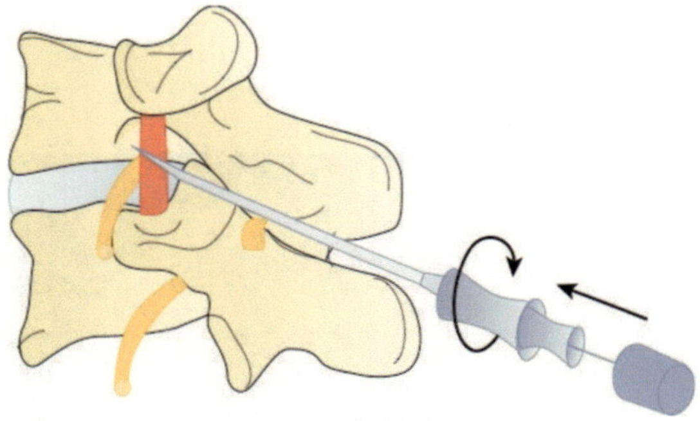

Fig. 17. Note the intertransverse ligament. The needle tip with the RX Coude 2 that has 1 mm protruding blunt stylet will pass through the ligament and will be less likely to damage the nerve.

As the needle is advanced slowly, a clear "pop" is felt as the needle penetrates the inter transverse ligament. Obtain a lateral fluoroscopic image. The tip of the needle should be just past the SAP in the posterior foramen. In the AP plane, the tip of the needle under continuous AP fluoroscopy, insert the catheter slowly into the foramen and advance until the tip should be just short of the middle of the spinal canal (Fig 18 to 20).

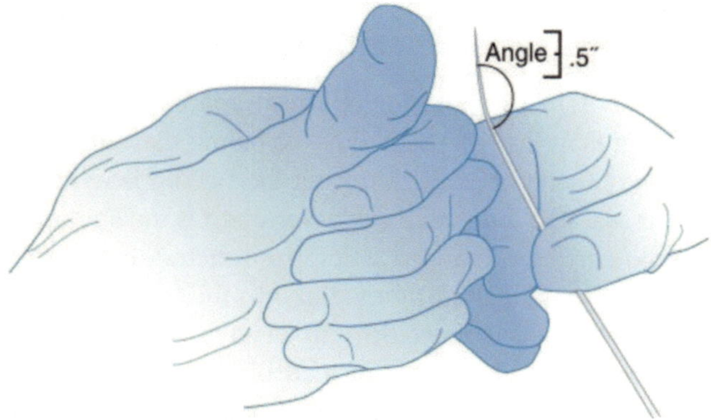

Fig. 18. The distal tip of the catheter may be bent 15-degrees, 3/4 inch length.

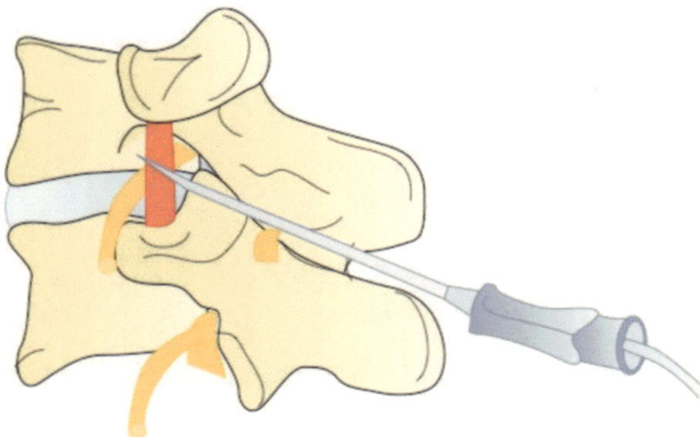

Fig. 19. Once the intertransverse ligament is perforated, the catheter is steered to the ventral lateral epidural space (lateral view).

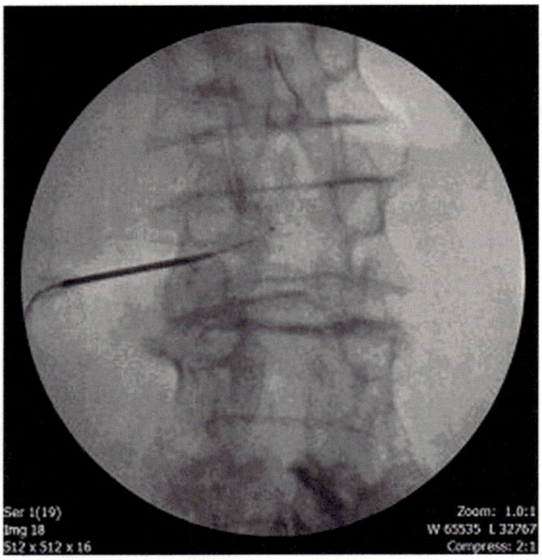

Fig. 20. Transforaminal 15-gauge RX-Coude 2 (Epimed International, Johnstown, NY) catheter at left L3-4 threaded almost to near *midcanal* position (anteroposterior view).

Confirm that the catheter is in the anterior epidural space with a lateral image (Fig 21). Anatomically, the catheter is in the foramen above or below the exiting nerve root (Fig 22). If the catheter cannot be advanced, it usually means the needle is either too posterior or too lateral to the foramen. It can also indicate that the foramen is too stenotic to allow passage of the catheter. The needle can be advanced a few millimeters anteriorly in relation to the foramen, and that will also move it slightly medial into the foramen. If the catheter still will not pass, the initial insertion of the needle will need to be more lateral. Therefore the fluoroscope angle will be about 20 degrees instead of 15 degrees. The curve of the needle usually facilitates easy catheter placement. The final position of the catheter tip is just short of the midline.

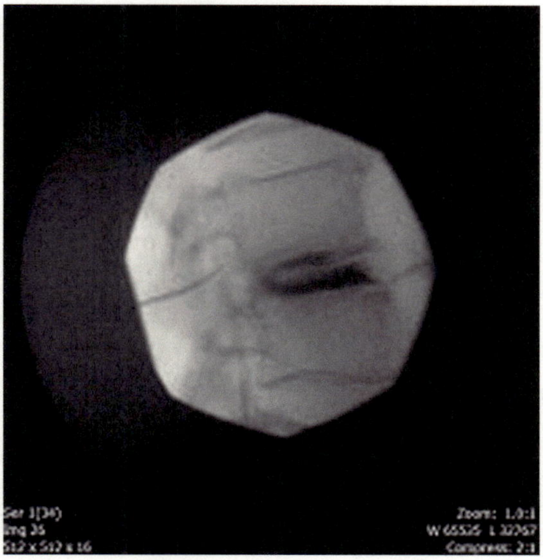

Fig. 21. Lateral view of Fig. 169-13 . Transforaminal-ventral-anterior catheter dye spread to epidural and L3-4 intradiscal area (through annular tear).

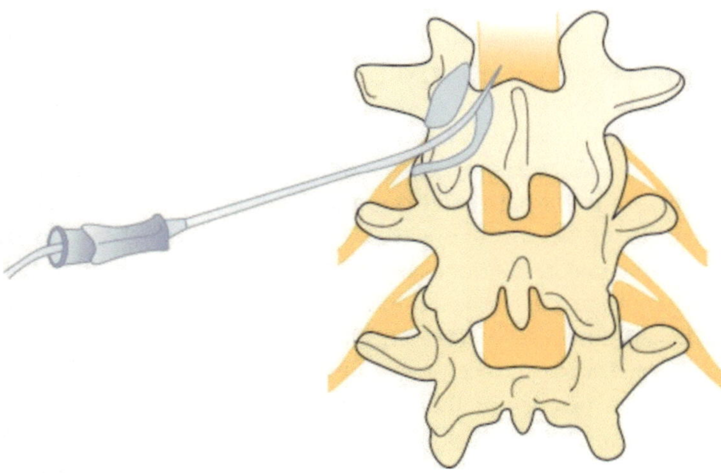

Fig. 22. Anteroposterior view. The catheter is in optimal position near midline via the transforaminal placement.

Inject 1 to 2 mL of contrast to confirm epidural spread. When a caudal and a transforaminal catheter are placed, the 1500 U of hyaluronidase are divided evenly between the two catheters (5 mL of the hyaluronidase/saline solution into each). The LA/S solution is also divided evenly, but a volume of 15 mL (1 mL steroid and 14 mL 0.2% ropivacaine; of the total volume, 5 mL is transforaminal and 10 mL is caudal) is used instead of 10 mL. Remove the needle under fluoroscopic guidance to make sure the catheter does not move from the original position in the epidural space. Secure and cover the catheter as described previously. The hypertonic saline solution is infused at a volume of 4 to 5 mL per transforaminal and 8 to 10 mL per caudal catheter over 30 minutes. The hypertonic saline injection volume should always be less than or equal to the local anesthetic volume injected to avoid pain from injection. It behooves the practitioner to check the position of the transforaminal catheter under fluoroscopy before performing the second and third infusions. The catheter may advance across the epidural space into the contralateral foramen or paraspinous muscles or more commonly back out of the epidural space into the ipsilateral paraspinous muscles.

This results in deposition of the medication in the paravertebral tissue rather than in the epidural space. As with the caudal approach, remove the transforaminal catheter after the third infusion. A recent development is the R-X Coude 2 needle in which a second protruding stylet may allow closer needle placement and less chance of nerve injury.

14. Cervical lysis of adhesions

The success of the caudal approach for lysis of adhesions led to the application of the same technique to the cervical epidural space. The indications and preprocedure workup are the same as those for the caudal lysis technique, but there are a few differences in technique and volumes of medication used.

The epidural space should be entered via the upper thoracic interspaces using a paramedian approach on the contralateral side. The most common levels are T1-2 and T2-3. Entry at these levels allows for a sufficient length of the catheter to remain in the epidural space after the target level has been reached. If the target is the lower cervical nerve roots, a more caudal interspace should be selected. We place the patient in the left lateral decubitus position, but use a prone approach in larger patients.

A technique referred to as the "3-D technique" is used to facilitate entry into the epidural space. The "3-D" stands for *direction, depth,* and *direction.* Using an AP fluoroscopic image, the initial *direction* of the 15- or 16-gauge RX Coudé needle is determined. Using a modified paramedian approach with the skin entry one and a half levels below the target interlaminar space, advance and direct the needle toward the midpoint of the chosen interlaminar space with the opening of the needle pointing medial. Once the needle engages the deeper tissue planes (usually at 2 to 3 cm), check the depth of the needle with a lateral image. Advance the needle toward the epidural space and check repeat images to confirm the *depth.* The posterior border of the dorsal epidural space can be visualized by identifying the junction of the base of the spinous process of the vertebra with its lamina. This junction creates a distinct radiopaque "straight line." Once the needle is close to the epidural space, obtain an AP fluoroscopic image to recheck the *direction* of the needle. If the tip of the needle has crossed the midline as defined by the spinous processes of the vertebral bodies, pull the needle back and redirect. The "3-D" process can be repeated as many times as is necessary to get the needle into the perfect position.

Using loss-of-resistance technique, advance the needle into the epidural space with the tip of the RX-Coudé needle, pointed caudally. Once the tip is in the epidural space, rotate the tip cephalad, and inject 1 to 2 mL of contrast to confirm entry. Rotation or movement of any needle in the epidural space can cut the dura. This technique has been improved with the advent of the RX Coudé 2 needle, which has a second interlocking stylet that protrudes slightly beyond the tip of the needle and functions to push the dura away from the needle tip as it is turned 180 degrees cephalad (Fig. 23 A-E).

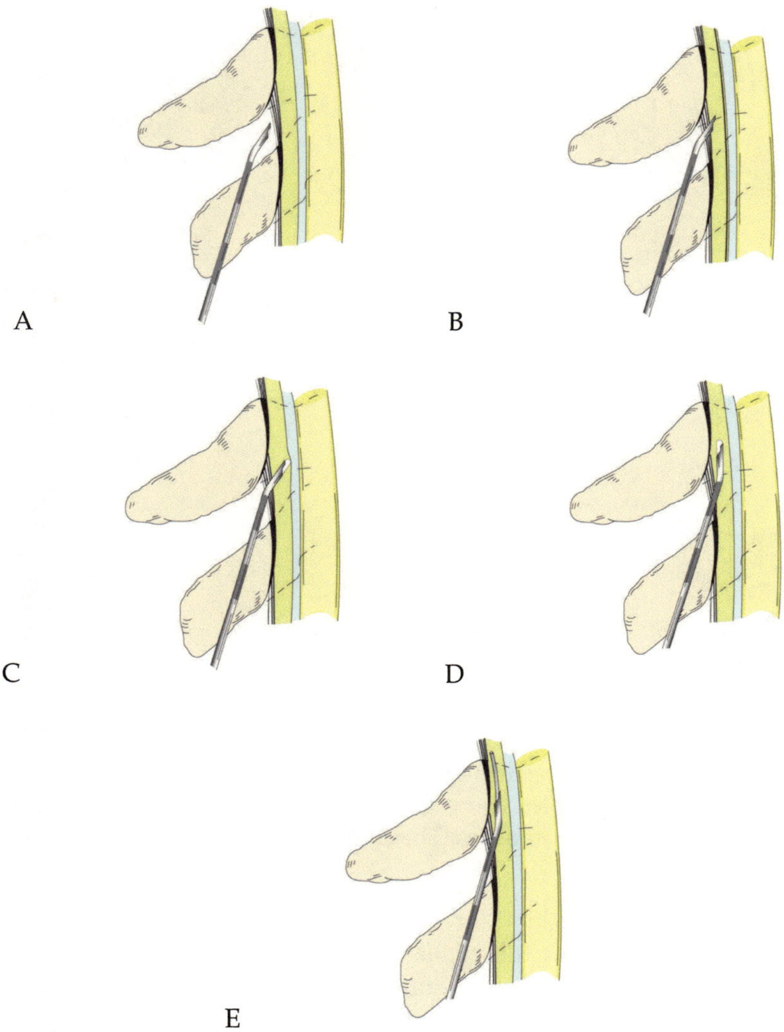

Fig. 23. Sequence of stages to place a catheter using the R-X Coude. **A** and **B.** The needle is inserted into the epidural space with the tip directed as shown. **C.** The protruding stylet is inserted. **D.** Then the needle is rotated so the tip is parallel to the dura. **E.** The catheter is inserted.

Inject an additional small volume as needed to complete the epidurogram. If there is no free flow of injected contrast, pressure may build up in the lateral epidural space. Characteristic fluid spread by the path of least resistance can be recognized as *perivenous counter spread* (PVCS). Presence of PVCS means pressure builds up in the lateral epidural space that is unable to spread laterally to decompress. The dye spread picks the path of least resistance to the opposite side. Pressure may build up and lead to ischemic spinal cord injury. Flexion and rotation of the head and neck can open up lateral runoff and release the pressure through the enlarged neural foramina (Fig 24)[34]

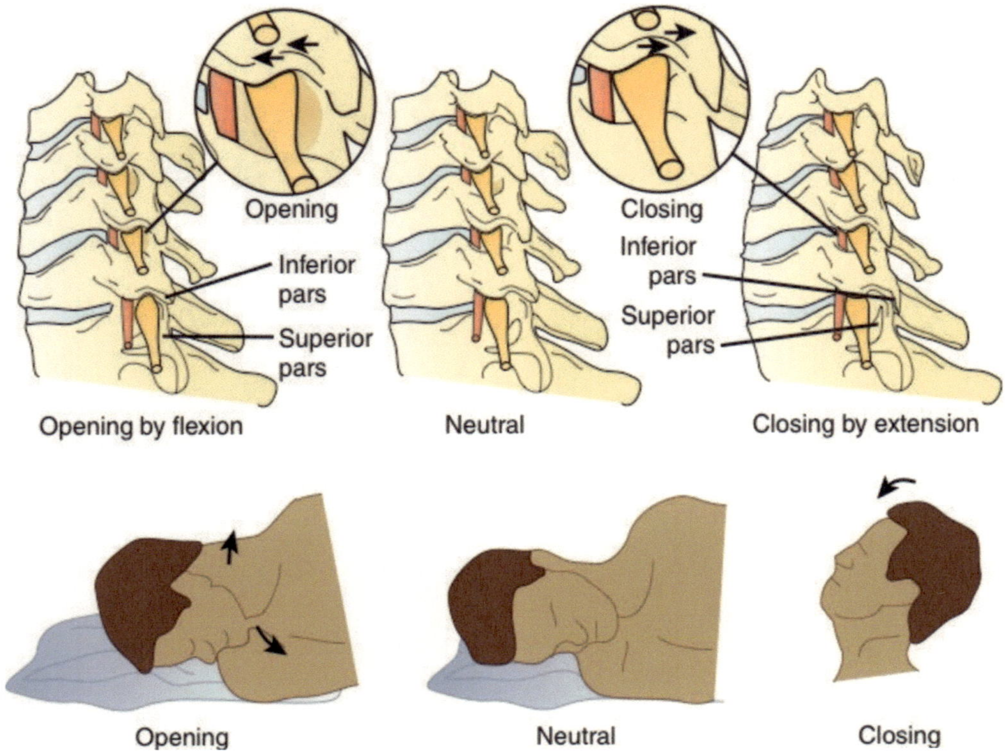

Fig. 24. Flexion rotation, left to right regardless patient position. The neural foramen enlarges on flexion rotation and gets smaller with extension. The inferior pars slides forward over the superior pars to enlarge the foramen. This allows lateral run off and pressure release with PVCS.

As with the caudal epidurogram, look for filling defects. It is extremely important to visualize spread of the contrast in the cephalad and caudal directions. Loculation of contrast in a small area must be avoided as this can significantly increase the pressure in the epidural space and can compromise the already tenuous arterial blood supply to the spinal cord. Place a bend on the catheter as previously described for the caudal approach and insert it through the needle (Fig 23E). The opening of the needle should be directed toward the target side. Slowly advance the catheter to the lateral gutter and direct it cephalad. Redirect the catheter as needed and once the target level has been reached, turn the tip of the catheter toward the foramen (Fig 25A). Inject 0.5 to 1 mL of contrast to visualize the target nerve root. Make sure there is runoff of contrast out of the foramen (Fig 25B). Slowly instill 150 U of Hylenex dissolved in 5 mL of preservative-free normal saline. Follow this with 1 to 2 mL of additional contrast and observe for "opening up" of the "scarred in" nerve root. Give a 2 mL test dose of a 6 mL solution of LA/S. Our combination is 5 mL of 0.2% ropivicaine and 4 mg of dexamethasone. If after 5 minutes there is no evidence of intrathecal or intravascular spread, inject the remaining 4 mL. Remove the needle, and secure and dress the catheter as previously described. Once 20 minutes have passed since the last dose of LA/S solution and there is no evidence of a subarachnoid or subdural block, start an infusion of 5 mL of hypertonic saline over 30 minutes. At the end of the infusion, flush the catheter with 1 to 2 mL of preservative-free normal saline and cap the catheter.

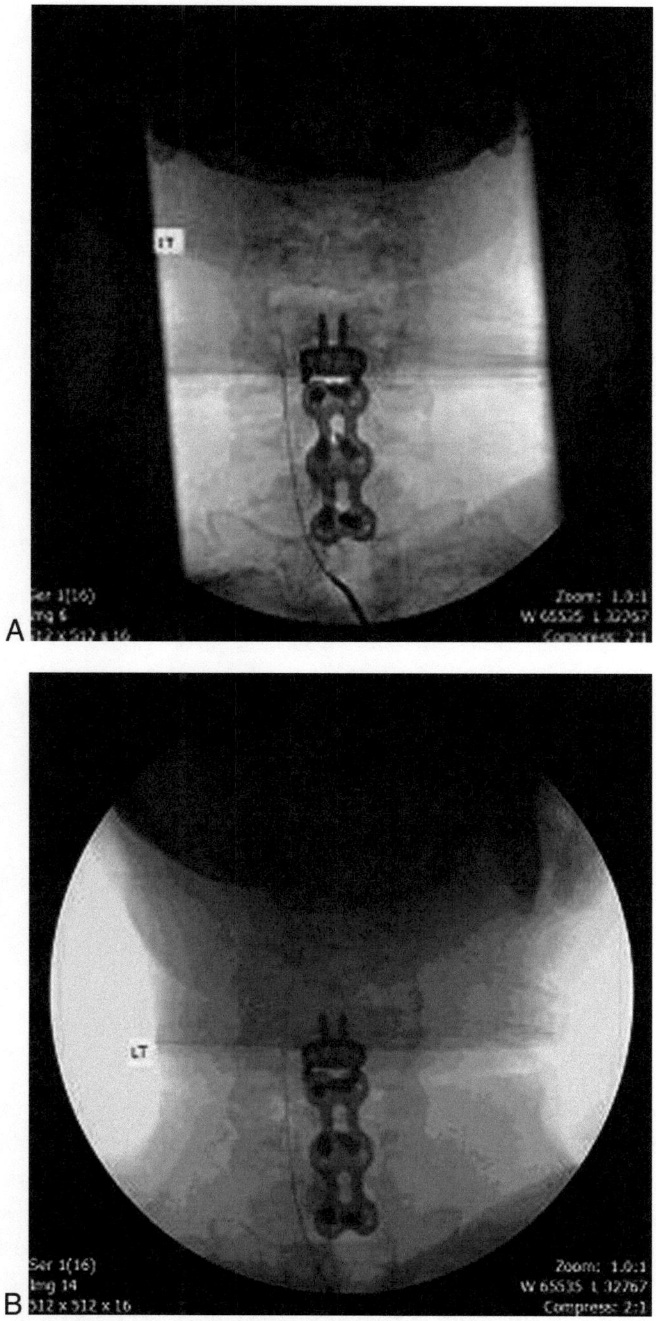

Fig. 25. A & B. **A** Cervical left ventral lateral catheter to the upper level of fusion C5-7. **B** Cervical-left ventral lateral catheter threaded to above level of fusion of C4. The dye injection spreads cephalad and lateral.

The second and third infusions are performed on the next day with 6 mL of 0.2% ropivacaine without spread and 5 mL of hypertonic saline using the same technique and precautions described for the first infusion. The catheter is removed and prophylactic antibiotics are prescribed. Clinic follow-up is 30 days.

15. Thoracic lysis of adhesions

The technique for entry into the thoracic epidural space for adhesiolysis is identical to that for the cervical region. Always remember the 3-D technique. Make sure to get a true lateral when checking the depth of the needle. This can be obtained by superimposing the rib shadows on one another. The target is still the ventrolateral epidural space with the tip of the catheter in the foramen of the desired level. The major difference for thoracic lysis compared to the caudal and cervical techniques is the volumes of the various injectates. Volumes of 8 mL are used for the contrast, Hylenex, LA/S, and hypertonic saline. (Table 1) lists typical infusion volumes for epidural adhesiolysis.

	Contrast	Hyaluronidase and Normal Saline	Local Anesthetic and Steroid	10% Hypertonic Saline Infusion
Caudal	10 mL	10 mL	10 mL	10 mL
Caudal and transforaminal	5 mL in each catheter	5 mL in each catheter	5 mL in each catheter	8 mL in caudal catheter and 4 mL in transforaminal catheter
Thoracic	8 mL	8 mL	8 mL	8 mL
Cervical	5 mL	6 mL	6 mL	5 mL

Table 1. Typical Infusion Volumes for Epidural Adhesiolysis

16. Neural flossing

The protocol for epidural adhesiolysis has been aided by neural flossing exercises that were designed to mobilize nerve roots by "sliding" them in and out of the foramen (Fig 26). This breaks up weakened scar tissue from the procedure and prevents further scar tissue deposition. If these exercises are done effectively three to four times per day for a few months after the procedure, the formation of scar tissue will be severely restricted.

In patients with multilevel radiculopathy and complex pain, it can be difficult to determine from where the majority of the pain is emanating. We have been using a technique that we have termed *mapping* to locate the most painful nerve root with stimulation and then carry out the adhesiolysis at that level. There are several references in the literature regarding the use of stimulation to confirm epidural placement of a catheter and for nerve root localization.[35] The TunL Kath and the TunL-XL catheter can be used as stimulating catheters to identify the nerve root(s).

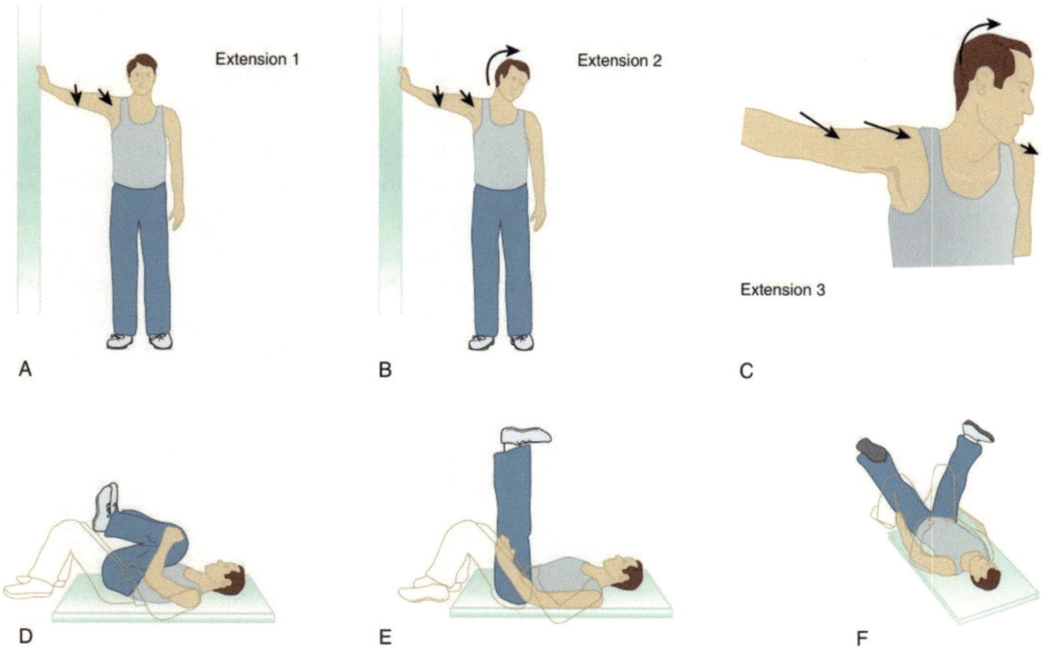

Fig. 26. **A-F Neural flossing exercises. A,** Standing erect, firmly grasp a stable surface (e.g., a door frame) with outstretched arm. Press elbow and shoulder forward. **B,** Next, slowly tilt head in opposite direction from outstretched arm to achieve gentle tension. **C,** Finally, rotate chin toward opposite shoulder as is comfortable. Hold this final position for approximately 20 to 30 seconds. **D,** Lay down supine on an exercise mat without a pillow. Slowly bring both knees close to the chest with bent legs and hold this position for 20 seconds. Release and assume a neutral position. **E,** Again in supine position, raise both legs to 90 degrees, with knees straight while laying flat on a firm surface. Hold for 20 seconds. Assume a neutral position and rest briefly. **F,** Bring both legs to a 90-degree angle while lying supine. Slowly spread legs in a V shape, as much as is comfortable, and hold for 20 seconds.**Epidural Mapping**

After entering the epidural space, advance the catheter into the ventrolateral epidural space past the suspected target level. Make sure the tip of the catheter is pointing laterally toward the foramina, just below the pedicle. Pull the catheter stylet back approximately 1 cm. Using alligator clips, attach the cathode to the stylet and ground the anode on the needle or ground pad or a 22-gauge needle inserted into the skin. Apply electrical stimulation with a stimulator box with a rate of 50 pulses per second and a pulse width of 450 milliseconds, dialing up the amplitude until a paresthesia is perceived in small increments, usually less than 2 or 3 volts. Inquire of the patient as to whether or not the paresthesia is felt in the area of the patient's recognized greatest pain. This process is repeated at each successive level until the most painful nerve root is identified. Once identified, the adhesiolysis is carried out at that level. The mapping procedure is also useful to identify the optimal site of surgery either before the first surgery or when surgery has failed one or more times.

17. Complications

As with any invasive procedure, complications are possible. These include bleeding, infection, headache, damage to nerves or blood vessels, catheter shearing, bowel/bladder dysfunction, paralysis, spinal cord compression from loculation of the injected fluids or hematoma, subdural or subarachnoid injection of local anesthetic or hypertonic saline, and reactions to the medications used. We also include on the consent form that the patient may experience an increase in pain or no pain relief at all. Although the potential list of complications is long, the frequency of complications is very rare. However, there is clearly a learning curve, and recent studies reflect this by the significantly improved long-term outcome and the very rare publications of complications and medicolegal consequences when one considers the ever-increasing clinical experience.
Subdural spread is a complication that should always be watched for when injecting local anesthetic. During the caudal adhesiolysis, particularly if the catheter is advanced along the midline, subdural catheter placement is a risk (Figs 27 and 28). Identification of the subdural motor block should occur within 16 to 18 minutes. Catheters used for adhesiolysis should never be directed midline in the epidural space.

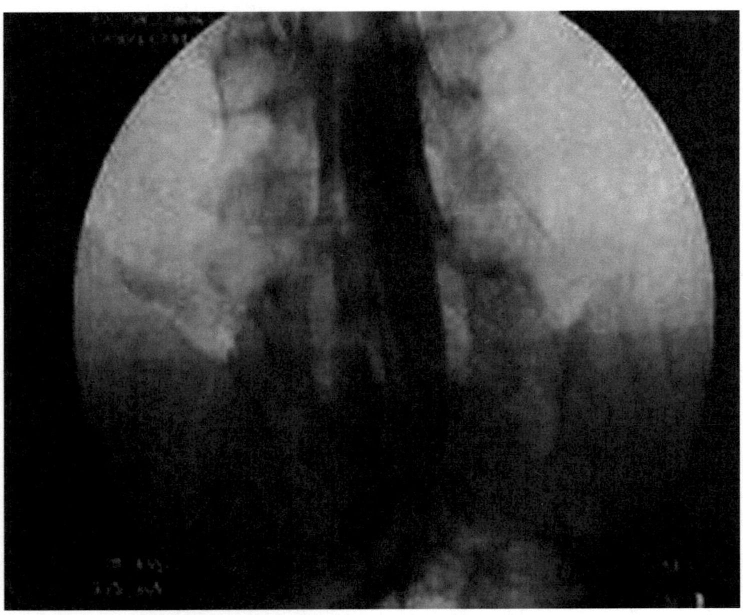

Fig. 27. Midline catheter placement enters subdural space. There is also some epidural dye spread. But the patient starts to complain of bilateral leg pain.

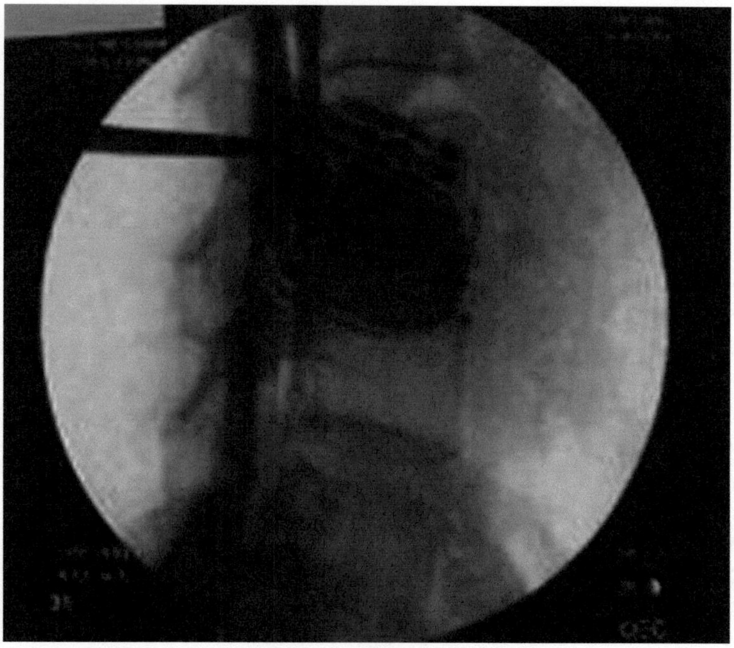

Fig. 28. A 22-gauge spinal needle and extension set with syringe placed in the subdural space and 12 mL fluid aspirated. The patient reported immediate reversal of bilateral leg pain. Note the dye in the extension tubing and syringe at the 7-o'clock position.

18. Outcomes

Initially in the early 1980s the protocol was designed to direct site-specific medication onto the dorsal root ganglion; however, after performing a number of the procedures, it was found that the dorsal root ganglion was exceptionally hard to reach secondary to developing scar tissue or adhesions. In the early days, our understanding was coming from the use of local anesthetics for surgery giving a 2- to 4-hour block for the surgeon to operate. It was gratifying to see chronic pain patients get months and years of pain relief following the placement of the new steerable x-ray visible catheter. The early report in 1985 by Racz et al[36] described the use of phenol at the dorsal root ganglion followed by an observational listing of outcomes that were clearly not as good as the latest studies on failed back surgery and spinal stenosis showing 75% to 80% improvement at 12 months' follow-up by Manchikanti.[34] Initially we were pleased to see some patients getting 3 to 4 months of relief and report seeing recovery of footdrops. This philosophy still proves to be true even in studies in 2008 by Sakai et al [37] in which they found that adhesiolysis with catheter-directed steroid and local anesthetic injection during epiduroscopy alleviated pain and reduced sensory nerve dysfunction in patients with chronic sciatica. The evolution of these findings has changed the process into what it is today.[38] Racz and Holubec first reported on epidural adhesiolysis in 1989.[39] There were slight variations in the protocol compared to today's protocol, namely the dose of local anesthetic and the fact that hyaluronidase was not used. Catheter placement was lesion-specific (i.e., the tip of the catheter was placed in the foramen corresponding to the vertebral level and side of the suspected adhesions). The retrospective analysis conducted 6 to 12 months after the procedure reported initial pain relief in 72.2% of patients ($N = 72$) at time of discharge. Relief was sustained in 37.5% and 30.5% of patients at 1 and 3 months, respectively. Forty-three percent decreased their frequency and dosage of medication use and 16.7% discontinued their medications altogether. In total, 30.6% of patients returned to work or returned to daily functions. In April 1990, at a presentation of the 7th IASP World Congress on Pain in Adelaide, Austraila, Arthur et al[40] reported on epidural adhesiolysis in 100 patients, 50 of whom received hyaluronidase as part of the procedure. In the hyaluronidase group, 81.6% of the participants had initial pain relief, with 12.3% having persistent relief; 68% of the no hyaluronidase group had relief of pain, with 14% having persistent relief at the end of the 3-year follow-up period from which the study sample was randomly selected.

In 1994 Stolker et al[41] added hyaluronidase to the procedure, but omitted the hypertonic saline. In a study of 28 patients, they reported greater than 50% pain reduction in 64% of patients at 1 year. They stressed the importance of the patient selection and believed that the effectiveness of adhesiolysis was based on the effect of the hyaluronidase on the adhesions and the action of the local anesthetic and steroids on the sinuvertebral nerve.

Devulder et al[42] published a study of 34 patients with failed back surgery syndrome in whom epidural fibrosis was suspected or proved with MRI.[42] An epidural catheter was inserted via the sacral hiatus to a distance of 10 cm into the caudal canal. Injections of contrast dye, local anesthetic, corticosteroid, and hypertonic saline (10%) were carried out daily for 3 days. No hyaluronidase was used. Filling defects were noted in 30 of 34 patients, but significant pain relief was noted in only 7 patients at 1 month, 2 patients at 3 months, and no patients at 12 months. They concluded that epidurography may confirm epidural filling defects for contrast dye in patients with filling defects, but a better contrast dye spread, assuming scar lysis does not guarantee sustained pain relief. This study was criticized for lack of lesion-specific catheter placement resulting in nonspecific drug delivery.[43] The catheter was never directed to the ventral lateral epidural space where the dorsal root ganglion is located and the lateral recess scarring occurs.

Heavner et al[44] performed a prospective randomized trial of lesion-specific epidural adhesiolysis on 59 patients with chronic intractable low back pain. The patients were assigned to one of four epidural adhesiolysis treatment groups: (1) hypertonic (10%) saline plus hyaluronidase, (2) hypertonic saline, (3) isotonic (0.9%) saline, or (4) isotonic saline plus hyaluronidase. All treatment groups received corticosteroid and local anesthetic. Overall, across all four treatment groups, 83% of patients had significant pain relief at 1 month compared to 49% at 3 months, 43% at 6 months, and 49% at 12 months. The hyaluronidase and the hypertonic saline study group had a much lower incidence of additional need for pain procedures than the placebo groups, showing that site-specific catheter placement is important. Active substances and preservative free normal saline were blinded for the placebo effect.

Manchikanti et al[45] performed a retrospective randomized evaluation of a modified Racz adhesiolysis protocol in 232 patients with low back pain. The study involved lesion specific catheter placement, but the usual 3-day procedure was reduced to a 2-day (group 1) or a 1-day (group 2) procedure. Group 1 had 103 patients and group 2 had 129 patients. Other changes included changing the local anesthetic from bupivacaine to lidocaine, substituting methylprednisolone acetate or betamethasone acetate and phosphate for triamcinolone diacetate, and reduction of the volume of injectate. Of the patients in groups 1 and 2, 62% and 58% had greater than 50% pain relief at 1 month, respectively, with these percentages decreasing to 22% and 11% at 3 months, 8% and 7% at 6 months, and 2% and 3% at 1 year. Of significant interest is that the percentage of patients receiving greater than 50% pain relief after four procedures increased to 79% and 90% at 1 month, 50% and 36% at 3 months, 29% and 19% at 6 months, and 7% and 8% at 1 year for groups 1 and 2, respectively. Short-term relief of pain was demonstrated, but long-term relief was not.

Manchikanti, in 1999, evaluated two groups of randomly pulled, 150 patients for a 2-day reinjection procedure, and a second 150 patients for a one-day procedure out of a pool of 536 patients. It was concluded that repeat use of the one-day procedure is also cost effective when evaluated on a 12-month follow-up. The cost effectiveness indicated the lysis procedure to be superior to surgery or the rehabilitation activity program.[45]

In a randomized, prospective study, Manchikanti et al[46] evaluated a 1-day epidural adhesiolysis procedure against a control group of patients who received conservative therapy. Results showed that cumulative relief, defined as relief greater than 50% with one to three injections, in the treatment group was 97% at 3 months, 93% at 6 months, and 47% at 1 year. The study also showed that overall health status improved significantly in the adhesiolysis group. Conservative therapy consisted of physical therapy and medications.

In 2004 Manchikanti et al[47] published their results of a randomized, double-blind, controlled study on the effectiveness of 1-day lumbar adhesiolysis and hypertonic saline neurolysis in treatment of chronic low back pain. Seventy-five patients whose pain was unresponsive to conservative modalities were randomized into one of three treatment groups. Group 1 (control group) underwent catheterization where the catheter was in the sacral canal without adhesiolysis, followed by injection of local anesthetic, normal saline, and steroid. Group 2 consisted of catheterization with site-specific catheter placement being ventral-lateral for adhesiolysis, followed by injection of local anesthetic, normal saline, and steroid. Group 3 consisted of site-specific catheter placement for adhesiolysis, followed by injection of local anesthetic, hypertonic saline, and steroid. Patients were allowed to have additional injections based on the response, either after unblinding or without unblinding after 3 months. Patients without unblinding were offered either the assigned treatment or another treatment based on their response. If the patients in group 1 or 2 received adhesiolysis and injection and injection of hypertonic saline, they were considered withdrawn, and no subsequent data were collected. Outcomes were assessed at 3, 6, and 12 months using visual analog scale pain scores, Oswestry Disability Index, opioid intake, range-of-motion measurement, and P-3. Significant pain relief was defined as average relief of 50% or greater. Seventy-two percent of patients in group 3, 60% of patients in group 2, and 0% of patients in group 1 showed significant pain relief at 12 months. The average number of treatments for 1 year was 2.76 in group 2 and 2.16 in group 3. Duration of significant relief with the first procedure was 2.8 + 1.49 months and 3.8 + 3.37 months in groups 2 and 3, respectively. Significant pain relief (>50%) was also associated with improvement in Oswestry Disability Index, range of motion, and psychologic status.

Manchikanti et al[48,49,] furthered this research using comparisons of percutaneous adhesiolysis versus fluoroscopically guided caudal epidural steroid injections. The first study involved a population of patients with chronic low back pain and known spinal stenosis. The results showed a 76% reduction in pain relief at 1 year with epidural adhesiolysis compared to 4% in the control group. The second study performed in a population of patients with post-lumbar surgery syndrome showed a reduction in pain and improvement in functional status in 73% of the epidural adhesiolysis group compared to 12% in the control group.

In 2006 a study by Veihelmann et al[50] evaluated patients with a history of chronic low back pain and sciatica. Inclusion criteria were radicular pain with a corresponding nerve root compressing substrate found on MRI or CT. All patients were randomized to receive physiotherapy, analgesics, or lysis of adhesions. The lysis group had statistically significantly better outcome than the physical therapy treatment group.

Two other prospective evaluations by Chopra et al and Gerdesmeyer et al[51, 52] evaluated patients with monosegmental radiculopathy of the lumbar spine. All the patients suffered from chronic disk herniations or failed back syndrome. All these randomized trials showed positive short-term and long-term relief. Two prospective evaluations also showed positive short- and long-term relief.[51,52]

19. Conclusion

Epidural adhesiolysis has evolved over the years as an important treatment option for patients with intractable cervical, thoracic, and low back and leg pain. Studies show that patients are able to experience significant pain relief and restoration of function. Manchikanti's studies show that the amount and duration of relief can be achieved by repeat procedures. Recent prospective randomized double-blind studies on failed back surgery and spinal stenosis show 75% and 80% improvement in visual analog scale scores and functional improvements at 12 months' follow-up. There have been no negative studies to date where the lysis target was the ventral-lateral epidural space. The one negative study used a 10 cm sacral mid-canal catheter placement which was non-target specific.[43] This negative study was subsequently used as the placebo group in a study performed by Manchikanti.[47] Manchikanti's study consisted of 3 treatment groups: placebo (sacral mid-canal catheter placement), target specific ventral-lateral epidural without hypertonic saline and target specific ventral-lateral epidural with hypertonic saline . The later two treatment groups had positive outcomes with the hypertonic saline group superior; whereas, the placebo group did not. [47] The evolution in the recognition of the site-specific importance of the catheter and medication delivery together with the fact that physicians need to acquire the skills to be able to carry out the procedure led to the improved outcomes seen in recent prospective randomized studies.

The management of failed back surgery syndrome and post laminectomy syndrome will likely continue to be controversial among the multitude of practitioners who treat these patients. However, in experienced hands, it is established as a reasonable option for many patients.

Percutaneous neuroplasty via a transforaminal approach evolved from the caudal approach. Lysis of adhesions via the caudal approach involves introducing a catheter through the sacral hiatus and advancing it to the affected nerve root in the ventral-lateral epidural space. On the other hand, transforaminal percutaneous neuroplasty achieves a midline catheter placement in the epidural space that is able to target the two most heavily innervated structures in the spine—the posterior annulus fibrosus and the posterior longitudinal ligament.[5] Apart from a surgical approach, the ventral epidural structures have been otherwise inaccessible.

Endoscopy offers direct visualization of the affected nerve roots in addition to mechanical adhesiolysis, and may become more mainstream as the technique is refined.

Facet pain is commonly associated with the postlysis period or after provocative testing a month or so later if two-facet diagnostic blocks show efficacy. In addition to epidural lysis of adhesions, the combined use of radiofrequency facet denervation gives us the best long-term outcome.

Epidural adhesiolysis has been accepted as a treatment for post laminectomy syndrome, failed back syndrome, and cervical and thoracic radicular syndromes. Additional studies are underway to further refine the technique and indications. The combined use of long term patient education for neural flossing exercises and the inclusion of the facet delayed treatment in the algorithm further improves patient outcome. The identification of back pain provocation by saline injection and the successful use of percutaneous neuroplasty in the treatment represents hopeful promise for a cost effective treatment of back pain.

20. Acknowledgements

Racz GB, Day MR, Heavner JE, Scott J. *Lysis of Epidural Adhesions.* In: Waldman S, ed. *Pain Management, 2nd Edition*. Elsevier; 2011: 1258-1272.

Racz GB, Day MR, Heavner JE, Smith JP. The Racz Procedure: Lysis of Epidural Adhesions (Percutaneous Neuroplasty). In: Deer T, ed. The AAPM Text of Pain Medicine. Springer; 2011.

The authors would also like to thank Marzieh N. Brown and Paula Brashear for their assistance in the editing of this chapter.

21. References

[1] Lawrence R., Helmick C., Arnett F., et al: Estimates of the prevalence of arthritis and selected musculoskeletal disorders in the United States. *Arthritis Rheum* 1998; 41(5):778-799.

[2] Straus B.: Chronic pain of spinal origin: the costs of intervention. *Spine* 2002; 27(22):2614-2619.

[3] National Center for Health Statistics : *National hospital discharge survey*, Washington, DC, US Department of Health and Human Services, Centers for Disease Control and Prevention, 1990. Report no. PB92-500818

[4] Van Zundert J.: *Personal communication*. 2005.

[5] Kuslich S., Ulstrom C., Michael C.: The tissue origin of low back pain and sciatica. *Orthop Clin North Am* 1991; 22:181-187.

[6] Racz G., Noe C., Heavner J.: Selective spinal injections for lower back pain. *Curr Rev Pain* 1999; 3:333-341.

[7] Anderson S.: A rationale for the treatment algorithm of failed back surgery syndrome. *Curr Rev Pain* 2000; 4:396-406.

[8] Pawl R.: Arachnoiditis and epidural fibrosis: the relationship to chronic pain. *Curr Rev Pain* 1998; 2:93-99.

[9] Cervellini P., Curri D., Volpin L., et al: Computed tomography of epidural fibrosis after discectomy: a comparison between symptomatic and asymptomatic patients. *Neurosurgery* 1988; 23(6):710-713.

[10] Manchikanti L., Staats P., Singh V.: Evidence-based practice guidelines for interventional techniques in the management of chronic spinal pain. *Pain Phys* 2003; 6:3-81.

[11] LaRocca H., Macnab I.: The laminectomy membrane: studies in its evolution, characteristics, effects and prophylaxis in dogs. *J Bone Joint Surg* 1974; 5613:545-550.

[12] Cooper R., Freemont A., Hoyland J., et al: Herniated intervertebral disc–associated periradicular fibrosis and vascular abnormalities occur without inflammatory cell infiltration. *Spine* 1995; 20:591-598.

[13] McCarron R., Wimpee M., Hudkins P., et al: The inflammatory effects of nucleus pulposus; a possible element in the pathogenesis of low back pain. *Spine* 1987; 12:760-764.

[14] Parke W., Watanabe R.: Adhesions of the ventral lumbar dura: an adjunct source of discogenic pain?. *Spine* 1990; 15:300-303.

[15] Viesca C., Racz G., Day M.: Special techniques in pain management: lysis of adhesions. *Anesthesiol Clin North Am* 2003; 21:745-766.

[16] Songer M., Ghosh L., Spencer D.: Effects of sodium hyaluronate on peridural fibrosis after lumber laminectomy and discectomy. *Spine* 1990; 15:550-554.

[17] Key J., Ford L.: Experimental intervertebral disc lesions. *J Bone Joint Surg Am* 1948; 30:621-630.

[18] Olmarker K., Rydevik B.: Pathophysiology of sciatica. *Orthop Clin North Am* 1991; 22:223-233.

[19] Ross J., Robertson J., Frederickson R., et al: Association between peridural scar and recurrent radicular pain after lumbar discectomy; magnetic resonance evaluation. *Neurosurgery* 1996; 38:855-863.

[20] Gilbert K., Brismee J., Collins D., et al: Lumbosacral nerve roots displacements and strain: part 1. A novel measurement technique during straight leg raise in unembalmed calavers. *Spine* 2007; 32(14):1513-1520.Phila Pa 1976

[21] Heavner JE, Chokhavatia S, Kizelshteyn G: Percutaneous evaluation of the epidural and subarachnoid space with a flexible fiberscope, *Reg Anesth* 1991;15:85.

[22] Bosscher HA, Heavner JE: Incidence and severity of epidural fibrosis after back surgery: an endoscopic study, *Pain Pract* 2010; 10: 18-24.

[23] Hatten Jr H.: Lumbar epidurography with metrizamide. *Radiology* 1980; 137:129-136.

[24] Stewart H., Quinnell R., Dann N.: Epidurography in the management of sciatica. *Br J Rheumatol* 1987; 26(6):424-429.

[25] Devulder J., Bogaert L., Castille F., et al: Relevance of epidurography and epidural adhesiolysis in chronic failed back surgery patients. *Clin J Pain* 1995; 11:147-150.

[26] Manchikanti L., Bakhit C., Pampati V.: Role of epidurography in caudal neuroplasty. *Pain Digest* 1998; 8:277-281.

[27] Day M., Racz G.: Technique of caudal neuroplasty. *Pain Digest* 1999; 9(4):255-257.

[28] Horlocker T., Wedel D., Benzon H., et al: Regional anesthesia in the anticoagulated patient: defining the risks (the second ASRA Consensus Conference on Neuraxial Anesthesia and Anticoagulation). *Reg Anesth Pain Med* 2003; 28:172-197.

[29] *Omnipaque product insert*, Princeton, NJ, Nycomed, Inc.

[30] *Isovue product insert*, Princeton, NJ, Bracco Diagnostics, Inc.

[31] *Hypaque product insert*, Princeton, NJ, Amersham Health, Inc.

[32] *Conray product insert*, Phillipsburg, NJ, Mallinckrodt, Inc.

[33] Racz G., Day M., Heavner J., et al: Hyaluronidase: a review of approved formulations, indications and off-label use in chronic pain management. *Expert Opin Biol Ther* 2010; 10(1):127-131.

[34] Racz G.B., Heavner J.E.: Cervical spinal canal loculation and secondary ischemic cord injury—PVCS—perivenous counter spread—danger sign!!. *Pain Pract* 2008; 8:399-403.

[35] Larkin T., Carragee E., Cohen S.: A novel technique for delivery of epidural steroids and diagnosing the level of nerve root pathology. *J Spinal Disord Tech* 2003; 16(2):186-192.

[36] Racz G.B., Sabonghy M., Gintautas J., et al: Intractable pain therapy using a new type of epidural catheter. *JAMA* 1985; 248:579-580.

[37] Sakai T., Aoki H., Hojo M., et al: Adhesiolysis and targeted steroid/local anesthetic injection during epiduroscopy alleviates pain and reduces sensory nerve dysfunction in patients with chronic sciatica. *J Anesth* 2008; 22(3):242-247.

[38] Anderson S., Racz G., Heavner J.: Evolution of epidural lysis of adhesions. *Pain Physician* 2000; 3(3):262-270.

[39] Racz G., Holubec J.: *Lysis of adhesions in the epidural space.* In: Raj P., ed. *Techniques of neurolysis*, Boston: Kluwer Academic; 1989:57-72.

[40] Arthur J., Racz G., Heinrich R., et al: *Epidural space: identification of filling defects and lysis of adhesions in the treatment of chronic painful conditions. Abstracts of the 7th World Congress on Pain*, Paris: IASP Publications; 1993.

[41] Stolker R., Vervest A., Gerbrand J.: The management of chronic spinal pain by blockades: a revew. *Pain* 1994; 58:1-19.

[42] Devulder J., Bogaert L., Castille F., et al: Relevance of epidurography and epidural adhesiolysis in chonic failed back surgery patients. *Clin J Pain* 1995; 11:147-150.

[43] Racz G., Heavner J.: In response to article by Drs. Devulder et al. *Clin J Pain* 1995; 11:151-154.

[44] Heavner J., Racz G., Raj P.: Percutaneous epidural neuroplasty: prospective evaluation of 0.9% saline versus 10% saline with or without hyaluronidase. *Reg Anesth Pain Med* 1999; 24:202-207.

[45] Manchikanti L., Pakanati R., Bakhit C., et al: Role of adhesiolysis and hypertonic saline neurolysis in management of low back pain: evaluation of modification of the Racz protocol. *Pain Digest* 1999; 9:91-96.

[46] Manchikanti L., Pampati V., Fellow B., et al: Role of one day epidural adhesiolysis in management of chronic low back pain: a randomized clinical trial. *Pain Phys* 2001; 4:153-166.

[47] Manchikanti L., Rivera J., Pampati V., et al: One day lumbar adhesiolysis and hypertonic saline neurolysis in treatment of chronic low back pain: a randomized, double-blinded trial. *Pain Phys* 2004; 7:177-186.

[48] Manchikanti L., Cash K., McManus C., et al: The preliminary results of a comparative effectiveness of adhesiolysis and caudal epidural injections in managing chronic low back pain secondary to spinal stenosis. *Pain Phys* 2009; 12(6):E341-E354.

[49] Manchikanti L., Singh V., Cash K., et al: A comparative effectiveness evaluation of percutaneous adhesiolysis and epidural steroid injections in managing lumbar post surgery syndrome. *Pain Phys* 2009; 12(6):E355-E368.

[50] Veihelmann A., Devens C., Trouiller H., et al: Epidural neuroplasty versus physiotherapy to relieve pain in patients with sciatica: a prospective randomized blinded clinical trial. *J Orthop Sci* 2006; 11(4):365-369.

[51] Gerdesmeyer L., Lampe R., Veihelmann A., et al: Chronic radiculopathy: use of minimally invasive percutaneous epidural neurolysis according to Racz. *Der Schmerz* 2005; 19:285-295.

[52] Gerdesmeyer L., Rechl H., Wagenpfeil S., et al: Minimally invasive epidural neurolysis in chronic radiculopathy: a prospective controlled study to prove effectiveness. *Der Orhopade* 2003; 32:869-876.

18

Chronic Pain in People with Physically Disabling Conditions: A Review of the Application of Biopsychosocial Models

Kathryn Nicholson Perry
University of Western Sydney, Australia

1. Introduction

There are a wide range of conditions which can result in physical disabilities, affecting more than a billion people or approximately 15% of the population worldwide (World Health Organisation, 2011). Disability is an umbrella term for the restrictions and impairments arising from the interaction between an individual with a health condition and the environment (World Health Organisation, 2011). The physical conditions from which disability arises are diverse and heterogeneous, but include both diseases, such as multiple sclerosis, as well as traumatic and non-traumatic injuries, including spinal cord injury and brain injuries. Research concerning the occurrence of chronic pain (defined as pain persisting beyond the period of healing, usually operationalized as three or six months) among people with physical disabilities, and the impact upon those individuals affected, is relatively limited compared to that focusing on primary pain conditions, such as low back pain. Within the available literature the focus is largely biomedical, with the majority of available research exploring biological factors and medical interventions. A great deal has been gained in the management of primary pain conditions through investigating psychological and social factors, and developing interventions such as cognitive behavioural pain management programs to target these factors. This chapter will describe the current understanding of the role of psychological and social factors in understanding the experience of chronic pain in the context of a physically disabling condition, and the use of interventions addressing these factors in this population.

2. The nature of chronic pain in people with physically disabling conditions

What is known about the nature of chronic pain among those with physically disabling conditions varies depending on the condition of interest. An examination of those publishing in the area suggests that often there are only a small number of groups involved in this research. Most of these research groups only work with one specific condition, with only a very small number working across a range of physically disabling conditions. As a result of these research silos, there are many inconsistencies in the approaches taken in investigating pain in the different conditions. Interpreting the findings of this body of work, particularly attempting to make comparisons across conditions, should therefore be done with caution keeping in mind some important caveats. First, there are variations across studies concerning the nature of the pain conditions which are the subject of investigation, including the duration of the pain condition being explored. Some studies focus on chronic pain (with various criterion applied, commonly either three or six months duration), where others report on episodic, procedural or acute pain or do not specify which type of pain participants are experiencing. Second, some studies restrict their attention to pain thought to be specific to the physically disabling condition in question (such as headaches in those with traumatic brain injury), putting aside those deemed to be general (such as low back pain) which may be overlooked by teams specialising in a specific disabling condition rather than pain itself (Ivanhoe & Hartman, 2004). Finally, studies draw samples from a number of different populations including community samples, membership organisations for people with the physically disabling condition in question, and clinical services, including tertiary services for either pain or a specific physically disabling condition. There are also the usual methodological issues associated with the use of cross-sectional designs and the inevitable reliance upon self-report measures which is a hallmark of this area of research. Despite these issues, there is increasing evidence of a significant prevalence of chronic pain among those with physically disabling conditions.

2.1 Injury related conditions

Injury related conditions for which there is data regarding the nature of chronic pain includes those with a traumatic onset, such as traumatic brain injury and spinal cord injury, and those with a non-traumatic onset, such as cerebral palsy which is thought to be due to an injury to the developing brain. The kinds of traumatic events from which these injuries arise, such as motor vehicle accidents and sporting injuries, may mean that the individual has acquired multiple injuries which may complicate the assessment of the relationship between specific pain conditions and the physically disabling condition of interest.

2.1.1 Traumatic brain injury

Specific pain conditions of interest among those with traumatic brain injury include headaches of various types, but others noted include complex regional pain syndrome (CRPS), heterotopic ossification, and pain due to spasticity (Ivanhoe & Hartman, 2004; Nampiaparampil, 2008). A recent systematic review of chronic pain among those with traumatic brain injury identified 23 studies meeting their criteria, from which they estimated the overall prevalence of chronic pain in people with traumatic brain injury at 51.5% among civilians, with 57.8% reporting chronic headache (Nampiaparampil, 2008). An interesting aspect of findings among this group is that prevalence of chronic headaches differs depending on the severity of the traumatic brain injury (Lahz & Bryant, 1996; Nampiaparampil, 2008), with higher prevalence reported among those with mild traumatic brain injury. It has been observed that those with traumatic brain injury may have other traumatic injuries, and studies regarding the pain conditions in this poly-trauma group are very limited (Dobscha, et al., 2009). The assessment of pain in those with traumatic brain injury, particularly those with severe enough injuries to result in significant impairments to cognition, language or behaviour, may be challenging and so result in less accurate estimates than in some other groups with physically disabling conditions.

2.1.2 Spinal cord injury

Relative to other conditions, there have been a larger number of studies examining chronic pain among those with spinal cord injury. Classifying the pain conditions associated with spinal cord injury has been undertaken by a number of groups, with more concordance among the groups in relation to some pain types than others, such as neuropathic pains (Cardenas, Felix, Cardenas, & Felix, 2009; Finnerup, Baastrup, & Jensen, 2009; Siddall, Yezierski, & Loeser, 2000). A recent systematic review of the prevalence of chronic pain of all causes among those with traumatic spinal cord injury have identified more than forty high quality studies from across the world, but the authors note that despite this there are many contradictions and unanswered questions about the nature of chronic pain in this group (Dijkers, Bryce, & Zanca, 2009). Prevalence rates of the studies included ranged from 26 to 98 percent, but the authors cautioned that the heterogeneity of the studies involved precluded calculation of an overall prevalence rate. It should be noted that co-morbid traumatic brain injury are not uncommon among this group, often within the mild range (Bradbury, et al., 2008). While spinal cord injury has been included in the section on traumatic injuries, some spinal cord injuries develop as a result of disease activity, such as cancer, which may mean the individual experiences other chronic pain conditions. As with many other physically disabling conditions, pain is only one of many troublesome complications. However, a recent study found that relative to others it is the most common and is closely associated with functioning (Jensen, Kuehn, Amtmann, & Cardenas, 2007).

2.1.3 Amputation

Studies of pain post-amputation are largely related to either upper or lower limb amputations. Most studies report on traumatically acquired amputations, although those related to vascular or other conditions are also relatively common. The most common type of pain problems reported in these studies is phantom limb pain and residual (or stump) pain, although it is also possible for people to develop musculoskeletal pain following amputation, for example in the back (Hammarlund, Carlström, Melchior, & Persson, 2011; Kooijman, Dijkstra, Geertzen, Elzinga, & van der Schans, 2000). Prevalence estimates suggest that phantom limb pain occurs in approximately 45 to 80% of people post-amputation, depending partly upon whether those with upper or lower limb amputations are considered, with rates of residual pain similarly high but varying (Behr, et al., 2009; Desmond & Maclachlan, 2010; Dijkstra, et al., 2002; Ehde, et al., 2000; Kooijman, et al., 2000; Schley, et al., 2008).

2.1.4 Cerebral palsy

In contrast to many of the other physically disabling conditions upon which this chapter focuses, research on cerebral palsy related pain is not confined to studies of adults. The common use of registries in a number of countries also means that the populations from which samples are drawn are more complete than in many other conditions. A French study of adults with cerebral palsy found that 75% reported pain of any sort (Gallien, et al., 2007). Musculoskeletal pain has been the subject of most investigation among this population. Prevalence estimates range from approximately one third to two thirds, with the pattern of distribution across the body different depending on the type of cerebral palsy (Engel, Jensen, Hoffman, & Kartin, 2003; Jahnsen, Villien, Aamodt, Stanghelle, & Holm, 2004; Schwartz, Engel, & Jensen, 1999; Vogtle, 2009). Although studies of children are more common in this group, they are limited by a number of factors regarding the measurement of pain and often rely on parental report. However, the available studies suggest 50 to 75 % of children are affected by pain, with approximately one third experiencing moderate to severe pain (Parkinson, Gibson, Dickinson, & Colver, 2010; Russo, Miller, Haan, Cameron, & Crotty, 2008).

2.2 Disease related conditions

Chronic pain has been investigated in the context of a range of diseases which are associated with physical disability. Some of the central pains, such as central post-stroke pain, associated with these conditions have only been recognized relatively recently, and have been subject to intense investigation.

2.2.1 Multiple sclerosis

A range of pain conditions, both general and specific, have been reported in people with multiple sclerosis. These include those related to spasm, neuropathic pains of various types (including trigeminal neuralgia and L'hermitte's sign), back pain and headaches. A recent systematic review of pain among people with multiple sclerosis found twenty-one studies reporting pain prevalence, with an overall range of 29 to 86%, and with few consistent findings related to the relationship between the report of pain and multiple sclerosis characteristics (O'Connor, Schwid, Herrmann, Markman, & Dworkin, 2008). Further, this study reported that between 11 and 23% of people reported pain as a symptom at the onset of their multiple sclerosis. Central pain, including trigeminal neuralgia, has been reported in approximately one third of people with MS (Osterberg, Boivie, & Thuomas, 2005).

2.2.2 Stroke

A number of chronic pain conditions are observed in people who have had a stroke, including shoulder pain, spasticity related pain and headaches, and central post-stroke pain is a uncommon condition particular to stroke. Estimates of the prevalence of chronic pain between studies are variable. Approximately 11 to 21% of people following a first stroke have been reported to have a stroke related pain condition up to 16 months following the stroke (Appelros, 2006; Jonsson, Lindgren, Hallstrom, Norrving, & Lindgren, 2006; Lundstrom, Smits, Terent, & Borg, 2009), whereas 42% of people following stroke attending an out-patient rehabilitation clinic had chronic musculoskeletal pain (Kong, Woon, & Yang, 2004). Neuropathic and central pain conditions occur at a significant level among those who have had a stroke, including estimates of complex regional pain syndrome in 15% of those undergoing inpatient post-stroke rehabilitation and 7% with central poststroke pain (Kitisomprayoonkul, Sungkapo, Taveemanoon, & Chaiwanichsiri, 2010; Klit, Finnerup, Andersen, & Jensen, 2011).

2.2.3 Parkinson's Disease

Relatively little is known about the prevalence and nature of pain in people with Parkinson's Disease, although clinically it is reported to be observed frequently (Beiske & Loge, 2009). Ford (2010) has classified pain problems associated with Parkinson's Disease in five categories: musculoskeletal pain; radicular or neuropathic pain; dystonia-related pain; akathitic discomfort; and central or primary pain. Overall estimates of the prevalence of pain in this group range between and 40 and 83% (Beiske & Loge, 2009; Ford, 2010). Pain has been reported to be the first reported symptom of Parkinson's Disease among a significant minority of those who initially present with non-motor symptoms (O'Sullivan, et al., 2008).

2.2.4 Muscular dystrophy

Duchenne muscular dystrophy, myotonic muscular dystrophy, type I and facioscapulohumeral muscular dystrophy have all been found to be associated with chronic pain (Engel, Kartin, Carter, Jensen, & Jaffe, 2009; Jensen, Abresch, Carter, & McDonald, 2005; Jensen, et al., 2008; Miro, et al., 2009) although there are limited studies with these groups. More than half of the respondents in these studies reported the presence of chronic pain, with pain in the back and legs most commonly reported but with a large number of sites reported to be involved.

2.3 Summary

Although not a comprehensive review of all of those physically disabling conditions which may result in the experience of chronic pain, the above summary suggests that chronic pain is a relatively common but perhaps neglected consequence of physically disabling conditions (Osterberg, et al., 2005). The specific causes and the nature of chronic pain experienced may differ between physically disabling conditions, but its high prevalence indicates that it is a legitimate concern for health practitioners and researchers. Awareness of the likelihood of pain is a necessary, although not sufficient, condition for the effective management of such pain. There is evidence that there are misconceptions among health professionals about the likely occurrence of pain in those with physically disabling conditions (Piwko, et al., 2007). Indeed, studies of people with pain associated with various conditions, including spinal cord injury, cerebral palsy, and multiple sclerosis, indicate that those affected perceive the available treatments and access to them to be inadequate (Cardenas, et al., 2009; Henwood & Ellis, 2004; Kennedy, Lude, & Taylor, 2006; Pollmann, Feneberg, & Erasmus, 2004; Wartan, Hamann, Wedley, & McColl, 1997). In addition, the economic costs of pain among those with physically disabling conditions appears to be large, with a Canadian study estimating that the cost of pain among people multiple sclerosis over a 6 month period was Can$80 million (Piwko, et al., 2007).

3. Psychological and social factors in chronic pain among those with physically disabling conditions

Biopsychosocial models of pain, which are characterized by a focus on the interaction between biological, psychological and social variables in the pain experience, dominate the contemporary understanding of primary pain conditions, such as headache and low back pain (Gatchel, Peng, Peters, Fuchs, & Turk, 2007). The use of biopsychosocial models has also been promoted as the most appropriate framework for the understanding and management of disability of all types (World Health Organisation, 2011).The importance of these models is that they broaden the focus of health professionals to consider psychological and social factors which affect the course of a chronic pain condition. Crucially, where many chronic pain conditions were resistant to the available medical interventions, resulting in a significant proportion of the population living with chronic pain, biopsychosocial models offered a new treatment target focused on reducing the psychological distress and functional disability experienced by those with persisting pain (Blyth, et al., 2001).

Within the broad category of biopsychosocial models, those informed by cognitive behavioural theories are most common. These models particularly address the role of cognitions and behaviours in the development and maintenance of pain, as well as associated pain-related distress and disability. A wide range of cognitive and behavioural constructs have been investigated to determine their relationship with the experience of pain and associated disability and distress (Vlaeyen & Linton, 2000). There is some support for many of these constructs in individual studies. However, among these constructs, pain catastrophizing, pain self-efficacy, and avoidance have all been found to be consistently related to the experience of pain and associated disability or distress across different populations and methodologies. In addition, the presence of altered mood, such as symptoms of depression and anxiety, or the co-existence of psychiatric disorders such as post-traumatic stress disorder, all seem to be important in influencing the course of a chronic pain condition.

The application of biopsychosocial models to chronic pain among those with physically disabling conditions has lagged significantly behind its use among primary pain conditions, where it has long been acknowledged that presence of pain or the intensity of pain does not fully explain pain-related disability or distress (Heneweer, et al., 2007). Among the physically disabling conditions outlined above with documented, significant rates of associated chronic pain there were no peer-reviewed publications available addressing psychosocial variables in the case of Parkinson's Disease. In addition, the investigation of variables has been patchy across the different conditions, and there are few specific models proposed for those with chronic pain in the context of physically disabling conditions. Some of the reasons for this are unclear, although it may be suggested that the obvious presence of pathology among those with physically disabling conditions results in a tendency to discount the possible role of other factors in causing pain-related disability or distress. This is despite repeated findings across a number of diagnoses that condition-related variables, such as severity of injury or illness, are frequently not at all or only weakly related to pain intensity and related disability or distress (Hoffman, et al., 2007).

It is notable that while biopsychosocial models do not dictate that only negative or adverse outcomes are possible following development of pain, much of the available research focuses on factors associated with poor outcomes. In contrast, a study of people with spinal cord injuries or multiple traumas examined factors which differentiated different adjustment trajectories and identified three: the resilience trajectory, characterized by low levels of mental health symptoms at both early and late stage of admission following injury, the recovery trajectory where the individual shows an improving pattern of mental health symptoms, and the distress trajectory, where higher levels of mental health symptoms at the early stage are sustained in the longer term (Quale & Schanke, 2010). The study reports that the latter accounted for only one fifth of the participants in their study, and that maximum pain at admission differentiated those in the resilience vs the distress trajectory.

Studies investigating the relationship between psychosocial factors and chronic pain in people with physically disabling conditions fall into two main categories. First, psychosocial factors are examined as predictors of chronic pain or pain-related disability, for example does a particular way of thinking about pain have an impact on how much pain is experienced. Second, chronic pain is examined as a contributor to adjustment following onset of a physically disabling condition, for example do those with chronic pain as a result of a physically disabling condition have higher levels of depressive symptomatology. The rapid development of theory and research related to biopsychosocial models of chronic pain has led to some overlap of concepts. A good example of this being that pain catastrophizing first appeared as one of many unhelpful coping strategies, but has now been reframed as a belief alongside others such as self-efficacy or helplessness. It is therefore somewhat difficult to categorize the current literature into particular themes. The purpose of this section is to describe the current evidence regarding the relationship between psychological and social factors and chronic pain in people with physically disabling conditions, and to identify gaps in the current literature which require further investigation.

3.1 Psychological factors

Under the category psychological factors, the main variables to consider are mood and mental health, cognitive responses to pain, and behavioural responses to pain. The extent of the literature in these three areas varies markedly across the various physically disabling conditions under consideration.

3.1.1 Mood and mental health

The association between chronic pain and changes in mood and mental health, including symptoms of depression and anxiety, is perhaps the most frequently explored aspect of biopsychosocial models among those with physically disabling conditions. In some physically disabling conditions, a clear relationship between chronic pain and psychological distress has been consistently demonstrated, whereas in others the findings are more mixed. Pain has been found to be associated with psychological distress in most of the studies identified in cerebral palsy, traumatic brain injury, multiple sclerosis, amputation, spinal cord injury, and muscular dystrophy (Engel, et al., 2003; Engel, Schwartz, Jensen, & Johnson, 2000; Hoffman, et al., 2007; Kalia & O'Connor, 2005; Kratz, et al., 2010; Middleton, Tran, & Craig, 2007; Miro, et al., 2009; Motl, McAuley, Snook, & Gliottoni, 2009; Nicholson Perry, Nicholas, & Middleton, 2009; Nicholson Perry, Nicholas, Middleton, & Siddall, 2009; Norrbrink Budh, Hultling, & Lundeberg, 2005; Stormer, et al., 1997; Turner, Jensen, Warms, & Cardenas, 2002), although the strength of the relationship has varied across studies and conditions. In addition, studies in people with spinal cord injury pain found that continuous pain, as opposed to intermittent pain, was associated with higher levels of depression and anxiety, and conversely more stress among women with spinal cord injuries was associated with consistent reports of pain over a ten year period (Norrbrink Budh & Osteraker, 2007; Rintala, Hart, & Priebe, 2004). Negative mood has also been reported to be a trigger to exacerbations in chronic pain among people with spinal cord injury (Widerstrom-Noga & Turk, 2004). Some studies have presented exceptions to this general rule in the case of cerebral palsy, multiple sclerosis and stroke (Hirsh, Gallegos, Gertz, Engel, & Jensen, 2010; Kong, et al., 2004; Newland, Naismith, & Ullione, 2009; Newland, Wipke-Tevis, Williams, Rantz, & Petroski, 2005). Moderators of this relationship include gender, with the relationship not being found in males with multiple sclerosis in one study, and aetiology (traumatic versus non-traumatic) for amputation in one study moderating the relationship at early time points (Kalia & O'Connor, 2005; Kratz, et al., 2010). Physically disabling conditions in which findings are mixed in this regard include those with phantom limb pain and stump pain following amputation (Fisher & Hanspal, 1998). While most of these studies have been conducted with adults with physically disabling conditions, a study with a large sample of older children with cerebral palsy suggests that children with moderate or severe pain are significantly more likely to have higher levels emotional and behavioural problems (Parkes, et al., 2008). One study in people with multiple sclerosis found that affective memory biases, a measure of vulnerability to depression, may mediate the relationship between chronic pain and depressive symptoms in this group (Bruce, Polen, & Arnett, 2007).

Most studies of the relationship between pain and depression in physically disabling conditions solely report on cross-sectional associations. In some studies, however, they specifically examine pain as a predictor of depression, or in other cases the reverse. Determining the direction of the relationship have proved problematic, although there is some evidence among people with spinal cord injury to support the hypothesis than persisting pain is a driver of depression rather than the converse (Cairns, Adkins, & Scott, 1996; Putzke, Richards, Hicken, & DeVivo, 2002).The presence of depression at one time point has been reported to be a risk factor for pain at a later time point among those with multiple sclerosis and spinal cord injury (Buchanan, Wang, Tai-Seale, & Ju, 2003; Putzke, et al., 2002).

Depression is associated with pain-related interference in a number of physically disabling conditions, including amputation, multiple sclerosis and spinal cord injury (Kratz, et al., 2010; Nicholson Perry, Nicholas, & Middleton, 2009; Nicholson Perry, Nicholas, Middleton, et al., 2009; Norrbrink Budh, et al., 2005; Norrbrink Budh & Osteraker, 2007; Osborne, et al., 2006; Turner, et al., 2002). There is evidence of a similar moderating effect of depression upon the relationship between pain and disability among those with spinal cord injury as is seen in other chronic pain populations (Borsbo, Peolsson, & Gerdle, 2009), and a similar but less clear interaction between these variables in those with traumatic brain injury (Hoffman, et al., 2007). The impairment to quality of life attributable to chronic pain has been reported to be related to depressive symptoms among individuals with spinal cord injury (Cruz-Almeida, Alameda, & Widerstrom-Noga, 2009). In addition, negative moods, boredom and stress reported in a large sample of older children with cerebral palsy was found to be significantly predicted by the presence of pain, although only to contribute a relatively small proportion of variation in this aspects of quality of life and interestingly overall quality of life was found to be consistent with other children without cerebral palsy (Dickinson, et al., 2007).

Studies of the relationship between chronic pain and anxiety among people with physically disabling conditions are less common. However, in studies of people with multiple sclerosis, anxiety has been found to be positively associated with pain severity, particularly among women (Kalia & O'Connor, 2005; Motl, et al., 2009). Studies among people with spinal cord injury have also shown a significant relationship between anxiety and pain severity (Nicholson Perry, Nicholas, & Middleton, 2009; Nicholson Perry, Nicholas, Middleton, et al., 2009; Norrbrink Budh, et al., 2005; Norrbrink Budh & Osteraker, 2007). There are a few studies examining the relationship between pain and post-traumatic stress disorder (PTSD). In a study of people with both traumatic and non-traumatic amputation, pain and pain-related interference was positively correlated with PTSD symptoms in both groups (Kratz, et al., 2010). Pain-related anxiety, often measured as a combination of cognitions, behaviours and emotion, has also been found to moderate the relationship between chronic pain and disability among those with spinal cord injury, with those reporting higher levels of pain related anxiety experiencing greater disability (Borsbo, et al., 2009). Anger has been less well investigated, although it has been shown to moderate the perception of pain in people with spinal cord injury (Conant, 1998; Summers, Rapoff, Varghese, Porter, & Palmer, 1991).

3.1.2 Cognitive responses to pain

The relationship between cognitive responses to pain, or beliefs, and pain-related disability and distress has been explored in those with a number of the physically disabling conditions of interest. Pain catastrophizing, characterized by a tendency to negative and unrealistic beliefs in response to pain, and is the cognitive factor with the greatest body of evidence supporting its role. While pain catastrophizing has often been measured in questionnaires designed to measure coping strategies, it is best considered alongside other beliefs, and so will be reported on in this section.

Pain catastrophizing has been found to be associated with pain intensity among people with chronic phantom limb pain post-amputation, multiple sclerosis and spinal cord injury (Hill, Niven, & Knussen, 1995; Nicholson Perry, Nicholas, & Middleton, 2009; Osborne, Jensen,

Ehde, Hanley, & Kraft, 2007; Turner, et al., 2002; Vase, et al., 2011; Wollaars, Post, van Asbeck, & Brand, 2007). In a study of people with phantom limb pain, pain catastrophizing was also shown to significantly contribute to wind-up-like pain when anxiety and depression were controlled for (Vase, et al., 2011)

Pain catastrophizing has been found to be positively associated with pain-related disability among those with spinal cord injury, cerebral palsy, phantom limb pain, muscular dystrophy and multiple sclerosis (Borsbo, et al., 2009; Douglas, Wollin, & Windsor, 2008; Engel, et al., 2000; Hill, et al., 1995; Miro, et al., 2009; Molton, et al., 2009; Nicholson Perry, Nicholas, & Middleton, 2009; Nicholson Perry, Nicholas, Middleton, et al., 2009; Osborne, et al., 2007). Psychological functioning among people with spinal cord injury, multiple sclerosis, phantom limb pain, muscular dystrophy and cerebral palsy has been found to be negatively associated with pain catastrophizing (Douglas, et al., 2008; Engel, Jensen, & Schwartz, 2006; Engel, et al., 2000; Hanley, et al., 2004; Hill, et al., 1995; Miro, et al., 2009; Molton, et al., 2009; Nicholson Perry, Nicholas, & Middleton, 2009; Nicholson Perry, Nicholas, Middleton, et al., 2009; Osborne, et al., 2007; Smedema, Catalano, & Ebener, 2011; Ullrich, Jensen, Loeser, & Cardenas, 2007; Wollaars, et al., 2007). Pain catastrophizing has also been shown to mediate the relationship between pain severity and psychological distress and pain-related disability among people with spinal cord injury (Ullrich, et al., 2007). It has been suggested that pain catastrophizing may, in fact, be a function of disturbed mood. This suggestion is brought into question by findings in both phantom limb pain and spinal cord injury related chronic pain which shows that pain catastrophizing is associated with pain intensity when mood is controlled for (Ullrich, et al., 2007; Vase, et al., 2011). Among the many studies of individuals with spinal cord injury pain, veterans with the condition appear to have higher levels of pain catastrophizing than non-veterans (Ullrich, Jensen, Loeser, Cardenas, & Weaver, 2008).

While most of these studies are cross-sectional in nature, a prospective study of people with spinal cord injury with chronic pain found that over a six month period decreases in pain catastrophizing were associated with decreased pain interference and improved psychological functioning (Hanley, Raichle, Jensen, & Cardenas, 2008). Conversely, a similar study in phantom limb pain found that pain catastrophizing at one month following amputation (that is, before chronic pain had developed) was predictive of decreased depressive symptoms and pain-related interference at both 12 and 24 months (Hanley, et al., 2004). While this may appear counter-intuitive, the authors suggest that the function of pain catastrophizing soon after amputation may be different to that in those with established chronic pain, who are the subject of most other studies on the subject.

Perceived control over pain has also been investigated, and there is less extensive evidence to support its role in relation to psychological functioning and disability in those with chronic pain secondary to physically disabling conditions. A study of people with spinal cord injury related chronic pain found that increases in perceived control over pain in a six month period was related to decreased pain intensity and pain interference, as well as increased psychological functioning, although the former was a non-significant finding (Hanley, et al., 2008). External locus of control in relation to pain as also been positively associated with depression among people with spinal cord injury related pain (Wollaars, et al., 2007). In addition, two studies of people with phantom limb pain, including a prospective study of people with phantom limb pain from one to 24 months, demonstrated some weak evidence for its influence on pain intensity, psychological functioning, and pain-related disability (Hanley, et al., 2004; Hill, et al., 1995).

Other findings related to pain-related beliefs have also been noted but with much less consistency. A belief that pain is constant or enduring has been found to significantly predict both pain intensity and interference to activities due to pain among those with multiple sclerosis (Douglas, et al., 2008). The lower endorsement of the belief that others should be solicitous in response to pain behaviours was associated with better psychological functioning among people with muscular dystrophy (Miro, et al., 2009)

3.1.3 Behavioural responses to pain

Comparison of the use of behavioural responses to pain, also commonly referred to as coping strategies, among people with chronic pain secondary to physically disabling conditions to those with chronic primary pain conditions has revealed both similarities and differences. In people with cerebral palsy, use of behavioural coping strategies such as guarding and rest was reported to be less common and task persistence more common (Engel, et al., 2000). Conversely, cognitive coping strategies, such as diverting attention, reinterpreting sensations, and praying and hoping, were reportedly used more commonly. The authors suggest that some of these differences may be attributable to different background levels of the use of behavioural strategies such as resting and guarding, which may already be employed for non-pain related reasons among those with physically disabling conditions, and increased reliance on cognitive strategies over which they may be hypothesized to have more control.

The association of particular coping strategies with pain intensity or associated psychological distress or disability has been explored in a number of physically disabling conditions, including spinal cord injury, but with few significant relationships detected (Hanley, et al., 2008; Turner, et al., 2002). In some other studies, however, significant relationships have been found. In a study of people with phantom limb pain, behavioural activity was found to be associated with higher levels of pain, in contrast with findings in those with chronic primary pain conditions (Hill, et al., 1995). Passive coping strategies, including guarding, resting, asking for assistance, seeking social support and pacing, were found to be predictive of pain interference but not psychological functioning among people with spinal cord injury and muscular dystrophy (Miro, et al., 2009; Molton, et al., 2009). Reduction of activity, through resting or avoidance, has been associated with positively associated with pain interference in people with cerebral palsy and muscular dystrophy, and with symptoms of depression in people with cerebral palsy (Engel, et al., 2000; Miro, et al., 2009).

Seeking social support has been found to be positively associated with pain-related disability among people with cerebral palsy and muscular dystrophy (Engel, et al., 2006; Miro, et al., 2009), a finding that may initially appear counter-intuitive. The authors of the cerebral palsy study identified the fact that the items on the scale potentially reflect both adaptive and maladaptive aspects of social support seeking (Engel, et al., 2006). However, operant models of chronic pain suggest that pain contingent social support would result in increased disability, which may also provide a parsimonious explanation of the findings.

The extent to which respondents with multiple sclerosis believed they were able to control or decrease their pain through use of their coping strategies has been found to be associated with decreased pain intensity, however no specific coping strategy was predictive (Douglas, et al., 2008). Further, in the same study no coping strategy was found to be predictive of life interference due to pain and only coping by increasing activities was found to be associated with improved psychological functioning.

3.2 Social factors

Although clearly identified as part of the various biopsychosocial models of pain proposed, social factors have been relatively less well represented in the literature. Studies examining social factors most often report on perceived social support and partner responses to pain behaviours.

3.2.1 Social support

Studies examining the associations between social support and pain are available in people with limb loss, spinal cord injury, multiple sclerosis and muscular dystrophy.

Social support was found to be negatively associated with pain in studies among people with traumatic limb loss, whereas no relationship was found in people with spinal cord injury pain (Kratz, et al., 2010; Stroud, Turner, Jensen, & Cardenas, 2006). Studies of people with multiple sclerosis have resulted in mixed findings, with negative associations with pain in one study and no association in the other (Motl, et al., 2009; Osborne, et al., 2007). A study designed to identify factors which were predictive of consistency of pain over ten years among people with spinal cord injury found that among male respondents, receiving less social support during the first phase of the study was predictive of continuing pain over the life of the study (Rintala, et al., 2004)

Associations between lower levels of social support and greater pain-related disability has been found in people with non-traumatic limb loss, multiple sclerosis and muscular dystrophy, but not in people with spinal cord injury (Kratz, et al., 2010; Miro, et al., 2009; Motl, et al., 2009; Osborne, et al., 2007; Stroud, et al., 2006). In one study, greater social support at one month post amputation was predictive of greater reduction in pain interference at 12 and 24 months (Hanley, et al., 2004). In addition, increased social support has been found to be associated with lower levels of anxiety and depression in people with multiple sclerosis and with depression in people with spinal cord injury (Motl, et al., 2009; Stroud, et al., 2006). Among people with muscular dystrophy, social support was associated positively with psychological functioning (Miro, et al., 2009). Hanley et al. (2004) also looked at the relationship between social constraint, which is the need to hide one's feelings about the amputation from others, and pain and pain-related interference. Increased need for social constraint was associated with pain intensity and interference in both those with traumatic and non-traumatic limb loss in the 6 to 12 month period.

3.2.2 Partner responses to pain behaviours

The most common maladaptive form of partner response to pain behaviours reported in the general chronic pain literature is that of solicitous responding, which is a key mechanism in operant models of pain, hypothesized to increase pain-related disability. A study in people with spinal cord injury chronic pain found perceived solicitous responding from partners were unrelated to pain intensity, pain-related disability, or depression (Stroud, et al., 2006). One study in people with limb loss found that less frequent solicitous responding at one month post amputation was predictive of greater reductions in pain interference at 12 and 24 months (Hanley, et al., 2004). Other forms of partner responses to pain behaviour measured in people with spinal cord injury related chronic pain are negative and distracting responses (Stroud, et al., 2006). Negative responses, such as criticism, and distracting responses were both associated with higher depression, but not pain intensity or pain related disability. Most studies which report upon partner responses to pain behaviours in the context of physically disabling conditions provide information about participants perception of their significant others solicitous responses to their pain behaviours. One study in people with spinal cord injury reported on partner's ratings of their own responses to pain behaviour, and it was notable that these were unrelated to pain intensity, depression or pain-related disability in their partner (Stroud, et al., 2006).

3.3 Summary

Reviewing the evidence presented here, a number of issues are apparent. First, that there is a great deal of variation across physically disabling conditions in the extent to which biopsychosocial factors have been investigated. Second, that over all the conditions considered, social factors are relatively less well explored and this remains a significant omission in the literature. Despite this, and the variation in the patterns in each specific physically disabling condition, across the majority of the conditions for which data is available it is clear that there is evidence to suggest that psychological and social factors are broadly related to pain intensity, as well as associated disability and distress. Across all the factors which have been investigated thus far, it appears that the findings related to pain catastrophizing and its association with pain intensity and related disability and distress are the most consistent. This suggests that pain catastrophizing should be explored as part of assessment protocols for people with chronic pain associated with physically disabling conditions. Further research in the area is clearly needed, particularly prospective studies that begin prior to the development of chronic pain, and which are sufficiently large to permit demographic and medical factors to be controlled for in the analyses.

4. Interventions focused on psychological and social factors

There are two major reasons why psychosocial interventions for pain might be considered for people with chronic pain secondary to physically disabling conditions. The first, that psychosocial variables are important contributors to variance in pain itself, as well as pain related distress or disability, and the second, that existing interventions based on biomedical models of pain are insufficient. The evidence presented in the previous section suggests that, while there are gaps in the literature, there is sufficient reason to think that psychosocial variables do make a significant contribution to pain and associated distress and disability. In addition, there is evidence that people with chronic pain secondary to a range of physically disabling conditions, including cerebral palsy, stroke and multiple sclerosis, are unlikely to be receiving treatment for their pain, are dissatisfied with the pain treatment available to them or report limited improvement in pain despite treatment (Engel, et al., 2003; Hirsh, et al., 2010; Kalia & O'Connor, 2005; Kong, et al., 2004).

Psychosocial interventions for people with chronic pain, predominantly behavioural and cognitive behavioural in origin, are well-established and supported by an extensive evidence base (Meldrum, 2007). A series of systematic reviews and meta-analyses attest to the efficacy of these programs among child and adults with primary chronic pain conditions, as well as early interventions designed to reduce the development of pain-related disability (Eccleston, Morley, Williams, Yorke, & Mastroyannopoulou, 2002; Eccleston, Yorke, Morley, Williams, & Mastroyannopoulou, 2003; Linton & Nordin, 2006; Morley, Eccleston, & Williams, 1999).

4.1 The nature of psychosocial interventions

A very small number of studies have been published that specifically report on the use of psychosocial interventions among people with physically disabling conditions. The majority of these have involved group-based cognitive behavioural pain management programs, but they also include cognitive restructuring and hypnosis. The potential use of such interventions in people with spinal cord injury was identified in the early 1990's (Umlauf, 1992), but a review of the literature concerning the application and evaluation of these programs among any group with a physically disabling condition reveals a disappointingly small number of studies and little translation into standard practice.

4.2 Feasibility and acceptability of psychosocial interventions

A study undertaken in the US specifically examined the issue of the feasibility and acceptability of psychosocial interventions, with a mixed sample of individuals with chronic pain of more than six months duration occurring secondary to multiple sclerosis, amputations, spinal cord injury and cerebral palsy (Ehde & Jensen, 2004). The study found that both the cognitive restructuring intervention, and the control condition which was an educational intervention, were both rated positively by the participants. A study of a cognitive behavioural pain management program for people with spinal cord injury neuropathic pain reported that attendance at the group was high and participants reported that they were very satisfied with the program (Norrbrink Budh, Kowalski, & Lundeberg, 2006). Authors of another study, examining the effectiveness of a cognitive behavioural pain management program for people with spinal cord injury, provide an analysis of the issues encountered in the implementation of the program (Nicholson Perry, Nicholas, & Middleton, 2010; Nicholson Perry, Nicholas, & Middleton, 2011). These findings suggest that these interventions are potentially acceptable, at least to people with spinal cord injury related pain.

4.3 Use and effectiveness of psychosocial interventions

Psychosocial interventions for pain either described for use with or evaluated with people with physically disabling conditions are extremely few. They are mainly cognitive behavioural, group-based pain management programs, but examples of the use of cognitive restructuring alone and hypnosis are also reported.

4.3.1 Cognitive behavioural group-based pain management programs

Four group-based, cognitive behavioural pain management program of various sorts are described in the literature (Cundiff, Blair, & Puckett, 1995; Gironda, 2004; Nicholson Perry, et al., 2010; Norrbrink Budh, et al., 2006). The main components of such interventions are represented in Table 1. The earliest reports in the literature of cognitive behavioural pain management programs in physically disabling conditions were for spinal cord injury pain and were descriptive. Cundiff and colleagues (1995) described the development of a group-based cognitive behavioural pain management program for people with spinal cord injury pain of all types. This involved many of the common components of pain management programs for primary pain diagnoses, including: the explanation of the self-management model, relaxation (including diaphragmatic breathing, guided imagery), the role of self-talk, and pain behaviours and their impact. Gironda (2004) reported on an intervention which was characterized as an interdisciplinary pain management program for spinal cord injury shoulder pain. It was described as a functional preservation approach aimed at enabling individuals to maintain and improve functional capacities where injuries had already been sustained. The program was provided during a two week in-patient stay and comprised of:

medication adjustment; an exercise regimen designed to increase range of motion, endurance and stretch in upper limbs; biomechanical education; a psychoeducational component designed to enhance understanding of the self-management approach, promote problem-solving and implementation of strategies at home, raise awareness of compensatory responses that may be impacting upon psychological or physical well-being; and recreation therapy to encourage return to social and leisure interests. Preliminary data from eight participants in the program suggested improvements across a range of domains, including mood, sleep and pain intensity during shoulder range of motion testing.

Component	Description
Education regarding pain	Information is presented about the underlying pain mechanisms relevant to chronic pain, including central sensitization, as well as the limitations of medical treatment for chronic pain.
Goal-setting	Collaborative goal-setting related to a variety of goals across a wide spread of domains, including physical activities or mood, emphasizing the identification of short-term goals building towards long-term goals that are challenging but achievable in order to increase a sense of mastery.
Activity pacing	Adoption of quota or time based activities, systematically upgraded over time and linked to goals.
Relaxation	Applied relaxation to reduce muscle tension and improve sleep.
Functional exercise	Whole body reconditioning exercise programme related functional physical goals.
Stretch	Whole body daily stretch programme.
Cognitive therapy	Identification and modification of unhelpful thoughts regarding pain, such as catastrophizing.
Medication reduction	Gradual reduction of inappropriate or excessive pain medications using an agreed schedule.
Flare-up management & relapse prevention	Development of a plan to manage temporary increases in pain (flare ups) or other situations likely to trigger relapse.

Table 1. Common components of cognitive behavioural pain management programs

Two controlled studies have been published which have examined the effectiveness of cognitive behavioural group pain management programs for people with physically disabling conditions, both in those with spinal cord injury (Nicholson Perry, et al., 2010; Norrbrink Budh, et al., 2006). The first controlled study in the literature described a cognitive behavioural pain management program for people with neuropathic pain arising from a spinal cord injury (Norrbrink Budh et al., 2006). The program developed was very like the pain management programs described for people with primary pain diagnoses in content, although of shorter duration (totalling 50 hours over ten weeks). Compared with those in the no-treatment control group, those participating in the program showed significant improvements in depression and sense of coherence (a concept comprising comprehensibility, manageability and meaningfulness of the injury) over 12 months. While there were no other significant differences between the groups, the treatment group showed improvements in anxiety symptoms, emotional reaction and sleep from baseline to the 12-month evaluation, but no significant changes over time were observed in the other outcome measures (including pain intensity and unpleasantness, health-related quality of life and life satisfaction). An Australian study compared a cognitive behavioural pain management program with standard care in a tertiary pain management service in Australia. The program was a modification of an existing program, the design and implementation of which is reported in depth elsewhere, which was approximately half of the usual number of contact hours (Nicholson Perry, et al., 2011). The group attending the pain management program showed an overall improved in mood and pain-related disability at the end of the program compared with the controlled group. This was associated with significant decreases in pain catastrophizing and anxiety in the pain management program group. Three-quarters of people completing the pain management program reported a clinically significant improvement, in contrast to less than a third in the usual care comparison group, however long-term follow up data in this group suggested that benefits were not maintained at six months. Both programs were approximately half of the optimal dose (100 hours) recommended for the management of patients with heterogeneous, disabling chronic pain in a pain management program (Guzman, et al., 2001). While it may appear at first sight that there is a degree of inconsistency in providing an intervention incorporating pacing, where other evidence suggests pacing is an unhelpful strategy among those with chronic pain due to physically disabling conditions, this may be a matter of definition; pacing as taught in cognitive behavioural pain management programs takes a systematic approach to continuing to build up quotas of activity which it may be hypothesized is absent in what respondents would endorse as pacing in surveys of pain-related coping strategies. However, the findings from the evaluation of the programs suggested that there was merit in pursuing the use of cognitive behavioural pain management programs in the context of refractive spinal cord injury pain.

4.3.2 Cognitive restructuring

A pilot program exploring the use of a cognitive restructuring intervention targeting catastrophizing for a heterogeneous group of people with disability related chronic pain has recently been reported (Ehde & Jensen, 2004). The authors compared eight 90-minute sessions of cognitive restructuring with an education control intervention among 18 people with disability-related chronic pain (including those with amputations, spinal cord injury, cerebral palsy and multiple sclerosis). The cognitive restructuring intervention included: the role of negative cognitions; how to identify maladaptive thinking; thought-stopping and cognitive restructuring techniques; and use of reassuring self-statements. The education control intervention included pain education (underlying mechanisms and theories of pain), sleep problems in pain and common pain treatments. The authors report that nine of those who attended the first session did not return, but of the eighteen who did continue with their treatment all reported benefiting from the intervention regardless of the group attended. The preliminary results reported by the authors, describing mean pain intensity on a range of 0 to 10 before and after attendance, suggested that whereas pain intensity was unchanged in those attending the education group there was a reduction of approximately 0.2 of a standard deviation among those participating in the cognitive intervention. The authors conclude that a properly powered controlled trial would be required to establish the effectiveness of this approach, but that it was certainly feasible to provide and regarded as acceptable by at least half the patients. Although the literature on the use of psychosocial interventions in people with physically disabling conditions is limited, there is some evidence of similar therapeutic mechanisms operating in these populations as in chronic primary pain conditions (Burns,

Kubilus, Bruehl, Harden, & Lofland, 2003). In particular, the observation of the association between decreased pain catastrophising and improvements in mood and disability in those who participate in the interventions is consistent with findings in other chronic pain populations (Jensen, et al., 2011; Nicholson Perry, et al., 2010). This cognitive restructuring intervention therefore has particular promise as it targets pain catastrophizing, but requires implementation of a smaller range of treatment strategies than traditional cognitive behavioural pain management programs as described above.

4.3.3 Hypnosis

Hypnosis has also been applied to spinal cord injury related pain in a series of studies (Ehde & Jensen, 2007) using individual hypnosis treatments with 10 sessions over four weeks and daily practice. The suggestions used were reported to include imagery, changing sensations and ignoring pain, with associated post-hypnotic suggestions that a relaxed state and the ability to ignore pain will become increasingly easy. The case studies found that a sub-group of individuals with disability-related pain were able to obtain decreases in pain severity, with associated improvements in mood, sleep and general well-being in individual cases. However, in the absence of randomized controlled trials, no firm conclusions can be drawn about the effectiveness of hypnosis in this context.

In a variation of the more common cognitive behavioural interventions reported in the literature, a cognitive restructuring approach combined with self-hypnosis training was reported in people with multiple sclerosis (Jensen, et al., 2011). This intervention was intended to target pain catastrophising as well as pain intensity. When compared with either cognitive restructuring or hypnosis alone, or the control condition, the combined approach resulted in a decrease in the frequency of pain catastrophising and increase in the frequency of reassuring cognitions, as well as improved average and worst pain intensity.

4.4 Barriers to the use of psychosocial interventions

While access to specialist pain management services of any type is problematic, there are some additional reasons to think that access to psychosocial pain interventions will be particularly difficult for those with physically disabling conditions. Broadly, these include the demands of providing such services and accessibility of such services. Health professionals specialising in the provision of psychosocial interventions for chronic pain, such as clinical psychologists, tend to be limited in supply and concentrated in specialist services in major cities. The skills and expertise required to provide psychosocial pain management interventions to those with physically disabling conditions requires expertise in both pain and some of the specific aspects of the physically disabling condition which may impact upon the delivery of the intervention. This includes having an understanding of the physically disabling conditions and its associated symptoms, such as motor function or fatigue, and how these may impact upon the relevance or implementation of the strategies taught. The additional challenges to mobility from having a physically disabling conditions, as well as chronic pain, in combination with environmental barriers which must be overcome to attend a specialist pain management service reduces the chances that an individual with a chronic pain problem due to a physically disabling condition will be able to attend. The costs of living with a physically disabling condition may result in limited financial resources available to fund travel or accommodation in locations where specialist pain management services are available.

Service delivery models which are able to overcome some of these barriers are yet to be designed, and many of the interventions with a research pedigree to support them have not generalized to routine care due to the lack of support to assist with translation into routine clinical practice. The increased availability of high speed internet may permit the use of online interventions to provide at least some access to some of the components of effective psychosocial interventions for chronic pain, either for use alone or with the support of a health professional, and this may be of particular benefit to those with pain secondary to physically disabling conditions.

4.5 Summary

Despite the limited evidence available about the effective of psychosocial interventions in people with physically disabling conditions, the findings suggest that there is merit in further research to evaluate their usefulness in a broader range of conditions. Intervention studies in this area are notoriously difficult, due to the many barriers to participation and retention in trials. National and international collaborations are likely to be necessary to ensure a sufficient sample size for such studies to be adequately powered. Provision of these services is impeded by a number of practical barriers, some of which might at least partially addressed by making more effective use of information technology (World Health Organisation, 2011). While there is currently insufficient evidence to support a wholesale recommendation to use these interventions in all physically disabling conditions, in light of the dissatisfaction with pain treatment among many with chronic pain secondary to physically disabling conditions they may be considered for use on an individual basis.

5. Conclusion

It can be concluded based upon the data presented that the application of biopsychosocial models to the understanding, assessment and management of chronic pain associated with physically disabling conditions is at an early stage of development. There is a well-established body of research in some conditions, such as spinal cord injury, whereas almost nothing is known about the application of these models to other conditions, notably Parkinson's Disease. Many of the patterns observed in primary pain conditions are replicated in these conditions, but the exceptions noted underscore the importance of caution in generalising findings from one condition to another. Relatively, research concerning the use of psychosocial interventions is less well-developed that research examining the relationships between psychosocial and pain variables in physically disabling conditions. Despite this, the findings generally are suggestive of an important role of including psychosocial variables in our conceptualization of individual differences in the experience of chronic pain and its consequences in people with physically disabling conditions, and the possibility of improved outcomes through the use of psychosocial interventions.

6. Acknowledgement

Much of what I have learned about this area has resulted from the conversations I have been privileged to have with people with physically disabling conditions, and I thank them for their willingness to educate me. I am continually grateful for the opportunity to work with many wise colleagues who have taught me a great deal about pain and some of the physically disabling conditions which have formed the subject of this chapter. In particular, I would like to thank Associate Professor Michael Nicholas, Associate Professor James

Middleton, Professor Ashley Craig and Associate Professor Philip Siddall. I would also like to express my gratitude to the School of Psychology, University of Western Sydney for the support provided in the writing of this chapter, particularly the continuing support of Professor Jane Ussher, as well as the able assistance of Rio Yamaguchi.

7. References

Appelros, P. (2006). Prevalence and predictors of pain and fatigue after stroke: a population-based study. *International Journal of Rehabilitation Research, 29*(4), 329-333.

Behr, J., Friedly, J., Molton, I., Morgenroth, D., Jensen, M. P., & Smith, D. G. (2009). Pain and pain-related interference in adults with lower-limb amputation: Comparison of knee-disarticulation, transtibial, and transfemoral surgical sites. *Journal of Rehabilitation Research and Development, 46*(7), 963-972.

Beiske, A., & Loge, J. (2009). Pain in Parkinson's disease: prevalence and characteristics. *Pain, 141*(1-2), 173-177.

Blyth, F. M., March, L. M., Brnabic, A. J., Jorm, L. R., Williamson, M., & Cousins, M. J. (2001). Chronic pain in Australia: a prevalence study. *Pain, 89*(2-3), 127-134.

Borsbo, B., Peolsson, M., & Gerdle, B. (2009). The complex interplay between pain intensity, depression, anxiety and catastrophising with respect to quality of life and disability. *Disability and Rehabilitation, 31*(19), 1605-1613.

Bradbury, C. L., Wodchis, W. P., Mikulis, D. J., Pano, E. G., Hitzig, S. L., McGillivray, C. F., et al. (2008). Traumatic brain injury in patients with traumatic spinal cord injury: Clinical and economic consequences. *Archives of Physical Medicine and Rehabilitation, 89*(12, Supplement 12), S77-84.

Bruce, J. M., Polen, D., & Arnett, P. A. (2007). Pain and affective memory biases interact to predict depressive symptoms in multiple sclerosis. *Multiple Sclerosis, 13*(1), 58-66.

Buchanan, R. J., Wang, S., Tai-Seale, M., & Ju, H. (2003). Analyses of nursing home residents with multiple sclerosis and depression using the Minimum Data Set. *Multiple Sclerosis, 9*(2), 171-188.

Burns, K., Kubilus, A., Bruehl, S., Harden, R., & Lofland, K. (2003). Do changes in cognitive factors influence outcome following multidisciplinary treatment for chronic pain? A cross-lagged panel analysis. *Journal of Consulting and Clinical Psychology, 71*, 81-91.

Cairns, D. M., Adkins, R. H., & Scott, M. D. (1996). Pain and depression in acute traumatic spinal cord injury: Origins of chronic problematic pain? *Archives of Physical Medicine & Rehabilitation., 77*(4), 329-335.

Cardenas, D. D., Felix, E. R., Cardenas, D. D., & Felix, E. R. (2009). Pain after spinal cord injury: a review of classification, treatment approaches, and treatment assessment. *PM and R, 1*(12), 1077-1090.

Conant, L. L. (1998). Psychological variables associated with pain perceptions among individuals with chronic spinal cord injury pain. *Journal of Clinical Psychology in Medical Settings, 5*(1), 71-90.

Cruz-Almeida, Y., Alameda, G., & Widerstrom-Noga, E. G. (2009). Differentiation between pain-related interference and interference caused by the functional impairments of spinal cord injury. *Spinal Cord, 47*(5), 390-395.

Cundiff, G. W., Blair, K. L., & Puckett, M. J. (1995). Group pain management therapy for persons with spinal cord injury. *SCI Psychosocial Process, 8*(2), 61-66.

Desmond, D. M., & Maclachlan, M. (2010). Prevalence and characteristics of phantom limb pain and residual limb pain in the long term after upper limb amputation. *International Journal of Rehabilitation Research, 33*(3), 279-282.

Dickinson, H. O., Parkinson, K. N., Ravens-Sieberer, U., Schirripa, G., Thyen, U., Arnaud, C., et al. (2007). Self-reported quality of life of 8-12-year-old children with cerebral palsy: a cross-sectional European study. *Lancet, 369*(9580), 2171-2178.

Dijkers, M., Bryce, T., & Zanca, J. (2009). Prevalence of chronic pain after traumatic spinal cord injury: a systematic review. *Journal of Rehabilitation Research and Development, 46*(1), 13-29.

Dijkstra, P. U., Geertzen, J. H., Stewart, R., van der Schans, C. P., Dijkstra, P. U., Geertzen, J. H. B., et al. (2002). Phantom pain and risk factors: a multivariate analysis. *Journal of Pain and Symptom Management, 24*(6), 578-585.

Dobscha, S. K., Clark, M. E., Morasco, B. J., Freeman, M., Campbell, R., & Helfand, M. (2009). Systematic review of the literature on pain in patients with polytrauma including traumatic brain injury. *Pain Medicine, 10*(7), 1200-1217.

Douglas, C., Wollin, J. A., & Windsor, C. (2008). Biopsychosocial correlates of adjustment to pain among people with multiple sclerosis. *Clinical Journal of Pain, 24*(7), 559-567.

Eccleston, C., Morley, S., Williams, A., Yorke, L., & Mastroyannopoulou, K. (2002). Systematic review of randomised controlled trials of psychological therapy for chronic pain in children and adolescents, with a subset meta-analysis of pain relief. *Pain, 99*(1-2), 157-165.

Eccleston, C., Yorke, L., Morley, S., Williams, A. C., & Mastroyannopoulou, K. (2003). Psychological therapies for the management of chronic and recurrent pain in children and adolescents. *Cochrane Database of Systematic Reviews, 1*.

Ehde, D. M., & Jensen, M. P. (2004). Feasibility of a cognitive restructuring intervention for treatment of chronic pain in persons with disabilities. *Rehabilitation Psychology, 49*(3), 254-258.

Ehde, D. M., Czerniecki, J. M., Smith, D. G., Campbell, K. M., Edwards, W. T., Jensen, M. P., et al. (2000). Chronic phantom sensations, phantom pain, residual limb pain, and other regional pain after lower limb amputation. *Archives of Physical Medicine & Rehabilitation, 81*(8), 1039-1044.

Ehde, D. M., & Jensen, M. P. (2004). Feasibility of a cognitive restructuring intervention for treatment of chronic pain in persons with disabilities. *Rehabilitation Psychology, 49*(3), 254-258.

Ehde, D. M., & Jensen, M. P. (2007). Psychological treatment for pain management in persons with spinal cord injury: cognitive therapy and self-hypnosis training. *Topics in Spinal Cord Injury Rehabilitation, 13*(2), 72-80.

Engel, J. M., Jensen, M. P., Hoffman, A. J., & Kartin, D. (2003). Pain in persons with cerebral palsy: extension and cross validation. *Archives of Physical Medicine and Rehabilitation, 84*(8), 1125-1128.

Engel, J. M., Jensen, M. P., & Schwartz, L. (2006). Coping with chronic pain associated with cerebral palsy. *Occupational Therapy International, 13*(4), 224-233.

Engel, J. M., Kartin, D., Carter, G. T., Jensen, M. P., & Jaffe, K. M. (2009). Pain in youths with neuromuscular disease. *American Journal of Hospice & Palliative Medicine, 26*(5), 405-412.

Engel, J. M., Schwartz, L., Jensen, M. P., & Johnson, D. R. (2000). Pain in cerebral palsy: the relation of coping strategies to adjustment. *Pain, 88*(3), 225-230.

Finnerup, N. B., Baastrup, C., & Jensen, T. S. (2009). Neuropathic pain following spinal cord injury pain: mechanisms and treatment. *Scandinavian Journal of Pain, 1*(S1), 3-11.

Fisher, K., & Hanspal, R. S. (1998). Phantom pain, anxiety, depression, and their relation in consecutive patients with amputated limbs: case reports. *BMJ (Clinical Research Ed.), 316*(7135), 903.

Ford, B. (2010). Pain in Parkinson's disease. *Movement Disorders, 25*(S1), S98-S103.

Gallien, P., Nicolas, B., Dauvergne, F., Petrilli, S., Houedakor, J., Roy, D., et al. (2007). Pain in adults with cerebral palsy. *Annales de Readaptation et de Medecine Physique, 50*(7), 558-563.

Gatchel, R. J., Peng, Y. B., Peters, M. L., Fuchs, P. N., & Turk, D. C. (2007). The biopsychosocial approach to chronic pain: scientific advances and future directions. *Psychological Bulletin, 133*(4), 581-624.

Gironda, R. J. (2004). An interdisciplinary, cognitive-behavioral shoulder pain treatment program. *SCI Psychosocial Process, 17*(4), 247-252.

Guzman, J., Esmail, R., Karjalainen, K., Malmivaara, A., Irvin, E., & Bombardier, C. (2001). Multidisciplinary rehabilitation for chronic low back pain: systematic review. *British Medical Journal, 322*(7301), 1511-1516.

Hammarlund, C. S., Carlström, M., Melchior, R., & Persson, B. M. (2011). Prevalence of back pain, its effect on functional ability and health-related quality of life in lower limb amputees secondary to trauma or tumour: a comparison across three levels of amputation. *Prosthetics and Orthotics International, 35*(1), 97-105.

Hanley, M. A., Jensen, M. P., Ehde, D. M., Hoffman, A. J., Patterson, D. R., & Robinson, L. R. (2004). Psychosocial predictors of long-term adjustment to lower-limb amputation and phantom limb pain. *Disability & Rehabilitation, 26*(14-15), 882-893.

Hanley, M. A., Raichle, K., Jensen, M., & Cardenas, D. D. (2008). Pain catastrophizing and beliefs predict changes in pain interference and psychological functioning in persons with spinal cord injury. *The Journal of Pain, 9*(9), 863-871.

Heneweer, H., Aufdemkampe, G., van Tulder, M. W., Kiers, H., Stappaerts, K. H., & Vanhees, L. (2007). Psychosocial variables in patients with (sub)acute low back pain: an inception cohort in primary care physical therapy in The Netherlands. *Spine, 32*(5), 586-592.

Henwood, P., & Ellis, J. A. (2004). Chronic neuropathic pain in spinal cord injury: the patient's perspective. *Pain Research and Management, 9*(1), 39-45.

Hill, A., Niven, C. A., & Knussen, C. (1995). The role of coping in adjustment to phantom limb pain. *Pain, 62*(1), 79-86.

Hirsh, A. T., Gallegos, J. C., Gertz, K. J., Engel, J. M., & Jensen, M. P. (2010). Symptom burden in individuals with cerebral palsy. *Journal of Rehabilitation Research and Development, 47*(9), 863-876.

Hoffman, J. M., Pagulayan, K. F., Zawaideh, N., Dikmen, S., Temkin, N., & Bell, K. R. (2007). Understanding pain after traumatic brain injury: impact on community participation. *American Journal of Physical Medicine and Rehabilitation, 86*(12), 962-969.

Ivanhoe, C. B., & Hartman, E. T. (2004). Clinical caveats on medical assessment and treatment of pain after TBI. *Journal of Head Trauma Rehabilitation, 19*(1), 29-39.

Jahnsen, R., Villien, L., Aamodt, G., Stanghelle, J. K., & Holm, I. (2004). Musculoskeletal pain in adults with cerebral palsy compared with the general population. *Journal of Rehabilitation Medicine, 36*(2), 78-84.

Jensen, M. P., Abresch, R. T., Carter, G. T., & McDonald, C. M. (2005). Chronic pain in persons with neuromuscular disease. *Archives of Physical Medicine & Rehabilitation, 86*(6), 1155-1163.

Jensen, M. P., Ehde, D. M., Gertz, K. J., Stoelb, B. L., Dillworth, T. M., Hirsh, A. T., et al. (2011). Effects of self-hypnosis training and cognitive restructuring on daily pain intensity and catastrophizing in individuals with multiple sclerosis and chronic pain. *International Journal of Clinical and Experimental Hypnosis, 59*(1), 45-63.

Jensen, M. P., Hoffman, A. J., Stoelb, B. L., Abresch, R. T., Carter, G. T., & McDonald, C. M. (2008). Chronic pain in persons with myotonic dystrophy and facioscapulohumeral dystrophy. *Archives of Physical Medicine and Rehabilitation, 89*(2), 320-328.

Jensen, M. P., Kuehn, C. M., Amtmann, D., & Cardenas, D. D. (2007). Symptom burden in persons with spinal cord injury. *Archives of Physical Medicine and Rehabilitation, 88*(5), 638-645.

Jonsson, A. C., Lindgren, I., Hallstrom, B., Norrving, B., & Lindgren, A. (2006). Prevalence and intensity of pain after stroke: a population based study focusing on patients' perspectives. *Journal of Neurology, Neurosurgery and Psychiatry, 77*(5), 590-595.

Kalia, L. V., & O'Connor, P. W. (2005). Severity of chronic pain and its relationship to quality of life in multiple sclerosis. *Multiple Sclerosis, 11*(3), 322-327.

Kennedy, P., Lude, P., & Taylor, N. (2006). Quality of life, social participation, appraisals and coping post spinal cord injury: a review of four community samples. *Spinal Cord, 44*(2), 95-105.

Kitisomprayoonkul, W., Sungkapo, P., Taveemanoon, S., & Chaiwanichsiri, D. (2010). Medical complications during inpatient stroke rehabilitation in Thailand: a prospective study. *Journal of the Medical Association of Thailand, 93*(5), 594-600.

Klit, H., Finnerup, N. B., Andersen, G., & Jensen, T. S. (2011). Central poststroke pain: A population-based study. *Pain, 152*(4), 818-824. doi: 10.1016/j.pain.2010.12.030

Kong, K.-H., Woon, V.-C., & Yang, S.-Y. (2004). Prevalence of chronic pain and its impact on health-related quality of life in stroke survivors. *Archives of Physical Medicine and Rehabilitation, 85*(1), 35-40.

Kooijman, C. M., Dijkstra, P. U., Geertzen, J. H. B., Elzinga, A., & van der Schans, C. P. (2000). Phantom pain and phantom sensations in upper limb amputees: an epidemiological study. *Pain, 87*(1), 33-41.

Kratz, A. L., Williams, R. M., Turner, A. P., Raichle, K. A., Smith, D. G., & Ehde, D. M. (2010). To lump or to split? Comparing individuals with traumatic and nontraumatic limb loss in the first year after amputation. *Rehabilitation Psychology, 55*(2), 126-138.

Lahz, S., & Bryant, R. A. (1996). Incidence of chronic pain following traumatic brain injury. *Archives of Physical Medicine and Rehabilitation, 77*(9), 889-891.

Linton, S. J. P., & Nordin, E. M. A. (2006). A 5-year follow-up evaluation of the health and economic consequences of an early cognitive behavioral intervention for back pain: A randomized, controlled trial. *Spine, 31*(8), 853-858.

Lundstrom, E., Smits, A., Terent, A., & Borg, J. (2009). Risk factors for stroke-related pain 1 year after first-ever stroke. *European Journal of Neurology, 16*(2), 188-193.

Meldrum, M. L. (2007). Brief history of multidisciplinary management of chronic pain, 1990-2000. In M. Schatman & A. Campbell (Eds.), *Chronic pain management: guidelines for multidisciplinary program development*: Informa Healthcare.

Middleton, J. W., Tran, Y., & Craig, A. (2007). Relationship between quality of life and self-efficacy in persons with spinal cord injuries. *Archives of Physical Medicine and Rehabilitation, 88*(12), 1643-1648.

Miro, J., Raichle, K. A., Carter, G. T., O'Brien, S. A., Abresch, R. T., McDonald, C. M., et al. (2009). Impact of biopsychosocial factors on chronic pain in persons with myotonic and facioscapulohumeral muscular dystrophy. *American Journal of Hospice & Palliative Medicine, 26*(4), 308-319.

Molton, I. R., Stoelb, B. L., Jensen, M. P., Ehde, D. M., Raichle, K. A., & Cardenas, D. D. (2009). Psychosocial factors and adjustment to chronic pain in spinal cord injury:

replication and cross-validation. *Journal of Rehabilitation Research and Development, 46*(1), 31-42.

Morley, S., Eccleston, C., & Williams, A. (1999). Systematic review and meta-analysis of randomized controlled trials of cognitive behaviour therapy and behaviour therapy for chronic pain in adults, excluding headache. *Pain, 80*(1-2), 1-13.

Motl, R. W., McAuley, E., Snook, E. M., & Gliottoni, R. C. (2009). Physical activity and quality of life in multiple sclerosis: Intermediary roles of disability, fatigue, mood, pain, self-efficacy and social support. *Psychology, Health and Medicine, 14*(1), 111-124.

Nampiaparampil, D. E. (2008). Prevalence of chronic pain after traumatic brain injury: A systematic review. *JAMA: Journal of the American Medical Association, 300*(6), 711-719.

Newland, P. K., Naismith, R. T., & Ullione, M. (2009). The impact of pain and other symptoms on quality of life in women with relapsing-remitting multiple sclerosis. *Journal of Neuroscience Nursing, 41*(6), 322-328.

Newland, P. K., Wipke-Tevis, D. D., Williams, D. A., Rantz, M. J., & Petroski, G. F. (2005). Impact of pain on outcomes in long-term care residents with and without multiple sclerosis. *Journal of the American Geriatrics Society, 53*(9), 1490-1496.

Nicholson Perry, K., Nicholas, M. K., & Middleton, J. W. (2009). Spinal cord injury-related pain in rehabilitation: a cross-sectional study of relationships with cognitions, mood and physical function. *European Journal of Pain: Ejp, 13*(5), 511-517.

Nicholson Perry, K., Nicholas, M. K., & Middleton, J. W. (2010). Comparison of a pain management program with usual care in a pain management center for people with spinal cord injury-related chronic pain. *The Clinical Journal of Pain, 26*(3), 206-216.

Nicholson Perry, K., Nicholas, M. K., & Middleton, J. W. (2011). Multidisciplinary cognitive behavioural pain management programmes for people with a spinal cord injury: design and implementation. *Disability and Rehabilitation, 33*(13-14), 1272-1280. doi: doi:10.3109/09638288.2010.524276

Nicholson Perry, K., Nicholas, M. K., Middleton, J. W., & Siddall, P. (2009). Psychological characteristics of people with spinal cord injury-related persisting pain referred to a tertiary pain management center. *Journal of Rehabilitation Research and Development, 46*(1), 57-67.

Norrbrink Budh, C., Hultling, C., & Lundeberg, T. (2005). Quality of sleep in individuals with spinal cord injury: a comparison between patients with and without pain. *Spinal Cord, 43*(2), 85-95.

Norrbrink Budh, C., Kowalski, J., & Lundeberg, T. (2006). A comprehensive pain management programme comprising educational, cognitive and behavioural interventions for neuropathic pain following spinal cord injury. *Journal of Rehabilitation Medicine, 38*(3), 172-180.

Norrbrink Budh, C., & Osteraker, A. L. (2007). Life satisfaction in individuals with a spinal cord injury and pain. *Clinical Rehabilitation, 21*(1), 89-96.

O'Connor, A. B., Schwid, S. R., Herrmann, D. N., Markman, J. D., & Dworkin, R. H. (2008). Pain associated with multiple sclerosis: systematic review and proposed classification. *Pain, 137*(1), 96-111.

O'Sullivan, S. S., Williams, D. R., Gallagher, D. A., Massey, L. A., Silveira-Moriyama, L., & Lees, A. J. (2008). Nonmotor symptoms as presenting complaints in Parkinson's disease: a clinicopathological study. *Movement Disorders, 23*(1), 101-106.

Osborne, T. L., Jensen, M. P., Ehde, D. M., Hanley, M. A., & Kraft, G. (2007). Psychosocial factors associated with pain intensity, pain-related interference, and psychological functioning in persons with multiple sclerosis and pain. *Pain, 127*(1-2), 52-62.

Osborne, T. L., Turner, A. P., Williams, R. M., Bowen, J. D., Hatzakis, M., Rodriguez, A., et al. (2006). Correlates of pain interference in multiple sclerosis. *Rehabilitation Psychology, 51*(2), 166-174.

Osterberg, A., Boivie, J., & Thuomas, K. A. (2005). Central pain in multiple sclerosis--prevalence and clinical characteristics. *European Journal of Pain, 9*(5), 531-542.

Parkes, J., White-Koning, M., Dickinson, H. O., Thyen, U., Arnaud, C., Beckung, E., et al. (2008). Psychological problems in children with cerebral palsy: a cross-sectional European study. *Journal of Child Psychology and Psychiatry and Allied Disciplines, 49*(4), 405-413.

Parkinson, K. N., Gibson, L., Dickinson, H. O., & Colver, A. F. (2010). Pain in children with cerebral palsy: a cross-sectional multicentre European study. *Acta Paediatrica, 99*(3), 446-451.

Piwko, C., Desjardins, O. B., Bereza, B. G., Machado, M., Jaszewski, B., Freedman, M. S., et al. (2007). Pain due to multiple sclerosis: analysis of the prevalence and economic burden in Canada. *Pain Research and Management, 12*(4), 259-265.

Pollmann, W., Feneberg, W., & Erasmus, L. P. (2004). Pain in multiple sclerosis--a still underestimated problem. The 1 year prevalence of pain syndromes, significance and quality of care of multiple sclerosis inpatients. *Nervenarzt, 75*(2), 135-140.

Putzke, J. D., Richards, J. S., Hicken, B. L., & DeVivo, M. J. (2002). Interference due to pain following spinal cord injury: important predictors and impact on quality of life. *Pain, 100*(3), 231-242.

Quale, A. J., & Schanke, A. (2010). Resilience in the face of coping with a severe physical injury: A study of trajectories of adjustment in a rehabilitation setting. *Rehabilitation Psychology, 55*(1), 12-22.

Rintala, D. H., Hart, K. A., & Priebe, M. M. (2004). Predicting consistency of pain over a 10-year period in persons with spinal cord injury. *Journal of Rehabilitation Research and Development, 41*(1), 75-88.

Russo, R. N., Miller, M. D., Haan, E., Cameron, I. D., & Crotty, M. (2008). Pain characteristics and their association with quality of life and self-concept in children with hemiplegic cerebral palsy identified from a population register. *Clinical Journal of Pain, 24*(4), 335-342.

Schley, M. T., Wilms, P., Toepfner, S., Schaller, H.-P., Schmelz, M., Konrad, C. J., et al. (2008). Painful and nonpainful phantom and stump sensations in acute traumatic amputees. *Journal of Trauma-Injury Infection & Critical Care, 65*(4), 858-864.

Schwartz, L., Engel, J. M., & Jensen, M. P. (1999). Pain in persons with cerebral palsy. *Archives of Physical Medicine & Rehabilitation, 80*(10), 1243-1246.

Siddall, P. J., Yezierski, R. P., & Loeser, J. D. (2000). Pain following spinal cord injury: clinical features, prevalence and taxonomy. *IASP Newsletter, 3*.

Smedema, S. M., Catalano, D., & Ebener, D. J. (2011). The relationship of coping, self-worth, and subjective well-being: A structural equation model. *Rehabilitation Counseling Bulletin, 53*(3), 131-142.

Stormer, S., Gerner, H. J., Gruninger, W., Metzmacher, K., Follinger, S., Wienke, C., et al. (1997). Chronic pain/dysaesthesiae in spinal cord injury patients: results of a multicentre study. *Spinal Cord, 35*(7), 446-455.

Stroud, M. W., Turner, J. A., Jensen, M. P., & Cardenas, D. D. (2006). Partner responses to pain behaviors are associated with depression and activity interference among persons with chronic pain and spinal cord injury. *The Journal of Pain, 7*(2), 91-99.

Summers, J. D., Rapoff, M. A., Varghese, G., Porter, K., & Palmer, R. E. (1991). Psychosocial factors in chronic spinal cord injury pain. *Pain, 47*(2), 183-189.

Turner, J. A., Jensen, M. P., Warms, C. A., & Cardenas, D. D. (2002). Catastrophizing is associated with pain intensity, psychological distress, and pain-related disability among individuals with chronic pain after spinal cord injury. *Pain, 98*(1-2), 127-134.

Ullrich, P. M., Jensen, M., Loeser, J. D., & Cardenas, D. D. (2007). Catastrophizing mediates associations between pain severity, psychological distress, and functional disability among persons with spinal cord injury. *Rehabilitation Psychology, 52*(4), 390-398.

Ullrich, P. M., Jensen, M. P., Loeser, J. D., Cardenas, D. D., & Weaver, F. M. (2008). Pain among veterans with spinal cord injury. *Journal of Rehabilitation Research and Development, 45*(6), 793-800.

Umlauf, R. L. (1992). Psychological interventions for chronic pain following spinal cord injury. *Clinical Journal of Pain, 8*, 111-118.

Vase, L., Nikolajsen, L., Christensen, B., Egsgaard, L. L., Arendt-Nielsen, L., Svensson, P., et al. (2011). Cognitive-emotional sensitization contributes to wind-up-like pain in phantom limb pain patients. *Pain, 152*(1), 157-162.

Vlaeyen, J. W., & Linton, S. J. (2000). Fear-avoidance and its consequences in chronic musculoskeletal pain: a state of the art. *Pain, 85*(3), 317-332.

Vogtle, L. K. (2009). Pain in adults with cerebral palsy: impact and solutions. *Developmental Medicine and Child Neurology, 51 Suppl 4*, 113-121.

Wartan, S. W., Hamann, W., Wedley, J. R., & McColl, I. (1997). Phantom pain and sensation among British veteran amputees. *British Journal of Anaesthesia, 78*(6), 652-659.

Widerstrom-Noga, E. G., & Turk, D. C. (2004). Exacerbation of chronic pain following spinal cord injury. *Journal of Neurotrauma, 21*(10), 1384-1395.

Wollaars, M. M., Post, M. W. M., van Asbeck, F. W. A., & Brand, N. (2007). Spinal cord injury pain: the influence of psychologic factors and impact on quality of life. *Clinical Journal of Pain, 23*(5), 383-391.

World Health Organisation. (2011). World report on disability 2011. Geneva: World Health Organisation.

19

The Role of Peripheral Nerve Blocks in the Interdisciplinary Care of Children with Chronic Pain: A Case Series and Review of the Literature

Gillian R. Lauder[1] and Nicholas West[2]
[1]*Department of Anesthesia, British Columbia Children's Hospital (BCCH),*
[2]*Pediatric Anesthesia Research Team, University of British Columbia (UBC),*
Canada

1. Introduction

Chronic pain of childhood is an extremely complex condition which can lead to damaging effects on physical and social wellbeing. Some children with severe chronic pain embark on a downward spiral of decreased physical, psychological and social functioning. This includes loss of mobility and inability to participate in physical and sporting activities, poor sleep, difficulty concentrating on school work, school absenteeism, social isolation and family stress. As chronic pain persists the child can experience increased pain intensity, distress, anxiety and depression. When enmeshed in this disordered lifestyle the child and their family require coordinated integrated care. The interdisciplinary team management approach, based on pharmacology, physiotherapy and psychology, is now well established to be the standard of care for children with chronic pain. Treatment goals are targeted to individual children after careful consideration of the history and examination. In appropriately selected children peripheral nerve blocks can provide immediate and effective pain relief. This chapter will present a referenced review of the literature on interdisciplinary paediatric chronic pain management whilst highlighting the role of peripheral nerve blocks. The case histories of eight paediatric patients with chronic pain who gained significant relief from peripheral nerve blocks will be presented.

The International Association for the Study of Pain (IASP) defines pain as "an unpleasant sensory or emotional experience associated with actual or potential tissue damage, or described in terms of such damage" (1986). One defining characteristic of pain is its duration. Acute pain is relatively short-term pain that typically lasts until the underlying cause has been identified and treated. On the other hand, chronic pain is understood to mean prolonged pain or "pain that extends beyond the expected period of healing" (Turk & Okifuji, 2001) and while defined time frames that determine a diagnosis of chronic pain vary, the definition adopted by most studies, including those cited here, is pain lasting longer than three months.

Chronic pain can have its roots in one or a combination of types of pain mechanism. Types of pain include nociceptive, inflammatory, neuropathic or psychogenic pain (DSM-IV "Pain Disorder"). Extreme caution is required before labelling a patient with a diagnosis of psychogenic pain, functional pain or somatisation disorder as the true prevalence of these conditions is extremely low. Most patients with chronic pain will have psychosocial elements to their suffering, but this does not mean that the pain is "psychogenic".

Nociceptive pain is felt in response to noxious stimuli, such as the trauma associated with injury, oncological and other disease processes as well as following surgery. This pain functions as a protective and interpretable symptom: 'it hurts here' means 'here is the damage' and can be a straightforward guide to what needs to be treated or allowed to heal. *Inflammatory pain* occurs as a result of inflammatory mediators in many disease processes or associated with healing following acute trauma or surgery. If either nociceptive or inflammatory pains are left unrecognised or undertreated they can lead to ongoing and then chronic pain. *Neuropathic pain* signifies some dysfunction in the nervous system itself and is a major cause of chronic suffering, occurring in about 6-7% of the population (Vinik, 2010).

Neuropathic pain may derive from some identifiable damage to the nerves, resulting from a disease process, inflammation or accidental damage during trauma or surgery, or may result from a failure of integration and function of the peripheral and central nervous systems. Many conditions previously labelled as functional pain are now known to have peripheral and central nervous elements, which would re-class them as neuropathic pain. Complex regional pain syndrome (CRPS) is an immuno-neurological disorder (Fechir et al, 2008). It may be associated with no nerve lesion (type I) or may be related to some identifiable nerve lesion (type II). Chronic conditions like functional abdominal pain syndrome (FAPS) and CRPS have been under-recognised by physicians, but are experienced by a significant number of adolescents (Clouse et al, 2006; Kachko et al, 2008). In summary, a combination of pain mechanisms may be involved in the development of chronic pain conditions.

1.1 The epidemiology of paediatric chronic pain

The epidemiology of chronic pain in children is less well understood than it is in adults, but some useful studies have been published in the last decade that help us to understand the overall scale of the problem and to elicit some socio-demographic particulars of the affected population. A survey of over 5,000 children aged 0 – 18 years in the Netherlands reported that 25% had experienced some form of chronic or recurrent pain (Perquin et al, 2000). A Spanish study, of 561 schoolchildren aged 8 – 16 years, reported an incidence of 37%, but concluded that only 5% suffer moderate or severe chronic pain (Huguet & Miró, 2008). In a Canadian study of 495 schoolchildren aged 9 - 13, more than half reported having experienced at least one recurrent pain, typically characterised as a headache, stomach pain or 'growing pain'. Although 46% reported a 'long-lasting' pain, the researchers judged that in many cases this represented a recurrent pain condition; nonetheless, 6% of children were classified as having possible, probable or definite chronic pain (van Dijk et al, 2006).

While these studies highlight the methodological difficulties in distinguishing acute, recurrent and chronic pain from children's responses to questionnaire and interview questions, these statistics clearly also demonstrate that childhood chronic pain is a significant problem: slightly more than one child in every twenty is a chronic pain sufferer; that is, at least one child in every average-sized classroom in every school. Perquin et al (2000) conclude that childhood chronic pain is 'a common experience' and that the incidence of severe chronic pain amongst adolescents should provoke both concern and further research from the healthcare community.

Previous pain experiences, cognitive, emotional and behavioural factors, family background, environment, peer group and culture have an influence on the impact, perception and biopsychosocial outcomes of chronic pain. Children living in lower educated, lower income families have been found to be at a greater risk of suffering recurrent pain, which is consistent with adult studies (Grøholt et al, 2003). Children suffering chronic pain themselves are quite likely to be living with another chronic pain sufferer, whether parent or sibling, and further investigation suggests that pre-existing chronic pain in the family environment is a predictor of both physical and psychological effects on the child (Lynch et al, 2006). Ethnicity and area of residence also appear to affect prevalence rates. For example, in Canada, the incidence of chronic pain is higher among Aboriginal people and, for males, is higher in rural areas (Ramage-Morin & Gilmour, 2010). There may also be cultural differences in the perception and reporting of pain (Mailis-Gagnon et al, 2007).

While chronic pain is clearly not confined to the developed world, most published studies provide figures for European or North American children, which may not be generalisable to different environments. A US study found that 13% of 12-13 year-olds and 17% of 15-16 year-olds experience abdominal pain every week (Hyams et al, 1996), while Dutta et al (1999) reported a considerably higher incidence (74%) in India. However, with gastrointestinal infections more widespread than the inflammatory bowel disease seen in developing countries, these figures probably represent the outcome of different disease processes (Ganesh et al, 2010). Abu-Saad Huijer (2010) considers the effects of war and traumatic events. Despite an absence of research in this area, he argues that chronic pain has been linked with post-traumatic stress disorders and that, as a consequence, we may expect to see a different profile of chronic pain among children affected by armed conflict.

In developed countries, headache, abdominal and musculoskeletal pain form the primary foci of chronic and recurrent pain among the paediatric population. In their study of Canadian 9-13 year olds, van Dijk et al (2006) received reports of recurrent headaches (32%), growing pains (21%), stomach pains (19%) and muscle aches (2%). Perquin et al (2000) had published similar findings from their survey of Dutch schoolchildren, in which they also analysed reports of pain at multiple locations. They found that the single location pain was most often reported. The combination of headache and abdominal pain was the most commonly reported multiple pain, found in 25% of all children. This greater than one pain profile was significantly more prevalent in adolescent girls.

Recent figures from a Statistics Canada health report identify chronic pain among 2.4% of males and 5.9% of females aged 12 to 17 years (Ramage-Morin & Gilmour, 2010). It has been reported that girls are as much as three times more likely to report chronic pain than boys (Martin et al, 2007). Perquin et al (2000) also showed a significant increase in the prevalence of chronic pain in girls. These girls were aged between 12 and 14 which may well be linked with the onset of menstruation. In general, abdominal pain is significantly more likely to be reported by girls and limb pain (or growing pains/muscle aches) is significantly more likely to be reported by boys (Perquin et al, 2000; van Dijk et al, 2006). A review on gender and pain suggests potential mechanisms within social and psychological processes, such as coping processes and catastrophising, are likely to contribute to the repeatedly observed sex differences in pain (Fillingim et al, 2009).

Aetiology and predisposition to chronic pain in children is largely unknown and depends on the type of pain. Factors associated with the development of chronic pain include surgery, trauma, emotional distress and chronic disease. In many cases, a definitive aetiology is difficult to establish. Even chronic post-surgical pain (CPSP) can be difficult to diagnose and consequently remains under-recognised. However, it represents a significant clinical problem. A 2006 review suggests that CPSP occurs after 10-50% of operations and results in severe chronic pain in 2-10% of these patients (Kehlet et al, 2006). This may, in fact, represent a significant portion of chronic pain sufferers. A UK study found that 22.5% of chronic pain patients developed their condition after surgery (Crombie et al, 1998). CPSP will often be neuropathic, resulting from nerve damage during surgery, though it could also be an ongoing inflammatory/nociceptive mechanism. The incidence of CPSP in the adult population is found to depend on a number of perioperative factors which include: genetic predisposition, degree of pre-operative anxiety, depression, pre-operative pain status, the surgical pain model, surgical technique, length of surgery and the quality of acute postoperative pain management (Kehlet et al, 2006; Macrae, 2008). The probability of an adult developing chronic pain after mastectomy or hernia surgery is decreased with increased age (Poleshuck et al, 2006; Poobalan et al, 2003). How this relationship to age translates to children and adolescents is not known as there is no published literature on CPSP in children. Six out of the eight paediatric cases presented in this chapter developed chronic pain following surgery.

Untangling factors to establish clear causality for the development of paediatric chronic pain is a challenge. Whether initiated by surgery or injury or other cause, it is a complex multi-factorial process. Understanding this mechanism requires not only a search for a cause, but also a clearer understanding of the effects of chronic pain. It is established that some paediatric chronic pain conditions have been under-diagnosed. Better recognition and early treatment of these conditions requires that healthcare providers understand the effects of chronic pain on a child and their family.

1.2 The impact of chronic pain on children and their families

Childhood chronic pain has a negative impact on physical, psychological and social function. It can prevent a child participating in sporting activities and other forms of exercise. It can cause sleep disruption and fatigue. It can contribute to depression and anxiety. It can affect school work through fatigue, poor memory and concentration and result in reduced school attendance. Friendships and family relationships are disrupted which may lead to varying degrees of social isolation. An Australian study of 207 children and adolescents attending a paediatric pain management clinic found that 95% had missed school, 90% had been unable to participate in some sporting activity and 71% had suffered some sleep disruption (Chalkiadis, 2001). Roth-Isigkeit et al (2005) found that 30-40% of children/adolescents with pain reported effects of their pain on school attendance, hobbies, social contacts, appetite, sleep, as well as increased utilization of health services because of their pain. An understanding of the range and interaction of all these different effects is crucial to the effective recognition and treatment of chronic pain in children.

These impacts on daily living can be bundled into the notion of Health-Related Quality of Life (HRQoL), which may be defined as *"an individual's subjective assessment of his or her functioning and emotional state"* (Gold et al, 2009) and can be used for comparative purposes. One such measurement instrument is the Pediatric Quality of Life Inventory (PedsQL), which contains items relating specifically to both physical and psychosocial function (the latter comprising emotional, social and school function) and can be completed by self-report or parent-proxy (Varni et al, 2001). Using this instrument, a US study of 100 patients, aged

2–21 years, attending a chronic pain clinic found that the HRQoL scores of these patients were not only considerably lower than scores obtained from normal healthy children, but were significantly lower than scores observed in children with rheumatological or cancer disease (Vetter, 2008). Another US study found that the mean PedsQL score for a cohort of 69 children and adolescents (aged 8 - 18 years) seeking outpatient pain management services, fell below the 'at-risk cut-off score' for all dimensions except social functioning, suggesting that the majority of these children were experiencing significant disruption in their day-to-day lives. The message from these studies is clear: the effects of chronic pain on a child's quality of life are wide-ranging and profound.

School functioning has received perhaps the most attention (Palermo, 2000). It demonstrates the most marked detriment of all the psychosocial dimensions of the PedsQL scale (Vetter, 2008; Gold et al, 2009) and clearly illustrates the complex effects of chronic pain on quality of life. A child with chronic pain may experience a range of problems which impact on their schooling: fatigue and/or poor sleep profile prevents early morning waking; pain inhibits physical ability to get to school, to sit in a classroom for long periods or to participate in physical activities; fear of pain by accidentally being knocked during recess times inhibits social interaction and imparts a sense of isolation, difference and not being involved with peers; poor memory and concentration affects schoolwork; as school work becomes missed or incomplete these unfinished projects become a barrier to return to school if workload is not controlled; and the school may represent an environment where their pain condition is not properly understood or tolerated.

For all these reasons school absences are common. In a survey of adolescent chronic pain sufferers aged 12-17 in Boston USA, 44% missed more than one-quarter of school days and 20% had missed more than half (Logan et al, 2008). Of course, schools typically offer only a limited degree of health-related support. In the Boston study, two-thirds of participants had received some form of accommodation from their school, such as being sent to the nurse's office, being sent home in pain, reduction in workload, extension on an assignment, and so on. Nonetheless, 44.3% of parents reported their child's grades had suffered (Logan et al, 2008) and missing school can clearly have negative consequences that extend beyond academic performance to a child's physical, emotional and social development. Six of the eight cases presented in this chapter had missed significant amounts of school.

Assessing the impact of chronic pain on a child's life is an important but problematic task. There are a number of reasons for this difficulty.

Firstly, the specific effects of chronic pain are not easily isolated from one another. For example, fatigue may be a mediating factor between pain and school functioning (Gold et al, 2009). Anxiety also plays a complex role in moderating the relationship between pain and function. Tsao et al (2007) studied anxiety sensitivity, or the fear of anxiety sensations, in 87 children aged 10-18 presenting at a US chronic pain clinic. Anxiety sensitivity was found to be linked with academic and/or social limitations, where those limitations arose from emotional rather than physical difficulties. Greater anxiety sensitivity was associated with lower self-esteem and perceived general and mental health, and with more behavioural problems and family disruption, but did not appear to affect physical functioning (Tsao et al, 2007). In a similar study of 222 adolescents aged 11 to 19 years attending two chronic pain clinics in the UK, Cohen et al (2010) found that in children with low anxiety, level of pain was a good predictor of physical and social function, but that high levels of anxiety prompted poorer function regardless of the level of pain.

Secondly, the impact of chronic pain on health and quality of life often extends beyond any immediate effects. For example, more than 50% of adolescents with chronic pain report some symptoms of insomnia (compared with less than 20% of healthy adolescents), and while these may initially be related directly to the experience of pain, behavioural patterns can transform this disruption into a primary sleep disorder (Palermo et al, 2010). Furthermore, chronic pain in childhood appears to increase the risk of developing further chronic conditions in adulthood. Adults, who have suffered recurrent headaches as children, are at an increased risk not only of headaches, but other physical and psychiatric symptoms (Fearon & Hotopf, 2001). Similarly, a longitudinal cohort study of paediatric FAPS patients, aged 6 to 18 at enrolment, found that, 15 years later, those with unresolved FAPS experienced higher levels of non-abdominal chronic pain (including migraine, tension-type headaches, and pelvic, back and limb pain) than those with resolved FAPS or normal controls (Walker et al, 2010).

Thirdly, the effects of chronic pain are felt not just by the child, but become a burden for the whole family. The child may no longer participate in shared physical activities, limiting family excursions and fun. Relationships with parents, siblings and other family members are put under strain resulting in anxiety and depression (Eccleston et al, 2004). A number of studies report associations between family functioning and the level of a child's pain-related disability, generally finding that the worse the disability, the greater the family dysfunction (Lewandowski et al, 2010). While it is difficult to interpret the causal relationship underpinning this association with confidence, it is likely that causation runs in both directions: a child's chronic pain has an adverse effect on family life; family problems make it more difficult for the child to cope and so worsen the experience of pain. The impact of chronic pain on the family matches the adverse impact experienced by families caring for children at home with severe cerebral palsy or birth defects (Vetter, 2008).

Daily care arrangements for the child/adolescent with chronic pain require additional support, which may cost money or require a parent to give up a job. The direct and indirect costs of caring for a child with chronic pain have been estimated. A UK study calculated, from a sample of 52 families, that the total annual cost, to a family living with a child in chronic pain, was as much as £14,160 or, approximately, $25,000 (Sleed et al, 2005). This figure included direct healthcare costs for the child and other family members and indirect costs such as loss of earnings, adaptations to housing, over-the-counter medications and care assistance. This is a potentially ruinous sum for low-income families.

Fourthly, physical and social effects of chronic pain carry another associated economic burden, which may be less easily identified and difficult to quantify. Diminished school function and educational achievement will have potential long-term career and economic cost for both the child and for society.

Finally, the immediate effects of chronic pain have the potential to feed back negatively on the physical and psychosocial health of children and their families. This further reduces their capacity to cope. Unremitting pain can cause sleep disruption and fatigue. Missing school leads to social isolation. The extra burden of stress and financial hardship on families makes them less able to provide the required care. The physical, psychological and social effects of chronic pain can lead the child and their family into a downward spiral, from which it is difficult to emerge without inter-disciplinary support. It is crucial that physicians not only identify the wider psychosocial effects of chronic pain, but recognise that these effects are contributory factors which play an important role in the ongoing pain and functioning of their patient (Jensen, 2011). With the goal of optimal patient care in mind, a clinician should consider including interventions that address these factors in their treatment strategies for children with chronic pain.

1.3 Interdisciplinary team management of children with chronic pain

Management of children and adolescents with severe suffering and extensive pain-related disability as a result of chronic pain requires an interdisciplinary approach (Eccleston et al, 2003). This includes the treatment modalities of pharmacology, physiotherapy and psychology running in parallel or, more importantly, enmeshed with one another. How these elements are balanced is dependant on each individual child and takes into consideration the type and duration of pain, as well as the impact of pain on particular biopsychosocial aspects of the child's life.

1.3.1 Pharmacology

The pharmacological approach to management of a child with chronic pain requires consideration of the type of pain, the impact of the pain on the child's biopsychosocial functions and the potential side effects of the medications. Medications need to be individualised to each child and continually re-assessed for efficacy and side effects. If medications are having no impact at therapeutic dosage they need to be discontinued and the child re-evaluated for consideration of other appropriate agents. Close liaison with psychiatry is advised prior to and following up on prescription of mood stabilising medications. It is important to emphasise that pharmacological interventions are only one part of an interdisciplinary approach to improve function in children/adolescents with chronic pain. Table 1 provides a summary of the medications that may be considered in the pharmacological treatment of paediatric chronic pain.

Drug	Dose	Comments
Acetamin-ophen	**>3 months of age to adolescents:** 10-15 mg/kg/dose PO Q4H PRN (max 75 mg/kg/day)	Central analgesic action via cannabinoid or prostaglandin mechanism Hepatotoxic in acute overdose or with chronic long term use; risk factors for toxicity include fever, prolonged fasting (>48 hrs), concomitant interacting drugs, obesity, poorly controlled diabetes, liver disease, viral infections and malnutrition Doses apply to normal healthy children (i.e. no hepatic or renal compromise)
Ibuprofen	5-10 mg/kg/dose PO Q6-8H (max 40 mg/kg/day)	Non steroidal anti-inflammatory agent; should not be used concomitantly with other NSAIDs Use caution in patients with aspirin hypersensitivity, hepatic or renal insufficiency Administer with food or milk to lessen GI upset; contraindicated with active GI bleeding and ulcer disease
Naprosyn	**Children >2 years:** 5-7 mg/kg/dose PO/PR Q8-12H	Non steroidal anti-inflammatory agent; should not be used concomitantly with other NSAIDs Contraindicated with active GI bleeding and ulcer disease; administer with food or milk to avoid GI upset; common GI side effects include abdominal pain, appetite loss, stomatitis or constipation May cause photosensitive vesicular rash (pseudoporphyria)

Drug	Dose	Comments
Tramadol (Ultram, Ralivia)	**Immediate-release form:** **Children:** 1-2 mg/kg Q4-6H PRN (max: 400 mg/day or 8 mg/kg/day) **Adolescents:** 50-100 mg Q4-6H PRN (max: 400 mg/day) **Extended-release form:** **Adolescents:** Initial: 100 mg PO daily; titrate by 100 mg increments every 2-3 days PRN (max: 300 mg/day).	An opioid analgesic with norepinephrine and serotonin effects Side effects include nausea and vomiting; tolerability is improved by gradual dose titration. Caution in renal and/or hepatic impairment Tramadol is metabolized to active form (i.e. a prodrug) Inter-individual pharmacogenomic variations affect efficacy Serotonin syndrome reported with concurrent use of serotonergic drugs Seizures reported with concurrent TCAs, SSRIs, and opioids or with conditions that lower seizure threshold Withdrawal symptoms may develop if abruptly discontinued; do not suddenly stop long-term treatment; wean dose by 25% per week Extended release product given ONCE daily.
Topical Lidocaine	Topical: 5% under occlusive dressing for 12 hours (once per day)	Blockade of upregulated sodium channel receptors in injured nerves. Useful for very localised pain Minimal side effects (mild skin reactions)
Amitriptyline	Initial: 0.1 mg/kg/dose PO HS; increase as needed and tolerated over 2-3 wks to 0.5-2 mg/kg/dose HS	Tricyclic antidepressant agent (TCA) used in low dose for chronic neuropathic pain; prevents the re-uptake of serotonin and norepinephrine. Pretreatment ECG required to exclude arrhythmia potential. Drug interactions via cytochrome p450 system; contraindicated if MAO inhibitors used within 14 days; tricyclics have limited efficacy for treatment of depression in children and adolescents Side effects include: sedation, confusion, weakness, fatigue, tremor, sweating, headache, anticholinergic effects, cardiovascular effects (including orthostatic hypotension, tachycardia, prolonged QTc and arrhythmias at higher plasma levels), decreased seizure threshold. Sedative side effect used to help with improved sleep profile If one TCA not helpful due to intolerable side effects try another with a different SE profile before abandoning this modality of pharmacological therapy (Nortriptyline is less sedating, doxepin less anticholinergic). Analgesic effect may not occur for 2 weeks from commencement. A withdrawal syndrome is documented for Tricyclics (flu-like symptoms, dizziness, mood changes). Assess patient carefully and limit prescribed quantities to minimum effective dose; do not suddenly stop long-term treatment; wean dose by 25% per week.
Gabapentin	**Children:** titrate to effect over a few days, starting at 2 mg/kg once or twice daily, then increase to TID dosing to a maximum of 35 mg/kg/24hr (max 3600 mg/day)	Calcium channel α 2-δ ligand; calcium channel blocker when neuron hyperexcited Analgesic, anticonvulsant, anxiolytic, and sleep-modulating activities. Side effects may include somnolence, ataxia, fatigue and behaviour change. Gradual dose increase helps to minimize sedation; increased

Drug	Dose	Comments
		oral doses are associated with decreased bioavailability; do not administer with antacids; primarily excreted unchanged in the urine, therefore need to adjust dose in renal impairment Maximum dose often not be needed for maximum effect; do not suddenly stop long-term treatment; wean dose by 25% per week.
Pregabalin	**Children > 10 years:** Initial: 25 mg PO daily Titrate upward to effect to 2.5 mg/kg PO BID or max 300 mg/day	Calcium channel α 2-δ ligand; calcium channel blocker when neuron hyperexcited. Similar in mechanism to gabapentin Side effects may include somnolence, ataxia, fatigue and behaviour change. Gradual dose increase helps to minimize sedation; increased oral doses are associated with increased bioavailability; do not administer with antacids; primarily excreted unchanged in the urine, therefore need to adjust dose in renal impairment. Maximum dose often not be needed for maximum effect; do not suddenly stop long-term treatment; wean dose by 25% per week.
Opioids	For dosing of different agents see Compendium of Pharmaceuticals and Specialties	mu-opioid agonist Additive sedative effects with other medications and/or alcohol Side effects include sedation, nausea, vomiting, constipation, pruritis, tolerance dependance opioid induced hyperalgesia, addiction Long-term use rarely indicated in children; addiction potential should be assessed prior to commencement of opioids; opioid prescription should follow national guidelines for safe practice
Venlafaxine	**Initial Dose:** 37.5 - 75 mg PO Once DAILY **Increment:** 37.5-75 mg every 4-7 days **Usual Dose Range:** 75-225 mg/day	Serotonin/norepinephrine reuptake inhibitor (SNRI) Effective in the treatment of Depression, Generalized Anxiety Disorder, Social Anxiety Disorder, Panic Disorder. Also used to treat ADHD, Post-Traumatic Stress Disorder and Obsessive-Compulsive Disorder. Side effects include: headache, nausea, increased heart rate and blood pressure (more prominent at higher doses), anorexia/weight loss, drowsiness, dizziness, dry mouth, sweating, tremor and impaired sexual function (adolescents/adults). Administer with food or milk to decrease GI upset; full beneficial effects may not be seen until 4 weeks of therapy completed. ***Warnings issued by Health Canada regarding use of antidepressants in pediatric patients.***
Clonidine	1-4 micrograms/kg/dose PO Q4-6H	An alpha adrenergic receptor antagonist; metabolism is hepatic and renal (roughly 50:50); drug interactions with beta blockers, tricyclic anti-depressants Sedative, anxiolytic and analgesic effects; a useful adjunct used to minimise other analgesic drug doses such as opioids Side effects include sedation, dry mouth, hypotension Do not suddenly stop long-term treatment; wean dose by 25% per week to prevent rebound hypertension

Table 1. Modalities of medications that may be considered in outpatient paediatric chronic pain management

1.3.2 Physiotherapy

Chronic pain sufferers often experience some level of physical incapacity and many adopt activity patterns that can make their pain worse, such as alternating episodes of over-activity and under-activity (Birkholtz et al, 2004). Physiotherapy plays an important role in the interdisciplinary treatment of chronic pain in children and adolescents. Eccleston & Eccleston (2004) divide it into the following four components:

- *Exercise* – this is used to increase aerobic endurance, flexibility, strength and overall fitness, which all have potential benefits for pain reduction;
- *Education* – this helps the patient relate their pain to their anatomy, physiology and activity levels and to address issues such as fear of movement and the potential for re-injury;
- *Behavioural management* – this may involve physical retraining and activity pacing, aiming for a gradual increase in the range and extent of movement, including a steady return to any activities abandoned since the onset of pain (see also Harding et al, 1998);
- *Performance assessment* – there is a clear link between reduced pain and improved physical function; the physiotherapist is well-placed to assess treatment progress.

Other reports of physiotherapy interventions in the treatment of chronic pain stress the importance of the interdisciplinary approach. For example, a combination of physical therapy and CBT has been shown to be effective in treating CRPS in children (Lee et al, 2002). Harding et al (1998) also highlight the need to integrate behavioural and cognitive components in activity training to minimise distress and unhelpful beliefs.

1.3.3 Psychology

There are a number of psychological factors, which are directly involved in the perception, reporting and self-management of pain. These include fear, vigilance to the feeling and threat of pain, catastrophising, avoidance of pain-inducing activity, sadness, depression, anger and self-denigration. Psychological factors are also important in coping mechanisms, taking action, and being able to predict or make sense of pain and its consequences (Eccleston, 2001). Psychologists provide continual education/reassurance on the pathophysiology of the chronic pain condition and teach mind-body techniques like breathing, muscle relaxation exercises, self-hypnosis, imagery, and cognitive strategies. These techniques help reduce the impact of pain on daily living and mood.

Cognitive behaviour therapy (CBT) is central to the notion of interdisciplinary care. CBT refers to an *"integration of treatments aimed at reducing or extinguishing the influence of the factors that maintain patients' maladaptive behaviours, beliefs and patterns of thought... and is delivered by a team of pain therapists, including anaesthetists, clinical psychologists and physiotherapists"* (Eccleston, 2001). Interdisciplinary CBT programmes aimed at adolescents with chronic musculoskeletal pain have been found to improve physical function, reduce emotional distress, increase attendance at school and reduce medicine consumption (Eccleston et al, 2003; de Blécourt et al, 2008). Furthermore, there is evidence to suggest that an interdisciplinary framework is beneficial for the family members involved. Schurman & Friesen (2010) report that an 'integrative care' approach in a paediatric Abdominal Pain Clinic (that is, service delivered by a gastroenterologist and a psychologist) was acceptable to families, produced higher satisfaction scores and, crucially, improved receptivity to treatment recommendations.

Relaxation strategies and plans to improve sleep hygiene are a vital part of the psychologist's role. When schooling has been impacted by pain, the psychologist helps teachers become more aware of the condition and its impact on schoolwork. The psychologist helps to negotiate or advocate for any accommodations needed in order to help the child succeed at school. Psychologists help the child and their family identify and resolve stresses such as anxiety or depression that could be preventing return to function.

A Cochrane Review determined that there is strong evidence for psychological therapies being effective in the treatment of headaches in children and some evidence for their efficacy in the treatment of musculoskeletal and recurrent abdominal pain (Eccleston et al, 2009). Psychological interventions are often, and ideally, delivered as part of an interdisciplinary approach and consequently there are few randomized-controlled-trial (RCT) studies providing definite evidence for individual therapies (McGrath & Holahan, 2003). Nonetheless, psychological techniques are a vital component of the interdisciplinary approach and experienced therapists will select particular techniques according to the needs of the individual patient.

1.3.4 Interventional therapies

Interventional procedures offered at Canadian paediatric *multidisciplinary pain treatment facilities* (MPTFs) include continuous epidural infusions, single epidural injections, facet injections, stellate ganglion nerve blocks, peripheral nerve blocks, trigger point injections, sympathetic blocks with local anaesthetic, Botox injections, intravenous regional anaesthesia, paravertebral nerve blocks and radiofrequency lesioning (Peng et al, 2007). Nerve blocks are used widely among Canadian anaesthesiologists who specifically practice chronic pain management: of those, 84% perform nerve blocks, compared with 60% who use pharmacotherapy, and a majority of them estimated that more than 40% of their patients require some form of nerve block as part of their treatment programme (Peng & Castano, 2005).

However, there is very little evidence to demonstrate that interventions benefit a patient more than would be seen from a placebo response. The literature is comprised of case reports and small case series, along with a few randomized, placebo-controlled trials (RCTs). For example, therapeutic lumbar facet joint nerve blocks can provide effective pain relief and functional improvement (Manchikanti et al, 2010). However, epidural corticosteroid injections for sciatica appear to offer only transient benefit (Arden et al, 2005). Results of RCTs are not always consistent, however. For example, one RCT has shown that radiofrequency lesioning of the dorsal root ganglion for treatment of chronic lumbosacral radicular pain appears not to be more effective than control treatment with local anaesthetic (Geurts et al, 2003); on the the other hand, another RCT has shown that it is both safe and effective (Simopoulos et al, 2008). For some techniques, such as myofascial trigger point injections, it has not even been possible to establish a consensus on methods for diagnosis or treatment (Tough et al, 2007). Furthermore, any RCTs that have been done mainly comprise adult studies. The evidence of efficacy in children/adolescents is even more limited and more research is required. There are also rare but significant iatrogenic risks associated with some of these interventions. Injection therapies for lower back pain carry the risk of paraspinal, spinal end epidural abscesses or meningitis (Gaul et al, 2005).

Despite this negative portrayal of interventional medicine for chronic pain "absence of evidence is not evidence of absence" (Altman & Bland, 1995) and there are many pain physicians and patients, including those in this case series, who have derived enormous benefit from interventional treatments.

2. Case reports

The cases are described below and summarised in table 2.

No	Gender	Age	Weight	Site of pain	Duration (months)	Diagnosis	Block(s) performed
1	Male	16	60kg	Chest	5	Intercostal neuralgia related to Nuss bar	Intercostal nerve blocks (1 diagnostic and 3 therapeutic)
2	Male	14	56kg	Abdomen	9	Abdominal wall pain	Bilateral rectus abdominis sheath blocks (diagnostic and therapeutic)
3	Male	18	60kg	Groin	12	Ilioinguinal neuralgia following hydrocele repair	Ilioinguinal nerve blocks (1 diagnostic and 3 therapeutic)
4	Male	15	66kg	Abdomen	3	Neuropathic pain, *not* incisional hernia	Intercostal nerve block; rectus sheath block.
5	Male	9	25kg	Groin	4	Genitofemoral or ilioinguinal neuralgia following orchidopexy	Rectus abdominis sheath block
6	Female	15	45kg	Rib	8	Intercostal neuralgia, post-surgery	intercostal nerve blocks (diagnostic and therapeutic)
7	Female	9	33kg	Abdomen	2	Abdominal wall pain following laparascopic appendectomy	Bilateral rectus abdominis sheath blocks (diagnostic and therapeutic)
8	Female	17	66kg	Rib	7	Intercostal neuralgia	Intercostal nerve blocks (diagnostic and therapeutic)

Table 2. Summary of cases

2.1 Case 1: A 16-year-old adolescent with chest pain related to a Nuss bar

A 60kg 16-year-old male presented with a 5 month history of right sided chest wall pain. He had undergone a Nuss procedure for cosmetic repair of pectus excavatum one year prior to presentation and had received satisfactory acute pain management with epidural analgesia. He was referred to the Pain Service by his surgeon. His pain was precipitated by a sudden lateral movement, but aggravated by activity, laughter and bending down. The pain was described as "shooting". The pain was not relieved by ibuprofen and/or acetaminophen.

This young man, an active kick-boxer, was extremely fit and well. However, his pain was so unremitting that he had to stop all sporting activities and was completely sedentary. His sleep was not disrupted, nor was his school attendance or academic performance. However, he was very frustrated that his pain prevented him pursuing his kick-boxing and his ability to perform simple physical tasks. He was able to maintain friendships, but could not engage in some of the more physical social activities.

On examination, his pain was found to radiate laterally from the site of his Nuss bar on the right side, in one dermatomal level at the level of the 7th rib from midaxillary line to sternum. There was no pain on palpation or deep inspiration/expiration. There was no numbness, allodynia or skin changes. Palpation of the thoracic spines, costochondral junctions, and left side of chest were unremarkable and pain free. His chest X-ray (CXR) revealed that his Nuss bar had not moved, with no bony reaction or wire migration. The CXR was otherwise normal. The presumed diagnosis was intercostal neuralgia.

A diagnostic intercostal nerve block was performed, which provided effective short-term symptomatic relief so a follow-up therapeutic block was done 10 days later. For the therapeutic block, 5mls of 0.25% bupivicaine with 1/200,000 epinephrine and 10mg triamcinolone was injected at four sites: at the affected rib, one above, one below and at the right sided Nuss bar insertion scar site. This provided complete pain relief to allow the patient to return to his previous physical activities.

He required repeat therapeutic blocks at 3 months and 1 year from the initial block for resurgence of pain, but had no further pain up to and after the removal of the Nuss bar.

2.2 Case 2: A 14-year-old male with abdominal pain

A 56kg 14-year-old male presented with a 9 month history of abdominal pain. There was no apparent precipitating event. He was referred to the Pain Service after multiple referrals and investigations had excluded a remedial cause for his pain but drawn a blank on a diagnosis. The pain was described as a dull, aching pain, present all the time, but worse with exercise and on palpation. There was no pattern to his pain or any relation to his diet. There were no other symptoms related to the abdominal system. The pain was not relieved by ibuprofen, acetaminophen or homeopathic remedies.

This young man had been extremely fit and well. However his pain was such that he had to stop all his sporting activities, experienced difficulty getting to sleep, was depressed and grumpy with his family and had been absent from school for the preceding 6 months.

On examination, his abdomen was slim and soft, with normal bowel sounds, no masses and no organomegaly. There was tenderness in the midline above the umbilicus, which was worse on abdominal wall tensing (Carnett's test positive). The presumed diagnosis was chronic abdominal wall pain.

A diagnostic bilateral rectus sheath block was performed above the umbilicus under ultrasound control which provided effective short-term symptomatic relief so a follow-up therapeutic block was done two weeks later. For the therapeutic block 10mls of 0.25% bupivicaine with 1/200,000 epinephrine and 20mg triamcinolone was injected at each site. He did not require repeat therapeutic blocks.

Two weeks after his therapeutic block, he slowly returned to his normal activity levels, sleeping and eating patterns and resumed his previous happy demeanour. The following term, he returned to school and reported no subsequent absences.

2.3 Case 3: An 18-year-old with groin pain after hydrocele repair

A 60kg 18-year-old male presented with a 1 year history of a shooting pain in his groin, which was present all the time and radiated down the medial aspect of his thigh to his knee. There was no apparent precipitating event; however, he was a competitive fencer and had undergone a left hydrocele repair 6 months prior to the onset of pain. The pain was worse in morning, walking up stairs and mobilizing from lying down. He had episodes of severe pain 2-3 times per day, which lasted several hours.

He was referred to the Pain Service after multiple referrals and investigations had excluded a remedial cause for his pain, but drawn a blank on a diagnosis. The pain was not relieved by acetaminophen.

This young man had been extremely fit and well. However his pain was such that his appetite was reduced, he was losing weight and he had to stop all his physical activities to the point that his future competitive aspirations were severely compromised. He continued to attend school, but was under pressure to compete in the fencing team. His mood during this period was described as 'testy'.

On examination, he had pain on palpation of the hydrocele repair scar, but no pain on palpation underneath inguinal ligament. He had a full range of non-painful movements of his lumbar spine, hips and knees with normal bulk, tone & power in his lower limbs, and brisk but equal knee and ankle jerk reflexes. He exhibited a downgoing plantar reflex and bilateral abdominal reflexes. His abdomen was slim and soft, with normal bowel sounds, no masses and no organomegaly. There was no apparent numbness to light touch of his scar or thigh and no allodynia, skin or hair changes. There was no pain to palpation in his scrotum or penis. The presumed diagnosis was ilioinguinal neuralgia.

A diagnostic ilioinguinal nerve block was performing under ultrasound control which provided effective short-term symptomatic relief so a follow-up therapeutic block was done one week later. For the therapeutic block 20mls of 0.25% bupivacaine with 1/200,000 epinephrine and 20mg triamcinolone was injected between the internal oblique and transverse abdominis muscles; some was also injected under the scar site from his hydrocele repair. This provided complete pain relief.

His mood and eating pattern improved within the first month, but he did require repeat therapeutic blocks at 5 months and 11 months following the initial block. These provided good pain relief to allow the patient to make a graded return to competitive fencing.

2.4 Case 4: A 15-year-old male with a suspected incisional hernia

A 66kg 15-year-old male presented with a 3 month history of left upper quadrant pain associated with a bulge just lateral & inferior to the incision from a congenital diaphragmatic hernia repair when he was 14 months old. The pain was described as a burning, stabbing sensation. He exhibited no symptoms related to the respiratory, cardiovascular or abdominal systems.

He had been extremely fit and well. However his pain was such that he could not stand up straight, suffered pain with all activity and was unable to sleep soundly because he could not get comfortable. He had completely lost his appetite and had lost 10kg in weight. He became depressed and ceased to interact with friends. His suffering affected his family deeply: his parents' relationship suffered, his sister became depressed. He could not sit or concentrate and consequently missed 5 months of school.

An upper gastrointestinal endoscopy was normal. Surgical repair of the suspected incisional hernia revealed no hernia of the abdominal wall. Pain occurred in the immediate postoperative period. This pain did not respond to simple analgesics or hydromorphone. He was referred to the Pain Service and a diagnosis of neuropathic pain was made.

Intercostal nerve blocks were administered to the left sided 9th, 10th, and 11th ribs. This provided effective short-term symptomatic relief, so a follow-up therapeutic block was done a week later. For the therapeutic block, 5ml of 0.25% bupivacaine with 1/200,000 epinephrine & 10mg triamcinolone was injected at the same 3 intercostal spaces; in addition, the same amount was administered as a left rectus sheath block under ultrasound control, adjacent to the site of surgery. On awakening, the patient reported that his pain had gone.

This treatment provided immediate pain relief, which allowed the patient to return to his normal self. His appetite returned the next day. Within a few days, he was laughing again and was sleeping normally. Within 2 months he had started gym. He quickly caught up with most of his schoolwork and was now motivated to do additional study during the summer vacation. He resumed contact with friends and his family were able to return to normal. He did not require repeat therapeutic blocks.

2.5 Case 5: A 9-year-old with post-orchidopexy pain

A 25kg 9-year-old male presented with a 4 month history of left sided groin pain. He had been experiencing this pain for three years on and off, but it had been worse since his orchidopexy surgery 4 months prior to the consultation. He was referred to the Pain Service by his surgeon.

He continued to attend school, but had to visit the nurse twice a day and lie down to recover his strength. Often the school requested that he be collected and taken home early. He found it difficult to engage in physical or social activities and had to give up Tae Kwon Do. He was often woken with pain and cramps and cried as a result of his pain.

The pain was described as "stabbing". It was not relieved by ibuprofen and/or acetaminophen. On examination, there was no numbness, allodynia or skin changes and Carnett's test was positive. The presumed diagnosis was genitofemoral or ilioinguinal neuralgia.

A diagnostic rectus abdominis sheath block was performed, under ultrasound control: 15ml 0.25% bupivicaine, 1/200,000 epinephrine was injected into the rectus sheath and between the transverse abdominis and internal oblique; 10ml was injected at his flank at the anterior superior iliac spine; and some was injected at his orchidopexy scar site. On awakening, the patient reported the pain was gone.

A therapeutic block was not done in this case. He was able to resume a normal sleeping pattern within 2 weeks, was much happier and once again able to spend time with friends. He made a gradual return to Tae Kwon Do and normal schooling with no absences.

2.6 Case 6: A 15-year-old female with chest pain following removal of exostosis

A 45 kg 15-year-old female presented at the Complex Pain Clinic with post-surgical chest pain. Successful removal of an exostosis from her right rib cage was followed by the gradual emergence of a new, sharp pain, which was present every day. It worsened during the day and with sitting or physical activity.

It was 8 months since her surgery. She had missed some school, had stopped gymnastics classes and soccer training completely and had to limit her social activities. She was grumpy with friends and family. Physiotherapy had not helped, but ketorolac (10mg twice a day as needed), psychology, TENS and laser therapy were judged to have provided some benefit.

She was examined by the interdisciplinary team. Physical examination revealed that her pain was localised to the right anterolateral aspect of her 10th rib, close to the exostosis excision; there was no associated numbness, no allodynia and no skin colour change. The physiotherapist noted that her right waist crease and elevated iliac crest suggested a protective response, but that she had a full range of motion in spine and extremities. The psychologist determined that she was not overly anxious or depressed, despite some ongoing family conflicts. A preliminary diagnosis of intercostal neuralgia was made.

A diagnostic intercostal nerve block was performed. This provided effective short-term symptomatic relief so a follow-up therapeutic block was done 3 weeks later. The therapeutic block comprised: 5ml 0.25% bupivicaine with 1/200,000 epinephrine & 2mg/ml triamcinolone injected at 3 sites above & below the affected rib; and 4ml 0.25% bupivicaine with 1/200,000 epinephrine & 1mg/ml triamcinolone injected under the scar site.

Though she did not return to gymnastics, her tiredness was resolved and she was able to begin soccer refereeing a week later. She was more energetic, happier and able to spend time with friends again. Her concentration and focus improved which enabled her to achieve better grades at school.

2.7 Case 7: A 9-year-old female with persistent pain following appendectomy

A 33kg 9-year-old female presented with right-sided abdominal pain, which had begun 3 days after a laparoscopic appendectomy two months previously. The pain, present all the time, but varying in intensity, was described as 'stabbing'. It was worse with activity and at the end of the day.

She had experienced disturbed sleep and was often woken by pain. She had only attended school for only three or four days since her surgery and was completely unable to attend her rhythmic gymnastics classes. Her appetite was reduced and her pain was worse after eating. She became anxious and this period of uncertainty was a tremendously stressful time for her whole family. Tramadol, ibuprofen and acetaminophen had not helped her pain.

A physical examination revealed a positive Carnett's test and normal bowel sounds. Her femoral pulses were present and equal. There was no lymphadenopathy in the inguinal region or neck and no organomegaly. There was no allodynia, no numbness and no skin colour change at the site of her pain. Pain was increased by squatting, walking, use of upper extremities and right leg raises. Right hip flexor function and ability to do sit-ups were limited by pain. She was diagnosed with abdominal wall pain secondary to surgery for laparoscopic appendectomy.

A diagnostic abdominal wall block was performed, which provided effective short-term symptomatic relief so a follow-up therapeutic block was performed two weeks later. The therapeutic block was administered on the right side using ultrasound control, with a 22-gauge IV cannula. A total of 10ml 0.25% bupivicaine with 2mg/ml triamcinolone was injected: 4ml into rectus sheath and 6ml between the transverse abdominus and internal oblique muscles.

On awakening she reported her right side was numb. She experienced an achy bruising pain for 36 hours, which settled down. She was soon able to return to normal sleeping, eating and activity levels. She returned to gymnastics within 3 weeks and was back to her previous level of activity within 2 months. She was significantly happier and quickly re-established her relationships with friends. She returned to school within 2 weeks and was back to a full timetable within a month.

2.8 Case 8: A 17-year-old female with rib pain

A 66kg 17-year-old female presented with a 6 month history of right-sided lower rib pain. It may have been caused by an injury incurred playing volleyball. She described it as a 'stabbing', burning pain that sometimes radiated to the back or the epigastrum. She had no pain-free days. The pain was worse at night, with deep-breathing and with sitting for long periods of time.

She experienced considerable difficulty maintaining a normal sleep balance: she had trouble getting to sleep and was woken at least once a night in pain, often for long periods. As a consequence, she was often very fatigued, which she felt made her pain worse. She had a reduced appetite in the morning and had stopped all sporting activities. She showed some signs of depression and isolated herself from friends and family. She struggled to concentrate and missed approximately 40% of school.

A variety of therapies had been tried, including psychology, physiotherapy, acupuncture, TENS and two sessions with a chiropractor, but these had afforded only partial pain relief. Acetaminophen and non-steroidal anti-inflammatory agents were not effective. She obtained some relief from morphine, consuming up to 50mg each day. The presumed diagnosis was intercostal neuralgia.

A diagnostic intercostal nerve block was performed, which provided effective short term symptomatic relief so a follow-up therapeutic block was done three weeks later. For the therapeutic block, a total of 12ml 0.25% bupivicaine with 1/200,000 epinephrine was injected at 3 sites; one above & below and at the site of the affected rib on the right side.

This treatment allowed her to make a gradual return to normal. She began exercising again after 2 weeks, started sleeping deeper and longer and was generally in much better mood. She was able to sit and concentrate once again and resumed social activities with friends.

3. Discussion

3.1 Diagnosis and selection criteria for the use of peripheral nerve blocks

The cases described in this chapter demonstrate that, in properly selected children and adolescents, a peripheral nerve block can be an extremely beneficial component of interdisciplinary care. The case histories demonstrate the effective use of targeted nerve blocks for specific pain conditions such as ilioinguinal block for ilioinguinal neuralgia. The children and adolescents affected are often extremely physically active prior to the first reports of pain. They are usually previously fit and well with no previous pain or medical problems. There is typically an inciting event. The pain is characteristically neuropathic in description with sharp shooting elements and allodynia. The pain distribution is often dermatomal but not necessarily associated with numbness. The pain is not responsive or resolved with simple medications. The impact of the pain is considerable in its effects on physical function, schooling, mood and family dynamics.

3.2 Effective techniques in the use of peripheral nerve blocks

Peripheral nerve blockade in paediatric chronic pain has previously been described specifically for chronic abdominal wall pain (Skinner & Lauder, 2007). Due to the lack of evidence to guide therapy, the following recommendations are the opinion of the author (GL). Peripheral nerve blocks are done under sedation or general anesthesia to minimise further stress and pain to children and adolescents. Strict sterile procedure is followed. Plain local anaesthetic is used for the initial block to ensure that the diagnosis is correct prior to installation of steroids. Peripheral nerve blocks are done whenever possible under ultrasound control to maximise the chance of an effective block by ensuring the local anaesthetic is deposited in the correct plane or near the correct nerve. A diagnostic peripheral nerve block is considered to have worked if the local anaesthetic provided numbness in the dermatomal region to be blocked and also resulted in a clinically significant reduction in pain (>50% reduction). A therapeutic block is only performed after a positive diagnostic block. To achieve a therapeutic peripheral nerve block the same block is performed under ultrasound control with local anaesthetic and steroid (1-2mg/ml of trimcinolone to a maximum dose of 40mg). Peripheral nerve blocks are only offered if children and adolescents are willing to participate in the whole team approach with adherence to paced activity and integration with psychology. The duration of effect of a therapeutic block is extremely varied and may be related to time from diagnosis as well as to the degree in which paced return to activity is adhered to following successful block. Subsequent therapeutic blocks tend to last longer than the previous.

3.2.1 Pharmacology

The steroid element of the therapeutic peripheral nerve block is considered to either reduce inflammation or result in thinning of the connective tissue around painful nerves (Suleiman & Johnston, 2001). There is no consensus on the correct dose of steroid that should be used for peripheral nerve blocks in children. Steroids have local and systemic side effects. The local effect of fascial thinning may have detrimental effects with repeat injections (Suleiman & Johnston, 2001). Side effects of ongoing or chronic systemic steroids include carbohydrate intolerance, hypothalamic-pituitary-adrenal suppression, growth failure (Hochberg, 2002) and others such as immunosuppression, cataracts, pseudomotor cerebri, pancreatitis steroid psychosis, and steroid myopathy (Rimsza, 1978). The incidence of major systemic side effects to infrequent intermittent steroid injections is not known.

3.3 The mechanism and effects of the treatment

The specific effects of peripheral nerve blocks rely on the action of pharmacological agents such as local anaesthetics and triamcinolone. However, broader elements of care are also significant. In the context of an ongoing treatment regime, it is particularly important to consider the psychosocial dynamics of the diagnosis and treatment processes, including development of trust in the healthcare team and springboard effects from the realization of interim treatment goals. It is presumed that the combination of these effects creates/initiates a break or change in the pain cycle and reverses the changes that occurred within the peripheral and central nervous system to cause chronic pain.

3.3.1 Nonspecific treatment effects

We may like to think that when a patient gets better, it is the direct and intentional result of medical intervention, but it may not be quite so straightforward. Jamison (2011) identifies three mechanisms, which may contribute to any improvement in a patient's pain or functioning - (i) the specific or intended effects of any treatment, (ii) natural history and (iii) nonspecific effects of treatment - and there may be some interaction between these elements. Nonspecific treatment effects are the outcomes of patient encounters with healthcare providers. These include attention, stimulation of the desire to get better, reduced anxiety, increased understanding, trust, hope, optimism and improved ability to cope (Jamison, 2011). One important nonspecific treatment effect with children and adolescents is for others, including healthcare providers, to believe that they have pain. These non-specific treatment effects represent a complex array of psychosocial variables that, when utilized correctly, can bestow huge benefit to the patient's sense of wellbeing and outcomes.

The team's attention to the broader effects of pain on daily functioning and quality of life is crucial. What does the child's pain mean to them? What does it mean to their family? What are the patient goals of therapy and are they achievable? As discussed, psychosocial effects of pain such as sadness, frustration, anxiety or depression can become contributory factors to the continuation or worsening of pain in a vicious circle that is hard to escape without effective support. If they remain unrecognized and untreated, these factors may hinder the progress of any management plan.

It has been established that the style of communication adopted by a physician can have a dramatic effect on patient patient's health outcomes (Di Blasi et al, 2001; Griffin et al, 2004;

Verheul et al, 2010). Meaningful two-way communication between healthcare provider and patient is crucial. However, a patient-centred dialogue may depend on circumstances, as physicians appear to adopt a more patient-centred style of communication with patients who participate actively in the discussion (Cegala & Post, 2009). In paediatric care, the communication is, typically, three-way between provider, patient and parent or caregiver which makes adopting a patient-centred approach will often be more challenging. Effective communication, in this context, means using appropriate terminology and actively listening to both patient and parent as well as giving attention to their body language. Factors which have to be considered include: identifying patient and parental expectations, i.e. goal directed therapy; devoting enough time to acquire the whole pain-related history; interpreting non-responsiveness; identifying hidden messages conveyed in what's being said and not said; understanding family beliefs, hopes and fears; asking potentially embarrassing questions separately and in confidence; conveying empathy; introducing appropriate humour into the dialogue; conveying expertise and credibility in pain management; establishing trust; not causing more pain on examination; providing an agreed workable goal-directed and achievable management plan.

3.3.2 Placebo response to peripheral nerve block intervention

Without the evidence of a randomized double blind placebo controlled trial, it is not easy to stipulate that the interventional blocks are the overriding therapeutic modality in this case series. Many would argue that this represents a placebo response. A placebo response refers to the psychobiological response seen after administration of a placebo (a non therapeutic modality) in an individual or groups of patients. Placebo treatments have known effects on the endogenous pharmacology, cognitive and conditioning systems in humans (Fields & Levine, 1981; de la Fuente-Fernandez et al, 2001; Meissner et al, 2007; Wager et al, 2007; Benedetti, 2008; Scott et al, 2008; Eippert et al, 2009; Finniss et al, 2009).

Expectations have the strongest evidence for contributing to the placebo response, especially placebo analgesia. Within the neuro-pharmacological aspect of an analgesic placebo response, there is evidence for the role of endogenous endorphins as some placebo analgesic responses are reversed with naloxone. The respiratory centres, serotonin secretion, hormone secretion, immune responses and heart function are also involved in the biological response to placebo analgesic treatments (Finniss et al, 2009).

Whatever the mechanism of therapeutic benefit, placebo responses are potentially embedded in every intervention for pain relief (Robinson, 2009). The key message from our case series is that plain local anaesthetic nerve block provided only temporary relief for 7 out of 8 cases. Only when local anaesthetic and steroid was used, in conjunction with their ongoing interdisciplinary care, did these children and adolescents turn their lives around to their pre-pain level of functioning. If only a placebo response, it would be expected to last 1-3 months only. Only 2 of the cases required repeat therapeutic blocks which were performed greater than three months after the initial therapeutic block. This all points to a mainly therapeutic effect, but would have to be supported by a properly conducted study.

4. Conclusion

Chronic pain of childhood is an extremely complex condition which can have devastating effects on physical, psychological and social functioning. The interdisciplinary team management approach, based on pharmacology, physiotherapy and psychology, is the standard of care for children with severe or ongoing chronic pain. However, in a small proportion of appropriately selected children peripheral nerve blocks can provide immediate, effective and long-term pain relief. The case histories outlined in this chapter demonstrate the enormous impact that pain can have on a child, their functioning and their families. The significant relief received from peripheral nerve blockade indicates that this is a modality that must be considered when the history and examination findings match those presented. However, formal studies are required to definitively evaluate the effectiveness of the peripheral nerve block intervention.

5. Acknowledgement

The authors would like to thank UBC's *Pediatric Anesthesia Research Team* and the children and adolescents reported in this chapter for allowing us to detail their pain journey.

6. References

Abu-Saad Huijer, H. (2010) 'Chronic pain in children and adolscents: a review', *Lebanese Medical Journal*, Vol. 58, No. 2, pp. 105-10, ISSN 0023-9852

Altman, D. & Bland, J. (1995) 'Statistics notes: Absence of evidence is not evidence of absence', *British Medical Journal*, Vol. 311, No. 7003, p.485, ISSN 0007-1447

Arden, N., Price, C., Reading, I., Stubbing, J., Hazelgrove, J., Dunne, C., Michel, M., Rogers, P. & Cooper, C. (2005) 'A multicentre randomized controlled trial of epidural corticosteroid injections for sciatica: the WEST study', *Rheumatology* , Vol. 44, No. 11, pp. 1399-406, ISSN 1462-0324

Benedetti F. (2008) 'Mechanisms of placebo and placebo-related effects across diseases and treatments', *Annual Review of Pharmacology and Toxicology*, Vol. 48, pp. 33–60, ISSN 0362-1642

Birkholtz, M., Aylwin, L. & Harman, R. (2004) 'Activity pacing in chronic pain management: one aim, but which method? Part one: introduction and literature review', *British Journal of Occupational Therapy*, Vol. 67, No. 10, pp. 447-452, ISSN 0308-0226

Cegala, D. & Post, D. (2009) 'The impact of patients' participation on physicians' patient-centered communication', *Patient Education and Counseling*, Vol. 77, No. 2, pp. 202-8, ISSN 0738-3991

Chalkiadis, G. (2001) 'Management of chronic pain in children', *The Medical journal of Australia*, Vol. 175, No. 9, pp. 476-9, ISSN 0025-729X

Clouse, R., Mayer, E., Aziz, Q., Drossman, D., Dumitrascu, D., Mönnikes, H. & Naliboff, B. (2006) 'Functional abdominal pain syndrome', *Gastroenterology*, Vol. 130, No. 5, pp. 1492-7, ISSN 0016-5085

Cohen, L., Vowles, K. & Eccleston, C. (2010) 'The impact of adolescent chronic pain on functioning: disentangling the complex role of anxiety', *The Journal of Pain*, Vol. 11, No. 11, pp. 1039-46, ISSN 1526-5900

Crombie, I., Davies, H. & Macrae, W. (1998) 'Cut and thrust: antecedent surgery and trauma among patients attending a chronic pain clinic ', *Pain*, Vol. 76, No. 1-2, pp. 167-71, ISSN 0304-3959

de Blécourt, A., Schiphorst Preuper, H., Van Der Schans, C., Groothoff, J., Reneman, M. (2008) 'Preliminary evaluation of a multidisciplinary pain management program for children and adolescents with chronic musculoskeletal pain', *Disability and Rehabilitation*, Vol. 30, No. 1, pp. 13-20, ISSN 0963-8288 de la Fuente-Fernandez, R., Ruth, T., Sossi, V., Schulzer, M., Calne, D. & Stoessl, A. (2001) 'Expectation and dopamine release: mechanism of the placebo effect in Parkinson's disease', *Science,* Vol. 293, No. 5532, pp.1164-6, ISSN 0036-8075

Di Blasi, Z., Harkness, E., Ernst, E. Georgiou, A. & Kleijnen, J. (2001) 'Influence of context on health outcomes: a systematic review', *The Lancet,* Vol. 357, No. 9258, pp. 757-62, ISSN 0140-6736

Dutta, S., Mehta, M. & Verma, I. (1999) 'Recurrent abdominal pain in Indian children and its relation with school and family environment', *Indian Pediatrics,* Vol. 36, No. 9, pp. 917-20, ISSN 0019-6061

Eccleston, C. (2001) 'Role of psychology in pain management', *British Journal of Anaesthesia,* Vol. 87, No. 1, pp. 144-52, ISSN 0007-0912

Eccleston, C., Malleson, P., Clinch, J., Connell, H. & Sourbut, C. (2003) 'Chronic pain in adolescents: evaluation of a programme of interdisciplinary cognitive behaviour therapy', *Archives of Disease in Childhood,* Vol. 88, No. 10, pp. 881–885, ISSN 0003-9888

Eccleston, C., Crombez, G., Scotford, A., Clinch, J. & Connell, H. (2004) 'Adolescent chronic pain: patterns and predictors of emotional distress in adolescents with chronic pain and their parents', *Pain,* Vol. 108, No. 3, pp. 221-229, ISSN 0304-3959

Eccleston, Z. & Eccleston, C. (2004) 'Interdisciplinary management of adolescent chronic pain: developing the role of physiotherapy', *Physiotherapy,* Vol. 90, No. 2, pp. 77-81, ISSN 0031-9406

Eccleston, C., Palermo, T., Williams, A., Lewandowski, A. & Morley, S. (2009) 'Psychological therapies for the management of chronic and recurrent pain in children and adolescents', *The Cochrane Database of Systematic Reviews,* Vol. 15, No. 2, CD003968, ISSN 1469-493X

Eippert, F., Bingel, U., Schoell, E., Yacubian, J., Klinger, R., Lorenz, J. & Büchel, C. (2009) 'Activation of the opioidergic descending pain control system underlies placebo analgesia', *Neuron,* Vol. 63, No. 4, pp. 533-43, ISSN 0896-6273

Fearon, P. & Hotopf, M. (2001) 'Relation between headache in childhood and physical and psychiatric symptoms in adulthood: national birth cohort study', *British Medical Journal,* Vol. 322, pp. 1145, ISSN 0959-8138

Fechir, M., Geber, C. & Birklein, F. (2008) 'Evolving understandings about complex regional pain syndrome and its treatment', *Current Pain and Headache Reports,* Vol. 12, No. 3, pp. 186-191, ISSN 1531-3433

Fields, H. & Levine, J. (1981) 'Biology of placebo analgesia', *The American Journal of Medicine,* Vol. 70, No. 4, pp. 745-6, ISSN 0002-9343

Fillingim, R., King, C., Ribeiro-Dasilva, M., Rahim-Williams, B. & Riley 3rd, J. (2009) 'Sex, gender, and pain: a review of recent clinical and experimental findings', *The Journal of Pain, Vol.* 10, No. 5, pp. 447-485, ISSN 1526-5900

Finniss, D., Nicholas, M. & Benedetti, F. (2009) 'Placebo analgesia - understanding the mechanisms and implications for clinical practice', *Reviews in Pain,* Vol. 3, No. 2, pp. 15-19

Ganesh, R., Arvind Kumar, R., Suresh, N. & Sathiyasekeran, M. (2010) 'Chronic abdominal pain in children', *The National Medical Journal of India,* Vol. 23, No. 2, pp. 94-9, ISSN 0970-258X

Gaul, C., Neundörfer, B. & Winterholler, M. (2005) 'Iatrogenic (para-) spinal abscesses and meningitis following injection therapy for low back pain', Pain, Vol. 116, No. 3, pp. 407-10, ISSN 0304-3959

Geurts, J., van Wijk, R., Wynne, H., Hammink, E., Buskens, E., Lousberg, R., Knape, J. & Groen, G. (2003) 'Radiofrequency lesioning of dorsal root ganglia for chronic lumbosacral radicular pain: a randomised, double-blind, controlled trial', *The Lancet*, Vol. 361, No. 9351, pp. 21-6, ISSN 0140-6736

Gold, J., Mahrer, N., Yee, J. & Palermo, T. (2009) 'Pain, fatigue and health-related quality of life in children and adolescents with chronic pain', *The Clinical Journal of Pain*, Vol. 25, No. 5, pp. 407-412, ISSN 0749-8047

Griffin, S. , Kinmonth, A., Veltman, M., Gillard, S., Grant, J. & Stewart, M. (2004) 'Effect on health-related outcomes of interventions to alter the interaction between patients and practitioners: a systematic review of trials', *Annals of Family Medicine*, Vol. 2, No. 6, pp. 595-608, ISSN 1544-1709

Grøholt, E., Stigum, H., Nordhagen, R. & Köhler, L. (2003) 'Recurrent pain in children, socio-economic factors and accumulation in families', *European Journal of Epidemiology*, Vol. 18, No. 10, pp. 965-75, ISSN 0393-2990

Harding, V. & Williams, A. (1998) 'Activities training: Integrating behavioural and cognitive methods with physiotherapy in pain management', *Journal of Occupational Rehabilitation*, Vol. 8, No. 1, pp. 47-60, ISSN 1053-0487

Hochberg, Z. (2002) 'Mechanisms of steroid impairment of growth', *Hormone Research*, Vol. 58, Suppl. 1, pp. 33–38, ISSN 0301-0163

Huguet, A. & Miró, J. (2008) 'The severity of chronic pediatric pain: an epidemiological study', *The Journal of Pain*, Vol. 9, No. 3, pp. 226-36, ISSN 1526-5900

Hyams, J., Burke, G., Davis, P., Rzepski, B. & Andrulonis, P. (1996) 'Abdominal pain and irritable bowel syndrome in adolescents: a community-based study', *The Journal of Pediatrics*, Vol. 129, No. 2, pp. 220-6, ISSN 0022-3476

International Association for the Study of Pain (1986) 'Pain terms: a current list with definitions and notes on usage', *Pain*, Vol. 24, Supplement 1, pp. S215-21, ISSN 0167-6482

Jamison, R. (2011) 'Nonspecific treatment effects in pain medicine', *Pain Clinical Updates*, Vol. 19, No. 2, pp. 1-7, ISSN 1083-0707

Jensen, M. (2011) 'Psychosocial approaches to pain management: an organisational framework', *Pain*, Vol. 152, No. 4, pp. 717-725, ISSN 0304-3959

Kachko, L., Efrat, R., Ben Ami, S., Mukamel, M. & Katz, J. (2008) 'Complex regional pain syndromes in children and adolescents', *Pediatrics International*, Vol. 50, No. 4, pp. 523-7, ISSN 1328-8067

Kehlet, H., Jensen, T. & Woolf C. (2006) 'Persistent postsurgical pain: risk factors and prevention', Lancet. 2006, Vol. 367, No. 9522, pp. 1618-25, ISSN 0140-6736

Lee, B., Scharff, L., Sethna, N., McCarthy, C., Scott-Sutherland, J., Shea, A., Sullivan, P., Meier, P., Zurakowski, D., Masek, B. & Berde, C. (2002) 'Physical therapy and cognitive behavioural treatment for complex regional pain syndromes', *Journal of Pediatrics*, Vol. 141, No. 1, pp. 135-40, ISSN 0022-3476

Lewandowski, A., Palermo, T., Stinson, J., Handley, S. & Chambers, C. (2010) 'Systematic review of family functioning in families of children and adolescents with chronic pain', *The Journal of Pain*, Vol. 11, No. 11, pp. 1027-38, ISSN 1526-5900

Logan, D., Simons, L., Stein, M. & Chastain, L. (2008) 'School impairment in adolescents with chronic pain', *The Journal of Pain*, Vol. 9, No. 5, pp. 407-416, ISSN 1526-5900

Lynch, A., Kashikar-Zuck, S., Goldschneider, K. & Jones, B. (2006) 'Psychosocial risks for disability in children with chronic back pain', *The Journal of Pain*, Vol . 7, No. 4, pp. 244-51, ISSN 1526-5900

Macrae, W. (2008) 'Chronic post-surgical pain: 10 years on', *British Journal of Anaesthesia*, Vol. 101, No. 1, pp. 77-86, ISSN 0007-0912

Mailis-Gagnon, A., Yegneswaran, B., Nicholson, K., Lakha, S., Papagapiou, M., Steiman, A., Ng, D., Cohodarevic, T., Umana, M. & Zurowski, M. (2007) 'Ethnocultural and sex characteristics of patients attending a tertiary care pain clinic in Toronto, Ontario', *Pain Research & Management*, Vol. 12, No. 2, pp. 100-6, ISSN 1203-6765

Manchikanti, L., Singh, V., Falco, F., Cash, K. & Pampati, V. (2010) 'Evaluation of lumbar facet joint nerve blocks in managing chronic low back pain: a randomized, double-blind, controlled trial with a 2-year follow-up', *International Journal of Medical Sciences*, Vol. 7, No. 3, pp. 124-35, ISSN 1449-1907

Martin, A., McGrath, P., Brown, S. & Katz, J. (2007) 'Children with chronic pain: impact of sex and age on long-term outcomes', *Pain*, Vol. 128, No. 1-2, pp. 13-9, ISSN 0304-3959

McGrath, P. & Holahan, A-L. (2003) 'Psychological Interventions with children and adolescents: evidence for their effectiveness in treating chronic pain', *Seminars in Pain Medicine*, Vol. 1, No. 2, pp. 99-109, ISSN 1537-5897

Meissner, K., Distel, H. & Mitzdorf, U. (2007) 'Evidence for placebo effects on physical but not on biochemical outcome parameters: a review of clinical trials', *BMC Medicine*, Vol. 5, No. 3, ISSN 1741-7015

Palermo, T. (2000) 'Impact of recurrent and chronic pain on child and family daily functioning: a critical review of the literature', *Developmental and Behavioral Pediatrics*, Vol. 21, No. 1, pp. 58-69, ISSN 0196-206X

Peng, P. & Castano, E. (2005) 'Survey of chronic pain practice by anaesthesiologists in Canada', *Canadian Journal of Anesthesia*, Vol. 52, No. 4, pp. 383-9, ISSN 0832-610X

Peng, P., Stinson, J., Choiniere, M. & Dion, D. (2007) 'Dedicated multidisciplinary pain management centres for children in Canada: the current status', *Canadian Journal of Anesthesia*, Vol. 54, No. 12, pp. 985-91, ISSN 0832-610X

Perquin, C., Hazebroek-Kampschreur, A., Hunfeld, J., Bohnen, A., van Suijlekom-Smit, L., Passchier, J. & van der Wouden, J. (2000) 'Pain in children and adolescents: a common experience', *Pain*, Vol. 87, No. 1, pp. 51-8, ISSN 0304-3959

Poleshuck, E., Katz, J., Andrus, C., Hogan, L., Jung, B., Kulick, D. & Dworkin, R. (2006) 'Risk factors for chronic pain following breast cancer surgery: a prospective study', *The Journal of Pain*, Vol. 7, No. 9, pp. 626-34, ISSN 1526-5900.

Poobalan, A., Bruce, J., Smith, W., King, P., Krukowski, Z., Chambers, W. (2003) 'A review of chronic pain after inguinal herniorrhaphy', The Clinical Journal of Pain, Vol. 19, No. 1, pp. 48-54, ISSN 0749-8047

Ramage-Morin, P. & Gilmour H. (2010) 'Chronic pain at ages 12 to 44', *Health reports / Statistics Canada* , Vol. 21, No. 4, pp 53-61, ISSN 0840-6529

Rimsza, M. (1978) 'Complications of corticosteroid therapy', *American Journal of Diseases of Children*, Vol. 132, No. 8, pp. 806–810, ISSN 0002-922X

Robinson, M. (2009) 'Placebo analgesia: Widening the scope of measured influences', *Pain*, Vol. 144, No. 1-2, pp. 5-6, ISSN 0304-3959

Roth-Isigkeit, A., Thyen, U,. Stöven, H., Schwarzenberger, J. & Schmucker, P. (2005) 'Pain among children and adolescents: restrictions in daily living and triggering factors', *Pediatrics*, Vol. 115, No. 2, pp. 152-62, ISSN 0031-4005

Schurman, J. & Friesen, C. (2010) 'Integrative treatment approaches: family satisfaction with a multidisciplinary paediatric Abdominal Pain Clinic', *International Journal of Integrated Care*, Vol. 10, July-Sept2010, pp. 1-9, ISSN 1568-4156

Scott, D., Stohler, C., Egnatuk, C., Wang, H., Koeppe, R. & Zubieta, J. (2008) 'Placebo and nocebo effects are defined by opposite opioid and dopaminergic responses', *Archives of General Psychiatry*, Vol. 65, No. 2, pp. 220–31, ISSN 0003-990X

Simopoulos, T., Kraemer, J., Nagda, J., Aner, M. & Bajwa, Z. (2008) 'Response to pulsed and continuous radiofrequency lesioning of the dorsal root ganglion and segmental nerves in patients with chronic lumbar radicular pain', *Pain Physician*, Vol. 11, No. 2, pp. 137-44, ISSN 1533-3159

Skinner, A. & Lauder, G. (2007) 'Rectus sheath block: successful use in the chronic pain management of pediatric abdominal wall pain', *Paediatric Anaesthesia*, Vol. 17, No. 12, pp. 1203-11, ISSN 1155-5645

Sleed, M., Eccleston, C., Beecham, J., Knapp, M. & Jordan, A. (2005) 'The economic impact of chronic pain in adolescence: Methodological considerations and a preliminary costs-of-illness study', *Pain*, Vol. 119, pp. 183-190, ISSN 0304-3959

Suleiman, S. & Johnston, D. (2001) 'The Abdominal Wall: An Over- looked Source of Pain', *American Family Physician*, Vol. 64, No. 3, pp. 431–438, ISSN 0002-838X

Tough, E., White, A., Richards, S. & Campbell, J. (2007) 'Variability of criteria used to diagnose myofascial trigger point pain syndrome--evidence from a review of the literature', *The Clincal Journal of Pain*, Vol. 23, No. 3, pp. 278-86, ISSN 0749-8047

Tsao, J., Meldrum, M., Kim, S. & Zeltzer, L. (2007) 'Anxiety sensitivity and health-related quality of life in children with chronic pain', *The Journal of Pain*, Vol. 8, No. 10, pp. 814-23, ISSN 1526-5900

Turk, D. & Okifuji, A. (2001). 'Pain terms and taxonomies' In: *Bonica's Management of Pain*, Loeser, D. (ed.), 3rd edn., pp. 18–25, Lippincott Williams & Wilkins, ISBN 0683304623

van Dijk, A., McGrath, P., Pickett, W. & VanDenKerkhof, E. (2006) 'Pain prevalence in nine- to 13-year-old schoolchildren', *Pain Research & Management*, Vol. 11, No. 4, pp.234-40, ISSN 1203-6765

Varni, J., Seid, M. & Kurtin, P. (2001) 'PedsQL 4.0: reliability and validity of the Pediatric Quality of Life Inventory version 4.0 generic core scales in healthy and patient populations', *Medical Care*, Vol. 39, No. 8, pp. 800-12, ISSN 0025-7079

Verheul, W., Sanders, A. & Bensing, J. (2010) 'The effects of physicians' affect-oriented communication style and raising expectations on analogue patients' anxiety, affect and expectancies', *Patient Education and Counseling*, Vol. 80, No. 3, pp. 300-6, ISSN 0738-3991

Vetter, T. (2008) 'A clinical profile of a cohort of patients referred to an anesthesiology-based pediatric chronic pain medicine program', *Anesthesia and Analgesia*, Vol. 106, No. 3, pp. 786-94, ISSN 0003-2999

Vinik, A. (2010) 'The approach to the management of the patient with neuropathic pain', *The Journal of Clinical Endocrinology and Metabolism*, Vol. 95, No. 11, pp. 4802-11, ISSN 0021-972X

Wager, T., Scott, D. & Zubieta, J-K. (2007) 'Placebo effects on human μ-opioid activity during pain', *Proceedings of the National Academy of Sciences of the USA*, Vol. 104, No. 26, pp.11056-61, ISSN 0027-8424

Walker, L., Dengler-Crish, C., Rippel, S. & Bruehl, S. (2010) 'Functional abdominal pain in childhood and adolescence increases risk for chronic pain in adulthood', *Pain*, Vol. 150, No. 3, pp. 568-72, ISSN 0304-3959

20

Risk Factors in Opioid Treatment of Chronic Non-Cancer Pain: A Multidisciplinary Assessment

Renata Ferrari, Michela Capraro and Marco Visentin
Hospital Psychology Service, Pain Relief and Palliative Care Unit, Vicenza Hospital, Italy

1. Introduction

When pain becomes chronic it assumes an almost absolute central role in the disease experience: it characterises and qualifies it, and constantly interferes with the daily life of the patient (Bonica, 1992). It could be said that chronic pain becomes a disease in itself in the patient's perception; daily activities, interpersonal relationships, feelings, are profoundly disturbed by living with pain (Loeser, 2000).

While modern medicine has made notable progress in understanding, diagnosing and treating chronic pain, it continues to be a very widespread problem that significantly compromises the professional, social and family life of the patient, and is often not adequately managed (Manchikanti et al., 2010).

The problem of inadequately managed pain is still a considerable one (Breivik et al., 2006), although the World Health Organization [WHO] (1990) has stated that to be pain free should be considered a right of every patient. The consequences of inadequately treated pain not only have an impact in terms of the physical and psychological suffering of the patient and his family, they also have an enormous economic impact on society as a whole (Brennan et al., 2007; van Leeuwen et al., 2006).

Options for the treatment of chronic pain include both pharmacological treatments (e.g. non steroidal anti-inflammatory drugs, opioids) and non-pharmacological treatments (e.g. physical therapies, acupuncture, cognitive-behavioural therapy, surgical procedures). Choice of treatment should be guided by a complex initial assessment of the patient, which includes the collection of historical information (e.g. pain history and treatments tried, surgical procedures, psychosocial and family history), a physical examination and appropriate diagnostic tests (Passik, 2009).

Opioids are considered one of the most efficacious groups of drugs in treating medium-severe pain (Portenoy, 2000), and their use can result in a significant improvement in the patient's quality of life (Dillie et al., 2008); while there is unanimous agreement on their use in acute and cancer pain, their long-term use for non-cancer chronic pain remains controversial (Dews & Mekhail, 2004; Manchikanti et al., 2010; Rosenblum et al., 2008). The discovery of the properties of these substances, and their use as analgesics, is lost in the mists of time: the Sumerians were starting to cultivate poppies as early as 3400 B.C. (Booth, 1986, as cited in Dews & Mekhail, 2004). In 1803, Friedrich Serturner, a German pharmacist, isolated an alkaloid from opium that he named morphine, and in 1853 Scottish physician Alexander Wood introduced the hypodermic needle and successfully used injections of morphine to treat neuralgia. As Way (1982, as cited in Dews & Mekhail, 2004) highlighted, morphine was the "mainstay" of medical treatment in the United States throughout the nineteenth century, used to treat pain, anxiety and respiratory problems as well as "consumption" and "women's ailments". Opium cultivation was legal in some states, and opium-based products could be bought over the counter (Dews & Mekhail, 2004). Between 1875 and 1877, German physician Eduard Levinstein published a series of articles calling attention to the problem of morphine dependence: his was one of the first studies on the risk of dependence on narcotics, which he estimated to be 75% (White et al., 2001a). In 1914 Kennedy Foster wrote, in New York Medical Journal, *"...morphinism is a disease, in the majority of cases, initiated, sustained and left uncured by members of the medical profession"* (White et al., 2001b); in the same year the US Congress approved the Harrison Anti-Narcotic Act, the first federal law to limit the sale of any drug. Opioids and cocaine were included in the list of drugs that could only be obtained from a physician or authorised pharmacist. Physicians were authorised to prescribe these substances, but not to patients with dependence problem; given the likelihood of arrest or prosecution, physicians became increasingly cautious in prescribing opioids even for chronic pain (Dews & Mekhail, 2004). In 1969, the WHO abandoned the belief that the medical use of morphine led inevitably to dependence; the WHO clarified that tolerance and physical dependence did not in itself constitute "drug dependence", a diagnosis characterised by typical behaviours, including difficulty in controlling the assumption of drugs, compulsive use of the substance and inappropriate social behaviours (WHO, 1986). In 1970 the Harrison Anti-Narcotic Act and the other federal laws on drugs were replaced by the Comprehensive Drug Abuse and Control Act, which divided substances into six categories, according to their risk of addiction: category I includes heroin and marijuana, category II includes cocaine, opium and morphine, category III includes codeine, category IV includes diazepam and alprazolam, category V includes drugs with small quantities of codeine and category VI includes penicillin and ibuprofen (Dews & Mekhail, 2004). This law established that there were no impediments to prescribing drugs in categories II, III or IV provided there were indications for their use, including chronic non-cancer pain. There was a further development when the WHO Expert Committee on Essential Drugs recognised morphine, codeine and other opioids as "essential drugs," defining them as: *"those that satisfy the health care needs of the majority of the population; they should therefore be available at all times in adequate amounts and in the appropriate dosage forms..."* (WHO, 1998). The WHO also introduced the "pain analgesia scale" (figure 1) which distinguishes between strong and weak opioids, and establishes their clear roles in pain relief. In Italy, which is one of the countries with the lowest morphine consumption in Europe, several measures have been developed to eliminate the bureaucratic obstacles to the use of opioid analgesics, starting with Law no. 12 of 2001. With Law no. 38 of 2010, opioids may finally be prescribed for pain relief in the same way as other prescription-only drugs.

As illustrated, the use of opioids has historically been subject to cycles of liberalisation and prohibition in clinical practice that account for their still-limited use today (WHO, 1998).

The potential barriers to treatment with opioids may be due to inadequate beliefs of both medical personnel and the patients themselves (Garcia & Altman, 1997).

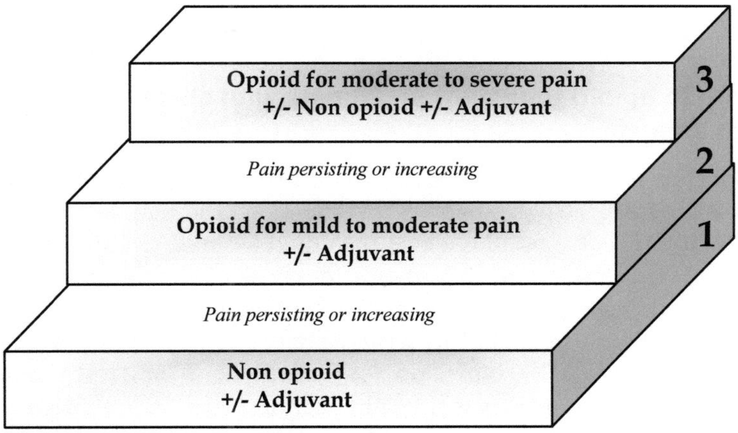

Fig. 1. The WHO pain analgesia scale

Physicians may not prescribe opioids at adequate doses because they do not know how to use them effectively, because they do not assess the pain or effects of treatment systematically, because of fear of sanctions by medical commissions. But some data lead one to believe that the overestimation of the risk of addiction is a significant problem (Dews & Mekhail, 2004); in this respect, the term *opiophobia* has been coined, to refer to the practice of under-prescription of opioid medication due to the fear of inducing addiction in patients (Collett, 1998). By interviewing over 248 US physicians, Bhamb et al. (2006) recently reported that just over half of those interviewed (55.9%), had specific clinical protocols for the prolonged use of opioids in patients with chronic non-cancer pain. 35.1% believed they prescribed opioids less frequently than their colleagues; while the most frequent concerns about starting treatment with opioids were the fear of abuse (84.2%) and addiction (74.9%). Concerns of patients should also be considered: they may not communicate their pain symptoms to their physicians, or may not take the drugs as instructed for fear of becoming dependent on "narcotics" (Dews & Mekhail, 2004). Furthermore, both physicians and patients may develop unjustified anxiety about the side effects of opioid use, believing that these drugs must therefore be reserved for cancer pain (Brennan et al., 2007). Finally, a further barrier to the use of these drugs may be due to overly restrictive national control laws and regulations. Because of this, the WHO has issued guidelines on legislative policies that enable Governments to check if their national laws ensure the availability of opioid analgesics to treat severe pain (WHO, 2002).

Given the importance of these drugs in pain management, as well as the concerns about their use, a series of investigations were carried out in the last twenty years to identify the risk factors that promote or exacerbate opioid misuse. In fact, for physicians, determining the patient's risk of addiction to opioids is of fundamental importance, so that a series of measures can be taken to limit the negative consequences of this (such as constantly monitoring the patient during treatment, planning interdisciplinary treatment or scheduling regular urine toxicology screening).

The intention of this chapter is to examine the principal risk factors for opioid misuse in patients with chronic non-cancer pain. It will also describe the principal tools for selecting patients who are candidates for opioid treatment and for stratifying the risk of misuse. This will be followed by a presentation of the preliminary results of our experience using a diagnostic protocol for patients undergoing long-term treatment with opioids in a multidisciplinary pain relief unit.

2. Risk factors in opioid treatment of patients with chronic pain: Theoretical and research aspects

Over the last twenty years, opioids have been used increasingly to treat chronic non-cancer pain (Ballantyne & Shin, 2008). A broad US investigation fund that, between 1980 and 2000, prescriptions of opioids for musculoskeletal pain doubled from 8% to 16%. Over the same two decades, the use of more powerful opioids for chronic pain (hydrocodone, oxycodone, morphine) increased from 2% to 9% (Caudill-Slosberg et al., 2004). However, if some patients benefit from such treatment in terms of reduction of pain and improvement in quality of life (Dillie et al., 2008), others do not (Ballantyne, 2007; Trescot et al., 2008). Side effects, the absence of any improvement in physical function, the excessive use of opioids, abuse and addiction are common problems that may present during the administration of opioid analgesics (Manchikanti et al., 2010). So in recent years experts and researchers have sought to answer many questions regarding risk factor for opioid misuse, selection of patients, efficacy of treatment particularly over time, whether opioids are able to improve physical function and quality of life. The clear and urgent need to answer these questions is reflected in the considerable increase in studies on this topic in the last decade (Ballantyne & Shin, 2008). Moreover, many guidelines for the use of opioids in patients with chronic non-cancer pain have been produced, which recommend their use for those patients who have not benefited from other pharmacological and non-pharmacological treatments (Chou, 2009; Chou et al, 2009a; Chou et al, 2009b; Chou et al, 2009c; Kalso et al., 2003; Trescot et al., 2006; Trescot at al., 2008).

The following section will provide some notes on pain, on the recommendations contained in the guidelines for the prolonged use of opioids and on the terminology used. The intention is to offer adequate context for the subsequent discussion of the risk factors related to abuse of opioids and the tools that have been developed to select patients to treat with these drugs.

Finally, the preliminary data of our experience using two of these tools, the *Pain Medication Questionnaire* (PMQ; Adams et al., 2004) and the *Diagnosis Intractability Risk and Efficacy Score* (DIRE; Belgrade et al., 2006) in the Italian population are presented.

2.1 The definition and classification of pain

Pain is an extremely complex and subjective phenomenon, defined by the International Association for the Study of Pain [IASP] as *"an unpleasant sensory and emotional experience, associated with real or potential tissue damage or described in terms of such damage"* (Merskey, 1986a). Whether acute or chronic, pain is above all a subjective and multidimensional experience, influenced by biological, psychological and socio-environmental factors.

Pain may be distinguished as acute or chronic based on its duration in time and underlying pathology. Acute pain is produced by lesions to body tissues and the activation of the nociceptive transducers at the site of the tissue damage. It may be consequent on a trauma, a surgical procedure or an inflammatory process, and generally lasts for a relatively short period of time (hours, days or weeks) and stops when the underlying pathology is resolved. Chronic pain lasts for a long period of time (continuously or recurring at intervals of months or years), and is generally accompanies by a low level of underlying pathology which fully explains neither the presence nor the intensity of the pain (Bonica, 1992). Disputes remain about the interval of time that needs to have elapsed since the trauma for pain to be defined as chronic; in clinical practice, a pain is generally described as chronic when it persists for more than 3-6 months (Bonica, 1991; Loeser & Melzack, 1999; Merskey, 1986b; Merskey & Bogduk, 1994).

From a pathogenic perspective, pain may be classified as nociceptive, neuropathic or mixed. Nociceptive pain (somatic or visceral pain) is determined by the activation of nociceptors located in the somatic and visceral structures. It may be further classified as superficial or deep, according to the structure involved, and is due to a tissue lesion that is often evident. Neuropathic pain is typically caused by a change or alteration in the transmission of impulses along the somato-sensorial pathways and is indicative of damage to the conduction systems or to the integration and transmission systems of the central or peripheral nervous system; often it is not accompanied by tissue damage. Finally, when these two types of pain (nociceptive and neuropathic) are both present, this is referred to as mixed pain (Mannion & Woolf, 2000).

Pain is physiological, i.e. it is a vital sign, and a defence system when it constitutes an alarm signal for tissue damage. It becomes pathological when it maintains itself, losing its initial meaning and becoming an illness in itself (pain syndrome) (Mannion & Woolf, 2000).

In biopsychosocial terms, the experience of pain and its impact on the individual are due to the complex interaction of somatic inputs (nociception), psychological processes (e.g. thoughts, coping strategies and emotions) and social contingencies (e.g. social context, significant others, roles and expectations) (Turk & Okifuji, 2002). In persistent pain syndromes, the weight of these three factors can change at different moments of the illness, and none alone can explain the pain situation as a whole. The biological factors can origin, maintain and modulate the physical disorder, the psychological factors influence perception and evaluation of body signals and the social factors give form to the patients' behavioural responses and their perception of their physical condition. Given this complexity, an adequate approach to chronic pain requires multidisciplinary intervention; the treatment aims in these patients are not only pharmacological treatment but also reduction of affective/emotional discomfort, functional recovery, return to work and improvement in family and social relationships.

2.1.1 The prevalence of chronic pain and its socio-economic impact

Chronic pain is a common and persistent problem in society, with a relatively high incidence and a low remission rate (Elliott et al., 2002). Verhaak et al. (1998), after reviewing 15 epidemiological studies on chronic pain in the adult population, concluded that its prevalence varied from 2% to 40%, with a mean value of 15%. Back pain is one of the most frequent forms of chronic pain, with a prevalence rate of approximately 48% (Gureje et al., 1998). Based on interviews of 2305 subjects aged between 35 and 45, Linton et al. (1998) showed that the prevalence of back pain is 66% with slightly higher incidence in women; in particular, 56% of the subjects complained of low back pain, 44% complained of neck pain, and 15% complained of pain in the thoracic spine.

A recent epidemiological study about the prevalence of chronic pain in European countries involving 46,394 subjects found that approximately 19% of adults suffer continuous pain of medium-high intensity that seriously compromises quality of their emotional, social and working life. The prevalence of chronic pain varies from 12% to 20%, and is highest in Norway, Poland and Spain. In Italy, people who suffer from chronic pain syndromes account for approximately 27% of the population. It also emerged that: 59% of those interviewed had been experiencing pain for at least 2-15 years, 21% had been diagnosed with depression consequent on pain, 61% reported great difficulty or incapacity in working outside home, 19% had lost their job and 13% had been forced to change jobs because of the pain. Just 2% of patients reported they were being treated by pain specialists, and about half of these were receiving inadequate treatment (Breivik et al., 2006).

Therefore chronic pain has serious negative effects on the quality of life of the millions of people who experience it, and on the quality of life of their families. In the absence of adequate treatments, patients with chronic pain are often unable to work or even to carry out their normal daily activities.

As well as causing unspeakable suffering to millions of people all over the world, chronic pain has high social cost too. Analysing data from the 1997 Medical Expenditures Panel Survey, which involved 14,147 families, Yelin et al.(2004) found that expenditure by patients with rheumatic disorders was US $ 4,865 per head, for a total of US $ 186.9 million. In 1998, US healthcare expenditure on lower back pain was US $ 90.7 billions (Luo et. al., 2004). A similar investigation found that in 2003 overall spending in the US on care for arthritis and other rheumatic disorders was approximately US $ 128 billion, equivalent to 1.2% of the US gross domestic product in 2003 (Centers for Disease Control and Prevention, 2007).

So far as Europe is concerned, a study of the socio-economic costs of pain syndromes in the United Kingdom estimated that the cost of direct healthcare was £ 1.6 billion in 1998. But this direct cost is insignificant compared to the indirect costs (e.g. days of work lost and loss of productivity) associated with back pain, totalling 10.7 billion (Maniadakis & Gray, 2000). Winkelmann et al. (2011) estimated the annual costs per fibromyalgia patient for 2008 as € 7,900 in France (of which €960 direct costs, €6,990 indirect costs), and € 7,256 in Germany (€ 1,756 direct costs, € 5,491 indirect costs).

2.2 Opioid treatment of chronic non-cancer pain

In recent years, many guidelines for the use of opioids in patients with chronic non-cancer pain have been drawn up. In general the objectives of such documents are: to bring consistency in opioid prescribing to the many diverse groups involved; to provide analysis of evidence to treat a chronic pain patient with opioids, thus, maintaining reasonable patient access while reducing the risk of drug diversion; to provide practical prescribing guidelines for physicians to reduce the risk of legal and regulatory sanctions; and to emphasize the need for systematic evaluation and ongoing care of patients with chronic or persistent pain (Trescot et al., 2006). The perceived benefits of these guidelines include: increased physician awareness about the current issues involving opioids and non-cancer pain; improved patient access; reduced level of opioid abuse; improved ability to manage patient expectations; reduced diversion; improved understanding by law enforcement about proper prescribing patterns; improved cooperation among patients, providers, and regulatory agencies; improved understanding by patients regarding their rights as well as their responsibilities when taking opioid medications (Trescot et al., 2008). These guidelines should be applied flexibly: every physician must establish a treatment plan that takes account of the specific medical conditions of the patient and his personal preferences and needs, and of the physician's own professional experience (Trescot et al., 2006; 2008). Based on a systematic review of the efficacy of treatment with opioids in chronic non-cancer pain by a multidisciplinary group of experts, the American Academy of Pain Medicine formulated a series of recommendations for: patient selection and the stratification of risk of abuse, informed consent to treatment with opioids, initiation and titration of chronic opioid therapy, the use of methadone, patient monitoring, the use of opioids in high risk patients, the assessment of the effectiveness of the drug and the aberrant drug-related behaviours, dose escalation and high dose therapy, opioid rotation, indications for discontinuation of therapy, prevention and management of opioid-related side effects and issues about driving and work safety during treatment with such drugs (Chou, 2009; Chou et al, 2009a; Chou et al, 2009b; Chou et al, 2009c). The recommendations of the American Pain Society and the American Academy of Pain Medicine are shown in table 1.

TOPIC AREA	RECOMENDATIONS
Patient selection and risk stratification	Prior to initiating chronic opioid therapy, clinicians should conduct a history, physical examination and appropriate testing, including an assessment of risk of substance abuse, misuse, or addiction (strong recommendation, low-quality evidence).
	Clinicians may consider a trial of chronic opioid therapy as an option if chronic non-cancer pain is moderate or severe, pain is having an adverse impact on function or quality of life, and potential therapeutic benefits outweigh or are likely to outweigh potential harms (strong recommendation, low-quality evidence).
	A benefit-to-harm evaluation including a history, physical examination, and appropriate diagnostic testing, should be performed and documented prior to and on an ongoing basis during chronic opioid therapy (strong recommendation, low-quality evidence).
Informed consent and opioid management plans	When starting chronic opioid therapy, informed consent should be obtained. A continuing discussion with the patient regarding chronic opioid therapy should include goals, expectations, potential risks, and alternatives to chronic opioid therapy (strong recommendation, low-quality evidence).
	Clinicians may consider using a written chronic opioid therapy management plan to document patient and clinician responsibilities and expectations and assist in patient education (weak recommendation, low-quality evidence).
Initiation and titration of chronic opioid therapy	Clinicians and patients should regard initial treatment with opioids as a therapeutic trial to determine whether chronic opioid therapy is appropriate (strong recommendation, low-quality evidence).
	Opioid selection, initial dosing, and titration should be individualized according to the patient's health status, previous exposure to opioids, attainment of therapeutic goals, and predicted or observed harms (strong recommendation, low-quality evidence). There is insufficient evidence to recommend short-acting versus long-acting opioids, or as-needed versus around-the-clock dosing of opioids.
Methadone	Methadone is characterized by complicated and variable pharmacokinetics and pharmacodynamics and should be initiated and titrated cautiously, by clinicians familiar with its use and risks (strong recommendation, moderate-quality evidence).
Monitoring	Clinicians should reassess patients on chronic opioid therapy periodically and as warranted by changing circumstances. Monitoring should include documentation of pain intensity and level of functioning, assessments of progress towards achieving therapeutic goals, presence of adverse events, and adherence to prescribed therapies (strong recommendation, low-quality evidence).
	In patients on chronic opioid therapy who are at high risk or who have engaged in aberrant drug-related behaviours, clinicians should periodically obtain urine drug screens or other information to confirm adherence to the chronic opioid therapy plan of care (strong recommendation, low-quality evidence).
	In patients on chronic opioid therapy not at high risk and not known to have engaged in aberrant drug-related behaviors, clinicians should consider periodically obtaining urine drug screens or other information to confirm adherence to the chronic opioid therapy plan of care (weak recommendation, low-quality evidence).

TOPIC AREA	RECOMENDATIONS
High-risk patients	Clinicians may consider chronic opioid therapy for patients with chronic non-cancer pain and history of drug abuse, psychiatric issues, or serious aberrant drug-related behaviours only if they are able to implement more frequent and stringent monitoring parameters. In such situations, clinicians should strongly consider consultation with a mental health or addiction specialist (strong recommendation, low-quality evidence).
Aberrant drug-related behaviours	Clinicians should evaluate patients engaging in aberrant drug-related behaviours for appropriateness of chronic opioid therapy or need for restructuring of therapy, referral for assistance in management, or discontinuation of chronic opioid therapy (strong recommendation, low-quality evidence).
Dose escalations and high-dose therapy	When repeated dose escalations occur in patients on chronic opioid therapy, clinicians should evaluate potential causes and re-assess benefits relative to harms (strong recommendation, low-quality evidence).
	In patients who require relatively high doses of chronic opioid therapy clinicians should evaluate for unique opioid-related adverse effects, changes in health status, and adherence to the chronic opioid therapy treatment plan on an ongoing basis, and consider more frequent follow-up visits (strong recommendation, low-quality evidence).
Opioid rotation	Clinicians should consider opioid rotation when patients on chronic opioid therapy experience intolerable adverse effects or inadequate benefit despite dose increases (weak recommendation, low-quality evidence).
Indications for discontinuation of therapy	Clinicians should taper or wean patients off of chronic opioid therapy who engage in repeated aberrant drug-related behaviours or drug abuse/diversion, experience no progress towards meeting therapeutic goals, or experience intolerable adverse effects (strong recommendation, low-quality evidence).
Opioid-related adverse effects	Clinicians should anticipate, identify, and treat common opioid-associated adverse effects (strong recommendation, moderate-quality evidence).
Use of psychotherapeutic co-interventions	As chronic noncancer pain is often a complex biopsychosocial condition, clinicians who prescribe chronic opioid therapy should routinely integrate psychotherapeutic interventions, functional restoration, interdisciplinary therapy, and other adjunctive non-opioid therapies (strong recommendation, moderate-quality evidence).
Driving and work safety	Clinicians should counsel patients on chronic opioid therapy about transient or lasting cognitive impairment that may affect driving and work safety. Patients should be counselled not to drive or engage in potentially dangerous activities when impaired or if they describe or demonstrate signs of impairment (strong recommendation, low-quality evidence).
Identifying a medical home and when to obtain consultation	Patients on chronic opioid therapy should identify a clinician who accepts primary responsibility for their overall medical care. This clinician may or may not prescribe chronic opioid therapy, but should coordinate consultation and communication among all clinicians involved in the patient's care (strong recommendation, low-quality evidence).
	Clinicians should pursue consultation, including interdisciplinary pain management, when patients with chronic non-cancer pain may benefit from additional skills or resources that they cannot provide (strong recommendation, moderate-quality evidence).
Breakthrough pain	In patients on around-the-clock chronic opioid therapy with breakthrough pain, clinicians may consider as-needed opioids based upon an initial and ongoing analysis of therapeutic benefit versus risk (weak recommendation, low-quality evidence).

Table 1. Guidelines recommended by the American Pain Society and the American Academy of Pain Medicine for the long-term treatment with opioids of patients with chronic non-cancer pain (adapted from Chou, 2009).

Trescot et al. (2006, 2008) confirmed the importance of an overall patient assessment (physical and psychological) before initiating long-term opioid therapy; this assessment must include an appropriate assessment of treatment efficacy at regular intervals (in terms of both pain reduction and recovery of physical function), the identification and treatment of side effects and the monitoring of any abuse or misuse of the drug. The authors proposed a ten step algorithm that physicians could use for this purpose during treatment with opioids.

2.2.1 Terminology of opioid abuse: Dependence, tolerance, addiction

To ensure effective communication between physicians, researchers and legislators, a clear common terminology is needed. Many drugs, including opioids, play an important role in the treatment of pain. However, as shown earlier, the use of opioids is often limited by concerns about abuse, dependence and their possible use for non-medical reasons. Addiction, tolerance and physical dependence are distinct and different phenomena that are often used in a confused way. Since their clinical implications and management are clearly different, it is important to establish uniform definitions based on current scientific and clinical knowledge, to improve the care of patients with chronic pain and encourage appropriate policies for the regulation and control of drugs. For this purpose, the American Academy of Pain Medicine, the American Pain Society and the American Society of Addiction Medicine (American Society of Addiction Medicine, 2001) have recognised the following definitions, and recommend their use:

Addiction is a primary, chronic, neurobiologic disease, with genetic, psychosocial, and environmental factors influencing its development and manifestations. It is characterized by behaviours that include one or more of the following: impaired control over drug use, compulsive use, continued use despite harm, and craving.

Physical dependence is a state of adaptation that is manifested by a drug class specific withdrawal syndrome that can be produced by abrupt cessation, rapid dose reduction, decreasing blood level of the drug, and/or administration of an antagonist.

Tolerance is a state of adaptation in which exposure to a drug induces changes that result in a diminution of one or more of the drug's effects over time.

Pseudoaddiction is a term that has been used to describe behaviour that can occur when the pain is undertreated. Patients with inadequately managed pain may in fact become excessively focused on obtaining drugs. In their intent to obtain relief, patients may also resort to trickery and the use of unlawful substances. Pseudoaddiction may be distinguished from true addiction by the fact that the behaviour disappears when the pain is treated efficaciously.

Misuse is defined as the use of any psychoactive substance in a way other than that for which it has been indicated or prescribed (Wasan et al., 2007). In practical terms, opioid misuse means: inadequate pain management, ineffective treatment, excessive focus on the drug and its effects which does not allow the patient to use other strategies efficaciously to cope with the pain, and finally, worsening of quality of life and altered social, working and psychological functioning.

The term *aberrant drug-related behaviours* has been used to indicate the broad array of problematic nonadherence behaviours (Passik et al., 2006), the nature of which is uncertain until a diagnosis can be developed based on astute clinical assessment (Rosenblum et al., 2008). Portenoy (1996; 2004) has listed a series of behaviours that should engender suspicion of addiction in patients with pain being treated with opioids (table 2). Moreover, Savage

(1993), suggested that the following aspects should also be considered: frequent cancellation of appointments; asking for medicines at the end of every appointment; a history of non-responsiveness to treatment, apart from opioids; a history of negative relationships with many physicians; many "drug allergies" that limit treatment options; finally, a degree of disability that is disproportionate to the basic disorder.
As described above, the use of opioids has raised many concerns; in fact, the use of analgesics without medical prescription, or just to test their effects ("non medical use") represents the second most frequent form of illicit substance use in the United States, after marijuana use (Office of Applied Studies, Substance Abuse and Mental Health Services Administration [SAMHSA], 2008). The National Survey on Drug Use and Health (Office of Applied Studies, SAMHSA, 2009) report on the use of opioids for non-medical purposes in the United States from 2002 to 2007 showed that: in 2007 approximately 5.2 million people of 12 years of age or more had used prescription-only analgesics for non-medical purposes in the previous month; from 2002 to 2007 the use of opioids for non-therapeutic purposes decreased among young people between 12 and 17 years of age (from 3.2% to 2.7%) , while it increased in young adults between 18 and 25 years of age (4.1% to 4.6%) and in adults over 26 (from 1.3% to 1.6%).

Behaviours probably more predictive of addiction
Selling prescriptions drugs
Prescription forgery
Stealing or "borrowing" drugs from others
Injection oral formulations
Obtaining prescription drugs from non-medical sources
Concurrent abuse of alcohol or illicit drugs
Multiple dose escalation or other non-compliance with therapy despite warnings
Multiple episodes of prescription "loss"
Repeatedly seeking prescription from other clinicians or from emergency rooms without informing prescriber or after warning to desist
Evidence of deterioration in the ability to function in work, in the family, or socially that appear to be related to the drug use
Repeated resistance to changes in therapy despite clear evidence of adverse physical or psychological effect from the drug
Behaviours probably less predictive of addiction
Aggressive complaining about the need for more drug
Drug hoarding during periods of reduced symptoms
Requesting specific drugs
Openly acquiring similar drugs from other medical sources
Unsanctioned dose escalation or other non-compliance with therapy on one or two occasions
Reporting psychic effects not intended by the clinician
Resistance to change in therapy associated with "tolerable" adverse effects with expression of anxiety related to the return of severe symptoms

Table 2. Behaviours predictive of addiction (adapted from Portenoy 1996, 2004).

Many studies have been carried out about the prevalence of opioid addiction in patients with chronic pain, but one of the limitations in interpreting their results is the fact that the researchers have used different criteria to establish problematic opioid use; some studies are based on behavioural observations, others on the results of urine toxicology screening, others again on the criteria Diagnostic and Statistical Manual of mental disorders - III or IV [DSM-III-IV] and yet other studies are based on definitions established by the authors themselves.

Based on an extensive literature review, Højsted & Sjøgren (2007) estimated that the prevalence of addiction in the population with chronic non-cancer pain varies from 0% to 50%. In particular, in the studies based on urine toxicology screening the prevalence varies from 17.2% to 39%; in the studies using the DSM-III or DSM-IV criteria it varied from 1.9% to 37%; and, finally, in the studies based on the various behavioural indicators, the prevalence varied from 0% to 50%. In a study of 100 patients with chronic pain in treatment with opioids, Manchikanti et al. (2001) found a prevalence of drug abuse, defined as the occurrence of obtaining a prescription of a controlled substance at least once a month from another physician without approval of the pain physician signing the controlled substance contract, of 24%. Fleming et al. (2007), considering 801 patients with non-cancer pain in chronic treatment with opioids, reported that 9.7% of the sample met the DSM-IV diagnostic criteria for opioid use disorder; the prevalence found by the authors was four times the prevalence in the general population.

Finally, a recent review of the prolonged use of opioids in patients with non-cancer pain estimated the prevalence of addiction indicators as 0.27% of the total number of patients examined (Noble et al., 2010); the authors also observed that minor unwanted effects (e.g. nausea, headache) are frequent during treatment with opioids, but more serious adverse events, such as addiction, are rare.

The hypothesis that short acting drugs such as hydrocodone may make patients more liable to ineffective pain management and misuse or abuse of the drugs than long acting drugs such as methadone was investigated by Manchikanti et al. (2005), who analysed 200 patients with chronic pain, half being treated with hydrocodone and the remainder with methadone. The study found no significant differences in the use of illegal substances and/or opioid abuse in patients treated with short- or long-acting drugs.

So addiction is a well documented problem in pain patients, although it is difficult to estimate its exact prevalence. It is therefore important that clinicians consider the risk of opioid addiction without this prejudicing their use where indicated. In fact, those who use opioids constitute a heterogeneous category that includes extreme cases of patients who abuse medical and non-medical substances, and patients who adhere to treatment (Passik, 2009). For adequate management and treatment of pain, physicians must balance the costs and benefits of opioid treatment; to maximise the benefits they can use different strategies, such as risk assessment and stratification, using specific tools, constant monitoring of treatment and any aberrant drug behaviours, regular urine screening and the possible involvement of another specialist (e.g. psychotherapist, addiction expert).

2.3 Risk factors for opioid abuse

Risk factors for opioid abuse and addiction may be divided into three categories: psychosocial factors, substance-related factors and genetic factors (figure 2). The risk of addiction is highest when the various categories of risk factor are combined. Pain patients without a genetic predisposition, without psychiatric comorbidity who take a stable dose of opioids for the treatment of severe pain in a controlled clinical setting are most unlikely to develop addiction. In contrast, patients with a personal or family history of substance abuse, and with one or more psychosocial issues are at greater risk of developing addiction, especially if the treatment is not carefully structured (Ballantyne, 2007).

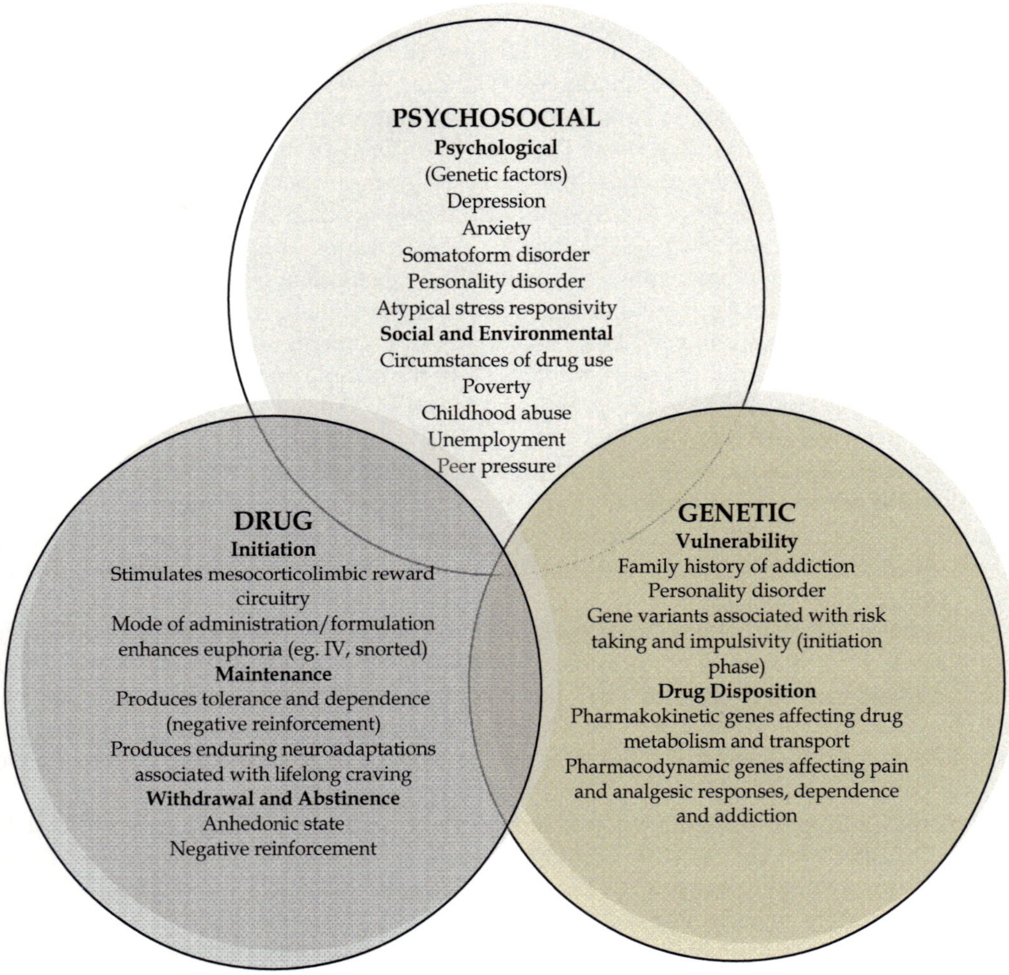

Fig. 2. Genetic, psychosocial and drug-related factors associated with the development of addiction. Adapted from Ballantyne (2007).

The psychosocial factors considered to be most predictive of opioid abuse are the presence of psychiatric disorders (Compton et al., 1998; Sullivan et al., 2006) and a personal and/or family history of substance abuse or drug abuse (Dunbar & Katz, 1996; Schieffer et al., 2005). A significant correlation has been found between chronic pain, mood disorders and aberrant drug use: patients with chronic pain report higher levels of anxiety and depression than patients with other medical conditions, and the incidence of mood disorders has been shown to be higher in patients at high risk of opioid misuse or dependence (Bair et al., 2003; Dersh et al., 2002; Fishbain, 1999).

Using logistic regression, the authors showed that panic attacks, high trait anxiety and the presence of a personality disorder are able to explain the 38% variance in potential abuse of prescribed opioids. To investigate the role of psychological adjustment and psychiatric symptoms in aberrant drug behaviours in pain patients, Wasan et al. (2007) divided the 228 patients enrolled into high-psychiatric and low-psychiatric morbidity, based on the responses to the psychiatric subscale of the Prescription Drug Use Questionnaire (PDUQ; Compton et al., 2008; see § 2.4.). Patients with high psychiatric comorbidity were significantly younger, with a longer mean opioid assumption time ($p<0.05$); altered urine toxicology screening results were also more frequent among these patients ($p<0.01$), and they often displayed aberrant drug-related behaviours.

Edlund et al. (2007) conducted a broad prospective study of the risk factors for opioid abuse and addiction using the South Central Veterans Affairs Health Care Network databank. The sample included 15.160 chronic users of opioids in 2002; 45.3% of the sample had a psychiatric diagnosis and 7.6% had a non-opioid substance abuse diagnosis. The results show that prior abuse of non-opioid substances is a strong predictor of abuse/addiction to opioid drugs, while mental disorders are moderately strong predictors. The authors also found that the risk of abuse decreases uniformly with age. Other risk factors for opioid abuse/addiction were male gender, being divorced/separated or single and, finally, being in treatment with opioids for longer. A broad retrospective cohort study that involved 704 patients with chronic pain being treated with opioids was carried out by Banta-Green et al. (2009a) to further comprehend the complex interaction between pain, mental health and addiction. The patients were initially assessed using a structured interview based on DSM-IV criteria for abuse and dependence on opioids, misuse of opioids, anxiety and depression. By regression analysis, the authors identified three distinct categories of patients which they called: a) Typical group (characterised by moderate pain symptoms and limited psychiatric problems); b) Addictive Behaviours group (high psychiatric symptoms, misuse of opioids and moderate pain symptoms); c) Pain Dysfunction group (high intensity and interference of pain, high psychiatric symptoms and consistent misuse of opioids). The patients in the last two groups took an average daily dose of opioids that was three times that of the typical group. The authors suggest that the use of high doses of drugs could constitute a simple indicator to identify those patients that might benefit from further medical or psychiatric assessment, or assessment of drug misuse behaviours.

To determine the incidence of opioid addiction, and the factors predictive for abuse, Ives et al. (2006) carried out a prospective cohort study of 196 patients with chronic pain being treated with opioids. Patients were monitored at regular intervals for an entire year. Opioid abuse was defined based on the presence of: negative urine toxicology screening for prescribed opioids; positive urine toxicology screening for non-prescribed drugs or opioids; supplies of opioids obtained from more than one provider; diversion of opioids, prescription forgery and positive urine toxicology screening for narcotics (cocaine or amphetamines). Opioid abuse was observed in 32% of patients; the most common form of misuse was the detection of cocaine or amphetamine in urine (40.3% of misusers). Abusers were found to be significantly younger ($p<0.001$); male ($p= 0.023$); with a history of abuse of alcohol ($p= 0.004$) and cocaine ($p<0.001$) than non-abusers. Ethnicity, income, education, levels of depression or disability and pain intensity were not found to be associated with drug misuse. Manchikanti et al. (2006) carried out a prospective longitudinal study of 500 patients with chronic pain to evaluate and correlate multiple variables with the abuse of opioids and illegal substances. Patients who obtained opioid drugs from sources other than the physicians at the clinic where the study was carried out were considered abusers; use of narcotics was ascertained through urine toxicology screening. Opioid abuse was observed in 9% of patients, while the use of illegal substances (e.g. cocaine, marijuana, metamphetamines) was detected in 16% of the sample. Opioid abuse was found to be more frequent in patients with pain due to road traffic accidents, pain in more than one region of the body and subjects with prior substance abuse. The use of illegal substances was more frequent among women and in patients under 45 years of age. The onset of pain after a road traffic accident and the presence of pain in more than one part of the body were also risk factors for narcotic substance abuse. To investigate the effect of gender on aberrant drug-related behaviours, Back et al. (2009) carried out a study on 121 patients (49 make and 72 female), who had to complete a set of tests designed to collect personal and clinical information and data on aberrant drug behaviours (e.g. prescription fraud, using other drug administration routes) and the use of nicotine, alcohol, marijuana, cocaine and hallucinogens. The results show that men were taking the prescribed drug significantly more regularly than women (91.7% v 77.8%, $p<0.05$), while women tend to keep unused drugs (67.6% v 47.7%; $p=0.04$) and to use other drugs (e.g. sedatives) to enhance the efficacy of analgesics (38.8% v 20%; $p=0.04$) more than men. Men tend to use other drug administration routes (e.g. crushing and snorting pills) than women, although this difference was not statistically significant. For men, there was an association between alcohol abuse, use of oxycodone or morphine and aberrant drug behaviours, while in women the aberrant drug behaviours were associated with the use of hydrocodone.

In conclusion, the presence of psychiatric disorders and a personal and/or family history of substance abuse seem to be the most predictive factors of risk of opioid misuse in patients with chronic pain. Other variables such as gender, age and marital status may influence the risk of abuse, although the relationship is less clear, and further investigation is required (Savage, 2002).

2.4 Tools to assess the risk of addiction and dependence

Guidelines suggest that the use of opioids in patients with chronic non-cancer pain must be preceded by an initial stratification of the risk of drug misuse; this evaluation should include even a psychological and psychiatric assessment (Chou, 2009; Chou et al, 2009a; Chou et al, 2009b; Chou et al, 2009c; Kalso et al., 2003; Trescot et al., 2006; Trescot at al., 2008). In recent years, many tools have been developed and examined for this purpose; most investigate the presence of a family and/or personal history of addiction and other factors correlated with opioid misuse, such as age, history of childhood sexual abuse and the presence of mental distress. Some of these tools, were created specifically for use in a population of patients with chronic pain, while others assess the addiction risk factors in general. Table 3 summarises the tools that will then be described in greater detail; however, it is important to bear in mind that none is able to produce an accurate diagnosis about the presence of addiction, abuse or dependence. Besides, many of these are self-assessment tools, and therefore potentially at risk of falsification by the respondent. It is therefore advisable to supplement the information obtained with such tools with data obtained from direct observation of the patient during medical appointments. Anyhow, for patients who are found to be at high risk of misuse of the drug from the initial assessment with one of these scales, it is advisable to provide for constant monitoring of treatment, with regular urine toxicology screening.

	Name	Abbreviated name	Authors	Year	Method of administration	Number of items
a	*CAGE- questions Adapted to Include Drugs*	CAGE-AID	Brown & Rounds	1995	Self-administered	4
b1	*Prescription Drug Use Questionnaire*	PDUQ	Compton et al.	1998	Interview	42
b2	*Prescription Drug Use Questionnaire – patient version*	PDUQp		2008	Self-administered	31
c	*Screening Tool for Addiction Risk*	STAR	Friedman et al.	2003	Self-administered	14
d	*Pain Medication Questionnaire*	PMQ	Adams et al.	2004	Self-administered	26
e1	*Screener and Opioid Assessment for Patients with Pain*	SOAPP	Butler et al.	2004	Self-administered	14
e2	*Screener and Opioid Assessment for Patients with Pain – Revised*	SOAPP-R		2008		24
f	*Opioid Risk Tool*	ORT	Webster et al.	2005	Self-administered	5
g	*Addiction Behaviour Checklist*	ABC	Wu et al.	2006	Interview	20
h	*Diagnosis Intractability Risk and Efficacy Score*	DIRE	Belgrade et al.	2006	Team assessment	7
i	*Drug Abuse Screening Test*	DAST	Yudko et al	2007	Self-administered	28

Table 3. Principal tools for the stratification of the risk of opioid addiction and abuse.

a. The *CAGE questions Adapted to Include Drugs* (CAGE-AID; Brown & Rounds, 1995) is an adaptation of the CAGE questionnaire, used for a short screening for alcohol abuse, which also includes substance use. The name CAGE is derived from 4 key words: "cut", "annoyed", "guilty" and "eye-opener". The questionnaire consists of the following 4 questions, to which the subject must reply "yes" or "no": 1) Have you felt you ought to cut down your drinking or drug use?; 2) Have people annoyed you by criticizing your drinking or drug use?; 3) Have you felt bad or guilty about your drinking or drug use?; 4) Have you ever had a drink or used drugs first thing in the morning to steady your nerves or to get rid of a hangover (eye-opener)?. The addiction screening is positive with at least 2 affirmative responses. The CAGE-AID has been validated on a sample of 124 pain patients, demonstrating high values of sensitivity (0.70) and specificity (0.85).

b1. *Prescription Drug Use Questionnaire* (PDUQ, Compton et al., 1998) is a tool, consisting of 42 items to be administered in the form of an interview, that assesses the degree of abuse / misuse of the drug in patients with chronic pain. Care staff trained in the use of the tool take about twenty minutes to complete the interview. The patient must answer yes/no to questions that investigate: pain condition (e.g. "Has the patient explored and/or tried non-opioid or non-pharmacological pain management techniques?"), the ways in which they use drugs (e.g. "Does the patient have more than one prescription provider?"), social/family factors (e.g. "Have family members expressed concerns that the patient is addicted?"), family history of chronic pain and/or addiction (e.g. "Is there a positive history of chronic pain in the patient's mother, father, sibling or blood relative?"), personal history of substance abuse (e.g. "Has the patient ever been diagnosed with addiction to any drug or alcohol") and psychiatric history (e.g. "Has the patient ever been diagnosed with a psychiatric disorder?"). The tool has good internal consistency (Cronbach's $\alpha = 0.79$). To identify a cut-off, the 52 patients with chronic pain who participated in the pilot study to validate the PDUQ were initially classified as addicted or non-addicted based on criteria developed by the American Society of Addiction Medicine (see § 2.2.2.). Patients with scores of less than 11 did not meet the criteria for a substance abuse disorder, while patients with scores of 15 or more reflected the criteria for a substance abuse disorder. So those who achieved scores of less than 11 use the drug in a suitable way. Moreover, positive answers to 3 specific items of the tool (notably "patient believes he/she is addicted"; "increases analgesic dose/frequency"; "specific drug or route of administration preference") have been identified as more predictive of addiction, with a 92.9% of correct classification. Banta-Green et al. (2009b) carried out a study of 704 patients who had been prescribed long-term treatment with opioids, aimed to examine the factorial structure of the PDUQ. The results show that the items may be grouped into three distinct types of factor "addictive behaviours", "addiction concerns" and "pain treatment problems". The limits of the PDUQ concern the fact that it relies solely on the sincerity of the patient and is difficult to use in an overloaded clinical context.

b2. The *Prescription Drug Use Questionnaire – patient version* (PDUQp) was created by Compton et al. (2008) to obviate the difficulty mentioned above. The PDUQp is a self-administered instrument which consists of 31 items and the total score can vary from 0 to 30. Analysis of the psychometric properties of the new self-administered version was carried out on 135 patients with chronic pain being treated with opioids, monitored for 12 months. The PDUQp proved to have good concurrent validity, calculated by comparing the scores obtained with the scores obtained with the PDUQ ($r = 0.64$). The tool also proved to have good test-retest reliability, assessed at 4, 8 and 12 months after its first administration ($r = 0.67$, $r = 0.61$ and $r = 0.40$ respectively). A cut-off of 10 is suggested as indicative of drug misuse.

c. The *Screening Tool for Addiction Risk* (STAR, Friedman et al., 2003) consists of 14 questions with true/false responses that investigate potential risk factors for drug. The items were developed based on a literature review carried out by a team of specialists in pain and addiction. Validation of the questionnaire was carried out on 48 patients with chronic pain, 14 of whom had a diagnosis of addiction based on the DSM-IV criteria. The authors found a close correlation between addiction and prior treatment in a rehabilitation unit for alcohol or drug dependence, smoking, and intensity of nicotine craving. In particular, the item on prior experience of alcohol and/or substance detoxification was able to identify correctly 93% of the patients who met the addiction criteria.

d. The Pain Medication Questionnaire (PMQ, Adams et al., 2004) is a self-administered questionnaire that describes a series of dysfunctional behaviours and characteristics that underlie the use of drugs for the treatment of pain. The tool consists of 26 items, for each of which the subject must indicate his degree of agreement or disagreement on a 5 point Likert scale, and a score is attributed to the selected response (disagree = 0, somewhat disagree = 1, neutral = 3, somewhat agree = 4, agree = 5). The sum of the scores of the single items gives a total score, which can vary from a minimum of 0 to a maximum of 104. High scores are correlated with a high risk of opioid misuse. In particular, scores of 25 or more are indicative of opioid misuse, while scores of 30 or more suggest that the patient should be constantly monitored during treatment (Dowling et al., 2007). The validity of the tool was investigated by Adams et al. (2004) on 184 patients with chronic pain, comparing the results obtained with the PMQ with a series of assessment of substance abuse, degree of psychosocial distress, and some indicators of psychological and physical functioning; the test-retest reliability coefficient is 0.85 and the internal consistency is acceptable (Cronbach's $\alpha = 0.73$). A further study to examine the psychometric characteristics of the PMQ in greater depth was carried out by Buelow et al. (2009). One of the aims was to examine the accuracy of the short form of the PMQ (from which items 5, 10 and 23 had been eliminated, since they had the lowest correlation coefficients) in predicting opioid misuse. Examining 4.182 subjects, of whom 1.813 were involved in an interdisciplinary treatment programme (that included physical, pharmacological and psychological therapy) the authors confirmed the adequate internal consistency of the abbreviated form (Cronbach's $\alpha = 0.70$) e and of test-retest reliability ($r = 0.77$). Significant differences also emerged in the mean PMQ score of patients with a history of substance abuse (mean = 24.39) and of patients without a history of abuse (mean = 21.95). Moreover, those patients who interrupted the treatment had mean scores that were significantly higher than those of patients who displayed good compliance. By logistic regression, the authors showed that early request of opioids is the only factor able to predict high or low questionnaire scores of those assessed (age, history of alcohol and/or substance abuse).

e1. The Screener and Opioid Assessment for Patients with Pain (SOAPP, Butler et al., 2004) is a self-administered tool with 14 items that investigate potential risk factors for opioid misuse (e.g. "How often do you take more medications than you are supposed to?"; "How often have others expressed concerns over your use of medication?"). These items were proposed and voted on by a team of experts; the patient must indicate the frequency of each behaviour on a 5 point Likert scale (0 = "never"; 4 = "very often"). The tool was administered to 175 patients with chronic pain and readministered 6 months later to 95 of these patients, to test its reliability over time. The SOAPP proved to have adequate internal consistency (Cronbach's $\alpha = 0.74$) and good test-retest reliability six months after its first administration ($r = 0.71$). Scores of 8 or more are indicative of high risk of abuse (sensitivity: 0.91; specificity: 0.69). In a study investigating the psychometric characteristics and clinical utility of the SOAPP in 397 patients, Akbik et al. (2006) found patients classified at high risk were significantly younger, with altered urine screening results ($p<0.05$) than low risk patients. The factor analysis also revealed the presence of 5 factors, called: 1) History of substance abuse; 2) Legal problems; 3) Craving medications; 4) Heavy smoking and 5) Mood swings. Moore et al. (2009), in a study to examine the efficacy of the SOAPP and other tools in predicting the risk of opioid misuse, found good sensitivity for the tool (0.72); combining the data from the SOAPP with those from a semi-structured clinical interview designed to investigate prior treatments used, the presence of emotional distress and prior substance abuse, the sensitivity increased to 0.90.

e2. *The Screener and Opioid Assessment for Patients with Pain – Revised* (SOAPP-R) is a 24-item version developed by Butler et al. (2008) in order to overcome some limitations of the original SOAPP. The new version, tested on a sample of 283 patients, proved to have good internal consistency (Cronbach's α = 0.88); the cut-off of 18 shows adequate sensitivity (0.81) and specificity (0.68). Patients with low SOAPP-R scores appear to be at less risk of developing a substance abuse disorder.

f. The *Opioid Risk Tool* (ORT, Webster et al., 2005) is a self-administered tool developed to estimate the probability that the patient displays aberrant drug behaviours during long-term opioid treatment. The ORT consists of 5 items which investigate the following risk factors: family history of substance abuse (alcohol, drugs or prescribed medicines); personal history of substance abuse (alcohol, drugs or prescribed medicines); age (if between 16 and 45 years); history of childhood sexual abuse; presence of psychological distress (attention deficit disorder, obsessive-compulsive disorder, bipolar disorder, schizophrenia and depression). Each factor has a different weight in determining the potential risk of drug misuse, and so a specific numerical value is assigned to each, which also varies according to the sex of the respondent. There are three risk levels: scores from 0 to 3 are indicative of low risk; scores from 4 to 7 determine moderate risk; finally, scores of 8 or more are indicative of a high risk of misuse. This questionnaire was validated on 108 women and 77 men with chronic pain, followed for a period of 12 months from the initial appointment. 94% of the patients classified as low risk based on the total ORT score did not display aberrant drug behaviours in the year in which they were monitored, while 90.9% of the patients with scores of the cut-off value of 8 or more displayed aberrant drug behaviours.

g. The *Addiction Behaviour Checklist* (ABC, Wu et al., 2006) consists of 20 items to be administered in the form of an interview. The items are grouped in two principal categories: 1) addicted behaviours noted during visit (e.g. "patient running out of medications early"; "receiving narcotics from other providers"); 2) addictive behaviours observed within the visit (e.g. "patient appearing sedated"; "patient expressing concern about the future availability of narcotics"). Finally, there is a further question that can be used if family members of the patient are present during the medical appointment ("significant others express concern over patient's use of analgesic"). The answer system is binary (yes/no): each affirmative answer is assigned a point and the total score can vary from 0 to 20. To investigate its psychometric characteristics, the ABC was administered to 136 patients with chronic pain prescribed long-term opioid treatment. The tool proved to have high inter-rater validity (0.94 - 0.95) and significant concurrent validity: a significant correlation ($r=0.40$; $p< .01$) was found between the ABC score and the Prescription Drug Use Questionnaire (PDUQ, Compton et al., 1998) score. A cut-off value of 3 on this tool is able to provide a good estimate of appropriate/inappropriate use that the patient will make of the drug. For scores of 3 or more, the authors suggest that the patient should be monitored frequently, including more frequent urine toxicology screening.

h. The *Diagnosis Intractability Risk and Efficacy Score* (DIRE, Belgrade et al., 2006) is a tool that is compiled by a multidisciplinary team of physicians and psychologists. It consists of 4 scales: Diagnosis, Intractability, Risk (4 subcategories) Efficacy. Each class requires assessment on a 3 point scale, where a score of 1 corresponds to characteristics and behaviours that are indicative of a negative prognosis, and a score of 3 is indicative of suitability for treatment with opioids. The Diagnosis factor requires the clinician to determine the extent to which the patient's diagnosis is sufficiently compelling or advanced to warrant an aggressive pharmacological approach. The Intractability factor requires a determination of how many appropriate treatments the patient has undergone and how he or she is involved in the treatment, i.e. if they play a passive or an active role in managing their pain. The Risk factor was created to estimate the extent to which the patient would adhere to the instructions of the clinician during treatment. As stated above, it comprises four categories: Psychological health assesses the psychiatric and psychological status of the patient; Chemical health assesses the patient's relationship with substances with potential risk of abuse; Reliability assesses compliance with treatment in the past, whether or not the patient attends appointments and following the physician's recommendations fully; Social support assesses the patient's support network and his or her ability to function in life roles, such as work, school, parenting, etc. Efficacy assesses the analgesic effectiveness of opioids, based on physical functionality and patient's pain self-report. When efficacy cannot be assessed because the patient has not yet started to take opioids, or takes them in quantities that are too low (less than the equivalent of 30 mg/day of morphine) a score of 2 is attributed. All the scales and subscales of the Risk factor are firstly assessed individually and then added together to obtain the DIRE score. The total score can vary from a minimum of 7 to a maximum of 21; scores between 14 and 21 are indicative of a greater degree of patient compliance and, in general, greater treatment efficacy. The psychometric analyses of the original version, carried out on a group of 61 patients with chronic pain, shown an internal consistency alpha coefficient of 0.80 and an inter-rater validity of 0.95.

i. The Drug Abuse Screening Test (DAST, Yudko et al., 2007) is a self-administered questionnaire consisting of 28 items with binary (yes/no) answers. Scores of 6 or more indicate the presence of substance dependence or abuse. In addition to the complete version of the questionnaire, which can be too time-consuming in some clinical contexts, there are various short versions of the DAST, based on 10 items instead of 28. The 28-item DAST has proved to have high test-retest reliability ($r = 0.85$) and good internal consistency (Cronbach's α 0.92-0.94). The tool has shown good sensitivity, between 81% and 96%, and good specificity (from 71% to 94%). One limitation of the tool is the fact that it is susceptible to falsification and may therefore not identify those people who, while abusing the drug, intentionally give false answers. Moreover, the tool is predictive of substance abuse but does not specifically examine the aberrant drug behaviours.

2.4.1 Ways of monitoring treatment

A number of different tools have been created for clinicians to monitor opioid treatment and as checklists for the systemic observation of aberrant drug behaviours. The tools most widely mentioned in the literature are described briefly below.

The *Prescription Opioid Therapy Questionnaire* (POTQ; Michna et al., 2004) is a tool with 11 items to which the clinician must answer yes or no to assess opioid misuse. The items reflect the behaviours suggested by Chabal et al. (1997) as indicative of substance abuse. These behaviours include multiple unauthorised dosage increases, episodes of lost or stolen prescriptions, frequent unplanned visits to the clinic or emergency room, excessive telephone calls and inflexibility about treatment options. Patients who were positively rated on two or more of the items met criteria for prescription opioid misuse.

The *Pain Assessment and Documentation Tool* (PADT; Passik et al., 2004; Passik et al., 2005) is a brief (takes between 10 to 20 minutes to complete) clinician-directed interview. The clinician asks the patients questions that are organized in four primary areas called the "Four A's" and are notably: Analgesia - focuses on pain intensity (numeric rating scales) and pain relief; Activities of Daily Living - focuses on whether the patient's functioning since the last assessment is better, same, or worse; Adverse Events - identifies whether the patient is experiencing side effects from current pain relievers, and if so, what they are; potentially Aberrant Drug-Related Behaviours - assesses 17 aberrant behaviours. The availability of this checklist is likely to improve the ability of clinicians to capture problematic behaviours and implement appropriate actions in response. In addition, there is a fifth section on "Assessment" which identifies a specific analgesic plan.

The *Current Opioid Misuse Measure* (COMM, Bultler at al., 2007) is a tool with 17 items, asking the patient how he or she currently uses pain medication. For each behaviour listed (e.g. "how often have you needed to take pain medications belonging to someone else?"), the patient must indicate the frequency of each behaviour on a 5 point Likert scale (0 = "never"; 4 = "very often"). The current 17-item version of COMM was created from the 40-item version produced from the concept mapping work carried out by 26 pain and addiction professionals. Validation of the tool was carried out on 227 patients with chronic pain. Scores of 9 or more (sensitivity=0.77; specificity=0.68) are considered to be indicative of high risk of drug abuse. The tool has excellent internal consistency (Cronbach's α= 0.86) and very good test-retest reliability one week after its first administration (r = 0.86).

As well as the tools mentioned above, urine drug screens and other laboratory tests can help the clinician to understand if the patient is using illegal substances or non-prescribed drugs. It is important to supplement the observation-based tools with laboratory tests. In fact, Katz et al. (2003) showed that even if a clinician has been very careful to detect aberrant drug behaviours, some signals may be missed: approximately 20% of patients considered compliant with the treatment prescribed by expert clinicians actually tested positive in urine toxicology screening. Urine screening is an economical and non-invasive monitoring strategy that enables most drugs to be identified between 1 and 3 days after they were taken (Heit & Gourley, 2004). In addition, urine screening may be very useful in preventing opioid abuse, detecting the presence of illegal substances, identifying those patients who are not taking the prescribed drugs, or those who are using non-prescribed opioids (Atluri & Sudarshan, 2003). However, the results of urine toxicology screening must be interpreted with caution, since they may not always be correct, and in some cases can produce false positives and false negatives. Moreover, some substances are not detected by standard urine screening, and so clinicians must result to more specific or costly urine tests (or to blood or hair analysis). For this reason the results of urine drug screen should be considered a further piece of the puzzle in assessing patients with problematic opioid use behaviours (Ballantyne, 2009).

2.5 The research

This section describes the preliminary results of a prospective longitudinal study to identify some procedures that allow the risk of opioid misuse to be determined in patients with chronic non-cancer pain. Specifically, the study examines the efficacy and clinical utility of the Pain Medication Questionnaire - PMQ (Adams et al. 2004) and the Diagnosis, Intractability, Risk and Efficacy - DIRE (Belgrade et al. 2006). The PMQ was selected because it is a self-administered scale that can easily be integrated into clinical-care routine, and the DIRE because it is an assessment tool used in a multidisciplinary setting that requires a medical and psychological assessment of the patient. In addition, both tools have been shown to possess characteristics that make them suitable for use in clinical practice: good psychometric properties in their original version, easy to complete, and sufficiently short to administer and score.

The specific aim of the study is to identify and examine the efficacy of a clinical protocol for the systematic assessment of patients who are candidates for starting opioid treatment. As a preliminary step, the predictive validity of the Italian versions of the PMQ and the DIRE was investigated: until now the Italian versions of these instrument are not available. Besides, the capacity of the two tools to predict opioid misuse was compared to the subjective estimate made by the physician based on his or her clinical experience. Furthermore, the presence of possible relationships between aberrant drug behaviours and the presence of risk factors for treatment compliance was examined, as was any use of illegal substances established by urine drug tests. Finally, the efficacy of the treatment was analysed the patient's perceived quality of life and pain experience after 2 and 4 months after the start of treatment.

2.5.1 Subjects

The preliminary data presented below refer to 25 patients treated in the Pain Relief and Palliative Care Unit. The inclusion criteria were: age between 18 and 70 years; presence of non-cancer pain for at least 6 months; pain intensity assessed on an 11 point Numerical Rating Scale of at least 4 in the last month; good knowledge/understanding of Italian; absence of cognitive deficit; use of fixed regime weak opioids insufficiently efficacious; other pharmacological and non-pharmacological treatments used for at least 3 months not sufficiently efficacious; no significant decrease in life expectancy; informed consent to participation in the study obtained.

	Descriptives (mean SD or % frequency)
Age	56.2 (10.6)
Sex	
- Women	17 (68.0%)
- Men	8 (32.0%)
Education (years)	
- 5	5 (20.0%)
- 8	10 (41%)
- 9-13	9 (35%)
- >13	1 (4%)
Marital status	
- Never married	2 (8%)
- Married	13 (52%)
- Divorced	3 (11%)
- Widowed	7 (27%)
Occupation	
- Employed	6 (24%)
- Housewife	7 (28%)
- Unemployed	1 (4%)
- Retired	11 (44%)
Type of pain	
- Nociceptive	10 (40%)
- Neuropathic	5 (20%)
- Mixed	10 (40%)
Duration of pain (months)	88.2 (57.7)

Table 4. Socio-demographic characteristics.

The socio-demographic and clinical characteristics of the group of subjects are represented in table 4. The mean age is 56.2 years (±10.6) and 68% are women. Most subjects were not working at the time of the study due to their pain condition. Regarding the characteristics of their pain symptoms, the most prevalent types were nociceptive (40%) or mixed (40%); the average duration of the pain condition was 88.2 months (±57.7). There were no statistically significant differences between men and women in any of the descriptive variables considered.

2.5.2 Instruments

The *Checklist for medical selection* is a tool constructed ad hoc that enabled physicians to collect information needed to check the suitability of the patient for inclusion in the study. It includes the collection of personal data (age, sex, nationality), clinical data (disorder causing the pain, characteristics of the pain, prior pharmacological and non-pharmacological treatments) and the assessment of pain intensity (in the last month) using the *11-point Numerical Rating Scale* (NRS-11). The doctor must also indicate the drug administration route (oral or transdermal) and the initial dosage.

The *11-point Numerical Rating Scale* (NRS-11) is a pain assessment scale in which the patient is asked to report the intensity of the pain, over a specific time interval, with a number from 0 to 10, where 0 indicates no pain and 10 the worst possible pain.

The risk opioid misuse was assessed using the Pain Medication Questionnaire- PMQ (Adams et al., 2004) and the Diagnosis Intractability Risk and Efficacy Score - DIRE; Belgrade et al. 2006): see § 2.4 for a detailed description of these tools. The Italian version of the tools elaborated for this study was authorised and approved by the original Authors.

The *Medical risk prediction* requires the physician to provide an estimate, based on his or her clinical experience, of the risk of opioid misuse, answering 3 questions on an 11 point numerical scale: compliance with medical treatment (0=no compliance; 10=maximum compliance), risk of abuse and/or underuse of the drug (0=no risk, 10=maximum risk) and expected efficacy of treatment (0=no efficacy, 10=maximum efficacy).

The *Medical control form* was designed to collect clinical information about the progress of the treatment, any side effects, and the intention to continue or suspend treatment. It contains also a list of aberrant drug behaviours, based on the reference literature; the physician must tick those behaviours displayed by the patient (e.g. The patient uses other opioids in addition to those prescribed, The patient displays little interest in managing himself and his rehabilitation).

Urine toxicology screening was performed with fast immunodosages that could be read visually, allowing the qualitative determination of the pharmacological substances and their metabolites present in the urine. For opiates, marijuana and buprenorfin, QuikStrip™ OneStep immunodosages were used; QuikPac II™ OneStep were used to detect the presence of amphetamines, metamphetamines and cocaine.

Regarding the psychological assessment the following tools were used.

The *Initial pain interview* is a semi–structured interview designed to reconstruct the clinical history of the pain, and its progress over time. The interview is used to gather a wide range of personal information (e.g. marital status, level of education, employment status, etc.) and other information about the pain and its interference in daily activities. The habits and behaviours that, based on the literature, are considered risk factors for aberrant opioid use were also investigated (smoking, alcohol consumption patterns, use of drugs, family history of alcohol and/or drug abuse, sexual abuse).

The *Visual Analogue Scale* (VAS) consists of a 10 cm long horizontal line, the start and end points of which are labelled "no pain" and "worst possible pain". The patient is asked to mark the precise points corresponding to his or her maximum, minimum and habitual pain in the last month.

The *Minnesota Multiphasic Personality Inventory II* (MMPI-2; Hataway e McKinley, 1989; Italian adaptation by Pancheri et al., 1996) is a self-administered questionnaire used to assess personality characteristics. It consists of 567 items to be answered "true" or "false". Scores are obtained referred to three control scales and ten clinical scales (Hypochondria, Depression, Hysteria, Psychopathic Deviate, Masculinity - Femininity, Paranoia, Psychasthenia, Schizophrenia, Hypomania and Social Introversion).

The *Beck Depression Inventory II* (BDI-II; Beck et al., 1996; Italian adaptation by Ghisi et al., 2006) is a 21-item self-administered questionnaire commonly used among chronic pain patients to determine their depressive reaction, assessing both the cognitive component (e.g. sadness, pessimism) and the somatic component (e.g. loss of appetite, sleep disorders).

The *State Trait Anxiety Inventory-Y* (STAI-Y, Spielberger,1983; Italian adaptation by Pedrabissi and Santinello, 1989) is a 40-item questionnaire that assesses the level of patient anxiety. Two scores can be obtained, referring to two subscales that assess state anxiety (i.e. the anxiety experienced by the patient at the time they complete the questionnaire) and trait anxiety (i.e. the anxiety that the patient habitually experiences).

The *Pain Related Self-Statement Scale* (PRSS; Flor and Turk, 1988; Italian adaptation by Ferrari et al., 2004) is a self-administered scale developed to assess the cognitions specifically triggered in the pain situation that might inhibit or promote coping responses. The tool consists of 18 items, from which two total scores can be obtained for the subscales called Catastrophizing and Coping.

The *Nottingham Health Profile* (NPH, Hunt et al., 1985; Italian adaptation by Bertin et al, 1992) was used to assess quality of life. It consists of 38 items covering 6 content areas: physical mobility, energy, sleep, pain, social isolation, emotional reactions. The scores are expressed on percentage scales and correspond to the level of compromise perceived by the subject in the quality of life area considered.

The *Multidimensional Pain Inventory* (MPI, Kerns et al., 1985; Italian adaptation by Ferrari et al., 2000) is a 61-item self-administered questionnaire that allow a multidimensional assessment of the pain experience. The tool is divided into 3 parts: the first focuses on assessing the intensity of the pain, its interference in the life of the patient, the patient's perceived control of the pain and of events in his or her life (it consists of the following subscales: pain severity, interference, life-control, affective distress and support). The second part investigates the patient's perception of the responses of his or her significant others to his or her pain communications (negative/solicitous and distracting responses). The third part examines the frequency with which the patient carries out common daily activities (household chores, outdoor work, distant activities, social activities and general activity).

Finally, the *McGill Pain Questionnaire* (MPQ, Melzack, 1983; Italian adaptation by Maiani and Sanavio, 1985) is a tool consisting of a list of 78 adjectives related to pain grouped into 20 subclasses of homogeneous content; within each subgroup the descriptors are arranged in order of increasing intensity. The subject is invited to choose the adjective that best describes his or her pain in each category. The tool allows the pain to be assessed as an experience with three major dimensions: sensory-discriminative, motivational-affective and cognitive-evaluative.

2.5.3 Procedure

The study is observational prospective and longitudinal; patient selection, data collection and the subsequent follow-ups took place from December 2009 to March 2011 in the Pain Relief and Palliative Care Unit of Vicenza hospital. The study consisted of the following assessment phases: patient selection, collection of pre-treatment data, 2 and 4 month follow-ups (figure 3).

The specialist physician selected patients according to the personal and clinical criteria indicated above, as well as by using the numerical scale to assess pain intensity. Patients who were candidates for opioid treatment were asked to undergo psycho-clinical assessment in accordance with the multidisciplinary care diagnostic protocol, for patients with chronic non-cancer pain referred for opioid treatment at our Centre.

Pre-treatment data were collected in the two week period following selection. It consisted of the compilation of the questionnaire to determine the risk of opioid misuse (PMQ) by the patient, and the compilation of the DIRE by the team of pain specialists. Questionnaires to assess the intensity and experience of pain (VAS, MPI, MPQ, PRSS) and affective/emotional state (STAI-Y, BDI-II), quality of life (NHP) and personality characteristics (MMPI-2) were also administered. Medical and psychological follow-ups were scheduled 2 and 4 months after the start of treatment. At 2 months, medical data such as the presence of any side effects, changes in dosage, presence of aberrant drug behaviours and any intention to stop treatment were collected for treatment monitoring. The PMQ was administered again, to assess its reliability over time, and the questionnaires assessing quality of life and pain experience (VAS, MPI and NHP) were also administered. The same medical and psychological data were collected at 4 months, apart from the PMQ. At both follow-up appointment urine drug test was proposed. The study protocol was approved by the competent Ethics Committee.

PATIENT SELECTION	PRE-TREATMENT	2 MONTH FOLLOW-UP	4 MONTH FOLLOW-UP
• Checklist for medical selection • Intensity of pain in the last month ≥4/10 (NRS)	*Medical assessment* • Medical risk prediction *Psychological assessment* • Risk of opioid misuse (PMQ) • Initial pain interview • Pain intensity (VAS) • Personality characteristics (MMPI-II) • Affective-emotional state (STAI-Y,BDI-2) • Pain experience and coping strategies (MPI,MPQ,PRSS) • Quality of life (NHP) *Team assessment* • Risk of opioid misuse (DIRE)	*Medical assessment* • Medical control form • Urine drug tests	*Medical assessment* • Medical control form • Urine drug tests *Psychological assessment* • Pain intensity (VAS) • Experience of pain (MPI) • Quality of life (NHP)

Fig. 3. Study procedures

2.5.4 Statistical analysis

Continuous variables are expressed with mean, standard deviation, minimum and maximum and centiles into which the variables fall, when possible. Discrete and nominal variables are reported in frequency tables with the related percentages. To examine the differences between continuous variables, Student's parametric t test was used, with Chi squared for the comparison of frequency distributions.
The reliability of the PMQ was assessed using test-retest, and Cronbach's α, while the internal consistency of the DIRE was determined from Cronbach's α.
Correspondence Analysis was used to examine the relationship between the PMQ and DIRE scores obtained by the patients in the pre-treatment phase and the number of aberrant drug behaviours detected in the patients at the medical follow-ups recorded in the "Medical control form", the duration of treatment and the presence of the drug in the urine. Analysis of variance and correlational analysis with Spearman's non-parametric coefficient were used to analyse the relationship between the PMQ scores and the DIRE and the clinical variables related to pain, psychological function and quality of life.

2.5.5 Results

All the patients reported continuous pain; table 5 shows the mean values for pain intensity (assessed using the VAS) and the data on pharmacological treatment in the three assessment phases. No significant gender differences were found in maximum, minimum or habitual pain intensity. However, there was a statistically significant reduction in maximum and minimum pain intensity from the pre-treatment to the 2 month follow-up ($F_{1,24}$= 4.64; $F_{1,24}$= 6.75 respectively; both for p<0.05); from pre-treatment to the 4 month follow-up the only difference was in maximum VAS ($F_{1,24}$= 8.21; p<0.01). This variation was not influenced by the active substance administration route.
Analysing the type of pharmacological treatment, it may be noted that at both the start of the pharmacological treatment and at the subsequent follow-ups, the most frequently administered active substance was oxycodone. The administration route during the data collection phases remained primarily oral. The drug dosages were transformed into equivalent mg of morphine, and classified as mild/average/high based on the indications supplied by Bruera et al. (1995). Regarding the dosage, it showed a tendency to increase at the 4 month follow-up.
Approximately half (46%) of the patients reported the presence of at least one side effect at the follow-ups; the most frequently reported side effects were sleepiness (29%), constipation (29%) and nausea (21%). The drug administration route did not appear to have any effect on the number and type of side effects reported by the patients.
With respect to the psychological indicators investigated in the pre-treatment assessment, it was found that, based on the personality profile obtained with the MMPI-2, 56.2% of women and 33.3% of men had clinically significant scores in at least one of the clinical scales with psychopathological content (Paranoia, Schizofrenia, Hypomania). As for the affective-emotional variables, the mean total score at BDI-II in the initial treatment phase was 24.6 (SD= 13.40) in women and 18.2 (SD= 9.94) in men; the level of depression was clinically significant (scores higher than 95th percentile) in 61% of women and 50% of men. Considering trait anxiety, the mean score was 52.7 (SD= 11.97) in women and 46.2 (SD= 7.22) in men, with 27.7% clinically significant levels of anxiety only in women (scores higher than 95th percentile).
Regarding PRSS, the subjects reported a mean score of 3.20 (range 0-5, SD= 1.15) on the Catastrophizing scale and 2.76 on the Coping scale (range 0-5, SD= 0.88).

	Initial treatment	2 month follow-up	4 month follow-up
	Mean (SD)	Mean (SD)	Mean (SD)
Pain intensity	Mean (SD)	Mean (SD)	Mean (SD)
- maximum VAS	90.2 (12.9)	80.6 (16.4)	78.7 (28.3)
- minimum VAS	33.1 (22.4)	24.0 (18.7)	31.8 (19.6)
- habitual VAS	55.5 (20.6)	52.6 (13.8)	56.1 (24.5)
	Frequency (%)	Frequency (%)	Frequency (%)
Drug active substance			
- Oxycodone	12 (48%)	12 (48%)	15 (60%)
- Fentanyl	10 (40%)	6 (24%)	5 (20%)
- Hydromorphone	3 (12%)	4 (16%)	5 (20%)
- Buprenorphine	-	3 (12%)	-
Route of administration			
- Oral	15 (60%)	16 (64%)	20 (80%)
- Transdermal	10 (40%)	9 (36%)	5 (20%)
Dosage (mg morphine)	Frequency (%)	Frequency (%)	Frequency (%)
- Mild (<60 mg)	24 (96%)	11 (44%)	6 (24%)
- Average (60-300mg)	1 (4%)	14 (56%)	11 (44%)
- High (>300 mg)	-	-	8 (32%)

Table 5. Pain intensity, active medication taken, administration route and dosage in initial treatment and in subsequent follow-ups.

In the description of the pain characteristics at the MPQ, higher scores emerged in the evaluative and affective -evaluative dimensions (means 0.87 and 0.73, respectively) , while the lower scores referred to the affective and mixed-sensory dimensions (means 0.4 and 0.52, respectively).

In the MPI the subjects reported high mean on "Pain severity" (mean: 4.6; SD= 0.9), "Interference" (mean: 4.3; SD= 1.1) and "Affective distress" (mean: 3.6; SD= 1.1) in the pre-treatment assessment. Quality of life, measured using the NHP, appears more compromised in the following areas: "Emotional reactions" (mean: 80; SD= 56), "Pain" (mean: 77; SD= 26.2) and "Energy" (mean: 64; SD= 40). There were no statistically significant variations in the mean scores at the start of treatment and at the subsequent follow-ups for either the MPI or the NHP.

As for the tools to assess the risk of opioid misuse, the mean score at the PMQ was 24.59 (SD=9.43); there were no significant gender differences in the PMQ scores. Figure 4 shows the three different levels of the PMQ scores that, according to the cut-offs established by Dowling et al. (2007), identify a low/moderate or high risk of drug misuse. Overall, 36% of the subjects were found to be at high risk of misuse, 20% at moderate risk, and the remaining 44% at low risk. The distribution in the three risk levels between men and women was comparable.

The group was subsequently divided into patients with high PMQ scores (H-PMQ; n=9) and patients with low PMQ scores (L-PMQ; n=11) in order to analyse the presence of any significant differences in the psychological variables considered in the study. The patients with H-PMQ had a mean score of 3.78 on the Catastrophizing scale of the PRSS, statistically higher than that of the L-PMQ patients (mean 2.61) ($t=-3.16$; $p<0.01$); while on the Coping scale the H-PMQ subjects had mean scores that were significantly lower than those of the L-PMQ group ($t=-2.18$; $p<0.05$). Further statistical differences were found for the "HS" scale

(Hypocondria) of the MMPI-2, in which the H-PMQ subjects had scores that were significantly higher than the L-PMQ subjects (means 21 and 16.5 respectively, t=23.60; p<0.05) and for the total depression score in the BDI-II (H-PMQ mean =27.36; L-PMQ mean =17.88; t=26.18, p<0.05).

As for the predictive validity of the tool, a highly significant correlation was found between the total PMQ score (high risk of opioid misuse) and the number of aberrant drug-related behaviours noted by the physician at the 4 month follow-up (r=0.95; p<0.01). Significant correlations were also found between the PMQ score and the "HS" (Hypochondria) scale of the MMPI-2 (r=0.49; p<0.01), the total score in the BDI-II (r=0.43; p<0.05), the trait anxiety score of the STAI-Y (r=0.38; p<0.05) and the "emotional reaction" scale of the NHP (r=0.39; p<0.05). The mean time required by the patient to complete the tool was 12'02" (SD=6.35; range: 4-30). Finally, analysis of internal consistency produced an alpha coefficient of 0.82, indicating that the tool has excellent internal coherence; the test-retest reliability at 2 months was very high (r= 0.76; p<0.001).

In the DIRE, the mean score assigned by the multidisciplinary team was 15.35; in this case too there were no significant differences in the mean scores of men and women. Figure 5 shows the percentage of patients suitable or not suitable for treatment based on DIRE total Score according to the cut-offs established by Belgrade et al. (2006). Most women (81.2%) and men (87.5%) were found suitable to start chronic opioid treatment according to the DIRE score.

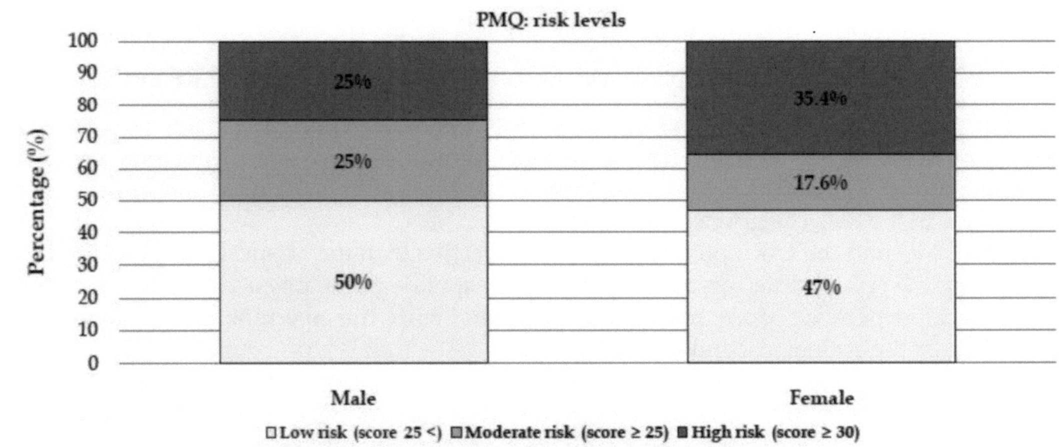

Fig. 4. Percentage of patients with low/moderate/high risk level for opioid misuse, based on PMQ scores.

The total DIRE score was not found to be significantly correlated with the number of aberrant drug behaviours recorded by the physician at 2 and 4 months; however, a significant negative correlation (r=0.83; p<0.05) was found between the scores in the "Risk" category of the DIRE (psychological risk, chemical health, reliability, social support) and the number of aberrant drug behaviours recorded by the physician at the 4 month follow-up.

The total DIRE score correlates negatively with the total BDI-II score (r=0.46, p<0.01) and with many of the MMPI-2 scales, and specifically: "PD" (Psychopathic Deviate) (r= 0.44; p<0.05), "PA" (Paranoia) (r= 0.40; p<0.05), "D" (Depression) (r= 039; p<005); "FAM" (Family Problems) (r= 044; p<005), "WRK" (Work Interference) (r= 040; p<005) and "TRT"(Negative Treatment Indicators) (r= 0.39; p<0.05).

The mean time required by the multidisciplinary team to complete the tool was 7'23" (SD=3.38; range: 1-16). The internal consistency of the Italian version of the tool was 0.48, which is very low; the item that contributed least to the internal consistency of the DIRE was Diagnosis (α if item deleted=0.51).

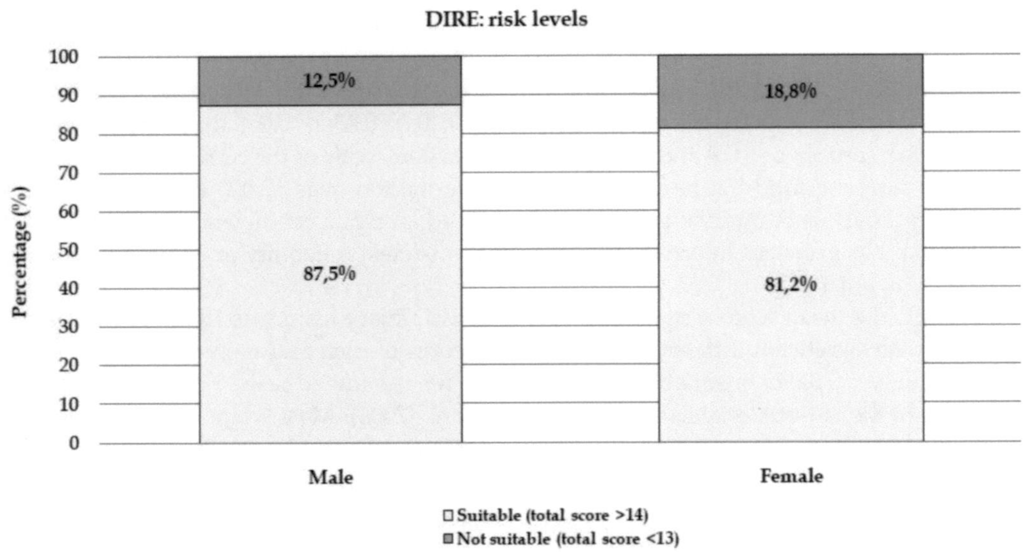

Fig. 5. Percentage of patients suitable or not suitable for treatment based on DIRE total Score.

As for the concurrent validity of the two tools, there were no significant correlations between the total scores of the PMQ and the DIRE. However, there was a moderate negative correlation ($r=0.36$; $p< 0.05$) between high total PMQ scores (high risk of opioid misuse) and low scores in the Risk category of the DIRE.

Both the PMQ and the DIRE proved to be more effective than the Medical risk prediction in estimating the risk of drug misuse: the subjective estimate of the physician based on his or her clinical experience does not in fact correlate with the aberrant drug behaviours displayed by the patient at 2 and 4 months.

In the urine toxicology screening, only one patient tested negative for the active principle at the two month follow-up, while all the patients were positive for the drug used at the four month follow-up. None of the patients tested positive for illegal substances.

In relation to aberrant drug behaviours, most of the subjects (71%) displayed no aberrant drug behaviour at the two month follow-up; there was a potential misuse indicator in 19%, and the remaining 10% displayed three or more. At the 4 month follow-up, 22% of the patients displayed three or more aberrant drug behaviours while no indicators of misuse were found in 56% of the subjects.

Regarding other factors that according to the literature might be predictive for improper use of opioids, none of the patients reported that they abused alcohol or narcotic substances at assessment; 4.9% reported a personal history of alcohol abuse and 5.4% stated that they had abused illegal substances in the past. 7.3% of the subjects had a family history of alcohol abuse and 2.4% had a family history of the use of narcotic substances. None of the patients reported that they had suffered sexual abuse in childhood or adolescence, 17.1% of the patients had a prior psychiatric diagnosis and 9.8% of the subjects were being treated by a psychiatrist at the time of the evaluation.

2.5.6 Discussion

The main purpose of this study was to identify clinical procedures that allow to estimate the risk of opioid misuse in patients with chronic non-cancer pain treated as outpatients in a pain relief centre. With this aim, two tools were selected and adapted in Italian - the Pain Medication Questionnaire (PMQ) and the Diagnosis, Intractability, Risk and Efficacy Score (DIRE). These tools examine the perspectives of the patient and the multispecialist team, respectively.

The preliminary results reported above show that the PMQ has a good capacity to predict the risk of drug misuse by the patient. A strong correlation was found between high PMQ scores and the number of aberrant drug behaviours reported by the physician 4 months after the start of the study.

From the PMQ scores, 36% of the subjects were found to be at high risk of misuse, 20% at moderate risk, and the remaining 44% at low risk. High PMQ scores (high risk of misuse) were found to be associated with higher levels of anxiety, depression and persistent body-related worries. Furthermore, those patients classified as high risk of misuse, based on the cut-offs suggested by Dowling et al. (2007), were found to be significantly more depressed, and with a greater tendency to somatise their emotional distress than those classified as low risk. High risk patients were also found to be less active in managing their pain condition, and to have a greater propensity to produce pessimistic and catastrophic thoughts about their pain symptoms. The association that emerged, between high PMQ scores and the presence of symptoms of depression, appears to be in line with the findings of Holmes et al. (2006) in their work assessing the long-term utility of the PMQ in 271 subjects. In this study the low risk patients had mean BDI scores that were significantly lower than those of the high risk of misuse group.

Furthermore, based on the initial results, the PMQ has demonstrated adequate internal consistency and good reliability over time. This suggests that the items composing it measure a single construct, and that the tool provides a reliable estimate of the risk of medication misuse. In addition, completing the PMQ requires just over ten minutes of the patient's time, and this makes it easy to incorporate into clinical practice.

To summarise, the tool seems to possess a good predictive capacity in relation to the use that the patient will make of the drug, and his or her compliance with treatment. The total score on the questionnaire, and the stratification of risk based on the cut-offs suggested by the authors therefore appear to be reliable indicators that the clinician can use to plan regular treatment monitoring. The strong association between high PMQ scores and the presence of symptoms of depression, tendency to somatisation and catastrophization, suggest that pharmacological treatment with opioids needs to be combined with psychological treatment to reduce the affective and emotional distress and modify the patient's dysfunctional convictions and behaviours in relation to use of the drug.

As for the Italian version DIRE, the preliminary results show that the total score for risk of drug misuse is a poor predictor with limited psychometric quality. The Risk category, which specifically assesses psychosocial aspects such as psychological adaptation, substance abuse, reliability in complying with previous treatments and perceived social support in life context, is an exception to this. The tool in fact has low internal consistency, which improves slightly when the Diagnosis factor is removed. This means that the items of which the tool is composed are very heterogeneous, and that the tool probably has a multifactorial structure. Our finding does not agree with the results reported by Belgrade et al. (2006) in the original validation study, in which the DIRE displayed a very high internal consistency. The total score of the DIRE - Italian version - is not at present predictive of the number of aberrant drug behaviours detected by the physician at the follow-ups. This seems to be in line with the work of Moore et al. (2007), who found that the DIRE had low sensitivity (0.17) in predicting aberrant drug behaviours. The authors suggest that the DIRE is more than simply an addiction risk tool and some of its items may not to be appropriate to predict drug misuse. However, as mentioned above, the score of the Risk category was found to be predictive of the number of aberrant drug behaviours at 4- months follow-up. This result is coherent with the findings of many studies on opioid abuse risk factors, which found that the factors considered to be most predictive of opioid abuse are the presence of psychiatric disorders (Compton et al., 1998; Sullivan et al., 2006) and a personal and/or family history of substance abuse or drug abuse (Dunbar & Katz, 1996; Schieffer et al., 2005). Our data indicate that a low score (not suitable for opioid treatment) is associated with depressive symptoms, the presence of paranoid personality traits and family and work difficulties. Completing the DIRE requires a few minutes of the team's time, but this must be preceded by an in-depth psychological assessment of the patient to determine if psychiatric disorders and past abuse, or current alcohol or substance abuse, are present.

The two tools selected do not appear to be correlated; instead, it is clear that there is an association between high PMQ scores (high risk of misuse) and low scores in the DIRE Risk category.

The prediction made by the physician based on his or her clinical experience was not found to be valid in estimating the risk of opioid misuse. This result highlights the need to use tools specifically created to assess the risk of opioid addiction in the chronic pain patient; clinical experience can be used to understand and contextualize the results obtained from these scales, but seems to be insufficient on its own.

So far as the experience of pain and the indicators of psychophysical function are concerned, the use of opioid drugs proved efficacious in reducing the maximum and minimum intensity of the perceived pain 2 months after the start of the treatment. A parallel improvement in the quality of life of the patients was not recorded by the questionnaire used in this study. This result seems to be in line with the data in the literature: despite ongoing research and the growing use of opioids in clinical practice, the effect of this treatment on the quality of life of the patient remains a subject of debate (Dillie et al., 2008). The reduction in pain, unaccompanied by an improvement in physical function and quality of life, indicates that these patients need psychological support, to examine their life habits, coping strategies and any secondary gain that might interfere with recovery of a state of psychophysical well-being. Quality of life is in fact a wide ranging concept, influenced by perception of one's health in a biopsychosocial sense, level of independence, social relationships and interaction with one's own specific environmental context in a complex way (Apolone et al., 1997).

As for the psychological variables considered in the study, half of the men and 60% of the women reported clinically significant levels of depression; and almost 30% of the women displayed high levels of anxiety. These data are in line with the findings of many authors, that clinically significant levels of depression and anxiety are very frequent in patients with chronic pain (Banks & Kerns, 1996; Boersma & Linton, 2006; Dersh et al., 2006; Gatchel, 2005; Vlayen & Linton, 2000). In addition, there was a high incidence of alterations in patients' personality profiles: over half of the women and approximately one third of the men reported high scores in at least one of the clinical content scales of the MMPI-2. This result too seems coherent with the reports in the literature, that the presence of psychiatric and personality disorders is more frequent in these patients (Banta-Green et al., 2009a; Haller & Acosta; 2010), and therefore it is advisable to involve a psychotherapist or psychiatrist in the treatment process (Chou, 2009; Chou et al, 2009a; Chou et al, 2009b; Chou et al, 2009c; Trescot et al., 2006; Trescot at al., 2008).

The analyses carried out to date have shown that only one patient in twenty five did not test positive to the prescribed drug; and no patients tested positive for illegal substances in the urine toxicology screening. These data seem very different to those of other studies, which found the prevalence of abuse of illegal substances in patients being treated with opioid to be 16% (Machikanti et al., 2006), 20% (Heit & Gourlay, 2004) or 40.3% (Ives et al., 2006). The preliminary results seem to suggest that in our context the more frequent problem may be the underuse of opioid analgesics rather than their compulsive use and abuse: this interpretation is supported by the difficulty, frequently expressed by our patient, in accepting these drugs for fear of dependence, loss of mental lucidity or being socially stigmatised as drug addicted. A further important objective of the management of patients who are candidates for opioid treatment in a multidisciplinary setting is thus to assess their convictions about the use of these drugs and their expectations of treatment, so as to be able to modify any dysfunctional beliefs and unrealistic hopes for the outcome of treatment.

The limitations of this study are primarily the small number of subjects examined and the differing distribution of men and women. In addition, the limited number of patients did not allow us to examine the effect of other variables that, based on the reference literature, can constitute risk factors for opioid addiction, such as a personal or family history of alcohol and/or substance abuse, or episodes of sexual abuse in childhood or adolescence.

Despite these limits, the high degree of correlation between risk of misuse and the psychological aspects supports the view that an in-depth assessment of the affective-emotional, cognitive and behavioural variables of the patient is crucial. So future research may be focused on understanding which psychological variables are most connected to the risk of opioid misuse (e.g. personality traits, anxiety, depression, etc.) so as to be able to develop tailored psychological interventions that maximise treatment efficacy, with positive outcomes for quality of life and overall well-being, as well.

Overall the results that have emerged so far highlight the need for a multidisciplinary assessment of patients who are candidates for opioid treatment so as to improve compliance and treatment benefits. The use of tools specifically designed to determine the risk of inappropriate use of the drug has proved to be more efficacious that the opinion expressed by the clinician based on his or her experience. The strong association between psychosocial distress and high risk of opioid misuse also suggests that pharmacological treatment should be combined with psychological interventions that can reduce the anxiety-depression symptoms and correct any irrational ideas about the use of these drugs. Furthermore, systemic monitoring of treatment and regular urine drug screen can contribute to improve adherence to treatment.

3. Conclusions

Chronic non-cancer pain remains a condition that affects a large number of people throughout the world, and is associated with significantly compromised quality of life. Although many pharmacological and non-pharmacological treatments have been proposed to manage chronic pain, the results have proved disappointing for a significant proportion of patients.

Opioid drugs seem promising for the management of chronic pain of medium-severe intensity, but many uncertainties remain about the long-term use of these drugs and the risk of dependence and abuse. In this respect, many guidelines and protocols with recommendations have been developed in recent years precisely to allow safer and more targeted use of opioid drugs in chronic non-cancer pain syndromes; these recommendations highlight, primarily, the importance of carrying out stratification of risk in the patient who is a candidate for pharmacological treatment with opioids. A number of standardised tools have been developed with the aim of identifying and objectively measuring the risk of abuse, dependence and aberrant drug behaviours.

This chapter has presented the preliminary results of a study that aims to analyse the clinical utility of the Italian adaptation of two tools for stratification of the risk: a self-administered patient questionnaire, the Pain Medication Questionnaire, and a team assessment tool, the Diagnosis Intractability Risk and Efficacy Score.

These tools have been used as part of a multidisciplinary medical and psychological assessment and treatment protocol; the data in the literature, confirmed in our study, clearly indicates that there is a frequent association between high risk of opioid misuse and the presence of psychological distress (Banta-Green et al., 2009a; Haller & Acosta; 2010). This emphasizes the importance of a physical, psychological and social assessment before starting treatment with opioids. In this respect, based on literature data and the preliminary results of the study described, we believe that an effective psychological assessment must consist of an initial clinical interview, specific tools to assess the risk of drug misuse, and questionnaires that investigate the patient's subjective experience of pain, perceived quality of life and personality characteristics. The interview, which may be more or less structured, is essential to understand the individual's experience of pain and its interference in the patient's family, professional, social and emotional life; it also allows the clinician to investigate behaviour habits related to opioid misuse (e.g. prior abuse of alcohol or illegal substances) and the presence of traumatic experiences such as sexual abuse in childhood or adolescence. During the interview the clinician may also identify any fears and worries about taking these drugs, the patient's expectations of the treatment and their reliability in following the indications of the therapist. Further areas of investigation concern the strategies that the patient uses to deal with the pain, and the possible presence of secondary gain that could compromise the efficacy of the treatment. Our results show that the indications provided by the specifically designed tools are more reliable than the clinical experience of the specialist physician in estimated aberrant drug behaviours. Investigation of the emotional-affective state of the patient, and his or her personality characteristics, always an important aspect of the multidimensional assessment of chronic pain, appears indispensable when long-term opioid therapy is initiated, since the presence of depression, anxiety or personality disorders has been found to be correlated with a greater risk of addiction. Pain coping strategies and any tendency to "catastrophize" must also be investigated using suitable questionnaires. Based on our experience, patients at greater risk of opioid misuse in fact seem to display a passive attitude to the management of their pain condition, and to have exaggeratedly pessimistic expectations of the progress of their symptoms. Finally, it is important to systematically assess the quality of life of these patients, as effective pain relief should always be accompanied by functional improvements in their physical, psychological and social area. The preliminary results of our study show that reduction in pain intensity of pain due to opioids does not seem to be accompanied by an improvement in physical and psychological functionality. This indicates that the patient needs to be monitored not only in medical term, but also from a psychological perspective, to be able to make cognitive, emotional and behavioural changes that can enhance and consolidate the efficacy of the treatment.

From our experience in the Italian context, the prevalence of addiction or misuse in patients with chronic pain in treatment with opioids appears to be low. The systematic assessment of risk using the tools created in recent years allows the clinician to overcome some biases, such as the overestimation of the risk of addiction, and hence avoid considering the entire population of chronic pain patients to be at risk of abuse.

The treatment of pain is a public health problem that is of such critical importance as to constitute an international imperative, as well as a fundamental human right (Brennan et al., 2007); opioid drugs appear as a potential resource to manage chronic pain efficaciously. However, their targeted use must be preceded by a suitable assessment of the patient by a multidisciplinary team that clarifies not only the causes of the pain, but also any risk factors or dysfunctional psychological aspects related to use of the drug, so as to increase the benefits of treatment and reduce the costs.

4. Acknowledgments

We would like to thank all the medical and nursing staff of the Pain and Palliative Care Unit from Vicenza Hospital for the precious contribution to the realization of this study.

5. References

Adams, L., Gatchel, R., Robinson, R., Polatin, P., Gajraj, N., Deschner, M. & Noe, C. (2004). Development of a self-report screening instrument for assessing potential opioid medication misuse in chronic pain patients. *Journal of Pain and Symptom Management*, Vol. 27, No. 5, (May), pp. 440-456.

Akbik, H., Butler, S., Budman, S., Fernandez, K. & Jamison R. (2006).Validation and clinical application of the Screener and Opioid Assessment for Patients with Pain (SOAPP). *Journal of Pain and Symptom Management*, Vol. 32, No. 3, (September), pp. 287-293.

American Society of Addiction Medicine (2001). *Definitions Related to the Use of Opioids for the Treatment of Pain: Consensus Statement of the American Academy of Pain Medicine, the American Pain Society, and the American Society of Addiction Medicine.* Last accessed June 2011, available from: http://www.pcssmethadone.org/pcss/documents2/ASAM_DefinitionsRelatedToUseOpioidsPain.pdf.

Apolone, G., Ballatori, E., Mosconi, P. & Roila, F. (Ed. Pensiero Scientifico) (1997). *Misurare la qualità di vita in oncologia: aspetti di metodo ed applicativi.* Il Pensiero Scientifico Editore, Roma, Italy. ISBN: 8870027880.

Atluri, S. & Sudarshan, G. (2003). Evaluation of abnormal urine drug screens among patients with chronic non-malignant pain treated with opioids. *Pain Physician.* Vol. 6, No. 4, (October), pp. 407-409.

Back, S.E., Payne, R.A., Waldrop, A.E., Smith, A., Reeves, S. & Brady, K.T. (2009). Prescription opioid aberrant behaviors: a pilot study of sex differences. *Clinical Journal of Pain.* Vol. 25, No. 6, (July-August), pp: 477-484.

Bair, M.J., Robinson, R.L., Katon, W. & Kroenke, K. (2003). Depression and pain comorbidity: a literature review. *Archives of Internal Medicine.* Vol. 163, No. 20, (November), pp. 2433-2445.

Ballantyne, J. (2007). Opioid analgesia : perspectives on right use and utility. *Pain Physician*, Vol. 10, No. 3, (May), pp. 479-491.

Ballantyne, J.C. & Shin, N.S. (2008). Efficacy of opioids for chronic pain: a review of the evidence. *Clinical Journal of Pain, Vol.* 24, No. 6, (July-August), pp. 469-478.

Ballantyne, J.C. (2009). U.S. opioid risk management initiatives International Association for the Study of Pain (IASP), Vol. XVII, No. 6, (November). Last accessed June 2011, available from: http://www.iasp-pain.org/AM/AMTemplate.cfm?Section=HOME,HOME,HOME,HOME&SECTION=HOME,HOME,HOME,HOME&TEMPLATE=/CM/ContentDisplay.cfm&CONTENTID=10419

Banks, S.M. & Kerns, R.D. (1996). Explaining high rates of depression in chronic pain: a diathesis-stress framework. *Psychological Bulletin*. Vol 119, No. 1, (January), pp. 95-110.

Banta-Green, C.J., Merrill, J.O., Doyle, S.R., Boudreau, D.M. & Calsyn, D.A. (2009a). Opioid use behaviors, mental health and pain development of a typology of chronic pain patients. *Drug and Alcohol Dependence*. Vol. 104, No. 1-2, (September), pp. 34-42.

Banta-Green, C.J., Merrill, J.O., Doyle, S.R., Boudreau, D.M. & Calsyn, D.A. (2009b). Measurement of opioid problems among chronic pain patients in a general medical population. *Drug and Alcohol Dependence*. Vol. 104, No. 1-2, (September), pp. 43-49.

Beck, A. T., Steer, R. A., & Brown, G. K. (1996). *Manual for the Beck Depression Inventory,* 2nd ed. San Antonio, TX: The Psychological Corporation.

Belgrade, M. J., Schamber, D. & Lindgren, B. R. (2006). The DIRE Score: predicting outcomes of opioid prescribing for chronic pain. *The Journal of Pain,* Vol. 7, No. 9, (September), pp. 671-681.

Bertin, G., Niero, M. & Porchia, S. (1992). L'adattamento del Nottingham health profile al contesto italiano. In *The european group for quality of life and health measurement,* European guide to the Nottingham Health Profile, Escubase, Montpellier.

Bhamb, B., Brown, D. Anderson, J., Balousek, S. & Fleming, M.F. (2006). Survey of select practice behaviors by primary care physicians on the use of opioids for chronic pain. *Current Medical Research & Opinion*, Vol. 22, No. 9, (September), pp. 1859-65.

Boersma, K. & Linton, S.J. (2006). Psychological processes underlying the development of a chronic pain problem: a prospective study of the relationship between profiles of psychological variables in the fear-avoidance model and disability. *The Clinical Journal of Pain*. Vol. 22, No. 2, (February), pp. 160-166.

Bonica, J.J. (1991) History of pain concepts and pain therapy. *The Mount Sinai Journal of Medicine*, Vol. 53, No. 3, (May), pp. 191-202.

Bonica, J.J. (Ed. Delphino). (1992). *Il Dolore: Diagnosi, prognosi e terapia.* Antonio Deplhino, ISBN 978-887-2870-48-8, Roma, Italia.

Breivik, H., Collett, B., Ventafridda, V., Cohen, R. & Gallacher, D. (2006). Survey of chronic pain in Europe: prevalence, impact on daily life, and treatment. *European Journal of Pain*. Vol. 10, No. 4, (May), pp. 287-333.

Brennan, F., Carr, D.B. & Cousins, M. (2007). Pain management: a fundamental human right. *Anesthesia & Analgesia*. Vol. 105, No. 1, (July), pp. 205-221.

Brown, R.L. & Rounds, L.A. (1995). Conjoint screening questionnaires for alcohol and other drug abuse: criterion validity in a primary care practice. *Wisconsin Medical Journal*. Vol. 94, No. 3, pp.135-140.

Bruera, E., Schoeller,T., Wenk, R., MacEachern, T., Marcelino, S., Hanson, J. & Suarez-Almazor, M. (1995). A prospective multicenter assessment of the Edmonton staging system for cancer pain. *Journal of Pain and Symptom Management*. Vol. 10, No. 5, (July), pp. 348-355.

Buelow, A.K., Haggard, R. & Gatchel, R.J. (2009). Additional validation of the pain medication questionnaire in a heterogeneous sample of chronic pain patients. *Pain Practice*. Vol. 9, No. 6, (November-December), pp. 428-434.

Butler, S.F., Budman, S.H., Fernandez, K. & Jamison, R.N. (2004). Validation of a screener and opioid assessment measure for patients with chronic pain. *Pain*. Vol. 112, No. 1-2, (November), pp. 65-75.

Butler, S.F., Budman, S.H., Fernandez, K.C., Houle, B., Benoit, C., Katz, N. & Jamison, R.N. (2007). Development and validation of the Current Opioid Misuse Measure. *Pain*. Vol. 130, No. 1-2, (July), pp. 144-156.

Butler, S.F., Fernandez, K., Benoit, C., Budman, S.H. & Jamison, R.N. (2008). Validation of the revised Screener and Opioid Assessment for Patients with Pain (SOAPP-R). *The Journal of Pain*. Vol. 9, No. 4, (April), pp. 360-372.

Caudill-Slosberg, M.A., Schwartz, L.M. & Woloshin, S. (2004). Office visits and analgesic prescriptions for musculoskeletal pain in US: 1980 vs 2000. *Pain*, Vol. 109, No. 3, (June), pp. 514-19.

Centers for Disease Control and Prevention (2007). National and state medical expenditures and lost earnings attributable to arthritis and other rheumatic conditions - United States, 2003. *Morbidity and Mortality Weekly Report*. Vol. 56, No. 1, (January), pp. 4-7.

Chabal, C., Erjavec, M.K., Jacobson, L., Mariano, A. & Chaney, E. (1997). Prescription opiate abuse in chronic pain patients: clinical criteria, incidence, and predictors. *The Clinical Journal of Pain*. Vol. 13, No. 2, (June), pp. 150-155.

Chou, R. (2009). 2009 clinical guidelines from the American Pain Society and the American Academy of Pain Medicine on the use of chronic opioid therapy in chronic noncancer pain. What are the key messages for clinical practice?. *Polskie Archiwem Medycyny Wewnętrznej*, Vol. 119, No. 7-8, (July-August), pp. 469-477.

Chou, R., Ballantyne, J.C., Fanciullo, G.J., Fine, P.G. & Miaskowski, C. (2009c). Research gaps on use of opioids for chronic noncancer pain: findings from a review of the evidence for an American Pain Society and American Academy of Pain Medicine clinical practice guideline. *The Journal of Pain*, Vol. 10, No. 2, (February), pp. 147-159.

Chou, R., Fanciullo, G.J., Fine, P.G., Adler, J.A., Ballantyne, J.C., Davies, P., Donovan, M.I., Fishbain, D.A., Foley, K.M., Fudin, J., Gilson, A.M., Kelter, A., Mauskop, A., O'Connor, P.G., Passik, S.D., Pasternak, G.W., Portenoy, R.K., Rich, B.A., Roberts, R.G., Todd, K.H. & Miaskowski C. (2009a). American Pain Society-American Academy of Pain Medicine Opioids Guidelines Panel. Clinical guidelines for the use of chronic opioid therapy in chronic noncancer pain. *The Journal of Pain*, Vol. 10, No. 2, (February), pp.113-130.

Chou, R., Fanciullo, G.J., Fine, P.G., Miaskowski, C., Passik, S.D. & Portenoy, R.K. (2009b). Opioids for chronic noncancer pain: prediction and identification of aberrant drug-related behaviors: a review of the evidence for an American Pain Society and American Academy of Pain Medicine clinical practice guideline. *The Journal of Pain*, Vol. 10, No. 2, (February), pp. 131-146.

Collett, B.J. (1998). Opioid tolerance: the clinical perspective. *British Journal of Anaesthesia*. Vol. 81, No. 1, (July), pp. 58-68.

Compton, P., Darakjian, J. & Miotto, K. (1998). Screening for addiction in patients with chronic pain and problematic substance use: evaluation of a pilot assessment tool. *Journal of Pain and Symptom Management*, Vol. 16, No. 6, (December), pp. 355-363.

Compton, P.A., Wu, S.M., Schieffer, B., Pham, Q. & Naliboff, B.D. (2008). Introduction of a self-report version of the Prescription Drug Use Questionnaire and relationship to medication agreement noncompliance. *Journal of Pain and Symptom Management*. Vol. 36, No. 4, (October), pp. 383-395.

Dersh, J., Gatchel, R.J., Mayer, T., Polatin, P. & Temple, O.R. (2006). Prevalence of psychiatric disorders in patients with chronic disabling occupational spinal disorders. *Spine*. Vol. 1, No. 31, (May), pp. 1156-1162.

Dersh, J., Gatchel, R.J., Polatin, P. & Mayer, T. (2002). Prevalence of psychiatric disorders in patients with chronic work-related musculoskeletal pain disability. *Journal of Occupational and Environmental Medicine*. Vol. 44, No. 5, (May), pp. 459-468.

Dews, T.E., Mekhail, N. (2004). Safe use of opioids in chronic noncancer pain. *Cleveland Clinic Journal of Medicine*. Vol. 71, No. 11, (November), pp. 897-904.

Dillie, K.S., Fleming, M.F., Mundt, M.P. & French, M.T. (2008). Quality of life associated with daily opioid therapy in a primary care chronic pain sample. *Journal of the American Board of Family Medicine*. Vol. 21, No. 2, (March-April), pp.108-17.

Dowling, L.S., Gatchel, R.J., Adams, L.L., Stowell, A.W. & Bernstein D. (2007). An evaluation of the predictive validity of the Pain Medication Questionnaire with an heterogeneous group of patients with chronic pain. *Journal of Opioid Management*, Vol 3, No. 5, (September-October), pp. 257-266.

Dunbar, S.A. & Katz, N.P. (1996). Chronic opioid therapy for nonmalignant pain in patients with a history of substance abuse: report of 20 cases. *Journal of Pain and Symptom Management*. Vol. 11, No. 3, (March), pp. 163-171.

Edlund, M.J., Steffick, D., Hudson, T., Harris, K.M. & Sullivan, M. (2007). Risk factors for clinically recognized opioid abuse and dependence among veterans using opioids for chronic non-cancer pain. *Pain*. Vol. 129, No. 3, (June), pp. 355-362.

Elliott, A.M., Smith, B.H., Hannaford, P.C., Smith, W.C. & Chambers, W.A. (2002). The course of chronic pain in the community: results of a 4-year follow-up study. *Pain*. Vol. 99, No. 1-2, (September), pp. 299-307.

Ferrari, R., Fipaldini, E. & Birbaumer, N. (2004). La valutazione del controllo percepito sul dolore: la versione italiana del Pain Related self-Statement Scale e del Pain Related Control Scale. *Giornale Italiano di Psicologia*. Vol. 1, No. 1, (March), pp. 187-208. ISSN : 0390-5349.

Ferrari, R., Novara, C., Sanavio, E. & Zerbini, F. (2000). Internal structure and validity of the Multidimensional Pain Inventory, italian language version. *Pain Medicine*. Vol. 1, No. 2, (June), pp. 123-30.

Fishbain, D.A. (1999). Approaches to treatment decisions for psychiatric comorbidity in the management of the chronic pain patient. *The Medical Clinics of North America*. Vol. 83, No. 3, (May), pp. 737-760.

Fleming, M.F., Balousek, S.L., Klessig, C.L., Mundt, M.P. & Brown, D.D. (2007). Substance use disorders in a primary care sample receiving daily opioid therapy. *Journal of Pain*, Vol. 8, No. 7, (July), pp. 573-582.

Flor, H., Turk, D.C. (1988). Chronic back pain and rheumatoid arthritis: predicting pain and disability from cognitive variables. *Journal of Behavioral Medicine*. Vol. 11, No. 3, (June), pp. 251-265.

Friedman, R., Li, V. & Mehrotra, D. (2003). Treating pain patients at risk: evaluation of a screening tool in opioid-treated pain patients with and without addiction. *Pain Medicine*. Vol. 4, No. 2, (June), pp. 182-185.

Garcia, J. & Altman, R.D. (1997). Chronic pain states: pathophysiology and medical therapy. *Seminars in Arthritis and Rheumatism*, Vol. 27, No. 1, (August), pp. 1–16.

Gatchel, R.J. (Ed. American Psychological Association) (2005). *Clinical essentials of pain management*. APA Press. Washington DC. ISBN: 1591471532

Ghisi, M., Flebus, G.B., Montano, A., Sanavio, E. & Sica, C. (Ed. Giunti Organizzazioni Speciali) (2006). *Beck Depression Inventory – second edition. Adattamento italiano: manuale*. Giunti O.S., pp. 1-79, Firenze, Italy.

Gureje, O., Von Korff, M., Simon, G.E. & Gater, R. (1998). Persistent pain and well-being: A World Health Organization study in primary care. *The Journal of the American Medical Association*. Vol. 280, No. 2, (July), pp. 147-151.

Haller, D.L. & Acosta, M.C. (2010). Characteristics of pain patients with opioid-use disorder. *Psychosomatics*. Vol. 51, No. 3, (May), pp. 257-66.

Hathaway, S.R. & McKinley, J.C. (1989). *MMPI-2: Manual for administration and scoring*, University of Minnesota Press, Minneapolis, MN

Heit, H.A. & Gourlay, D.L. (2004). Urine drug testing in pain medicine. *Journal of Pain and Symptom Management*. Vol., 27, No. 3, (March), pp. 260-267.

Højsted, J. & Sjøgren, P. (2007). Addiction to opioids in chronic pain patients: A literature review. *European Journal of Pain*, Vol. 11, No. 5, (July), pp. 490- 518.

Holmes, C.P., Gatchel, R.J., Adams, L.L., Stowell, A.W., Hatten, A., Noe, C. & Lou, L. (2006). An opioid screening instrument: long-term evaluation of the utility of the Pain Medication Questionnaire. *Pain Practice*. Vol. 6, No. 2, (June), pp. 74-88.

Hunt, S. M., McEwan, J. & McKenna, S. P. (1985). Measuring health status: a new tool for clinicians and epidemiologists. *Journal of the Royal College of General Practitioner*. Vol. 35, No. 273, (April), pp. 185-188.

Ives, T.J., Chelminski, P.R., Hammett-Stabler, C.A., Malone, R.M., Perhac, J.S., Potisek, N.M., Shilliday, B.B., DeWalt, D.A. & Pignone, M.P. (2006). Predictors of opioid misuse in patients with chronic pain: a prospective cohort study. *BMC Health Services Research*. Vol. 4, No. 6, (April), pp: 6:46.

Kalso, E., Allan, L., Dellemijn, P.L., Faura, C.C., Ilias, W.K., Jensen, T.S., Perrot, S., Plaghki, L.H. & Zenz, M. (2003). Recommendations for using opioids in chronic non-cancer pain. *European Journal of Pain*, Vol 7, No. 5, pp. 381-6.

Katz, N.P., Sherburne, S., Beach, M., Rose, R.J., Vielguth, J., Bradley, J. & Fanciullo, G.J. (2003). Behavioral monitoring and urine toxicology testing in patients receiving long-term opioid therapy. *Anesthesia and Analgesia*. Vol. 97, No. 4, (October), pp. 1097-1102.

Kerns, R.D., Turk, D.C. & Rudy, T.E. (1985). The West Haven-Yale Multidimensional Pain Inventory (WHYMPI). *Pain*. Vol. 23, No. 4, (December), pp. 345-356.

Linton, S.J., Hellsing, A.L. & Hallden, K. (1998). A population based study of spinal pain among 35-45-year old individuals. *Spine*. Vol. 23, No. 13, (July), pp. 1457-1463.

Loeser, J.D. & Melzack, R. (1999). Pain: an overview. *Lancet*, Vol. 8, No. 352, (May), pp. 1607-1609.

Loeser, J.D. (2000). Pain and suffering. *The Clinical Journal of Pain*, Vol. 16, No. 2, (June), pp. 2-6.

Luo, X., Pietrobon, R., Sun, S.X., Liu, G.G. & Hey, L. (2004). Estimates and patterns of direct health care expenditures among individuals with back pain in the United States. *Spine*. Vol. 29, No. 1, (January), pp. 79-86.

Maiani, G. & Sanavio, E. (1985). Semantics of pain in Italy: the Italian version of the McGill Pain Questionnaire. *Pain*. Vol. 22, No. 4, (August), pp. 399-405.

Manchikanti, L., Benyamin, R., Datta, S., Vallejo, R. & Smith, H. (2010). Opioids in chronic noncancer pain. *Expert Review of Neurotherapeutics*. Vol. 10, No. 5, (May), pp. 775-789, ISSN 1473-7175.

Manchikanti, L., Cash, K.A., Damron, K.S., Manchukonda, R., Pampati, V. & McManus, C.D. (2006). Controlled substance abuse and illicit drug use in chronic pain patients: an evaluation of multiple variables. *Pain Physician*. Vol. 9, No. 3, (July), pp: 215-225.

Manchikanti, L., Manchukonda, R., Pampati, V. & Damron, K.S. (2005). Evaluation of abuse of prescription and illicit drugs in chronic pain patients receiving short-acting (hydrocodone) or long-acting (methadone) opioids. *Pain Physician*. Vol. 8, No. 3, (July), pp. 257-261.

Manchikanti, L., Pampati, V., Damron, K.S., Fellows, B., Barnhill, R.C. & Beyer, C.D. (2001). Prevalence of opioid abuse in interventional pain medicine practice settings: a randomized clinical evaluation. *Pain Physician*. Vol. 4, No. 4, (October), pp. 358-365, ISSN 1533-3159.

Maniadakis, N. & Gray, A. (2000). The economic burden of back pain in the UK. *Pain*. Vol. 84, No. 1, (January), pp. 95-103.

Mannion, R.J. & Woolf, C.J. (2000) Pain mechanisms and management: a central perspective. *Clinical Journal of Pain*, Vol. 16 Supplement, pp. 144-156.

Melzack R. (Raven Press) (1983). *The McGill Pain Questionnaire*. In: Pain Measurement and Assessment. Raven Press, pp. 41-48, New York, USA.

Merskey, H. & Bogduk, N. (Ed.s Merskey & Bogduk) (1994). *Classification of Chronic Pain: descriptions of chronic pain syndromes and definitions of pain terms, II edition*. IASP press, Seattle, USA, ISBN 978-0931092053

Merskey, H. (1986a). Classification of chronic pain. Descriptions of chronic pain syndromes and definitions of pain terms. Prepared by the International Association for the Study of Pain, Subcommittee on Taxonomy. *Pain*, Suppl. 3, pp. 1-226

Merskey, H. (1986b). Variable meanings for the definitions of disease. *Journal of Medicine and Philosophy*, Vol. 11, No. 3, (August), pp. 215-232.

Michna, E., Ross, E.L., Hynes, W.L., Nedeljkovic, S.S., Soumekh, S., Janfaza, D., Palombi, D. & Jamison, R.N. (2004). Predicting aberrant drug behavior in patients treated for chronic pain: importance of abuse history. *Journal of Pain and Symptom Management*. Vol. 28, No. 3, (September), pp. 250-258.

Moore, T.M., Jones, T., Browder, J.H., Daffron, S. & Passik, S.D. (2009). A comparison of common screening methods for predicting aberrant drug-related behavior among patients receiving opioids for chronic pain management. *Pain Medicine*. Vol. 10, No. 8, (November), pp. 1426-1433.

Noble, M., Treadwell, J.R., Tregear, S.J., Coates, V.H., Wiffen, P.J., Akafomo, C. & Schoelles, K.M. (2010). Long-term opioid management for chronic noncancer pain. *Cochrane Database of Systematic Reviews*. Vol. 20, No. 1, (January), pp. 214-228.

Office of Applied Studies, Substance Abuse and Mental Health Services Administration (SAMHSA). (2009). *Trends in Nonmedical Use of Prescription Pain Relievers: 2002 to 2007*. Last accessed June 2011, Available from: http://oas.samhsa.gov/2k9/painRelievers/nonmedicalTrends.pdf.

Office of Applied Studies, Substance Abuse and Mental Health Services Administration (SAMHSA). (2008). *Results from the 2007 National Survey on Drug Use and Health: National findings*. Last accessed June 2011, Available from: http://oas.samhsa.gov/p0000016.htm.

Pancheri, P., Sirigatti, S., & Biondi, M. (1996). *Adaptation of the MMPI-2 in Italy*. In J. N. Butcher (Ed.), International adaptations of the MMPI-2: Research and clinical applications (pp. 416-441). Minneapolis, MN: University of Minnesota Press.

Passik, S.D. (2009). Issues in long-term opioid therapy: unmet needs, risks, and solutions. *Mayo Clinic Proceedings*. Vol. 84, No. 7, (July), pp. 593-601

Passik, S.D., Kirsh, K,L,, Whitcomb, L., Portenoy, R.K., Katz, N.P., Kleinman, L., Dodd, S.L. & Schein, J.R. (2004). A new tool to assess and document pain outcomes in chronic pain patients receiving opioid therapy. *Clinical Therapeutics*. Vol. 26, No. 4, (April), pp. 552-561.

Passik, S.D., Kirsh, K.L., Donaghy, K.B. & Portenoy, R.K. (2006). Pain and aberrant drug-related behaviours in medically ill patients with and without histories of substance abuse. *The Clinical Journal of Pain*. Vol. 22, No. 2, (February), pp. 173-181.

Passik, S.D., Kirsh, K.L., Whitcomb, L., Schein, J.R., Kaplan, M.A., Dodd, S.L., Kleinman, L., Katz, N.P. & Portenoy, R.K. (2005). Monitoring outcomes during long-term opioid therapy for noncancer pain: results with the Pain Assessment and Documentation Tool. *Journal of Opioid Management*. Vol. 1, No. 5, (November-December), pp. 257-266.

Pedrabissi, L. & Santinello, M. (Ed. Giunti Organizzazioni Speciali) (1996). STAI, State-Trait Anxiety Inventory, Forma Y: Manuale. Giunti OS, Firenze, Italy.

Portenoy, R.K. (1996) Opioid therapy for chronic nonmalignant pain: a review of the critical issues. *Journal of Pain and Symptom Management*. Vol. 11, No. 4, (April), pp. 203-217.

Portenoy, R.K. (2000). Current pharmacotherapy of chronic pain. *Journal of Pain and Symptom Management*. Vol. 19, No. 1 Suppl., (January), pp. 16-20.

Portenoy, R.K. (2004) Appropriate use of opioids for persistent non-cancer pain. *Lancet*. Vol. 364, No. 9436, (August-September), pp. 739-740.

Rosenblum, A., Marsch, L.A., Joseph, H. & Portenoy R.K. (2008). Opioids and the treatment of chronic pain: controversies, current status, and future directions. *Experimental and Clinical Psychopharmacology*.Vol. 16, No. 5, (October), pp. 405–416.

Savage S.R. (1993). Addiction in the treatment of pain: significance, recognition, and management. *Journal of Pain Symptom Management*. Vol. 8, No. 5, (July), pp. 265-278.

Savage S.R. (2002). Assessment for addiction in pain-treatment settings. *Clinical Journal of Pain*. Vol. 18, No. 4 Suppl, (July-August), pp: 28-38.

Schieffer, B.M., Pham, Q., Labus, J., Baria, A., Van Vort, W., Davis, P., Davis, F. & Naliboff, B.D. (2005). Pain medication beliefs and medication misuse in chronic pain. *The Journal of Pain*. Vol. 6, No. 9, (September), pp. 620-629.

Spielberger, C.D (Ed. Mind Garden) (1983). *State-Trait Anxiety Inventory for adults*. Mind Garden, Palo Alto, CA, USA.

Sullivan, M.D., Edlund, M.J., Zhang, L., Unützer, J. & Wells, K.B. (2006). Association between mental health disorders, problem drug use, and regular prescription opioid use. *Archives of Internal Medicine*. Vol. 166, No. 19, (October), pp. 2087-2093.

Trescot, A.M., Boswell, M.V., Atluri, S.L., Hansen, H.C., Deer, T.R., Abdi, S., Jasper, J.F., Singh, V., Jordan, A.E., Johnson, B.W., Cicala, R.S., Dunbar, E.E., Helm, S., Varley, K.G., Suchdev, P.K., Swicegood, J.R., Calodney, A.K., Ogoke, B.A., Minore, W.S. & Manchikanti, L. (2006). Opioid guidelines in the management of chronic non-cancer pain. *Pain Physician*, Vol. 9, No. 1, (January), pp. 1-39.

Trescot, A.M., Helm, S., Hansen, H., Benyamin, R., Glaser, S.E., Adlaka, R., Patel, S. & Manchikanti, L. (2008). Opioids in the management of chronic non-cancer pain: an update of American Society of the Interventional Pain Physicians (ASIPP) guidelines. *Pain Physician*, Vol. 11, No. 2 Suppl., (March), pp. 5-62.

Turk, D. & Okifuji, A. (2002). Psychological factors in chronic pain: evolution and revolution. *Journal of Consulting and Clinical Psychology*. Vol. 70, No. 3, (June), pp. 678-690.

van Leeuwen, M.T., Blyth, F.M., March, L.M., Nicholas, M.K. & Cousins, M.J. (2006). Chronic pain and reduced work effectiveness: the hidden cost to Australian employers. *European Journal of Pain*. Vol. 10, No. 2 (February), pp. 161-66.

Verhaak, P.F., Kerssens, J.J., Dekker, J., Sorbi, M.J. & Bensing, J.M (1998). Prevalence of chronic benign pain disorder among adults: a review of the literature. *Pain*. Vol. 77, No. 3, (September), pp. 231-239.

Vlaeyen, J.W. & Linton, S.J. (2000). Fear-avoidance and its consequences in chronic musculoskeletal pain: a state of the art. *Pain*. Vol. 85, No. 3, (April), pp. 317-332.

Wasan, A.D., Butler, S.F., Budman, S.H., Benoit, C., Fernandez, K. & Jamison, R.N. (2007). Psychiatric history and psychologic adjustment as risk factors for aberrant drug-related behaviour among patients with chronic pain. *Clinical Journal of Pain*. Vol. 23, No. 4, (May), pp. 307-315.

Webster, L. R. & Webster, R. M. (2005). Predicting aberrant behaviors in opioid-treated patients: preliminary validation of the Opioid Risk Tool. *Pain Medicine*, Vol. 6, No. 6, (November-December), pp. 432-442.

White, W., Ernest Kurtz, M.A., & Acker, C. (2001a). *Combined Addiction Disease Chronologies*. Last accessed June 2011, available from: http://silkworth.net/kurtz/Kurtz-1864-1879-OCR.pdf.

White, W., Ernest Kurtz, M.A., & Acker, C. (2001b). *Combined Addiction Disease Chronologies*. Last accessed June 2011, available from: http://silkworth.net/kurtz/Kurtz-1900-1919-OCR.pdf.

Winkelmann, A., Perrot, S., Schaefer, C., Ryan, K., Chandran, A., Sadosky, A. & Zlateva, G. (2011). Impact of fibromyalgia severity on health economic costs: results from a European cross-sectional study. *Applied Health Economics and Health Policy*. Vol. 9, No. 2, (March), pp. 125-136.

World Health Organization (1990). Cancer pain relief and palliative care: report of a WHO expert committee. *Technical Report Series 804*. Geneva, Switzerland.

World Health Organization (1998). The use of essential drugs: report of a WHO Expert Committee. *Technical Report Series No. 882*, Geneva, Switzerland.

World Health Organization (1986). Cancer pain relief, Geneva, Switzerland.

World Health Organization. (2002). Achieving balance in national opioids control policy: guidelines for assessment. Geneva, Switzerland.

Wu, S., Compton, P., Bolus, R., Schieffer, B., Pham, Q., Baria, A., Van Vort, W., Davis, F., Shekelle, P. & Naliboff, B. (2006). The Addiction Behaviors Checklist: validation of a new clinician based measure of inappropriate opioid use in chronic pain. *Journal of Pain and Symptom Management*, Vol. 32, No. 4, (October), pp. 342-351.

Yelin, E., Cisternas, M.G., Pasta, D.J., Trupin, L., Murphy, L. & Helmick, C.G. (2004). Medical care expenditures and earnings losses of persons with arthritis and other rheumatic conditions in the United States in 1997: total and incremental estimates. *Arthritis and Rheumatisms*. Vol. 50, No. 7, (July), pp. 2317-2326.

Yudko, E., Lozhkina, O. & Fouts, A. (2007). A comprehensive review of the psychometric properties of the Drug Abuse Screening Test. *Journal of Substance Abuse Treatment*. Vol. 32, No. 2, (March), pp. 189-198.

21

Psychological Strategies in Pain Management: Optimizing Procedures in Clinics

FuZhou Wang
Department of Anesthesiology and Critical Care Medicine,
The Affiliated Nanjing Maternity and Child Health Care Hospital,
Nanjing Medical University, Nanjing,
China

1. Introduction

Pain is the most awful sensory suffering that makes people exhausted. Although pain itself possesses protective role in keeping patients from further injury, it is still obliged to be treated for its negative effect on patients' physiological and psychological well-beings. Great progress has been made in our understanding of the therapeutic strategies with different agents and techniques on pain in the past decades, but the analgesic result is not as effective as we desired specifically when the acute process tends to be chronic (Li et al., 2011). As one of the important parts of somatosensory system, pain nets closely with spiritual and psychological feelings, which often results in analgesic failure when conventional pharmacological methods and means are used, and also raises questions on how to alleviate pain through psychotherapeutics (Manchikanti et al., 2011). Given the big difference in methods of psychological interventions and the association with the changing therapeutic context, the analgesic efficacy of psychosocial support fluctuates. Therefore, standardizing and optimizing the psychotherapeutic strategies in clinical practice would make it more effective in relieving pain. Here we review and prospect the psychological management of pain, and then give a recommendation of the therapeutic flow of the standardized optimal procedures.

2. Origins of psychological analgesia

Two hundreds years ago, the word "placebo" was defined by Robert Hooper in his dictionary to a more modern medical meaning as "any medicine adapted more to please than benefit the patient" (Hooper, 1811). In fact, this is the original description of psychological intervention in the field of medicine of which the meaning is broadened further during the following years. However, placebo therapies were becoming popular until the past century. To date, placebo medicine generally means (i) containing pharmacologically inactive ingredients, and (ii) the contents have pharmacological activity. The effect of placebo is mainly dependent on the psychological state of patients, therapeutic context and physicians' console. In contrast to placebo, nocebo was adapted to describe the negative effect (i.e. unpleasant consequence) occurs in expectation of a harmful occurrence when an inert substance was used. In pain medicine, both placebo and nocebo are also two majorities that can be used in psychological intervention. Therefore, psychological placebo (positive) or psychological nocebo (negative) are derived from the traditional conceptions of placebo or nocebo. Although the key patterns of psychological therapy is on the basis of the linguistic console from physicians or investigators, psychological analgesia with series of strategies of psychology is the result of the above-mentioned placebo or nocebo.

3. Mechanisms of psychological analgesia

Psychological analgesia is a broad concept that includes all aspects referring to the psychological intervention. Hypnosis, music therapy, preoperative education, and linguistic suggestion all belong to psychological approaches in pain control (Hobson et al., 2006; Patterson et al., 2010; Sen et al., 2010; Wang et al., 2008). Whatever psychological methods used in analgesia, common neurophysiological mechanisms exist and different models explain its function.

Functional magnetic resonance imaging (fMRI) verified an increase in neural activity during placebo associated psychological stimulation that is related to two major pain modulation mechanisms (Craggs et al., 2008): i) affective regulation which includes activation of the rostral anterior cingulate cortex, bilateral amygdala, and medial prefrontal cortex; and ii) higher cognitive regulation during which the posterior cingulate, pre-cuneus, rostral anterior cingulate cortex, perihippocampal gyrus, and the temporal lobes are activated. As the "gate theory" described that afferent inhibition blocks ascending signals from the periphery, psychological stimuli at the early period produce analgesic effect through a self-reinforcing feedback mechanism (Vase et al., 2005).

Several models give an in-depth understanding of the psychological stimulation associated analgesia. Conditioning, expectancy, motivation, and emotion are four psychological mediators involving in the process of analgesia. Conditioning model says that the interventional effect presented when the individual without knowing the stimulation would be and this process would not produce cognition (Williams & Rhudy, 2007). In this model, the perception of pain after psychological treatment largely depends on the learning history of the individual which determines the response variability under different context. The psychological conditioning as well as the verbal suggestion can turn tactile stimuli into pain and low-intensity pain into high-intensity pain. For this, the direct evidence was the conditioned pain reduction could be absolutely removed when the psychological stimuli were explained (Montgomery & Kirsch, 1997). Originally, conditioning is the primary response to psychological analgesia. Following conditioning, expectancy of the psychological stimuli to produce an effective analgesia takes place. Once the patients expect to have an improvement in pain management, the effect of psychological analgesia would play its role. Due to anxiety and fear to pain, patients generally want to have rapid and effective methods that can relieve their pain (Cornally & McCarthy, 2011; den Hollander et al., 2010; Kennedy et al., 2011), which consequently leads to an expectancy of their pain therapies. Under this condition, physicians' attitude and enthusiasm takes an important part in whether or not the psychological analgesia comes into play (Weintraub, 2005). Give patients the hope to conquer pain accompanying with a warmth care, the expected effect of psychological analgesia would be maximized. After expectancy, motivation of analgesia is another aspect in determining the effect of psychological interventions. If the patient desires for a relief of pain, the real analgesic role of psychological stimuli would be magnitude (Radat & Koleck, 2011). The motivation itself whether or not could predict the psychological effect on one type of pain needs to be explored at length, and could it be effective for different types of pain is also yet to be guaranteed. A body of literature has confirmed the role of emotions in pain perception and alleviation. Anxiety and stress are two main factors of emotion-associated psychological mediator. It is believed that anxiety is the cause of increased levels of pain, and reduction in anxiety produces analgesia (Luciano et al., 2011). Stress sometimes is related with increased levels of pain, but in some contexts, stress can produce analgesia (Donello et al., 2011; Wang et al., 2008). Therefore, the purpose of psychological suggestion in pain control is to alleviate patients' anxiety and stress, which in turn produces a feedback analgesia effect.

As described in the general model of the placebo-associated psychological analgesia, three consecutive stages exist when psychological treatment was given: the induction, psychophysiological mediation, and actualization (Goffaux et al., 2010). In the induction stage, three aspects compose the major contents including the introduction or initiation (therapeutic message; method of administration; follow-up and booster sessions; assessment of side effects), idiosyncratic variables (beliefs and values; personal history; innate predisposition) and therapeutic context (treatment objectives; therapeutic alliance; sociocultural factors). In the second stage, psychophysiological mediation composes of psychological and biological mechanisms. Psychological mechanisms include above-mentioned conditioning, expectancy, motivation, and emotion, and the biological mechanisms include neurochemical mediators (endorphins, dopamine, and other neurotransmitters/neuromodulators) and neurophysiology (activation of central modulatory mechanisms including descending inhibitory circuits). In the actualization stage, three main aspects exist including subjective experience (pain, emotions, quality of life, satisfaction, and related relief), behavioral markers (amount of analgesics consumed and overt pain behaviors), and physiological markers (physiological nociceptive activity, objective clinical indicators). As thus, when a psychological intervention is given, these three stages would be experienced. However, in consideration of the multiple phases of these stages, the actual effect of psychological analgesia may be variable in different individuals under different circumstances.

4. Efficacy of psychological analgesia

The analgesic effect of psychological approaches depends on types of pain, individual status, caregivers' attitude and contextual frame, which finally determines the efficacy of psychological analgesia. For postoperative pain, preoperative hypnosis could accelerate wound healing and alleviate pain intensity after mammoplasty (Ginandes et al., 2003), and reduce post-surgical pain and distress in patients undergone excisional breast biopsy (Schnur et al., 2008). However, in other surgical contexts, psychological interventions did not produce detectable difference compared with the control: relaxation training for spinal surgeries could not reduce postoperative pain (Gavin et al., 2006), and intraoperative music therapy also could not produce analgesia in Cesarean patients (Reza et al., 2007). Contrary to this, postoperative music can alleviate the pain and reduce the need for analgesics in patients who undergone Cesarean section (Ebneshahidi & Mohseni, 2008). Besides, in cardiac surgeries, music therapy produced effective role in alleviating anxiety and pain (Sendelbach et al., 2006). These different even controversial results raise questions on the real analgesia efficacy of psychological interventions. In fact, difference in interventional methods, types of surgeries, and professionals of investigators may all contribute to the changeable results of psychological analgesia. An attractive study performed to observe the influence of linguistic suggestion on postoperative pain management after abdominal surgeries, and found that negative words from nursing professionals results in therapeutic failure of patient-controlled analgesia, and suggested that a trusting psychological relationship between medical caregivers and patients should be established (Wang et al., 2008). Therefore, it is necessary to seek a standardized effective psychological method that can be employed at any time to alleviate pain and pain-associated psychological contributors.

Chronic pain, due to its multi-original property and hypo-responsiveness to traditional analgesics, is a complex pathological condition that needs to be cared with specific concentration. How to predict psychological problems in patients with chronic pain and then to take steps to overcome them plays pivotal role in alleviating this kind of pain. Modified Somatic Perception, Zung Questionnaires and Catastrophizing Scale are major means in predicting possible psychological factors in patients with chronic pain (Mannion et al., 1996; Meyer et al., 2008). These tools can help to identify psychological problems at early period that is crucial for understanding the development of acute pain into chronic and also possibly preventing its chronicity. Several studies considered psychological factors are contributors to patients' chronicity, but others did not find such a relationship (Roth et al., 2011a; Roth et al., 2011b; Roth et al., 2011c; Wallin et al., 2011; Xu et al., 2011). Various results in different studies questioned the real analgesic effect of psychological approaches in chronic pain management. Also, seek an optimized psychological procedure in chronic pain management is necessary for pain physicians.

5. Optimizing psychological analgesic procedure

Difference in methods of psychological interventions makes it difficult to reach a standardized uniform procedure that could be used for each individual at different pathological conditions. No matter what kind of methods employed, following four aspects are constant and also can be the interventional entry points: types of pain, individual expectancy status, therapeutic context, and professional level of physicians. Therefore, standardized psychological approach in analgesia should be based on these four factors. Besides, an optimized interventional flow of psychological analgesia from induction to performance to completion also will be standardized.

How to standardize the types of pain is so difficult because of its property of multiple originalities plus difference in its duration, intensity and responsiveness to pharmacological analgesics. To have a clear description and avoid an extra complexity of the standardization of the psychological procedure in the types of pain, here two major types of pain, acute and chronic, are discussed. First, acute pain is relatively easier to treat and generally resulted from traceable causes. So herein the acute pain is standardized on the basis of postoperative pain: surgical procedures → tissue injury → afferent fibers activation → dorsal root ganglion → spinal cord dorsal horn → ascending modulatory tracts → hypothalamus → cerebral cortex. However, chronic pain is refractory to pharmacological treatments and without assured causes. Here the standardization is based on chronic low back pain: regional chronic injury → persistent activation of peripheral fibers → spinal sensitization → reduction in pain threshold → activation of multiple brain regions. Although acute pain and chronic pain have different transduction pathways, they finally reach brain and then the perception is occur. This is the basis of the standardization when it is treated with psychological approaches.

Individual expectancy status is the second factor that needs to be standardized. Every one expects to have an effective method that can conquer the pain because of the unpleasant experience. Once a patient has such a hope, the psychological analgesia would play its role. However the psychological complexity makes people doubt the real efficacy of the analgesia. Therefore, give a timely psychological intervention along with patients' expectancy is the best way for analgesia through matching their different time windows. Under this condition, careful assessment of patients' psychological status with proper means would give physicians more information on what, how and when a psychological stimulation could be employed. In fact, psychological intervention if given appropriately at this moment exactly fills patients' psychological gap. If want take effective steps to control the pain, time communication with patients is the guarantee. So, the following flow is recommended: talk to confirm the expectancy → predisposition for psychological intervention → psychological preparation → increase confidence of conquering.

Therapeutic context is the environment where the patients go and seek for pain management. Whether clinics could provide proper and humanistic care or not determines the final conclusion of psychological analgesia. Due to big difference in the contextual background, it is hard to standardize the consulting environment. Here just give a proposal that should at least be followed when administering psychological interventions for pain control: i) avoiding negative stimuli; ii) establishing a warm setting; iii) patient-centered communication; iv) one-stop services. A trusting relationship between medical environment and patients could pave the way to a successful analgesia with psychological approaches.

Professional level of physician is the "software" that needs to be updated step by step and improved gradually with practice. Of course, personal morality is another crucial part that can give patients the "be-taken-seriously" feeling. Further, if the physician trained in psychological treatment, such professional knowledge in psychology would make the psychological analgesia more effective, and would produce the best efficacy in alleviating pain. This section, in fact, is the easiest one that can be improved after training and practice. Following is the suggestion on how to get better results in psychological analgesia: i) take patients' claim into heart; ii) build friend relationship with patients; iii) serve with the best professional knowledge; iv) psycho-language communication; v) unchangeable attitude and performance.

The changing window of man's mind is wide, and it is so easy to change when each above-mentioned part cannot satisfy the expectancy. Besides, the prone-to-be-broken psychological state would be shattered by improper intervention. Therefore, patients with different types of pain have various expectancy of analgesia that needs to be treated with optimal psychological procedures even at different clinics.

When performing psychological analgesia, following three-step procedure should be referred to. First step, induction: i) communicate without hint of psychological intervention; ii) confirm patient's psychological state; iii) predict patient's expectancy; iv) increase confidence that is bound to succeed. After this, the next step should be followed without interruption, i.e. performance: i) select a relatively quiet environment; ii) build a kind talking ambient; iii) give personalized linguistic intervention; iv) choose an interesting topic; v) talk without constraint; vi) observe psychological change during talking; vii) fine regulation in communication strategies. Following these procedures, the whole process of psychological intervention needs to be finalized, namely completion: i) conclude what have been talked; ii) thank patient's patience; iii) assess pain intensity with appropriate tools. Application of psychological linguistic suggestion should not be similar for one person at different visits, and the communicating environment should be changed time after time. The schematic flow of psychological intervention is presented in the Figure 1.

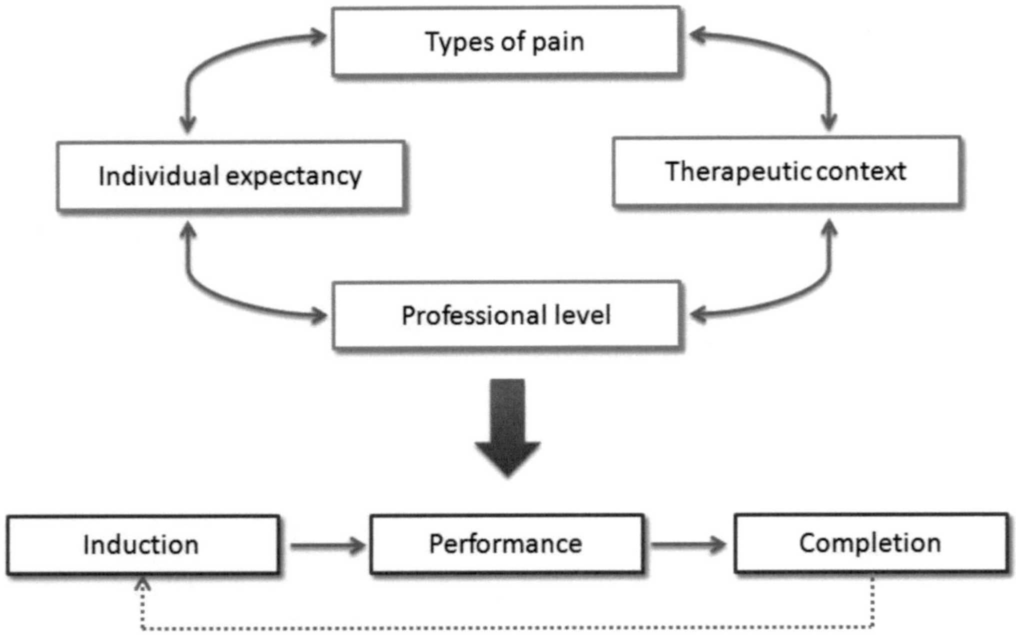

Fig. 1. Schematic flow of psychological analgesia.

6. Concluding remarks

Psychological activity is a complex emotional response that can be influenced by many factors. Psychological analgesia itself, however, is so complex that its efficacy is uncertain for different types of pain at different conditions. Therefore, how to select interventional methods and how to perform them for different patients with various psychological states is a thorny problem. Although here the optimized procedure of psychological analgesia is presented, it is necessary to be changed for different patients under different contextual conditions. Also this recommendation should favor the improvement of psychological intervention in pain management in future work.

7. References

Cornally, N. & McCarthy, G. (2011) Help-seeking behaviour for the treatment of chronic pain. *Br J Community Nurs* 16(2): 90-98.

Craggs, J.G.; Price, D.D.; Perlstein, W.M.; Verne, G.N. & Robinson, M.E. (2008) The dynamic mechanisms of placebo induced analgesia: Evidence of sustained and transient regional involvement. *Pain* 139(3): 660-669.

den Hollander, M.; de Jong, J.R.; Volders, S.; Goossens, M.E.; Smeets, R.J. & Vlaeyen, J.W. (2010) Fear reduction in patients with chronic pain: a learning theory perspective. *Expert Rev Neurother* 10(11): 1733-1745.

Donello, J.E.; Guan, Y.; Tian, M.; Cheevers, C.V.; Alcantara, M.; Cabrera, S.; Raja, S.N. & Gil, D.W. (2011) A peripheral adrenoceptor-mediated sympathetic mechanism can transform stress-induced analgesia into hyperalgesia. *Anesthesiology* 114(6): 1403-1416.

Ebneshahidi, A. & Mohseni, M. (2008) The effect of patient-selected music on early postoperative pain, anxiety, and hemodynamic profile in cesarean section surgery. *J Altern Complement Med* 14(7): 827-831.

Gavin, M.; Litt, M.; Khan, A.; Onyiuke, H. & Kozol, R. (2006) A prospective, randomized trial of cognitive intervention for postoperative pain. *Am Surg* 72(5): 414-418.

Ginandes, C.; Brooks, P.; Sando, W.; Jones, C. & Aker, J. (2003) Can medical hypnosis accelerate post-surgical wound healing? Results of a clinical trial. *Am J Clin Hypn* 45(4): 333-351.

Goffaux, P.; Léonard, G.; Marchand, S. & Rainville, P. (2010) Placebo analgesia. In: Beaulieu, P., Lussier, D., Porreca, F., Dickenson, A.H. (eds). *Pharmacology of Pain*. IASP Press, Seattle, pp. 451-473.

Hobson, J.A.; Slade, P.; Wrench, I.J. & Power, L. (2006) Preoperative anxiety and postoperative satisfaction in women undergoing elective caesarean section. *Int J Obstet Anesth* 15(1): 18-23.

Hooper, R. (1811) Quincy's Lexicon-Medicum. *A New Medical Dictionary*. London.

Kennedy, C.E.; Moore, P.J.; Peterson, R.A.; Katzman, M.A.; Vermani, M. & Charmak, W.D. (2011) What makes people anxious about pain? How personality and perception combine to determine pain anxiety responses in clinical and non-clinical populations. *Anxiety Stress Coping* 24(2): 179-200.

Li, A.; Montaño, Z.; Chen, V.J. & Gold, J.I. (2011) Virtual reality and pain management: current trends and future directions. *Pain Manag* 1(2): 147-157.

Luciano, J.V.; Martínez, N.; Peñarrubia-María, M.T.; Fernández-Vergel, R.; García-Campayo, J.; Verduras, C.; Blanco, M.E.; Jiménez, M.; Ruiz, J.M.; López del Hoyo, Y.; Serrano-Blanco, A. & FibroQoL Study Group. (2011) Effectiveness of a psychoeducational treatment program implemented in general practice for fibromyalgia patients: a randomized controlled trial. *Clin J Pain* 27(5): 383-391.

Manchikanti, L.; Giordano, J.; Fellows, B. & Hirsch, J.A. (2011) Placebo and nocebo in interventional pain management: a friend or a foe-or simply foes? *Pain Physician* 14(2): E157-E175.

Mannion, A.F.; Dolan, P. & Adams, M.A. (1996) Psychological questionnaires: do "abnormal" scores precede or follow first-time low back pain? *Spine (Phila Pa 1976)* 21(22): 2603-2611.

Meyer, K.; Sprott, H. & Mannion, A.F. (2008) Cross-cultural adaptation, reliability, and validity of the German version of the Pain Catastrophizing Scale. *J Psychosom Res* 64(5): 469-478.

Montgomery, G.H. & Kirsch, I. (1997) Classical conditioning and the placebo effect. *Pain* 72(1-2): 107-113.

Patterson, D.R.; Jensen, M.P.; Wiechman, S.A. & Sharar, S.R. (2010) Virtual reality hypnosis for pain associated with recovery from physical trauma. *Int J Clin Exp Hypn* 58(3): 288-300.

Radat, F. & Koleck, M. (2011) Pain and depression: Cognitive and behavioural mediators of a frequent association. *Encephale* 37(3): 172-179.

Reza, N.; Ali, S.M.; Saeed, K.; Abul-Qasim, A. & Reza, T.H. (2007) The impact of music on postoperative pain and anxiety following cesarean section. *Middle East J Anesthesiol* 19(3): 573-586.

Roth, R.S.; Punch, M. & Bachman, J.E. (2011a) Psychological Factors in Chronic Pelvic Pain due to Endometriosis: A Comparative Study. *Gynecol Obstet Invest* In press.

Roth, R.S.; Punch, M.R. & Bachman, J.E. (2011b) Patient beliefs about pain diagnosis in chronic pelvic pain: relation to pain experience, mood and disability. *J Reprod Med* 56(3-4): 123-129.

Roth, R.S.; Punch, M.R. & Bachman, J.E. (2011c) Psychological factors and chronic pelvic pain in women: a comparative study with women with chronic migraine headaches. *Health Care Women Int* 32(8): 746-761.

Schnur, J.B.; Bovbjerg, D.H.; David, D.; Tatrow, K.; Goldfarb, A.B.; Silverstein, J.H.; Weltz, C.R. & Montgomery, G.H. (2008) Hypnosis decreases presurgical distress in excisional breast biopsy patients. *Anesth Analg* 106(2): 440-444.

Sen, H.; Yanarateş, O.; Sızlan, A.; Kılıç, E.; Ozkan, S. & Dağlı, G. (2010) The efficiency and duration of the analgesic effects of musical therapy on postoperative pain. *Agri* 22(4): 145-150.

Sendelbach, S.E.; Halm, M.A.; Doran, K.A.; Miller, E.H. & Gaillard, P. (2006) Effects of music therapy on physiological and psychological outcomes for patients undergoing cardiac surgery. *J Cardiovasc Nurs* 21(3): 194-200.

Vase, L.; Robinson, M.E.; Verne, G.N. & Price, D.D. (2005) Increased placebo analgesia over time in irritable bowel syndrome (IBS) patients is associated with desire and expectation but not endogenous opioid mechanisms. *Pain* 115(3): 338-347.

Wallin, M.; Liedberg, G.; Börsbo, B. & Gerdle, B. (2011) Thermal detection and pain thresholds but not pressure pain thresholds are correlated with psychological factors in women with chronic whiplash-associated pain. *Clin J Pain* In press.

Wang, F.; Shen, X.; Xu, S.; Liu, Y.; Ma, L.; Zhao, Q.; Fu, D.; Pan, Q.; Feng, S. & Li, X. (2008) Negative words on surgical wards result in therapeutic failure of patient-controlled analgesia and further release of cortisol after abdominal surgeries. *Minerva Anestesiol* 74(7-8): 353-365.

Weintraub, M.I. (2003) Complementary and alternative methods of treatment of neck pain. *Phys Med Rehabil Clin N Am* 14(3): 659-674.

Williams, A.E. & Rhudy, J.L. (2007) The influence of conditioned fear on human pain thresholds: does preparedness play a role? *J Pain* 8(7): 598-606.

Xu, W.H.; Guo, C.B.; Wu, R.G. & Ma, X.C. (2011) Investigation of the Psychological Status of 162 Female TMD Patients with Different Chronic Pain Severity. *Chin J Dent Res* 14(1): 53-57.

Part 5

Cancer Pain

22

Radiation Mucositis

P. S. Satheesh Kumar
Department of Oral Medicine and Radiology,
Government Dental College, Trivandrum, Kerala
India

1. Introduction

Mucosal injury remains an undesirable, painful, and expensive side effect of cytotoxic cancer therapy and is disheartening for patients and frustrating for caregivers.[1,2] Mucositis and associated outcomes in patients receiving radiotherapy (RT) for head and neck cancer shows that the mean incidence was 80%.[3] Rates of hospitalization due to mucositis are reported to be 16% overall and 32% for RT-AF (altered fraction radio therapy) patients.[3 Patients in the high risk of developing oral mucositis group fall into the head and neck cancer population where the incidence of mucositis is high in this group.[3]

Oral mucositis is a distressing toxic effect of chemotherapy and radiotherapy. It can increase the need for total parenteral nutrition and opioids analgesics, prolong hospital stays, increase the risk of infection, and greatly affect the patient's quality of life [4]. All patients treated with high-dose chemotherapy requiring hematopoietic stem cell or bone marrow transplantation develop oral mucositis of varying severity. In addition, up to 80% of patients receiving radiotherapy for head or neck tumours and almost 90% of pediatric patients treated for cancer also develop oral mucositis[5,6]

2. Mechanism of development

Radiation induced mucositis is initiated by direct injury to basal epithelial cells and cells in the underlying tissue. DNA-strand breaks can result in cell death or injury. Non-DNA injury is initiated through a variety of mechanisms, some of which are mediated by the generation of reactive oxygen species. Radiation and chemotherapy are effective activators of several injury-producing pathways in endothelia, fibroblasts, and epithelia. In these cells, the activation of transcription factors such as nuclear factor-κB (NF-κB) and NRF-2 leads to the upregulation of genes that modulate the damage response. Immune cells (macrophages) produce pro-inflammatory cytokines, such as tumor-necrosis factor-α (TNF-α) and interleukin-6, which causes further tissue injury.[7] These signaling molecules also participate in a positive-feedback loop that amplifies the original effects of radiation and chemotherapy. For example, TNF-α activates NF-κB and sphingomyelinase activity in the mucosa, leading to more cell death. In addition, direct and indirect damages to epithelial stem cells result in a loss of renewal capacity. As a result, the epithelium begins to thin and patients start to experience the early symptoms of mucositis.[8]

An oropharyngeal epithelial surface has a rapid rate of cell turnover and appears to be at high risk of injury from ionizing radiation. A healthy oral mucosa serves to clear microorganism and provides a chemical barrier that limits penetration of many compounds into the epithelium. A damaged mucosal surface increases the risk of a secondary infection. Acute mucositis results from the loss of squamous epithelial cells owing to the sterilization of mucosal stem cells and the inhibition of transit cell proliferation. This leads to a gradual linear decrease in epithelial cell numbers. Normally, cells of the mouth undergo rapid renewal over a 7–14 day cycle. Radiation therapy interferes with cellular mitosis and reduces the ability of the oral mucosa to regenerate. [9]

As radiation therapy continues, a steady state between mucosal cell death and regeneration may occur because of an increased cell production rate from the surviving cells. Usually, however, cell regeneration cannot keep up with cell death, and therefore, partial or complete denudation develops. This presents as patchy or confluent mucositis. As the mucositis becomes more severe, pseudomembranes and ulceration develops. Poor nutritional status further interferes with mucosal regeneration by decreasing cellular migration and renewal. The loss of the epithelial barrier enhances insults from physical, chemical, and microbial agents.

Stages of mode l[10] for the pathogenesis of mucositis are based on the evidence available to date:

1. **Initiation of tissue injury:** Radiation and/or chemotherapy induce cellular damage resulting in death of the basal epithelial cells. The generation of reactive oxygen species (free radicals) by radiation or chemotherapy is also believed to exert a role in the initiation of mucosal injury. These small highly reactive molecules are by-products of oxygen metabolism and can cause significant cellular damage.
2. **Up-regulation of inflammation via generation of messenger signals:** In addition to causing direct cell death, free radicals activate second messengers that transmit signals from receptors on the cellular surface to the inside of cell. This leads to up-regulation of pro-inflammatory cytokines, tissue injury, and cell death.
3. **Signaling and amplification:** Up-regulation of pro-inflammatory cytokines, such as TNF-a, produced mainly by macrophages, causes injury to mucosal cells, and also activates molecular pathways that amplify mucosal injury.
4. **Ulceration and inflammation:** There is a significant inflammatory cell infiltrate associated with the mucosal ulcerations, based in part on metabolic by-products of the colonizing oral microflora. Production of pro-inflammatory cytokines is also further up-regulated as a result of this secondary infection.[10]
5. **Healing:** This phase is characterized by epithelial proliferation, as well as, cellular and tissue differentiation,[11] restoring the integrity of the epithelium.

A number of authors have reported that the oropharyngeal flora may contribute to radiation-induced mucositis. In health, the oral mucosa has a number of distinct habitats which are colonized by micro-organism that are able to establish a homeostatic community.[12] These homeostatic microbial communities are protective for the host by preventing or interfering with the colonization of exogenous pathogens; this potent defense mechanism is called "colonization resistance". When the oral tissues are irradiated, the colonization resistance is practically abolished. Irradiation mucositis is caused by a combination of alteration of the normal oral microflora with concomitant changes in the tissues. However, healing eventually occurs when cells regenerate from the surviving mucosal stem cells.

3. Clinical presentation

Clinically, mucositis presents with multiple complex symptoms. It begins with a symptomatic redness and erythema and progresses through solitary white elevated desquamative patches that are slightly painful to contact pressure. Following this, large, painful contiguous pseudo membranous lesions develop with associated dysphagia and decreased oral intake. The nonkeratinized mucosa is the most affected one. The most common sites include the labial, buccal, and soft palate mucosa, as well as, the floor of the mouth and the ventral surface of the tongue. Oral lesions usually heal within two to three weeks [Figure 1].

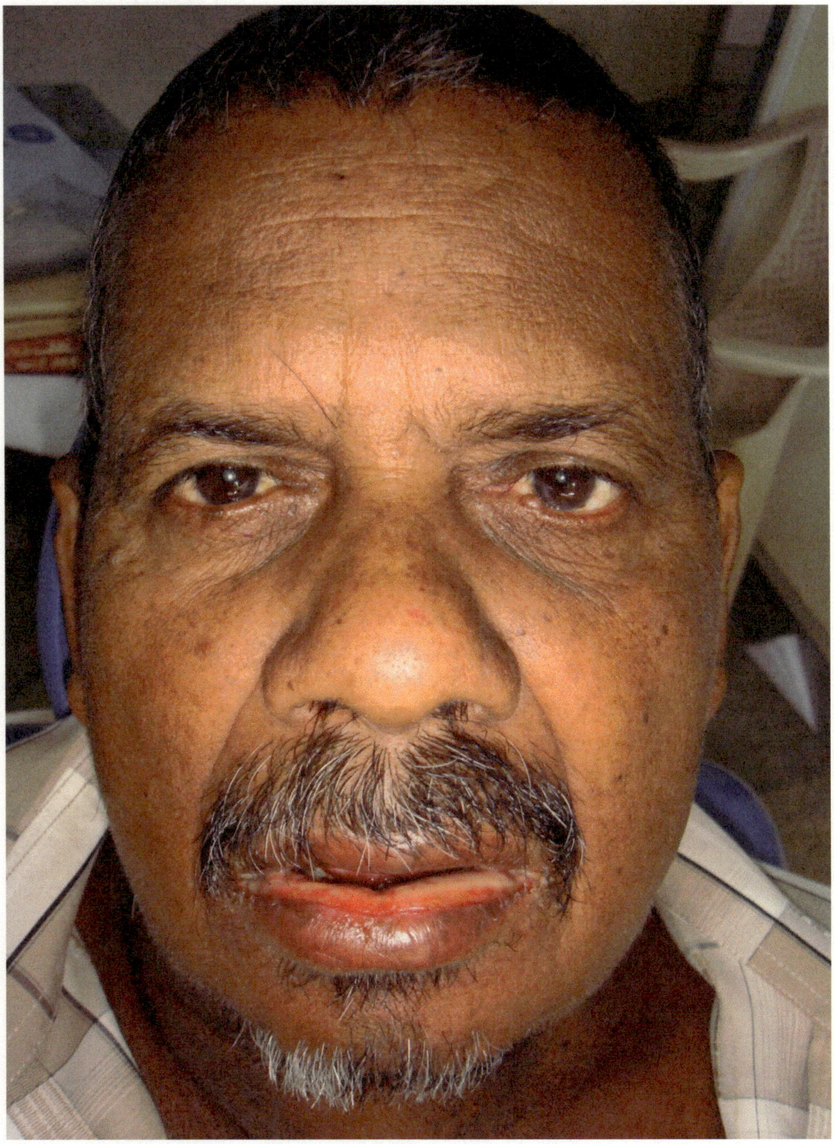

Fig. 1. Oral mucositis in a patient.

Mucositis is an inevitable side effect of radiation. Its severity is dependent on the type of ionizing radiation, the volume of irradiated tissue, the dose per day, and cumulative dose. It has been noted in a considerable number of clinical trials that the severity of acute normal tissue responses, particularly oral mucositis, is significantly increased when the overall treatment time is shortened.[12,13] The clinical course of oral mucositis may sometimes be complicated by local infection, particularly in immunosuppressed patients. Viral infections such as herpes simplex virus (HSV), and fungal infections such as candidiasis can sometimes be superimposed on oral mucositis. Although HSV infections do not cause oral mucositis, they can complicate its diagnosis and management.

Histopathologically, edema of the retepegs is noted, along with vascular changes that demonstrate a thickening of the tunica intima with concomitant reduction in the lumen size and destruction of the elastic and muscle fibers of the vessel walls. The loss of the epithelial cells to the basement membrane exposes the underlying connective tissue stroma with its associated innervations, which, as the mucosal lesions enlarge, contributes to increasing pain. If the patient develops both severe mucositis and thrombocytopenia, oral bleeding may occur, which is very difficult to treat.

4. Clinical management of oral mucositis

Management of oral mucositis can be divided into the following sections: pain control, nutritional support, oral decontamination, palliation of dry mouth, management of oral bleeding, and therapeutic interventions for oral mucositis.

4.1 Pain control

The most common symptom of oral mucositis is pain. Pain significantly affects the nutritional intake, the mouth care, and the quality of life. Thus, management of mucositis pain is a primary component of any mucositis management strategy. Many centers use saline mouth rinses, ice chips, and topical mouth rinses containing an anesthetic, such as 2% viscous lidocaine, which may be mixed with equal volumes of diphenhydramine and a soothing covering agent in equal volumes. Such topical anesthetic agents may provide short-term relief. Sucralfate is the most commonly used and widely studied, even though there is no significant decrease in the pain control.[14,15] In addition to the use of topical agents, most patients with severe mucositis require systemic analgesics, often including opioids, for satisfactory pain relief. Though, the so called '*magic mouthwash*' (lidocaine, diphenhydramine, magnesium aluminum hydroxide) has been observed to be beneficial, morphine mouth washes are preferable.[16,17] It was significantly better at reducing intensity and duration of pain and functional impairment, with fewer adverse effects.

4.1.1 Sucralfate

Sucralfate also has been tested in patients receiving radiation therapy. One study compared 21 patients who received standard oral care to the head and neck with 24 patients who received sucralfate suspension four times daily. Results revealed a significant difference in mucosal edema, pain, dysphagia, and weight loss in patients receiving sucralfate [18]. In a pilot study done by Pfeiffer et al. [19], sequential patients who received radiation therapy to the head and neck received sucralfate at the onset of mucositis. Most patients had a decrease in pain following the use of sucralfate. A double-blind, placebo-controlled study with sucralfate in 33 patients who received. irradiation to the head and neck reported no stastitically significant differences in mucositis; however, the sucralfate group reported less oral pain, and other topical and systemic analgesics were started later in the course of radiation [20]. A prospective double-blind study compared the effectiveness of sucralfate suspension versus diphenhydramine syrup plus kaolin-pectin on radiotherapy-induced mucositis. Data were collected daily, including perceived pain, helpfulness of mouth rinses, weekly mucositis grade, weight change, and interruption of therapy. Analysis of the two groups revealed no statistically significant differences between the two groups. In a retrospective review, 15 patients who had not used daily oral rinses were compared with the two groups, and the results suggested that the use of a daily oral rinse with a mouth-coating agent may result in less pain, reduce weight loss, and help prevent interruption of radiation because of severe mucositis[21].

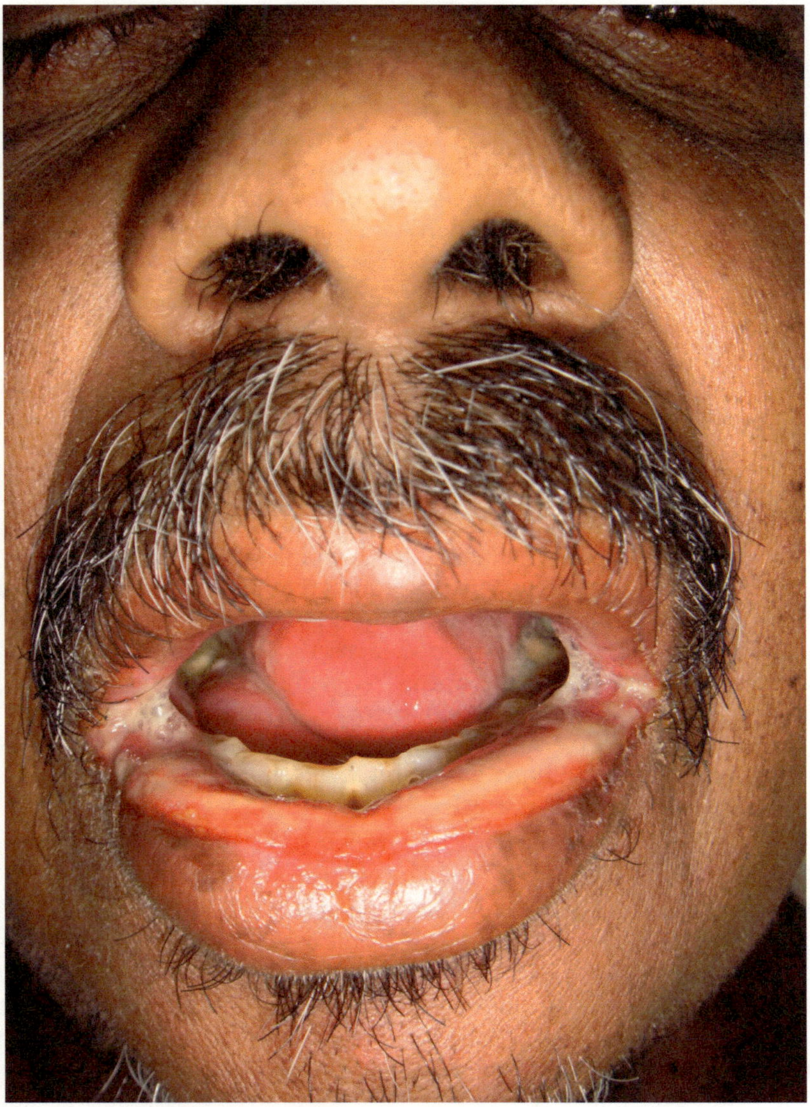

Fig. 2. Oral mucositis in a patient.

4.1.2 Morphine in pain control

In a study to compare the effect of locally applied morphine mouthwash(MO) with Magic mouth wash (MG) on mucositis-related oral pain and on the maintenance of oral intake in patients with tumors of the head and neck area treated with a chemoradiotherapy regimen[51]. Additional objectives were to evaluate the safety of MO by determining the frequency of treatment-emergent drug-related adverse events (local and systemic) or hematologic and biochemical abnormalities, the intensity of chemoradiotherapy administered, tumor response, weight loss, need of a nasogastric tube, and mucositis-related hospitalizations. The duration of severe pain was 3.5 days less in the Morphine group compared with the Magic mouth wash group (*P* _ 0.032). The intensity of oral pain was also significantly lower in the MO group compared with the MG group .More patients in the MG group needed supplementary (oral or parenteral) analgesia compared with the MO group (*P* _ 0.019). Nevertheless, the time elapsed before the first supplemental analgesic and the total amount of analgesics taken was similar for both groups. Of 12 patients in the MG group, 3 (25%) and none in the MO group required third-step opiates for alleviation of mouth pain. However, the differences in the maximum WHO step needed for control of pain were not statistically significant. There was a significant difference in duration of severe functional impairment. Nevertheless, the body weight change was similar for both groups. There were no significant differences in documented or highly suspected infections, change in performance status, tumor response rate, and intensity of the chemoradiotherapy delivered between the two treatment groups. No patients required hospitalization due to mucositis during the study. Patients in the MG group reported more local side effects [51].

4.2 Nutritional support

A soft diet or liquid diet was more easily tolerated than a normal diet, when oral mucositis is present; gastrostomy tube is more beneficial, when there is severe mucositis.

4.3 Selective oral decontamination

It has been hypothesized that microbial colonization of oral mucositis lesions exacerbates the severity of oral mucositis and, therefore, decontamination may help to reduce mucositis. Due to the fact that the oral cavity contains a high amount of Gram-negative bacilli and considering its etiological role in mucositis, the concept of 'Selective Decontamination' has been developed. In this regard, lozenges composed of polymyxin E, tobramycin, and amphotericin B have been studied in patients receiving radiation for cancers of head and neck in a randomized trial that compared lozenges with placebo or chlorhexidine rinses, the antimicrobial lozenges provided more effective mucositis prevention in patients receiving head and neck irradiation. Addition of ciprofloxacin or ampicillin with clotrimazole to Sucralfate has shown reduction in mucositis.[22]

4.4 Oral hygiene

Significant reduction in oral mucositis can be attained by proper oral hygiene measures.[23] It was noted that proper oral care also reduced oral toxicity of radiation therapy. Indeed, multiple studies have demonstrated that maintenance of good oral hygiene can reduce the severity of oral mucositis. Furthermore, oral decontamination can reduce infection of the oral cavity by opportunistic pathogens.[24] Therefore, a second function of oral decontamination can be to reduce the risk of systemic sepsis from resident oral and/or opportunistic pathogens. Intensive oral care protocol decreased risk of oral mucositis, but not the percentage of patients with a documented septicemia.[25]

The RTOG and MASCC/ISOO (Mucositis study group of the multinational association for supportive care in cancer and the International society of oral oncology) guidelines recommend use of a standardized oral care protocol, including brushing with a soft toothbrush, flossing, and the use of nonmedicated rinses (for example, saline or sodium bicarbonate rinses). Patients and caregivers should be educated regarding the importance of effective oral hygiene [26, 52, 53].

4.5 Palliation of dry mouth

In cancer therapy, patients often develop transient or permanent xerostomia and hyposalivation. Hyposalivation can further aggravate inflamed tissues, increase risk for local infection, and make mastication difficult. Many patients also complain of a thickening of salivary secretions, because of a decrease in the serous component of saliva. The following measures can be taken for palliation of a dry mouth:

- Sip water as needed to alleviate mouth dryness; several supportive products including artificial saliva are available.
- Rinse with a solution of half a teaspoon of baking soda half in one cup warm water several times a day to clean and lubricate the oral tissues and to buffer the oral environment.
- Chew sugarless gum to stimulate salivary flow.
- Use cholinergic agents as necessary.

4.6 Kaolin pectin

Kaolin pectin, combined with diphenhydramine, which is a H1-histamine antagonist and local anesthetic, was found to reduce oral pain without reducing the degree of mucositis in a double blind randomized and controlled study.[27]

5. Growth factors

One of the problem faced by the therapy is the loss of proliferation of the oral epithelial cells, it has seen that various growth factors that can increase epithelial cell proliferation have been studied for the management of oral mucositis. Recent evidence shows that intravenous recombinant human keratinocyte growth factor-1, Palifermin, significantly reduced incidence of WHO grades 3 and 4 oral mucositis in patients with hematologic malignancies (for example, lymphoma and multiple myeloma) receiving high-dose chemotherapy and total body irradiation before autologous hematopoietic cell transplantation.[28]

Human keratinocyte growth factor-2, Repifermin, was found to be ineffective in reducing the percentage of subjects who experienced severe mucositis.[29] Intravenous human fibroblast growth factor-20, Velafermin, is currently in clinical development for reduction of mucositis secondary to high-dose chemotherapy in autologous hematopoietic cell transplant patients.[30] The safety of this class of growth factors has not been established in patients with nonhematologic malignancies. There is a theoretical concern that these growth factors may promote growth of tumor cells, which may have receptors for the respective growth factor. However, one recent study found no significant difference in survival between subjects with colorectal cancer receiving Palifermin or placebo at a median follow-up duration of 14.5 months.[31] Further studies are ongoing to confirm the safety of epithelial growth factors in the solid tumor setting, including patients receiving radiation therapy for head and neck cancer.

Source	Grade 0	Grade 1	Grade 2	Grade 3	Grade 4
WHO	No change	Soreness/erythema	Erythema,ulcers, can eat solids	Ulcers; requires liquid diet only	Alimentation not possible
RTOG	No change over baseline	May experience mild pain not requiring analgesic	Patchy mucositis may have a serosanguinous discharge. May experience pain requiring analgesics. < 1.5 cm, noncontiguous	Confluent fibrinous mucositis/may include severe pain requiring narcotics, > 1.5 cm, contiguous	Necrosis or deep ulceration, ± bleeding .
NCI CTC	None	Painless ulcers, erythema or mild soreness	Painful erythema,oedema or ulcers, but can eat.	painful erythema, edema or ulcers can not eat.	Requires Parenteral or enteral support
Van der schueren *et al*	None	Slight erythema	Pronounced erythema	Spotted mucositis	Confluent mucositis patches >0.5cm.
Byfield *et al*	---	Minimal dysphasia, thinning but no overt break in mucosal integrity.	Significant dysphasia, semi soft foods only, focal mucosal vesicles or denuded patches.	Fluids only tolerated, obviously large confluent patches of mucosal denudation	Parenteral fluids only, severe confluent mucosal denudation with bleeding.
Seto *et al*	-----	Localized erythema with no pain	Generalized erythema without pain or localized erythema or ulcers with mild pain.	Multiple ulcers or generalized erythema with moderate pain	Generalized erythema or ulcers with moderate to severe pain.
Eilers *et al*	-----	Pink and moist	Reddened or white film without ulcerations	Ulceration with or without bleeding	-------
NCIC	None	Painless ulcers,erythema,or mild soreness.	Painful erythema,oedema,or ulcers, but can eat	Painful erythema,oedema,or ulcers, but can not eat	Mucosal necrosis and/or requires Parenteral or enteral support,dehydration.
Spijkervet *et al*	None	White discoloration	Erythema	Pseudomembrane	ulceration
Maceijewski	None	Type: mild erythematous area: <25%	Type : severe erythematous area: 25-50%	Type: spotted mucositis area >50%	Type:confluent mucosistis
Hickey *et al*	No stomatitis	Whitish gingival or slight burning sensation or discomfort.	Moderate erythema and ulcerations or white patches.pain, but can eat, drink and swallow.	severe erythema and ulcerations or white patches. Severe Pain and can not eat, drink or swallow.	-------

Table 1. Comparison of commonly used mucositis scoring system

6. Anti-inflammatory agents

6.1 Benzydamine hydrochloride

It is a nonsteroidal antiinflammatory drug that inhibits proinflammatory cytokines including TNF-a. In a Phase III trial, Benzydamine hydrochloride mouthrinse reduced the severity of mucositis in patients with head and neck cancer undergoing radiation therapy of cumulative doses up to 50-Gy radiation therapy.[32] Based on this and previous studies, the MASCC/ISOO guidelines recommends use of this agent in patients receiving moderate-dose radiation therapy.[33]

6.2 Saforis

It is a proprietary oral suspension of L-glutamine that enhances the uptake of this amino acid into epithelial cells. Glutamine may reduce mucosal injury by reducing the production of proinflammatory cytokines and cytokine-related apoptosis;[34,35] and may promote healing by increasing fibroblast and collagen synthesis.[36] In a Phase III study, this topical agent reduced the incidence of clinically significant chemotherapy-induced oral mucositis compared to placebo.[37] By comparison, the MASCC/ISOO guidelines recommend that systemically administered glutamine not be used for the prevention of GI mucositis because of lack of efficacy.[38]

6.3 Amifostine

It (phosphothiorate, radiation protection agent) is thought to act as a scavenger for harmful reactive oxygen species that are known to potentiate mucositis.[39] However, because of insufficient evidence of benefit, various guidelines could not be established regarding the use of this agent in oral mucositis in chemotherapy or radiation therapy patients. The use of amifostine has been recommended for the prevention of esophagitis in patients receiving chemoradiation for nonsmall-cell lung cancer.[40]

6.4 RK- 0202 (RxKinetix)

It consists of the antioxidant, *N-acetylcysteine*, in a proprietary matrix for topical application in the oral cavity. In a placebo-controlled phase II trial in patients with head and neck cancer, this agent significantly reduced the incidence of severe oral mucositis up to doses of 50-Gy radiation therapy.[41]

6.5 Beta carotene

Beta carotene, a vitamin A derivative, is a scavenger of singlet oxygen. Based on the findings of different randomized controlled study, it is of the view that supplemental dietary beta-carotene lead to a mild decrease in the severity of chemotherapy and radiotherapy-induced oral mucositis.[42]

7. Immunomodulatory drugs

7.1 Pentoxifylline

Oral pentoxiphylline reduced the frequency and severity of all major complications after BMT, including reduction of oral mucositis.[43] Contradictory to this, other workers reported a significant aggravation of symptoms when they studied the effect of IV Pentoxiphylline in 92 patients.[44] However, no difference in symptoms was noted in patients who undergone chemo radio therapy.

7.2 Indomethacin

Indomethacin, a nonsteroidal antiinflammatory drug inhibiting prostaglandin synthesis is noted to delay the onset of mucositis.

7.3 Immunoglobulin

Treatment with low-dose intra muscular immunoglobulin is said to decrease the severity and duration of radio therapy-induced oral mucositis. Immunoglobulin has also been tried as a therapeutic agent in radiation-induced mucositis in various clinical trials and the observations were promising.[45]

7.4 Cytokines

Preclinical models have been used to demonstrate that the cytokines interleukin-1, interleukin-2, epidermal growth factor, interleukin-11, and transforming growth factor-beta have direct effect on intestinal or oral mucosa. Interleukin-1 increases thymidine labeling, and protects oral and intestinal mucosa, when given to mice before radiation. Interleukin-11 can decrease mucositis, when given to hamster models.

7.5 G-CSF, GM-CSF

The mucosal protection effects of granulocyte colony stimulating factor G-CSF were observed in patients treated with various chemotherapy regimens by many authors.[46] But controversies to this exist in other clinical trials. In a recent preliminary report of a pilot study found significant reduction in oral mucositis.[47] The study was to evaluate the effect of GM-CSF in reduction of radiotherapy induced oral mucositis. At about second week of radiotherapy, when oral pain was experienced 400 μg of GM-CSF was administered locally once a day, until completion of radiotherapy. The patients were evaluated weekly for mucosal reaction and functional impairment. The result of the study was prompting with reduction and almost healing of oral mucositis in 14 out of 17 patients with completion of radiotherapy within the preplanned schedule. Moreover patients did not show a significant weight loss or functional impairment.

8. Anti-viral drugs

8.1 Acyclovir

Although acyclovir prophylaxis is effective in preventing oropharyngeal shedding of the virus in herpes simplex virus seropositive patients receiving intensive chemotherapy or BMT, it did not influence chemotherapy, radiotherapy and BMT-related oral toxicity.

9. Role of safe radiotherapy

Normal tissue reactions can be reduced in a substantial number of patients with head and neck cancer by the use of computed tomography (CT)-based target delineation, Intensity-Modulated Radiation Therapy (IMRT), and simple, custom-made, intraoral devices that are designed to exclude uninvolved tissues from the treatment portals or to provide shielding of tissues within the treatment area.[43] Stents can be useful in excluding the palate mucosa during treatment of the tongue or floor of the mouth. These shielding stents can decrease the amount of radiation that is delivered to the contra-lateral mucosa. More frequent use of electron-beam and/or sophisticated three-dimensional conformal, multibeam, wedged-pair, or oblique treatment plans will also help to exclude or minimize the radiation dose to uninvolved mucosa. Packing gauze between metallic dental restorations and mucosa of the lateral tongue and buccal area appears to be very beneficial in minimizing the dose from scattered radiation.

9.1 Antifungal therapy

The mucosa of patients undergoing radiation therapy to the oral cavity should be examined at least once a week, and antibiotic or antifungal medications should be prescribed when infections are documented. Clotrimazole troches, dissolved in the mouth five times a day for 14 days, generally works well for oral candidiasis. However, if significant mucositis, altered taste, or xerostomia has developed, the troches might not be tolerated. In this situation, nystatin oral suspension or Fluconazole in tablet or liquid form is often effective. Fluconazole is more effective than nystatin and might need to be given at a higher dose and/or for an extended period of time in patients who are receiving combined chemotherapy and radiation therapy due to infections with resistant species.[48]

9.2 Low-level laser therapy

The mechanism of low-level laser therapy is not understood, but many studies have proved the efficacy of the same in reducing the symptoms related to oral mucositis. Low-level laser therapy may reduce levels of reactive oxygen species and/or proinflammatory cytokines that contribute to the pathogenesis of mucositis.[49] The various guidelines suggest the use of low-level laser therapy for reducing the severity of chemotherapy and radiotherapy-induced oral mucositis.[50]

9.3 AMP-18 (Antral mucosal protein) 18

A study on AMP18 (AMP-18 is a protein constitutively expressed in epithelial cells of the gastric antrum that is cell protective, mitogenic and motogenic in cell culture and in vivo) shows, AMP peptide, by activating CCKBR (cholecystokinin-B/gastrin receptor), targets TJs(Tight Junctions) to maintain mucosal integrity, and sets in motion protective and cell regenerative mechanisms for the prevention and treatment of OM. Treatment with AMP peptide protected the surface epithelium of the mouse oral mucosa. AMP-18 peptide stimulates growth of diverse types of epithelial cells including HaCaT cells [54].

10. Summary

Mucositis is an inevitable side effect of radiation. The severity of the mucositis depends on the type of ionizing radiation, the volume of irradiated tissue, the daily dose, and the cumulative dose. As the mucositis becomes more severe, pseudomembranes and ulcerations develop. Poor nutritional status further interferes with mucosal regeneration by decreasing cellular migration and renewal. Radiation-induced oral mucositis affects the quality of life of the patients and the family concerned. The present day management of oral mucositis is mostly palliative and or supportive care. Management includes good oral hygiene, avoiding irritating or abrasive substances, use of bland rinses, topical anesthetic agents, and systemic analgesics. Though, the newer guidelines are suggesting Palifermin, which is the first active mucositis drug as well as Amifostine, for radiation protection and cryotherapy for symptoms related to high-dose melphalan; the role of safe radiotherapy remains the ultimate goal in reducing the symptoms of radiation-induced oral mucositis. Future research for the newer drugs in the field of radiation-induced oral mucositis is a must, and the current management should focus more on palliative measures, such as pain management, nutritional support, and maintenance, of good oral hygiene.

11. References

[1] Sonis ST. Is mucositis an inevitable consequence of intensive therapy for hematologic cancers? Nat Clin Pract Oncol 2005;2:134-5.

[2] Keefe DM. Mucositis guidelines: What have they achieved, and where to from here? Support Care Cancer 2006;14:489-91.

[3] Trotti A, Bellm LA, Epstein JB, Frame D, Fuchs HJ, Gwede CK, *et al.* Mucositis incidence, severity and associated outcomes in patients with head and neck cancer receiving radiotherapy with or without chemotherapy: A systematic literature review. Cancer 2008;113:2704-13.

[4] Satheesh Kumar PS, Balan A, Sankar A, Bose T. Radiation induced oral mucositis. Indian J Palliat Care 2009;15:95-102

[5] Satheeshkumar PS, Chamba MS, Balan A, Sreelatha KT, Bhatathiri VN, Bose T. Effectiveness of triclosan in the management of radiation-induced oral mucositis: A randomized clinical trial. J Can Res Ther 2010;6:466-72.
[6] P.S Satheeshkumar, A. Balan.Subjective response of pain on patients treated with aqueous base Hexidine and weekly dentist assisted oral hygiene maintenance for radiation induced oral mucositis- An interventional study." Oral Oncology, Volume 47, Supplement 1, July 2011, Page S82
[7] Logan RM, Gibson RJ, Sonis ST, Keefe DM. Nuclear factor-κappaB (NF-kappaB) and cyclooxygenase-2 (COX-2) expression in the oral mucosa following cancer chemotherapy. Oral Oncol 2007;43:395-401.
[8] Gibson RJ, Bowen JM, Cummins AG, Logan R, Healey T, Keefe DM. Ultrastructural changes occur early within the oral mucosa following cancer chemotherapy [abstract A-373]. Support Care Cancer 2004;12:389.
[9] Sonis ST, Elting LS, Keefe D, Peterson DE, Schubert M, Hauer-Jensen M, *et al*. Perspectives on cancer therapy-induced mucosal injury: Pathogenesis, measurement, epidemiology, and consequences for patients. Cancer 2004;100:1995-2025.
[10] Sonis ST, Elting LS, Keefe D, Peterson DE, Schubert M, Hauer-Jensen M, *et al*. Perspectives on cancer therapy-induced mucosal injury: Pathogenesis, measurement, epidemiology, and consequences for patients. Cancer 2004;100:1995-2025.
[11] Sonis ST, Peterson RL, Edwards LJ, Lucey CA, Wang L, Mason L, *et al*. Defining mechanisms of action of interleukin-11 on the progression of radiation-induced oral mucositis in hamsters. Oral Oncol 2000;36:373-81.
[12] Dorr W, Emmendorfer H, Haide E. Proliferation equivalent of 'accelerated repopulation' in mouse oral mucosa. Int J Radiat Biol 1994;66:157-67.
[13] Epstein JB, Gorsky M, Guglietta A, Le N, Sonis ST. The correlation between epidermal growth factor levels in saliva and the severity of oral mucositis during oropharyngeal radiation therapy. Cancer 2000;89:2258-65.
[14] Dodd MJ, Miaskowski C, Greenspan D, MacPhail L, Shih AS, Shiba G, *et al*. Radiation-induced mucositis: A randomized clinical trial of micronized sucralfate versus salt and soda mouthwashes. Cancer Invest 2003;21:21-33.
[15] Nottage M, McLachlan SA, Brittain MA, Oza A, Hedley D, Feld R, *et al*. Sucralfate mouthwash for prevention and treatment of 5-fluorouracil-induced mucositis: A randomized, placebo-controlled trial. Support Care Cancer 2003;11:41-7.
[16] Barclay L. Morphine mouthwash relieves pain of oral mucositis. Cancer 2002;95:2230-6.
[17] Spijkevet FK, van saene JJ, Panders AK, Vermy A, Mehta DM, Filder V. Effect of selective elimination of the oral flora on mucositis in irradiated head and neck cancer patients. J Surg Oncol 1991;46:167-73.
[18] Matthews RH, Ercal N. Prevention of mucositis in irradiated head and neck cancer patients. J Exp Ther Oncol 1996;1:135-8.
[19] Borowski B, Benhamou E, Pico JL, Laplanche A, Margainaud JP, Hayat M. Prevention of oral mucositis in patients treated with high-dose chemotherapy and bone marrow transplantation: A randomized controlled trial comparing two protocols of dental care. Eur J Cancer B Oral Oncol 1994;308:93-7.
[20] Yoneda S, Imai S, Hanada N, Yamazaki T, Senpuku H, Ota Y, *et al*. Effects of oral care on development of oral mucositis and microorganisms in patients with esophageal cancer. Jpn J Infect Dis 2007;60:23-8.
[21] McGuire DB, Correa ME, Johnson J, Wienandts P. The role of basic oral care and good clinical practice principles in the management of oral mucositis. Support Care Cancer 2006;14:541-7.

[22] Barker G, Loffus L, Cuddy P, Barker B. The effects of of sucralfate suspension and diphenhydramine syrup plus kaolin-pectin on radiotherapy-induced mucositis. Oral Surg Oral Med Oral Pathol 1991;71:288-93.

[23] Spielberger R, Stiff P, Bensinger W, Gentile T, Weisdorf D, Kewalramani T, *et al.* Palifermin for oral mucositis after intensive therapy for hematologic cancers. N Engl J Med 2004;351:2590-8.

[24] von Bultzingslowen I, Brennan MT, Spijkervet FK, Logan R, Stringer A, Raber-Durlacher JE, *et al.* Growth factors and cytokines in the prevention and treatment of oral and gastrointestinal mucositis. Support Care Cancer 2006;14:519-27.

[25] Scherlacher A, Beaufort-Spontin E. Radiotherapy of head-neck neo-plasms:prevention of inflammation of the mucosa by sucralafate treatment. HNO 1990;38:24-28.

[26] Pfeiffer P, Hansen O, Madsen el, et al. A prospective pilot study on the effect of sucralafate mouth-swishing in reducing stomatitis during radiotherapy of the oral cavity. Acta Oncol 1990;29:471-3.

[27] Epstein jb, Wong FLW The efficacy of sucralafate suspension in the prevention of oral mucositis due to radiation therapy. Int J Radiat Oncol Biol Phys 1994;28:693-698.

[28] Barker G, Loftus L, Cuddy P, et al. The effects of sucralafate suspension and diphenhydramine syrup plus kaolin-pectin on radiotherapy-induced mucositis. Oral Surg Oral Med Oral Pathol Oral Radiol Endod 1991;71:288-293.

[29] Lalla RV. Velafermin (CuraGen). Curr Opin Investig Drugs 2005;6:1179-85.

[30] Rosen LS, Abdi E, Davis ID, Gutheil J, Schnell FM, Zalcberg J, *et al.* Palifermin reduces the incidence of oral mucositis in patients with metastatic colorectal cancer treated with fluorouracil-based chemotherapy. J Clin Oncol 2006;24:5194-200.

[31] Epstein JB, Silverman S Jr, Paggiarino DA, Crockett S, Schubert MM, Senzer NN, *et al.* Benzydamine HCl for prophylaxis of radiation-induced oral mucositis: Results from a multicenter, randomized, double-blind, placebo-controlled clinical trial. Cancer 2001;92:875-85.

[32] Lalla RV, Schubert MM, Bensadoun RJ, Keefe D. Anti-inflammatory agents in the management of alimentary mucositis. Support Care Cancer 2006;14:558-65.

[33] Coeffier M, Marion R, Leplingard A, Lerebours E, Ducrotté P, Déchelotte P. Glutamine decreases interleukin-8 and interleukin-6 but not nitric oxide and prostaglandins e production by human gut in-vitro. Cytokine 2002;18:92-7.

[34] Evans ME, Jones DP, Ziegler TR. Glutamine prevents cytokine-induced apoptosis in human colonic epithelial cells. J Nutr 2003;133:3065-71.

[35] Bellon G, Monboisse JC, Randoux A, Borel JP. Effects of preformed proline and proline amino acid precursors (including glutamine) on collagen synthesis in human fibroblast cultures. Biochim Biophys Acta 1987;930:39-47.

[36] Peterson DE, Jones JB, Petit RG 2nd. A Randomized, placebo-controlled trial of Saforis for prevention and treatment of oral mucositis in breast cancer patients receiving anthracycline-based chemotherapy. Cancer 2007;109:322-31.

[37] Pytlik R, Benes P, Patorkova M, Chocenská E, Gregora E, Procházka B, *et al.* Standardized parenteral alanyl-glutamine dipeptide supplementation is not beneficial in autologous transplant patients: A randomized, doubleblind, placebo controlled study. Bone Marrow Transplant 2002;30:953-61.

[38] Mantovani G, Maccio A, Madeddu C, Mura L, Massa E, Gramignano G, *et al.* Reactive oxygen species, antioxidant mechanisms and serum cytokine levels in cancer patients, Impact of an antioxidant treatment. J Environ Pathol Toxicol Oncol 2003;22:17-28.

[39] Bensadoun RJ, Schubert MM, Lalla RV, Keefe D. Amifostine in the management of radiation induced and chemo-induced mucositis. Support Care Cancer 2006;14:566-72.

[40] Barasch A, Peterson DE, Tanzer JM, D'Ambrosio JA, Nuki K, Schubert MM, *et al.* Helium-neon laser effects on conditioning induced oral mucositis in bone marrow transplantation patients. Cancer 1995;76:2550-6.

[41] Mills EE. The modifying effect of beta-carotene on radiation and radiotherapy and chemotherapy induced oral mucositis. Br J Cancer 1988;57:416-7.

[42] Bianco JA, Appelbaum FR, Nemunaitis J, Almgren J, Andrews F, Kettner P, *et al.* Phase I-II trial of pentoxifyline for the prevention of transplant-related toxicities following bone marrow transplantation. Blood 1991;78:1205-11.

[43] Clift RA, Bianco JA, Appelbaum FR, Buckner CD, Singer JW, Bakke L, *et al.* A randomized controlled trial of pentoxifylline for the prevention of regimen-related toxicities in patients undergoing allogeneic marrow transplantation. Blood 1993;82:2025-30.

[44] Mose S, Adametz IA, Saran F, Thilmann C, Hayd R, Knecht R, *et al.* Can Prophylactic application of immunoglobulin decrease radiotherapy-induced oral mucositis. Am J Clin Oncol 1997;20:407-11.

[45] Hermann F, Schuiz G, Weser M, Kolbe K, Nicolay U, Noack M, *et al.* Effect of granulocyte-macrophage colony stimulating factor on neutropenia and related morbidity induced by myelotoxic chemotherapy. Am J Med 1990;88:619-24.

[46] Gluckman E, Lotsberg J, Devergie A, Zhao XM, Melo R, Gomez-Morales M, *et al.* Oral acyclovir prophylactic treatment of herpes simplex infection after bone marrow transplantation. J Antimicrob Chemother 1983;12:161-7.

[47] Kaanders JH, Fleming TJ, Ang KK, Maor MH, Peters LJ. Devices valuable in head and neck radiotherapy. Int J Radiat Oncol Biol Phys 1992;23:639-45.

[48] Dahiya MC, Redding SW, Dahiya RS, Eng TY, Kirkpatrick WR, Coco BJ, *et al.* Oropharyngeal candidiasis caused by non-albicans yeast in patients receiving external beam radiotherapy for head-and-neck cancer. Int J Radiat Oncol Biol Phys 2003;57:79-83.

[49] Bensadoun RJ, Franquin JC, Ciais G, Darcourt V, Schubert MM, Viot M, *et al.* Low-energy He/Ne laser in the prevention of radiation-induced mucositis: A multicenter phase III randomized study in patient's with head and neck cancer. Support Care Cancer 1999;7:244-52.

[50] Migliorati CA, Oberle-Edwards L, Schubert M. The role of alternative and natural agents, cryotherapy, and/or laser for management of alimentary mucositis. Support Care Cancer 2006;14:533-40.

[51] Cerchietti LC, Navigante AH, Bonomi MR, Zaderajko MA, Menéndez PR, Pogany CE, Roth BM. Effect of topical morphine for mucositis-associated pain following concomitant chemoradiotherapy for head and neck carcinoma. Cancer. 2002 Nov 15;95(10):2230-6.

[52] S.K. Poolakkad Sankaran, A. Balan. Neighbourhood Dental Clinic programme (NDCP) for oral care in patients undergoing head and neck cancer therapy. Support Care Cancer (2011) 19 (Suppl 2):S67–S370.

[53] S.K. Poolakkad Sankaran, A. Balan. The degree of discomfort due to mucositis is related to the prior patient awareness? Support Care Cancer (2011) 19 (Suppl 2):S67–S370.

[54] Chen P, Lingen M, Sonis ST, Walsh-Reitz MM, Toback FG. Role of AMP-18 in oral mucositis. Oral Oncol. 2011 Sep;47(9):831-9. Epub 2011 Jul 6

Part 6

Non Pharmacological Treatments

23

Non-Pharmacological Therapies in Pain Management

Yurdanur Demir
Abant İzzet Baysal University, Bolu Health Sciences High School, Turkey

1. Introduction

Pain is an unpleasant feeling and emotional experience that is related to real or potential tissue damage or a damage that is defined similarly. Pain is mostly subjective (Merskey, Bogduk 1986). From many points of view, the pain is a common symptom intended for seeking aid (Dickens et al. 2002). International Association for the Study of Pain (IASP) defines the pain as "an unpleasant emotional situation which is originating from a certain area, which is dependant or non-dependant on tissue damage and which is related to the past experience of the person in question" (Merskey, IASP 1986).

Although there is an increase of knowledge and developments in technological resources regarding the pain, many patients still experience pain (Nash et al. 1999). This situation causes for reduction in living quality and functional situation of the patients, increase in the fatigue levels (Kim et al. 2004) and impairments in daily life activities in working capacity and social interactions (McMillan et al., 2000; Allard et al., 2001). Also this situation will cause loss of workforce and will affect not only the patients but also his/her family members in economical terms thus causing undesired problems in psychological and social well being status (Uçan and Ovayolu 2007). All of these elements have directed both the patients and caregivers to seek for different searches in pain management (Evans and Rosner, 2005). For this reason in addition to the pharmacological treatment options for pain management, today, non-pharmacological treatment options and complementary medical attempts have started to be used (Kwekkeboom et al., 2003; Menefee and Monti, 2005). It is stated that such kind of therapies can be useful in pain management (Uçan and Ovayolu 2007). In a study conducted with the participation of 31.044 adults in United States, Barnes et al. (2004) determined that the usage rate of the complementary methods for the last year has been 36% and back pain and lumbago come first with 16.8% and neck pain comes third with 6.6% in terms of usage reasons of the complementary methods . Sherman et al. (2004) have stated that 24% of the patients with chronic lumbago used massage therapy.

2. Non-pharmacological therapies in pain management

It is considered that these therapies help the standard pharmacological treatment in pain management. While medical drugs are being used for treating the somatic (physiological and emotional) dimension of the pain non-pharmacological therapies aim to treat the affective, cognitive, behavioral and socio-cultural dimensions of the pain (Yavuz 2006).

These therapies can treat the pain as adjuvant or complementary at middle level and severe pain experiences as an adjuvant or complementary treatment. (Delaune & Ladner 2002).
Non-pharmacological methods,

- Increase the individual control feeling.
- Decrease the feeling of weakness.
- Improves the activity level and functional capacity.
- Reduces stress and anxiety.
- Reduces the pain behavior and focused pain level.
- Reduces the needed dosage of analgesic drugs thus decreasing the side effects of the treatment (Yıldırım 2006).

Non-pharmacological methods used in pain management can be classified in different ways. In general; they are stated as physical, cognitive, behavioral and other complementary methods or as invasive or -non-invasive methods. Meditation, progressive relaxation, dreaming, rhythmic respiration, biofeedback, therapeutic touching, transcutaneous electrical nerve stimulation (TENS), hypnosis, musical therapy, acupressure and cold-hot treatments are non-invasive methods (Black & Matassarin Jacobs, 1997). The most famous and common method among the invasive methods is acupuncture (Menifee and Monti, 2005). It is considered that these methods control the gates that are vehicles for pain to be transmitted to the brain and affect pain transmission or the release of natural opioids of the body such as endorphin (Black & Matassarin Jacobs, 1997; Menefee & Monti, 2005; Uçan & Ovayolu 2007).
Non-pharmacological methods used in pain management have been examined below in three groups such as peripheral therapies (physical agents/skin stimulation methods), cognitive-behavioral therapies and other therapies. Some of these methods require special training (Turan et al. 2010).

2.1 Peripheral therapies (physical agents/skin stimulation)

Skin stimulation that provides analgesia is defined as stimulating the patient's skin in a harmless manner to treat the pain (Yıldırım 2006). Skin stimulation attempts (physical therapies) can be classified as hot-cold treatments, exercise, positioning, movement restriction-resting, acupuncture, hydrotherapy, TENS, massage and therapeutic touch. If used in an appropriate manner these methods are effective on secondary pathologies such as inflammation, edema, progressive tissue damage, muscle spasm and function loss which takes part in acute pain. (Yıldırım 2006).

2.1.1 TENS (Transcutaneous Electrical Nerve Stimulation)

TENS has been defined by the American Physical Therapy Association as applying electrical stimulation to the skin to manage the pain (Sluka & Walsh 2003). Usually, it may be used in addition or instead of pharmacological agents to manage acute, chronic and post-operative pain. It is an electro-analgesia method (Mucuk and Başer, 2009). That is to say, thick and rapid transmitting nerve fibers are stimulated artificially with TENS and the pain transmission is tried to be stopped or reduced. TENS, which functions in that way, has an effect to reduce the narcotic drugs usage and pain level (Arslan & Çelebioğlu; Chen et al. 1998). TENS has various mechanisms of action regarding pain. Gate Control Theory is a theory used to define how TENS affects the pain perception which also has a part in improving TENS. Gate control theory regarding pain management is very commonly used by TENS in defining the process to

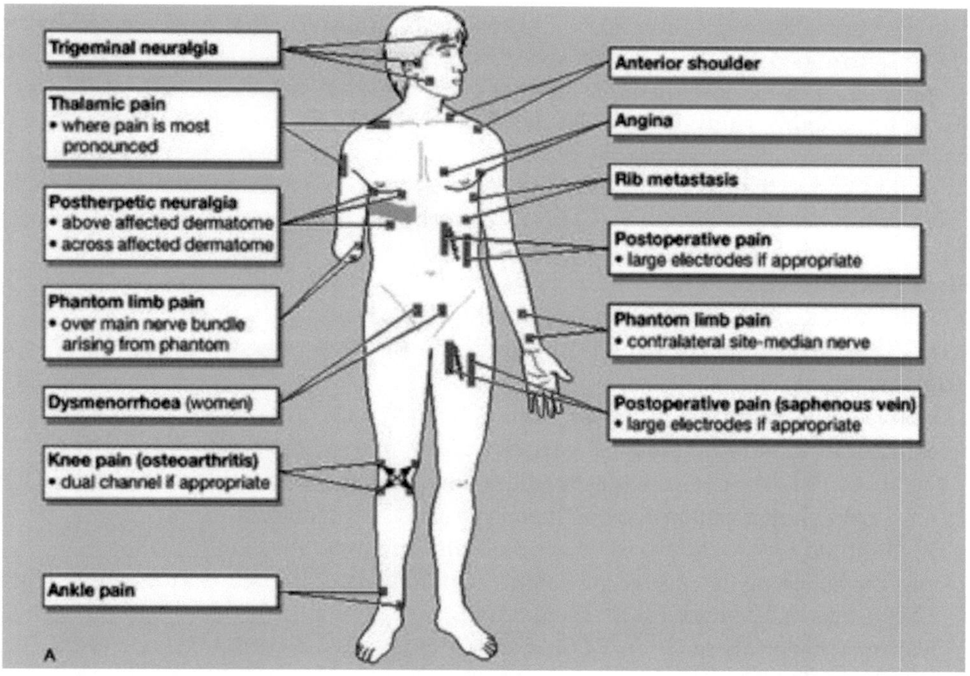

Fig. 1. a) *http://www.ib3health.com/products/TensandEMS/Literature/ApplicationChart.shtml* June/2011

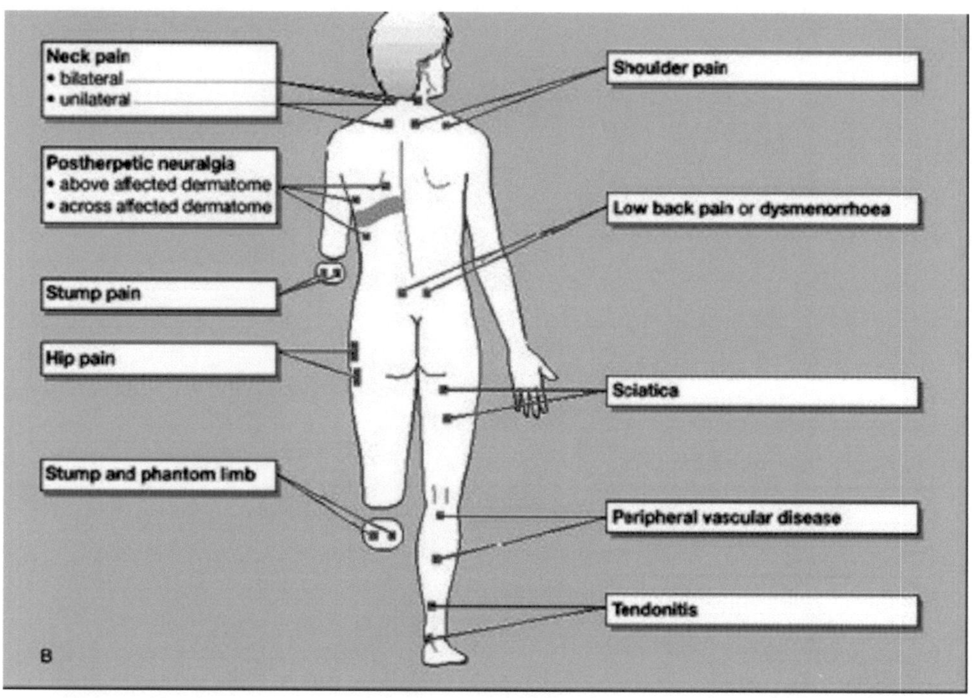

Fig. 1. b) *http://www.ib3health.com/products/TensandEMS/Literature/ApplicationChart.shtml* June/2011

prevent the pain (Sluka & Walsh 2003; Johnson 2002). In a study that has been conducted, it has been determined that the placebo group experienced 2-4 times less pain when TENS is used with pharmacological methods in post-operative pain management (Rakel & Frantz 2003), and in another study it has been determined that TENS usage in post-operative pain management has helped reducing the pain level and dosage of using analgesics (Bjordal et al. 2003). In addition to that, in some other studies it has been determined that first phase of labor in TENS group has been shorter and TENS treatment has been effective in relieving the pain (Kaplan et al. 1998; Simkin and Bolding 2004).

Points to Take into Consideration While Using Tens:

- TENS device should be used under the control of a health personnel.
- TENS devices should be used with caution in the areas where the pain could not be defined exactly.
- Device should be turned off while placing the materials.
- Electrical stimulation should not be used in front parts of the neck.
- You should use the device after controlling machine or motor vehicle producing TENS.
- This device should not be used on metal prostheses or monitors.
- TENS should be kept at places where the children cannot reach.
- People who are using cardiac pacemaker should consult to their doctors about whether TENS usage will be harmful for them or not.
- Electronic materials such as ECG monitors and ECG alarms may not work in full capacity while using TENS.
- It can cause damages on skin. That can be prevented by changing the type of gel and electrodes that are used.
- There are not reliable study results describing TENS usage during pregnancy (Yavuz 2006).

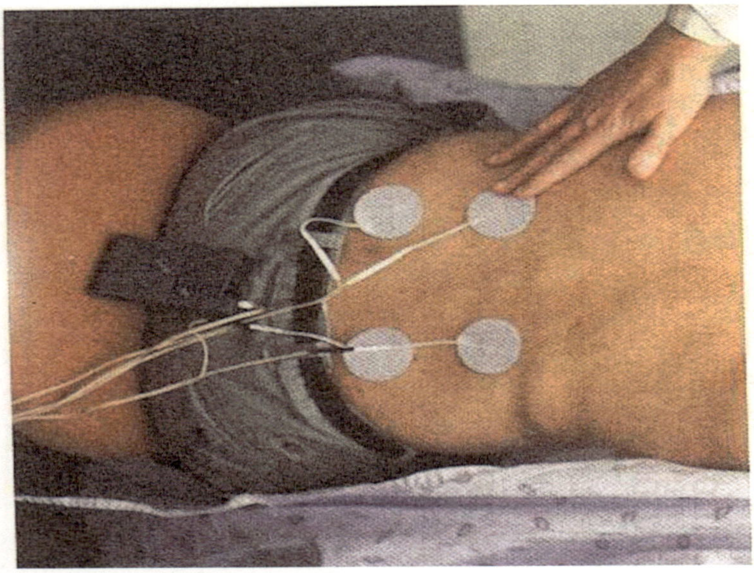

Dewit, S.C., (2009), *Fundamental concepts and skills for nursing,* 3rd Edition, W.B. Saunders Comp. Philadelphia, p.603-614.

Fig. 2. TENS Usage

2.1.2 Hot-cold treatment

Hot treatment moves the reflex arcs that inhibit the pain by means of heat receptors and reduces pain by vasodilatation effect. It is cheap and easy to use and it has a minimum amount of side effects when used regularly. It can be applied deeply or on surfaces. Application to the surface includes hot compresses, warm baths and paraphine usage. Deep applications such as ultrasound may increase the temperature of the tissues which are three to five centimeter deep (Arslan & Çelebioğlu, 2004).

On the other hand, cold treatment consists of applying a cooling material or device on any part of the body. Cold treatment which is a simple and cheap treatment method has an important place in non-drug therapies for pain management(Yavuz, 2006). Cold gel packages and ice packages commonly used in the application should be used by placing a tin towel/gauze between the skin and the package for being able to withstand extreme cold feeling during the first contact of the package, for having a homogenous cooling and providing hygiene. Cold treatment may be done for 15-30 minutes averagely until the anesthesia is felt on the area of application. The cold ice packs should be applied for at least 20 minutes. As a matter of fact, the affect of cold treatment on the human skin reveals itself in 4 stages. The patient will feel the cold within 1 to 3 minutes after the application, then feel a burning and pain sensation within 2 to 7 minutes and the pain and lethargy will decrease within 5 to 12 minutes, a breaking occurs for the pain-spasm vicious-circle and transmission of the nerve fibers in the area will decrease. An increase will occur for the metabolism within 12 to 15 minutes after cold treatment and a reflex vasodilatation occurs on the deep tissue. Thus, the edema and the pain will reduce and the tissue will be nourished with vasodilatation that will develop 15 minutes later (Karagözlüoğlu, 2001). Results of the studies made in the area have shown that the cold treatment has increased the pain threshold (Koç et al. 2006; Raynor et al. 2005; Sarifakioğlu & Sarifakioğlu 2004). So, the cold treatments that are applied locally are used to reduce the edema and treat the pain by taking the inflammation process under control (Saeki 2002; Sarifakioğlu & Sarifakioğlu 2004; Van der Westhuijzen et al. 2005).

It has been stated that cold treatment over the area where surgical sutures are found after lumbar disc surgery reduces both the pain during first 24 hours and the need for morphine (Brandner et al. 1996). Also, it has been shown that fluoromethane spray applications are a cheap method that are rapidly effective in managing the injection pain due to vaccination (Mawhorter et al. 2004) and cold package and ice applications have reduced the pain due to heparin injections (Kuzu ve Uçar 2001; Ross and Soltes 1995). In the study that they conducted, Demir and Khorshid (2010) have stated that cold treatment that is applied to the skin around the chest tube reduced the severity of the pain that is felt due to exclusion of chest tube and it has extended the time between exclusion of chest tube and taking an analgesic. It is stated that cold treatment is contraindicated for the situations such as urticaria/hypersensitivity, hypertension, Reynaud's phenomenon and sickle cell anemia which are related to cold (Mucuk & Başer, 2009).

2.1.3 Acupuncture and acupressure

Acupuncture which is one of the important components of traditional Chinese medicine has become a largely complementary in the West together with the conventional medicine. Acupuncture is accepted as a scientific treatment method that provides the body to restore its balance by means of stimulating some special points on the body with needles (Taşçı & Sevil 2007). Mechanism of action for the acupuncture could not be completely understood until now. Effect of the acupunctures is tried to be explained by Gate Control Theory. According to this theory, effect of a sensory stimulant (for example lumbago) can be suppressed with another stimulant (picking a needle) within a neural system. Another theory that explains the effect of acupuncture is Raising Pain Threshold Theory. That is a theory in which inhibitor effect of acupuncture is defined. In this theory, it is predicted to stimulate the analgesia mechanisms of the body by causing various pains on the area where an individual is feeling the pain to be treated. In addition to these, it has also been evidence that the acupuncture stimulates the production of endorphin, serotonin and acetyl choline within the central nerve system (Van Tulder et al. 2005). It has been shown in the studies that have been conducted that the acupuncture had positive effects on post-traumatic somatic pain, patella-femoral pain, rheumatoid arthritis and idiopathic head pain. (Snyder & Wieland 2003). It is sated in the literature that the acupuncture is especially useful in treating the lumbago but it is underlined that the patients should be informed in terms of increasing or carrying on the activities (Öztekin, 2005). Although there are some strong evidences showing the benefit of acupuncture in acute pain, the evidence regarding the cancer pain is limited (Black & Matassarin Jacobs, 1997; Filshie & Thompson 2004; Menefee & Monti, 2005). In spite of that, Alimi et al. (2003) stated that the acupuncture applied to cancer patient has decreased the pain level.

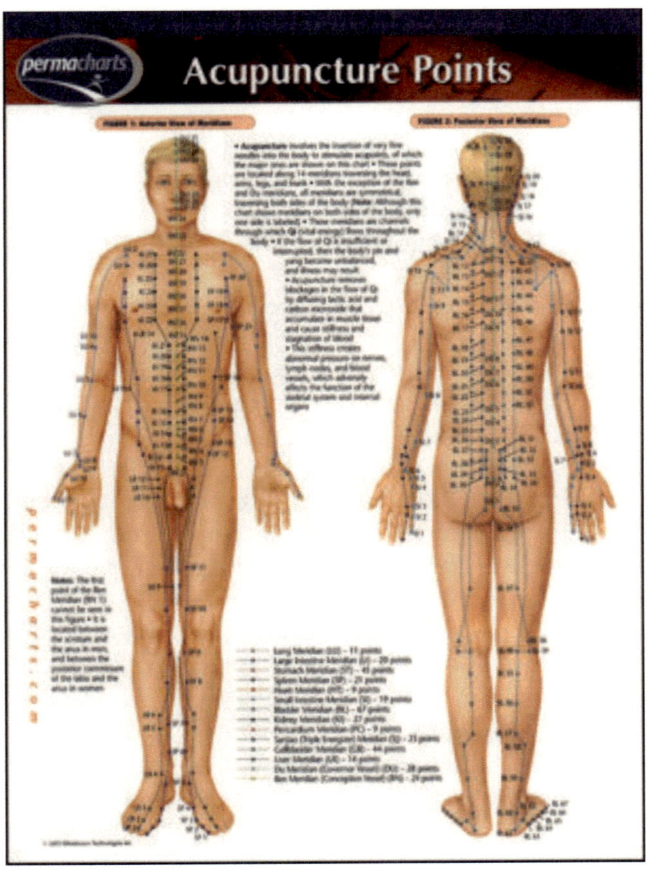

Fig. 3. http://suphecimelek.wordpress.com/2010/10/31/akupunktur June/2011

Acupressure is one of the traditional Chinese medicine approaches used for pain relief, diseases and injuries. Acupressure is a therapy that is conducted by applying physical pressure on various points on body surface by means of energy circulation and balance in cases of pain symptoms. This therapy is similar to the acupuncture and it is conducted by applying pressure on selected points of the body by fingers, hands, palms, wrists and knees in order to provide internal flow of energy. Acupressure technique is a noninvasive, safe and effective application (Hakverdioğlu, & Türk, 2006). It is suggested that acupressure reduces back, head, osteoarthritis, musculoskeletal and neck pains, pre-operative and post-operative pains, nausea-vomiting and sleeping problems (Tsay, Rong and Lin 2003; Tsay & Chen 2003; Hakverdioğlu, & Türk 2006).

2.1.4 Exercise

Exercise includes active-passive movements, bed movements and ambulation. Exercise increases the movement and provides continuity thus increasing the blood flow, preventing spasm and contractures of the muscles and relieving the pain (Musclow et al., 2002).

2.1.5 Positioning

It is applied to help or support the patient. This application can be supported by pillows, special beds and weight lifting. Position changes, which prevent the subsequent development of pain and reducing the acute pain, also increase the blood flow and prevent muscle contraction and spasms (Akdağ & Ovayolu, 2008). Positioning has been determined as the most common post-operative non-pharmacological method (Carroll 1999).

2.1.6 Restriction of movement /resting

These are applied for the patients who need certain bed rest and which are in traction. However, it should not be used alone for pain management. It can be used for fractures and back surgeries. Restriction of movement can also decrease edema development (Arslan & Çelebioğlu, 2004).

2.1.7 Massage

Massage is a manipulation applied on the soft tissue with various techniques (such as friction, percussion, vibration and tapotement) for recovery and supporting health. It is thought that the massage relieve the mind and muscles and increase the pain threshold (Karagöz 2006). Peripheral receptors on the body are stimulated with massage and stimulants reach the brain by means of spinal cord. In addition to pleasant feeling, a general relief is provided here (Turan et al. 2010). It is underlined that especially therapeutic massage is effective on chronic lumbago and that effect is stated to be a short term effect (Hsieh et al. 2004). Melancon and Miller (2005) draw attention to the fact that pain management in patient groups with lumbago that are treated with massage and pharmacological therapies are similar and they recommend the sue of massage as an alternative treatment option for the patients with lumbago within the framework of a integrated care. Nixon et al (1997) has stated that massage played a role in reducing the pain. In addition to that it is determined in some randomized controlled studies that massage made during labor decreases pain and anxiety; it also improves the general well being and progression of birth process and less reaction is given to the pain (Caton et.al 2002; Simkin & O'Hora 2002).

2.1.8 Hydrotherapy (Balneotherapy)

Using water for treatment by means of thermal springs, potable water resources and other methods is defined as "hydrotherapy" while using the water for therapy by means of temperature effect is defined as "hydrothermal treatment". Effect of hydrotherapy is related to its mechanical or thermal effect. Hot application stimulates the immune system, provides hormones that are suppressing the stress to be released, stimulates the circulation and digestion systems, increases the blood flow and provides muscle relaxation thus reducing the sensitivity developed against the pain (Karagöz, 2006). It is stated in the literature that hydrotherapy is effective while treating back and chronic lumbago (Balogh et al. 2005; Hartel & Volger 2004).

2.2 Cognitive-behavioral therapies

Cognitive-behavioral therapies are a part of multimodal approach in pain management. These attempts affect not only the pain level but also helps the patients to establish a management feeling of theirselves while dealing with pain and develop management behaviors and improved self-esteem. Cognitive-behavioral therapies can generally be applied by all members of the pain team. Most of the special techniques can be learned and applied by doctors, nurses, social service specialists and psychologists (Yıldırım 2006). These therapies should be thought and applied as early as possible before the patient experiences pain (Delaune & Ladner 2002).

2.2.1 Relaxation - respiration techniques and dreaming

Relaxation techniques cause an increase in slow brain waves in EEG by decreasing oxygen consumption, blood pressure, respiration amount and the number of pulse. Therefore, it is stated that the sensitivity developed against the pain should be prevented by means of these techniques (Karagöz, 2006).

Techniques used in providing the spiritual and physical relaxation are summarized below:

- *Respiration providing the relaxation:* It is provided to focus on the respiration and avoid disturbing thoughts by taking a deep breath slowly through the nose and giving it back in a long time through the mouth. These techniques can be applied for 5-10 minutes per day (Nordin 2002).
- *Advanced muscle relaxation treatment:* It is aimed to relax the unwanted contractions by determining them through making the patient contract and relax certain muscle groups on his body (Nordin 2002).
- *Dreaming:* After relaxation is provided, the patient is made to focus on a stimulant that makes the patient happy (light, color, sound, pattern etc.) in order to get the patient far away from his pain for a short period of time (Karagöz 2006). In a study made by Lewandowski et al (2005) it has been stated that an effective pain management can be obtained by directing the patients to dreaming for more than 4 days.

2.2.2 Distraction

Getting the attention away from the pain reduces its severity. The aim in using that technique is to increases the tolerance for pain and decrease the sensitivity for pain. This method includes listening to music, watching television, reading books and dreaming (Arslan & Çelebioğlu, 2004). There are some sources which supports that distraction is a method used in decreasing the pain (Seers & Carroll 1998; Petry 2002).

2.2.3 Praying

Most of the individuals with chronic pains use the praying method. It is indicated that praying has positive results for decreasing the body pain in old people and relieving their physical functional disorders and it is suggested to use the praying method in order to reduce the depression and anxiety that is caused by chronic pain (Meisenhelder & Chandler, 2000; Karagöz, 2006).

2.2.4 Meditation

In the traditional meaning, meditation is generally focusing on the moment. Meditation; can also be defined as focusing on the present. This act is realized with an individual focusing on his own respiration, a word or picture. Duration of the meditation can last from a few minutes to 30 minutes or take more (Snyder & Wieland, 2003; Gray, 2004). Considering the fact that meditation helps relaxation, it is thought to be effective in relieving the pain (Gray, 2004). Carson et al (2005) have stated that an 8-week meditation is useful for relieving the pain for patients with chronic lumbago.

2.2.5 Yoga

Yoga is providing relaxation by using respiration exercises and meditation with slow movements. It is considered that it can be useful against musculoskeletal pain in terms of using physical stretching moves and increasing strength (Dillard & Knapp, 2005). Individuals that use yoga have stated that they believe in the benefit of this method and it is a cost-effective method. It is stated in a study that applying yoga for 16 weeks has cured the chronic lumbago (Williams et al. 2005). Also, in a study conducted by Williams et al (2005) it has been stated that functional insufficiency experienced with chronic lumbago and use of pain killers have been reduced by means of yoga.

2.2.6 Hypnosis

Hypnosis; it is the state of conscious change similar to sleep. Hypnosis requires the body to relax and the patient to focus on an object, a stimulant or memory. Hypnosis is *"the deep physical relaxation state during which subconscious can be reached and important abilities are suspended"*. In this state, ability of people to be dominated increases (Taşçı & Sevil, 2007). Besides mechanism of action of hypnosis over the pain is not known exactly and it is mentioned that the pain is reduced with some physiological changes that occur as a result of hypnosis. Hypnosis has been used in a positive manner in terms of cancer pain, pains in head-neck region and phantom pain which is the sensations felt by amputees (Black & Matassarin Jacobs, 1997). Jensens and Patterson (2006) has stated that hypnotherapy/hypnosis is used for analgesia in various types of chronic pains and it has been stated that hypnosis has been effective for neck pain. Also Liossi et al (2006) has made a study with pediatric cancer patients in which it has been determined that hypnosis application has decreased pain and anxiety level in patients (Liossi et al. 2006).

2.2.7 Bio-feedback

Biological feedback is based informing the patient in order to help relaxation or control a physiological function. For example, in cases of tension type headache, it is provided for the electrical activity received by means of head muscles and facial muscles to be perceived as colors or sounds by the patient. Thus, observing the color changes or decreases in the sound, the patient understands whether the relaxation occurred or not (Uçan & Ovayolu 2007). Bio-feedback is used for treatment in the cases of pain, migraine pain, spinal cord injuries and movement disorders. It is aimed to control of physiological reactions such as muscle tension, body temperature, heart rate, brain wave activity and other vital parameters. Efficiency of the treatment depends on the desire that a patient shows for learning of how controlling of these functions and participation of patient in the process. Biofeedback appliers train the patient in terms of mental and physical exercises, visualization and deep breaths (Eidelson, 2005). In many types of chronic pain the bio-feedback has been shown to be effective (Moseikin 2003; Teyhen et al. 2005).

2.2.8 Behavioral therapy

Aim of this therapy is to increase the functional level of the patient decrease the maladaptive behaviors and firstly reduce and then completely stop painkiller usage. The family is trained by the treatment team; description of pain (grimacing, moaning, and remaining motionless) is avoided and well-adaptive behaviors such as physical activities are reinforced (Brietbart et al. 2004).

2.3 Other non-pharmacological therapies

2.3.1 Reflexology

Reflexology is a technique that is based on the principle that suggests there are reflex points on our feet corresponding to all parts of our bodies , all organs and systems and these points are the mirrors of the body anatomy. Pressure applied to these reflex points by special hand and finger techniques provides the stress to be relieved and cause physiological changes and a reduction in pain perception (Yıldırım, Fadıloğlu and Uyar, 2006). There are totally five pressurizing techniques to make massage on reflex areas: Thumb move, finger move, rubbing move, patting move and compressing move. These moves are applied to ears, hands and feet similarly. The important thing here is to know how this technique will be applied to whom. Physical structure of an individual, age and current health status are taken into consideration. Treatment consists of applying pressure with the side of a thumb or other fingers and turning it clockwise. This pressure is generally deep but it does not have to be painful. A good reflexologist prefers repetition of short and painless seances to a single but painful seances for the whole disease. Intensity of the pressure can be low at the beginning and increased as the treatment progresses. Each seance takes from 10 minutes to 30 minutes and it is decided according to the situation of the person how many seance will be necessary (Stephenson et al. 2000; Bolsoy 2008).

It is stated in the literature that reflexology is used especially for reducing migraine pain, back pain, muscle pain, end stage cancer pain and side effects of chemotherapy and to increase living quality (Long et al. 2001; McNeill et al. 2006; Mollart 2003; Quattrin et al.2006; Wringht et al.2002) In spite of that, it is stated that it is unfavorable to use reflexology in acute infections and fever situation, deep venous thrombosis, surgical situations and in cases of open scars, malign melanoma and during first trimester of the pregnancy or with the patients that has miscarriage or premature birth risks (Long et al. 2001; Lett 2002).

2.3.2 Herbal treatments

Herbal medicine is using the chemical materials obtained from inside, root, leave, seed and flower parts of the herbs for treatment (Karagöz 2006). Today, most individuals use herbal products in addition to their medical treatments with drugs without consulting to any professional (Turan et al. 2010 ; Deng et al. 2005). It is stated in the literature that herbal medicine has been commonly used to treat lumbago and back pains (Gray, 2004; Gagnier et al. 2006; Hartel & Volger 2004).

2.3.3 Aromatherapy

Aromatherapy is using the essential oils that are obtained from flowers, herbs and trees to improve health and well being. These oils are applied by being respired through oily gauze that is placed under the nostrils of the patient or as massage oils being applied on skin. It has been evidenced that the aroma oils reached the lymph system by means of blood circulation and provided recovery by means of intercellular fluids (Turan et al. 2010). It is thought that aromatherapy may be able to help reducing stress, treating cold, sniffles, skin and menstruation problems and relieving pain (Karagöz, 2006; Jennings, 2004; Yıldırım et al. 2006; Deng et al. 2005). It is known that lavender oil is used in treating migraine pain, osteoarthritis, rheumatoid arthritis and lumbago. It is also known that eucalyptus, black pepper, ginger, daisy, licorice, rosemary and myrrh oils are used in relieving pain. But it is stated that lavender oil can cause hypersomnia and using licorice for long time can cause hypertension (Delaune & Ladner 2002). Although the usage of aromatherapy within health system increases day by day it is seen that the researches in this meaning is quite insufficient. Data regarding the efficiency of essential oils depend only on individual experiences. For this reason, it is necessary to conduct studies with large samples and high level of evidence to determine the efficiency of essential oils in pain management (Snyder & Wieland 2003; Tseng 2005)

2.3.4 Chiropractics

Chiropractics is the neck-pulling movement used in treatment of the disorders in connective tissues and musculoskeletal system which consists of muscles, joints, bones, tendon, cartilage and ligaments. The main principle of this approach is the fact that to relieve the pain and to improve health with the applications made on spine and joints which have had a positive effect on neural system and natural defense mechanisms (Gray, 2004). Chiropractics have focused on the connection between body structure and the functions of the neural system and manipulation of bones and joints to regain the health. It is known that the application that is taken, decreases the amount of burden on the neck and relives the pain. However, the individuals who have serious disorders such as severe cervical disc hernia, complaints due to rheumatoid arthritis , tumors and infection have to avoid from these applications (Turan et al. 2010; Karagöz 2006; Deng et al. 2005).

2.3.5 Musical therapy

Many studies that have been conducted have sown that the music had positive effects on pain and anxiety and increased the living quality of the patient or healthy individuals. Music reduces heart rate, blood pressure, body temperature and respiration rate and it distraction the attention of the patient to another point thus reducing the pain perception and reducing especially the nausea due to chemotherapy so that increasing living quality of patients in terminal period of cancer (Chase, 2003; Hilliard, 2003; Deng et al. 2005; Stefano et al. 2004, Uçan & Ovayolu 2007). In a study that states listening to music stimulates the alpha waves of brain which have been determined as a stimulator for the release of endorphin and creates a relaxation state and therefore music has played a role not only in relieving the pain but also decreasing blood pressure, heartbeat rate and other physiological responses (Henry, 1995). A point to be taken into consideration here is to let the music type to be prefered by the patient (Delaune & Ladner, 2002). New studies show that slow music creates a relaxing effect. According to the literature musical therapy should not be used continuously to be an effective method. Applying musical therapy form 25 to 90 minutes per day will provide sufficient treatment period.

Attempt	Advantage	Disadvantage
Relaxation Bio-feedback Distraction	• It may reduce the pain and anxiety without having drug-related side effects. • It can be used more likely as an adjuvant therapy together with other methods. It may increase the management feeling of the patient. • Most of them are not expensive, they do not require special equipment and they are easily applicable.	• The patients should be aware of using the management strategies by theirselves. • An appropriate time zone is needed to teach the attempts.
Psychotherapy, Hypnosis	• It may reduce the pain and anxiety of the patients who have pains that are relatively difficult to manage. • It may increase the number of methods that the patient uses to manage.	• It requires an experienced therapist.
Skin Stimulation/Cutaneous Stimulation (superficial hot-cold application and massage)	• It may reduce muscle spasms, inflammation and pain. • It can be used more likely as an adjuvant therapy together with other methods. • It may increase the controlling ability of pain feeling of the patient. • It is so easy to use. • It may be applied by the patients or families. • It is a cheap method.	• Hot application can increase the bleeding or edema after acute injuries. • Cold application is contraindicate for the situations such as uritcaria/hypersensitivity, hypertension, Reynaud's phenomenon and sickle cell anemia which are related to cold.
Transcutaneous Electrical Nerve Stimulation (TENS)	• It reduces the pain without having any drug-related side effects. • It can be used more likely as an adjuvant therapy together with other methods. • It gives the feeling of pain management to the patient.	• It requires an experienced therapist. • There is a risk for bleeding and infection. • There are no reliable results for use in cases of pregnant women.
Aromatherapy	• It has an analgesic effect. • It has a sedative and relaxing effect.	• It may cause hypersomnia. • Some herbs should not be used with other anti-depressants and alcohol.
Acupuncture	• It may provide pain reduction without any side effects. • It can be used more likely as an adjuvant therapy together with other methods.	• It requires an experienced therapist.

Table 1. Advantages and Disadvantages of Some Non-pharmacological Methods

In a study they conducted, Nilsson et al (2003) have stated that listening to music for one hour in earl post-operative period may reduce post-operative pain and morphine consumption of the patients. In a study conducted by Sahler and Hunter (2003) with the patients who had bone marrow transplantation, the patients were made to listen music which has a relaxing effect, at least twice a week for 45 minutes and it has been determined that the group which was not included to music therapy has a higher pain score when compared to the one that has received musical therapy. It has been stated that the musical also has positive effects during labor period. In a study that is conducted by Browning (2000) related to the mother's pain and anxiety levels to evaluate the effect of musical therapy applied to primipar mothers before delivery, the mothers have stated that the musical therapy relives their pain and it made them feel themselves more comfortable and calm.
Advantages and disadvantages of some non-pharmacological methods used in pain management have been specified below (Table 1).

3. Conclusion

As a result, the pain can be managed in a more effective manner with the combination of pharmacological and non-pharmacological therapies. Developments in pain management may provide different opportunities to the patients and their families thus providing the patients to carry on a more comfortable and productive life. Both health personnel and caregivers need to have important responsibilities while following these developments. For an effective care to be provided to patients, developments regarding pain management and updated pharmacological and non-pharmacological approaches regarding pain management and pain should be followed. Also these techniques may help reducing pain and it must be encouraged as a part of the comprehensive pain management efforts. For this reason, abilities and preferences of the patient regarding the use of non-pharmacological methods should be taken into consideration; it should be underlined for the patients that these are used together with medical and pharmacological treatments and the use of non-pharmacological methods should be included to the care plan when patient is appropriate and willing. From this point of view, it is recommended to use various non-pharmacological methods for pain management but we need more study results that support the efficiency of these methods. For this reason, it will provide the evidence-based results to be put forward if randomized controlled experimental studies, which examine the efficiency of these methods in taking the pain under control, are conducted.

4. References

Akdağ, R. G. & Ovayolu, N. (2008). Hemşirelerin Ağrı Yönetimi ile İlgili Bilgi, Tutum ve Klinik Karar Verme Durumlarının Değerlendirilmesi. *Gaziantep Üniversitesi Sağlık Bilimleri Enstitüsü,* Master's Thesis.

Alimi, D.; Rubino, C.; Pichard-Leandri, E.; Fernand, B.S.; Dubreuil-Lemaire, M.L. & et al. (2003). Analgesic effect of auricular acupuncture for cancer pain: randomized, blinded, controlled trial. *Journal of Clinical Oncology,* 15;21(22): 4120-4126; Nov 2003.

Allard, P.; Maunsell, E.; Labbe, J. & Dorval, M. (2001). Educational interventions to improve cancer pain control: a systematic review . *Journal of Palliative Medicine,* Vol.4 , No:2 , pp.191-203.

Arslan, S. & Çelebioğlu, A. (2004). Postoperatif Ağrı Yönetimi ve Alternatif Uygulamalar. *International Journal of Human Sciences*, 1(1): 1-7.

Balogh, Z.; Ordogh, J.; Gasz, A.; Nemet, L. & Bender, T. (2005). Effectiveness of balneotherapy in chronic low back pain -- a randomized single-blind controlled follow-up study. *Forsch Komplementarmed Klass Naturheilkd*, 12(4): 196-201; Aug 2005.

Barnes, P.; Griner, E.; Mcfann, K. & Nahin, R.L.(2004). Complementary and alternative medicine use among adults: United States, 2002. *Adv Data.* , Vol.27, pp.1-19.

Bjordal, M.J.; Johnson, I.M. & Ljunggreen, A.E. (2003). Transcutaneous Electrical Nerve Stimulation (TENS) Can Reduce Postoperative Analgesic Consumption: A Meta-Analysis With Assesment Of Optimal Treatment Parameters For Postoperative Pain. *The European Journal Of Pain*, 7(2): 181-188.

Black, J.M. & Matassarin Jacobs, E. (1997). Pain , In: *Medical-Surgical Nursing: Clinical Management for Continuity of Care. 5.th edition,* J.M. Black, E.M. Jacobs & J. Luckmann(Edts.) pp: 342-365, W.B. Saunders Co., ISBN: 978-0721663999.

Bolsoy, N. (2008). Perimenstrüel Distresin Hafifletilmesinde Refleksolojinin Etkinliğinin İncelenmesi. Ege Üniversitesi Sağlık Bilimleri Enstitüsü, PhD Thesis.

Brandner, B.; Munro, B.; Bromby, L.M. & Hetreed, M. (1996). Evaluation of the Contribution to Postoperative Analgesia by Local Cooling of the Wound. *Anaesthesia,* 51(11): 1021-1025; Nov 1995.

Brietbart, W.; Payne, D. & Passik, S.D. (2004). Psychological and psychiatric interventions in pain control. In: *Oxford Textbook of Palliative Medicine. 3rd ed.* Doyle D, Hanks NC, Calman K (eds), pp: 424-438 NY: Oxford University Pres, New York; ISBN:9780198566984.

Browning, C.A. (2000) Using musiv during childbirth. *Birth*,27(4),272-276.

Carroll, C.et al.(1999). Pain Assessment and Management in Critically ill Postoperative and Trauma Patients: A Multisite Study . *American Journal of Critical Care.* Vol.8 (2),March 1999..

Carson, J.W.; Keefe, F.J.; Lynch, T.R.; Carson, K.M.; Goli, V.; Fras, A.M. & et. al. (2005). Loving-kindness meditation for chronic low back pain: results from a pilot trial.*J. Holist. Nurs.*, 23(3): 287-304; Sep 2005.

Caton, D.; Corry, M.P.; Frigoletto, F.D.; Hopkins, D.P.; Lieberman, E.; Mayberry, L.; Rooks, J.P.; Rosenfield, A.; Sakala, C.; Simkin, P. & Young, D. (2002). The nature and management of labor pain: executive summary. *American Journal of Obstetrics And Gynecology,* 186(5 Suppl Nature):S1-15;May 2002.

Chase, K.M. (2003). Multicultural music therapy: A review of literature. *Music Therapy Perspectives*, 21(2):84-88;ISSN : 0734-6875.

Chen, L.; Tang, J.; White, P. F.; Slonınsky, A.; Wender, R. H.; Naruse, R. & Kariger, R. (1998). The Effect of Location of Transcutaneous Electrical Nerve Stimulation on Postoperative Opioid Analgesic Requirement: Acupoint Versus Nonacupoint Stimulation. *Anesth Analg*, 87(5): 1129–34; Nov 1998.

Delaune, S.C.& Ladner, P.K. (Eds.) (2002). *Fundamental of Nursing : Standard And Practice (2nd Edition),* pp.916-941,Newyork, Thomson Delmar Learning. ISBN: 978-076824522.

Demir, Y. & Khorshıd, L. (2010). The Effect of Cold Application in Combination with Standard Analgesic Administration on Pain and Anxiety During Chest Tube Removal: A Single-Blinded, Randomized, Double-Controlled Study. *Pain Management Nursing*, (11)3: 186-196; Sep 2010.

Deng, G. & Cassileth, B.R. (2005). Integrative oncology: complementary therapies for pain, anxiety, and mood disturbance. *CA: A Cancer Journal for Clinicians*, 55(2):109-116;May/April 2005.

Dewit, S.C. (2009). *Fundamental concepts and skills for nursing, 3rd Edition*, p.603-614, W.B. Saunders Comp. Philadelphia,; ISBN : 978-1-4160-5228-9.

Dickens C, Jayson M, Creed F (2002) Psychological Correlates Of Pain Behavior in Patients With Chronic Low Back Pain. *Psychosomatics*, 43:42–48;February 2002.

Dillard, J.N. & Knapp, S. (2005). Complementary and alternative pain therapy in the emergency department. *Emerg Med Clin North Am*, 23(2): 529-549; May 2005.

Eidelson, S.G. (2005). *Advanced Technologies to Treat Neck and Back Pain, A Patient's Guide*; Eidelson's book; http://www.spineuniverse.com/displayarticle.php/article224.html; March 2005.

Evans, R. & Rosner, A. (2005). Alternative in cancer pain treatment: the application of chiropractic care . *Seminars in Oncology Nursing* , Vol.21 , No:3 , pp.184-189.

Filshie, J. & Thompson, J.W. (2004). Acupuncture; In: *Oxford Textbook of Palliative Medicine. 3rd ed,* D. Doyle ; NC. Hanks & K. Calman (eds), pp: 410-424.. NY: Oxford University Press, New York. ISBN-13: 978-0198510987

Gagnier, J.J.; Van Tulder, M.; Berman, B. & Bombardier, C. (2006). Herbal medicine for low back pain. *Cochrane Database Syst Rev*,19(2); CD004504 April 2006

Gray, D.P. (2004). Complementary and alternative therapies. In : *Medical Surgical Nursing,* S.M., Lewis, ; L. Heitkemper, & S.R. Dirksen, (Eds). pp:94-109, St. Louis : Mosby Inc; ISBN-13: 978-0323016100.

Hakverdioğlu G. & Türk, G. (2006). Acupressure. *Journal of Hacettepe University School of Nursing*,43-47.

Hartel, U.; Volger, E. (2004). Use and acceptance of classical natural and alternative medicine in Germany--findings of a representative population-based survey. *Forsch Komplementarmed Klass Naturheilkd*, 11(6): 327-334; Dec 2004.

Henry, L.L. (1995). Music therapy: a nursing intervention for the control of pain and anxiety in the ICU: a review of the research literature. Dimensions of Critical Care Nursing, 14(6):295-304.

Hilliard, R.E. (2003). The effect of music therapy on the quality and length of life people diagnosed with terminal cancer. *Journal of Music Therapy*, 40(2):113-117.

Hsieh, L.L.; Kuo, C.H.; Yen, M.F. & Chen, T.H.A. (2004). A Randomized controlled clinical trial for low back pain treated by acupressure and physical therapy. *Prev Med*, 39(1): 168-176; Jul 2004.

http://suphecimelek.wordpress.com/2010/10/31/akupunktur-ise-yarar-mi; June/2011

http://www.ib3health.com/products/TensandEMS/Literature/ApplicationChart.shtml, June 2011.

Jennings, W.M. (2004). Aromatherapy practice in nursing: literature review. *Journal of Advanced Nursing*, 48 (1): 93–103.

Jensen, M. & Patterson, D. (2006). Hypnotic treatment of chronic pain. *J. Behav. Med.*,29(1): 95-124;Feb 2006.

Johnson MI. (2002). Transcutaneous Electrical Nevre Stimulation. In: *Electrotherapy: Evidence-Based Practice(11th edition),* S. Kitchen.(Ed.), pp.:259-286; Edinburgh: Churchill Livingstone, ISBN : 0443072167.

Kaplan, B.; Rabinerson, D.; Lurie, S.; Bar, J.; Krieser, U.R. & Neri, A. (1998). Transcutaneous electrical nevre stimulation (TENS) for adjuvant pain-relief during labor and delivery. *International Journal of Gynecology & Obstetrics*, 60(3): 251-255; Mar 1998.

Karagöz, G. (2006). Sırt, boyun, bel ağrıları olan ve ameliyat programına alınan nöroşürurji hastalarının ağrı gidermede kullandıkları tamamlayıcı ve alternatif tedaviler. *İstanbul Üniversitesi Sağlık Bilimleri Enstitütüsü. İstanbul* Master's Thesis.

Karagözoğlu, Ş.A. (2001). Intravenöz Sıvı Tedavısı Komplikasyonu Olarak Gelişen Tromboflebitte Hemşirelik Bakımı Ve Sıcak - Soğuk Uygulamanın Yeri. *C.Ü. Hemşirelik Yüksekokulu Dergisi*, 5(1):18-25.

Kim, J.E.; Dodd, M. & West, C. (2004). The PRO-SELF Pain control program improves patients knowledge of cancer pain management. *Oncology Nursing Forum*, Vol. 31 , No:6 , pp.1137-1143.

Koç, M.; Tez, M.; Yoldaş, Ö.; Dizen, H. & Göçmen, E. (2006). Cooling for the Reduction of The Postoperative Pain. Prospective-Randomized Study. *Hernia*, 10(2):184-186; Apr 2006.

Kuzu, N. & Uçar, H. (2001). The Effect of Cold on The Occurence of Bruising, Haematoma and Pain at the Injection Site in Subcutaneous Low-Molecular Weight Heparin. *International Journal of Nursing Studies*, 38(1):51-59; Feb 2001.

Kwekkeboom, K.; Kneip, J. & Pearson, L. (2003). A pilot study to predict success with guided imagery for cancer paitent . *Pain Management Nursing*, Vol. 4 , No.3 , pp.112-123.

Lett, A. (2002). The Future of Reflexology. *Complementary Therapy in Nursing & Midwifery*, 8(2): 84-90; May 2002.

Lewandowski, W.; Good, M. & Draucker, C.B. (2005). Changes in the Meaning of pain with the use of Guided Imagery. *Pain Manag Nurs*, 6(2): 58-67; Jun 2005.

Liossi, C.; White, P. & Hatira, P. (2006). Randomized clinical trial of local anesthetic versus a combination of local anesthetic with self-hypnosis in the management of pediatric procedure-related pain. *Health Psychology*, 25(3):307-315; May 2006.

Long, L.; Huntley, A.& Ernst, E. (2001) Which Complementary and Alternative Therapies Benefit Which Conditions? A Survey of Opinions Of 223 Professional Organizations. *Complementary Therapy in Medicine*, 9: 178-185.

Mawhorter, S.; Daugherty, L.; Ford, A.; Hughes, R.; Metzger, D. & Easley, K. (2004). Topical Vapocoolant Quickly and Effectively Reduces Vaccine- Associated Pain: Results of Randomized Single-Blinded, Placebo-Controlled Study. *J. Travel Med*, 11(5), 267-272; Sep-Oct 2004.

McMillan, S.C.; Tittle, M.; Hagan, S. & Laughlin, J. (2000). Management of pain and pain-related symptoms in hospitalized veterans with cancer . *Cancer Nursing*, Vol. 23 , No:5 , pp.327-336.

McNeill, J.A.; Alderdice, F.A. & Mcmurray, F. (2006). A Retrospective Cohort Study Exploring the Relationship Between Antenatal Reflexology and İntranatal Outcomes. *Complementary Therapies in Clinical Practice*;12(2): 119-125; May 2006.

Meisenhelder, J.B. & Chandler, E.N. (2000). Prayer and health outcomes in church members. *Altern. Ther. Health Med.*, 6(4): 56-60; Jul 2000.

Melancon, B. & Miller, L.H. (2005). Massage therapy versus traditional therapy for low back pain relief: implications for holistic nursing practice. *Holist Nurs Pract*, 19(3): 116-21;May-Jun 2005.

Menefee, L.A. & Monti, D.(2005).Nonpharmacologic and complementary approaches to cancer pain management . *The Journal of the American Osteopathic Association*, Vol.105, No.11 , pp.15-20.

Merskey, H. & Bogduk, N. (editors.).(1986). Pain, In:*Classification of chronic pain : description of chronic pain syndromes and definition of pain terms , Prepared by the İnternational Association for the study of Pain,(IASP), Subcommittee on Taxonomy*. Pain Suppl 3:S1–226., IASP Press, ISBN-13: 978-0-931092-05-3

Mollart, L. (2003). Single-Blind Trial Addressing the Differential Effects of Two Reflexology Techniques Versus Rest, On Ankle and Foot Oedema in Late Pregnancy. *Complementary Therapy in Nursing & Midwifery*, 9(4): 203-208; November 2003.

Moseikin, I.A . (2003). Use of biofeedback in combined treatment of low spine pain. *Zh Nevrol Psikhiatr Im S S Korsakova*, 103, 32-6.

Mucuk, S. & Başer, M. (2009). Doğum ağrısını hafifletmede kullanılan tensel uyarılma yöntemleri. Journal of Anatolia Nursing and Health Sciences, 12(3),61-66.

Musclow, SL.;Sawhney, M. & Watt-Watson, J. (2002). The emerging role of advanced nursing practice in acute pain management throughout Canada. *Clinical Nurse Specialist* 16(2):63-67.

Nash, R.; Yates, P.; Edwards, H.; Fentiman, B.; Dewar, A; Mcdowell, J. & Clark, R. (1999). Pain and administration of analgesia: what nurses say. *Journal of Clinical Nursing*, 1999; 8(2):180.

Nilsson, U.; Rawal, N.; Enqvist, B.& Unosson, M.(2003) Analgesia following music and therapeutic suggestions in the PACU in ambulatory surgery; a randomized controlled trial. *Acta Anaesthesiol Scand*;47(3):278-83.

Nixon, M. et al.(1997). Expanding the nursing repertoire: The effect of massage on post-operative pain .*Australian Journal of Advanced Nursing*, 14(3):21-26,March-May 1997.

Nordin, M. (2002). Self-care techniques for acute episodes of low-back pain. *Best Practice & Research Clinical Rheumatology*, 16(1): 89-101;Jan 2002.

Öztekin, İ. (2005). Bel ağrısı: Primer tedavide bütünleyici yaklaşım. *Akupunktur Dergisi*, 15(55-56): 7-11.

Petry, JJ.(2002). Surgery and complementary therapies: A review. *Alternative Therapies in Health and Medicine*,6(5):64-74.

Quattrin, R.; Zanini, A.; Buchini, S.; Turello, D.; Annunziata, M.A.; Vidotti, C.; Colombatti, A. & Brusaferro, S. (2006). Use of Reflexology Foot Massage to Reduce Anxiety in Hospitalized Cancer Patients in Chemotherapy Treatment: Methodology and Outcomes. *Journal of Nursing Management*, 14(2): 96-105; March 2006.

Rakel, B. & Frantz, R.(2003). Effectiveness Of Transcutaneous Electrıcal Nerve Stimulation On Postoperative Pain With Movement. *The Journal of Pain*, 4(8); 455-464.

Raynor, M.C.; Pietrobon, R.; Guller, U. & Higgins, L.D. (2005). Cryotherapy After ACL Reconstruction: a Meta Analysis. *J. Knee Surgery*, 18(2),123-9; Apr 2005.

Ross, S. & Soltes, D. (1995). Heparin and Haematoma: Does Ice Make a Difference?. *Journal of Advanced Nursing*, 21(3), 434-439; Mar 1995.

Saeki, Y. (2002). Effect of Local Application of Cold or Heat for Relief of Pricking Pain. *Nursing and Health Sciences*. 4(3):97-105; Sep 2002.

Sarifakioğlu, N. & Sarifakioğlu, E. (2004). Evaluating the Efffect of Ice Application on The Pain Felt During Botilinum Toxin Type-a Injections: a Prospective, Randomized, Single-blind, Controlled Trial. *Ann Plast Surg*, 53(6),543-546; Dec 2004.

Seers, K.& Carroll, D.(1998) Relaxation techniques for acute pain management : a sistematic review. Australian *Journal of Advanced Nursing*, 27(3)466-475,March 1998.

Sherman, K.J.; Cherkin, D.C.; Connelly, M.T.; Erro, J.; Savetsky, J.B. & Davis, R.B.(2004). Complementary and alternative medical therapies for chronic low back pain:What treatments are patient willing to try? *BMC Complement Altern Med, Jul 19;4-9.*

Simkin, P. & Bolding, A. (2004). Update on nonpharmacologic approaches to relieve labor pain and prevent suffering. *Journal of Midwifery & Women's Health*, 49 (6), 489- 504; Nov-Dec 2004.

Simkin, P.P.& O'Hara, M. (2002). Nonpharmacologic relief of pain during labor: systematic reviews of five methods, *American Journal of Obstetrics and Gynecology,* 186 (5 Suppl Nature):S131-159; May 2002.

Sluka, K.A. & Walsh, D. (2003). Transcutaneous Electrical Nevre Stimulation: Basic Science Mechanism and Clinical Effectiveness. *The Journal of Pain,* 4(3): 109-121. Apr 2003.

Snyder, M. & Wieland, J. (2003). Complementary and alternative therapies: What is their place in the management of chronic pain? *Nurs Clin North Am.* 38(3): 495-508; Sep 2003.

Stefano, G.B.; Zhu, W.; Cadet, P.; Salamon, E. & Mantione, K.J. (2004). Music alters constitutively expressed opiate and cytokine processes in Listeners. *Medical Science Monitor,* 10(6):18-27.

Stephenson, N.L.N.; Weinrich, S.P. & Tavakoli, A.S. (2000). The Effects of Foot Reflexology on Anxiety and Pain in Patients with Breast and Lung Cancer. *Oncol Nurs Forum,* 27(1):67-72.

Taşçı, E. & Sevil, Ü. (2007). Doğum ağrısına yönelik farmakolojik olmayan yaklaşımlar. *Genel Tıp Dergisi,* 17(3): 181-186.

Teyhen, D.S.; Miltenberger, C.E.; Deiters, H.M.; Del Toro, Y.M.; Pulliam, J.N. & Childs, J.D. (2005). The use of ultrasound imaging of the abdominal drawing-in maneuver in subjects with low back pain. *J Orthop Sports Phys Ther,* 35(6): 346-355;Jun 2005.

Tsay, S.L. & Chen, M.L.(2003). Acupressure and quality of sleep in patients with end- stage renal disease-a randomized controlled trial. *International Journal of Nursing Studies;* 40(1): 1-7; Jan 2003.

Tsay, S.L. ; Rong, J.R. & Lin, P.F.(2003). Acupoints massage in improving the quality of sleep and quality of life in patients with end-stage renal disease. *Journal of Advanced Nursing;* 42 (2): 134-142; April 2003.

Tseng, Y.H. (2005). Aromatherapy in nursing practice. *Hu Li Za Zhi,* 52(4):11-5;PMID 16088776.

Turan, N.; Öztürk, A. & Kaya, N.(2010).Hemsirelikte Yeni Bir Sorumluluk Alanı: Tamamlayıcı Terapi. *Maltepe Üniversitesi Hemsirelik Bilim ve Sanatı Dergisi,* 3(1):.93-98.

Uçan, Ö. & Ovayolu, N. (2007). Kanser ağrısının kontrolünde kullanılan nonfarmakolojik yöntemler. *Fırat Sağlık Hizmetleri Dergisi,* Vol.2 , No:4 , pp.123-131.

Van der Westhuijzen, A. J.; Becker, P.J.; Morkel, J. & Roelse, J.A. (2005). A Randomized Observer Blind Comparison of Bilateral Facial Ice Pack Therapy with No Ice Therapy Following Third Molar Surgery. *Int J Oral Maxillofac Surg,* 34(3): 281-286; May 2005.

Van Tulder, M.W.; Furlan A.D. & Gagnier J.J. (2005). Complementary and alternative therapies for low back pain. *Best Pract Res Clin Rheumatol,* 19(4): 639-654; Aug 2005.

Williams, K.A.; Petronis, J.; Smith, D.; Goodrich, D.; Wu J.; Ravi, N.; Doyle, E.J.; Juckett, G.; Kolar, M.M.; Gross, R. & Steinberg, L. (2005).Effect of Iyengar yoga therapy for chronic low back pain. *Pain;*115(1-2):107–17; May 2005

Wringht, S.; Courtney, U.; Donnelly, C.; Kenny, T.; Lavin, C. (2002). Clients'perceptions of the benefits of reflexology on their quality of life. *Complementary Therapy in Nursing & Midwifery,* 8(2): 69-76; May 2002.

Yavuz, M.(2006). Ağrıda Kullanılan Nonfarmakolojik Yöntemler, In: *Ağrı Doğası ve Kontrolü,* 1st edition , F.E. Aslan (Editor), , Vol.42, pp.135-147., Avrupa Tıp Kitapçılık Ltd. Şti. Bilim Yayınları, ISBN: 975-6257-17-2.

Yıldırım, Y.K. (2006).Kanser Ağrısının Nonfarmakolojik Yöntemlerle Kontrolü, In: *Kanser ve Palyatif Bakım,* In M. Uyar, R. Uslu, YK. Yıldırım, (Eds), pp.97-126; Meta Press Matbaacılık, İzmir.

Yıldırım, Y.K.; Fadıloğlu, Ç.& Uyar, M. (2006). Palyatif Kanser Bakımında Tamamlayıcı Tedaviler. *Ağrı,* 18(1), 26–32.

24

Overview of Collateral Meridian Therapy in Pain Management: A Modified Formulated Chinese Acupuncture

Chih-Shung Wong[1], Chun-Chang Yeh[2] and Shan-Chi Ko[3]
[1]*Department of Anaesthesiology, Cathay General Hospital, Taipei,*
[2]*Department of Anaesthesiology, Tri-Service General Hospital, Taipei,*
[3]*Painless Hospital, Ginza, Tokyo,*
[1,2]*Taiwan*
[3]*Japan*

1. Introduction

The Western approach to pain management is focused on the use of pharmacotherapy, physical therapy, nerve blocks, nerve ablations, implantable devices. Even though increasing of understanding of the mechanisms of pain for the treatments; some pains remain intractable (Hariharan et al, 2007; Wagner et al, 2007; Laxmaiah et al, 2009). In contrast, traditional Chinese medicine (TCM) centres primarily on the energy relationship among the environment and the body and organs, without a clear understanding of pathophysiology or the mechanisms of diseases and its effects are varied and inconsistent. The collateral meridian therapy (CMT), offers an alternative treatment for different types of pain by taking a systematic approach to a variant of traditional Chinese acupuncture (TCA). Here, we highlight the recent development of CMT by describing the main theory, discussing the differences between CMT and TCA, defining abbreviations associated with CMT, explaining acupoint localization principles, and providing clinical reports for application in pain management.

2. The theory behind CMT

To achieve an understanding of CMT, it is necessary to revisit the modality on which it is based. In TCA, it is believed that the manipulation of certain points on the skin can affect the movement of energy, or "Qi", throughout the body. It is assumed that "Qi" flows in channels, or meridians, along the body, and that good health is maintained through balancing the circulation of Qi along these channels. In TCA, there are 12 established meridians. On these 12 meridians, a total 361 acupoints are located through which the flow of Qi can be manipulated. The selection of points for treatment, following the "one-needle effect", where therapeutic effect is obtained from manipulation of one strong acupoint, is based on the nature of the disease treated as defined by the five-element theory of TCM, and by a number of personal factors. As a result, the treatment for disease is changed on a case-by-case basis. There has no standard method; the effectiveness of TCA varies from patient to patient.

In CMT, however, two acuponts are manipulated, instead of one. The meridian lines are the same as in TCA, but each meridian has only nice standard acuponits (a total of 108). Two acupoints are used for redirection the flow of Qi from one meridian to another. As such, in CMT, the points selected for treatment are commonly on non-diseased meridians. CMT also follows the use of a standardized set of protocol for treatment, instead of the individual varied treatments given in TCA. The two points manipulated are known as control C-point and functional F-point. These points are specific to each meridian and allow the flow of Qi to be linked from the diseased meridian to a healthy one.

2.1 Two-point theory: C-point and F-point

The C-point is used to connect the diseased meridian and the healthy meridian. In treatment, practitioners manipulate the healthy meridian to relieve the pain or symptoms. Obstructed energy Qi is allowed to flow from the lesion site to the unobstructed healthy meridian, through which the disease will be discharged. Each meridian has its own C-point. For the location of C-points, please see figures 1 and 2. For the abbreviations and anatomical definition of C-points, please see table 1. The C-point is for linking the diseased meridian to the treatment meridian, and the F-point is for the treatment of the disease symptom or painful location. The F-points in the different regions of the body are shown in figure 3. Each region of pain or disease in the body is represented by its own F-point. For instance, if the patient had pain in the neck of shoulder, the practitioner should select "a" as an F-point for treatment (Fig. 3). If a patient has an acute lumbar strain, the F-point over the lumbar L4-5 region would be "4"; the F-point over the lumbar L3-4 region would be "5" (Fig. 3).

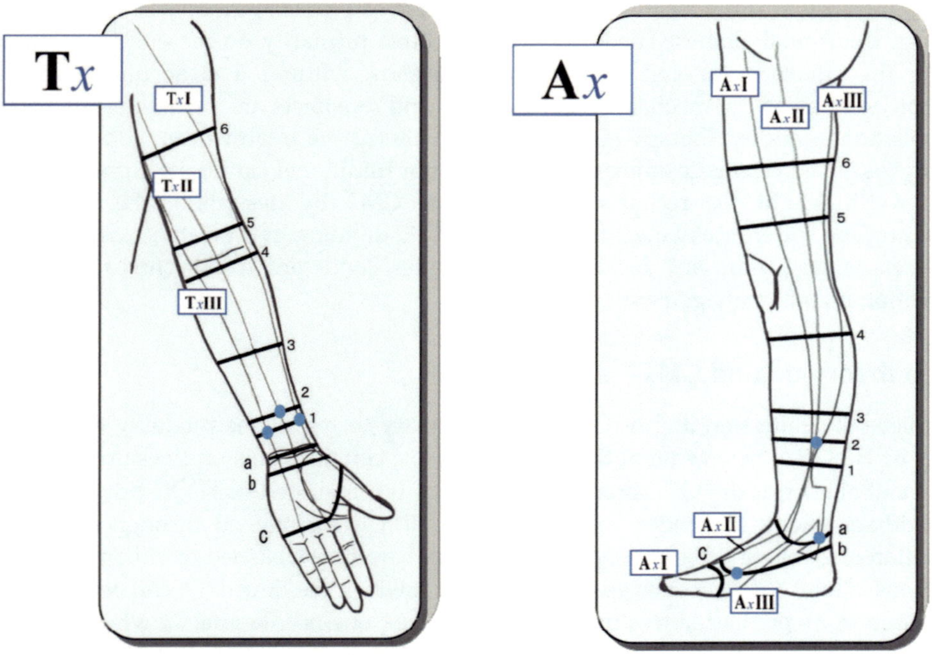

Fig. 1. The numbers 6, 5, 4, 3, 2, 1 and letters a, b, c are the treatment function points of six yin meridians. The blue points indicated control-point of each yin meridian (1, 2, and 1 for TxI, TxII, TxIII; b, 2 and a for AxI, AxII, AxIII).

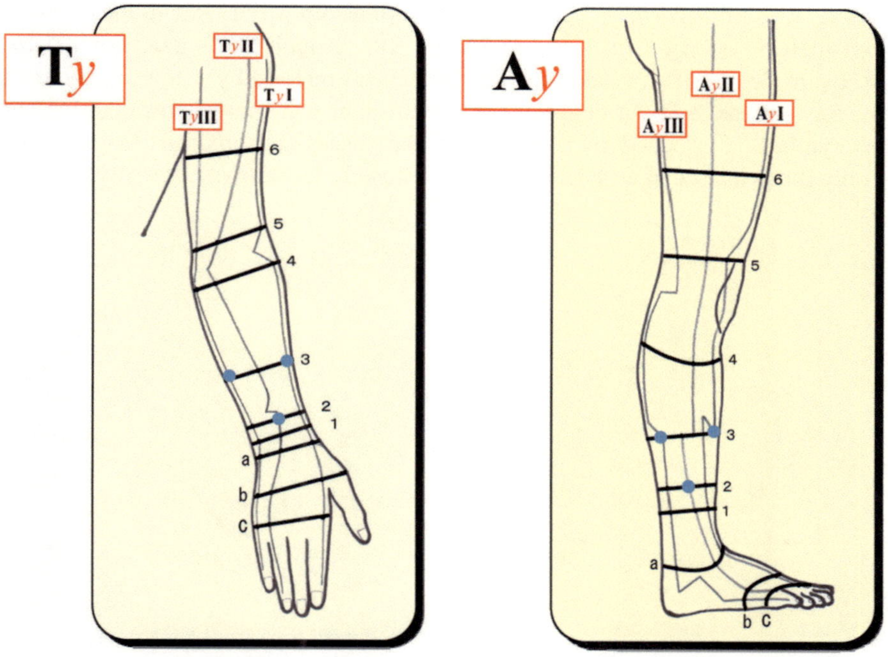

Fig. 2. The numbers 6, 5, 4, 3, 2, 1 and letters a, b, c are the treatment function points of six yin meridians. The blue points indicated control-point of each yang meridian (3, 2, and 3 for both TyI, TyII, TyIII and AyI, AyII, AyIII).

2.2 Abbreviations in CMT

The abbreviations used in CMT are defined as follows: "T" represents the upper extremity (Te is the pronunciation of "arm" in Japanese); "A" represents the lower extremity (Ashi is the pronunciation of "leg" in Japanese); the roman numerals, I, II and III represent the meridians on the radial, median and unlar side of the upper extremities, and the meridians on the anterior, medial (or lateral), and posterior aspect on the lower extremities, respectively. The use of "x" symbolizes the yin aspect, and use of "y" denotes the yang aspect of the extremities. Each extremity had nine acupoints in which point a, b and c are located on the hand or foot, and point 1 to 6 are located on the arm or leg (Figs. 1 and 2). The letters "r" and "l" represent the right and left side of the limb, respectively. For example, "lTyI" describes a meridian on the dorsal aspect (y) of the radial side (I) of the left (l) upper extremity (T) (see Fig. 8a).

2.3 How CMT identifies the diseased meridian and formulates a treatment protocol

For the purpose of simplicity, the symbols "/", "()" and "." are used to describe diseased or treatment meridians. For example, if the diseased region is over the right wrist (corresponding to "a", Fir. 3) of the TyI meridian, it is represented by rTyI/a. If the treatment meridian selected is lTxI/1:a, then constant pressure is applied on the C-point "1' of the lTxI meridian (Fig. 1), while a "remove" manoeuvre at the corresponding "a" point is simultaneously performed on the lTxI meridian. The letter "1" before ":" signifies the C-point of the lTxI meridian, while the letter "a" after ":" expresses the F-point "a". T denote a supplement or enhancement manoeuvre, place "()" around "a" to make the treatment formula lTxI/1:a); otherwise, "a" without "()" represents a removal manoeuvre on point "a". When there is no need to use the C-point, the symbol "0" is used for the treatment meridian. Examples of cases where no C-point is used included yin to yin or yang to yang meridians for namesake (T-A) links, or for the original meridian manipulation. Therefore, the colon symbol ":" is used to differentiate the diseased from the treatment meridian because only the presence of an F-point on the diseased meridian is necessary.

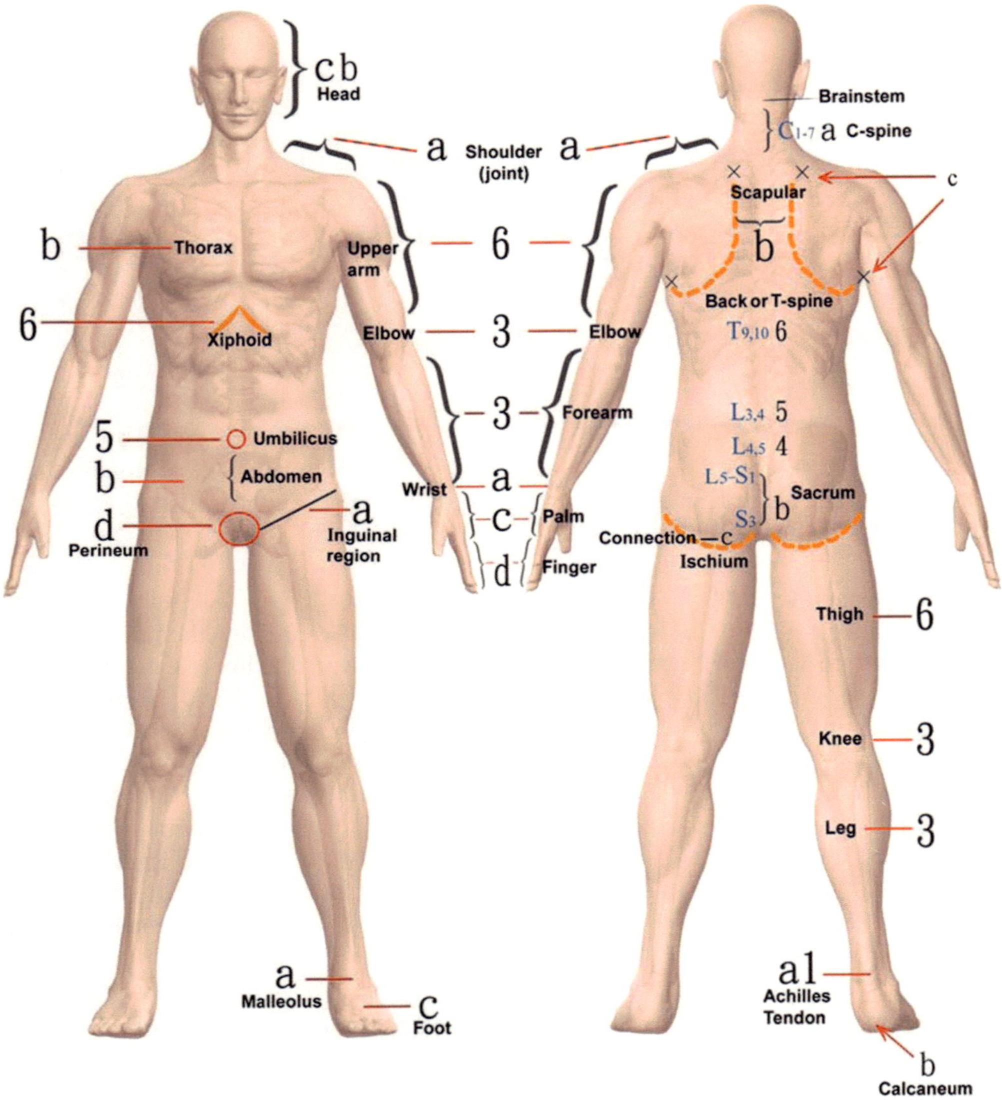

Fig. 3. This figure indicates specific body regions corresponding to F-points. The unique "d" system, different form the ordinary 9-point (6, 5, 4, 3, 2, 1, a, b, c) system on the treatment meridians, corresponds to intracranial, perineum and digits. al: the most painful point between point-a and point-1 on the treatment meridian, ac: the most painful point between point-c and point-b on the treatment meridian.

2.4 How CMT links to channel Qi and diverts the body flow in the meridians

The C-point ensures the link to channel Qi from the diseased meridian to the healthy one. Four different types of links are available to channel Qi: 1) Zang-Fu (TA-xy). 2) Exterior-Interior (x-y), 3) Namesake (T-A), and 4) Original meridian links (Fig. 4). The selection of treatment from the diseased meridian is shown in Figure 4. Zang-Fu (TA-xy) is the most common link for treatment. For example, if the diseased meridian is AxI, the treatment meridian is TyIII (TA-xy link) and vice versa. The determination of the treatment meridian, whether ipsilateral or contralateral, is based on the location of the lesion, as shown in Figure 5. For example, if the diseased meridian is rAyI, the treatment meridian is TxII (according to the TA-xy link in Fig. 4). Figure 5 shows that the treatment side for the TxII meridian is contralateral side to the diseased meridian; thus the left side is selected as the treatment side. Figure 6 illustrates the usage of the C-point to link the diseased meridian (rAyI) to the lTxII meridian by the TA-xy link (visceral Znag-Fu link) for treatment, acting as an area of energy discharge. By simultaneously manipulating the C-point and the F-point that corresponds to the painful site, the pain in rAyI will flow to lTxII, and the pain will be removed or reduced by manipulating the functional F-point pressed against the body flow direction (yin meridian). Similarly for the lAyIII or rAyIII problem in post-regional anesthesia/analgesia backache, the treatment meridian will be chosen as rTxI or lTxI (Yeh et al, 2009). Most acupoints are located along the edge of the bony shaft or on the tendinomuscular grooves. The accurate localization of the acupoint can be achieved through patient reports of soreness or painful sensation when the area is pressed deeply. For detailed anatomical localization of acupoints, please refer to 10b, and book by Ko and Chao (2007).

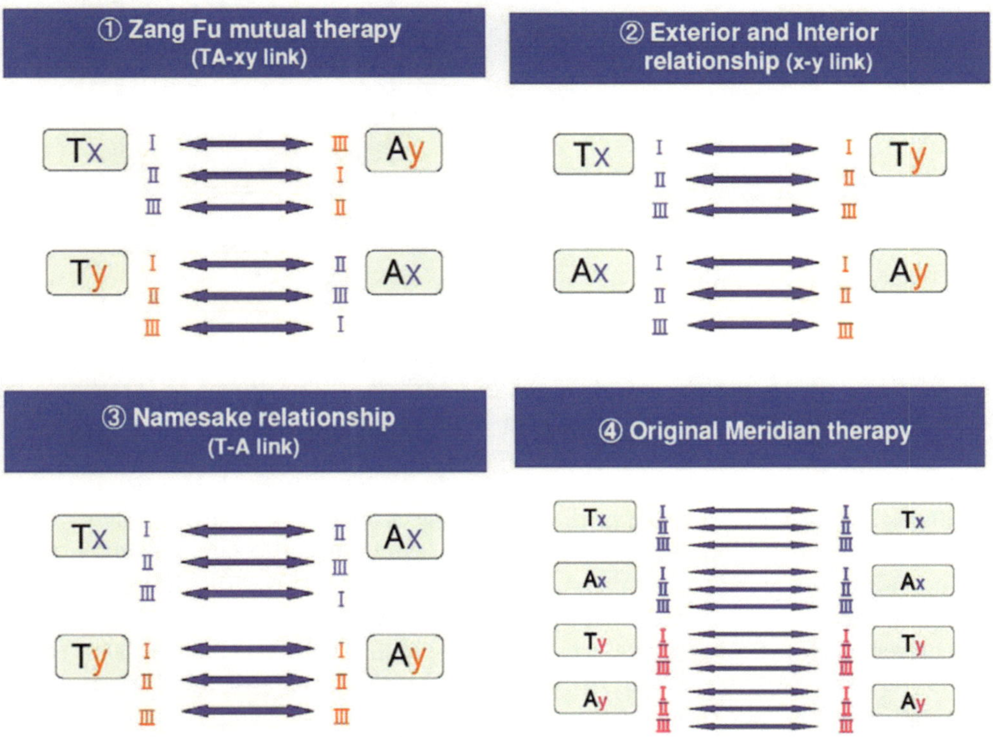

Fig. 4. The four types of links used to choose the treatment meridian.

<table>
<tr><th></th><th colspan="2">Yin (x)</th><th colspan="2">Yang (y)</th></tr>
<tr><td rowspan="3">T
Upper
limbs</td><td>I</td><td rowspan="2">contralateral</td><td>I</td><td>contralateral</td></tr>
<tr><td>II</td><td>II</td><td rowspan="5">ipsilateral</td></tr>
<tr><td>III</td><td>Ipsilateral</td><td>III</td></tr>
<tr><td rowspan="3">A
Lower
limbs</td><td>I</td><td rowspan="3">contralateral</td><td>I</td></tr>
<tr><td>II</td><td>II</td></tr>
<tr><td>III</td><td>III</td></tr>
</table>

Fig. 5. Determination to choose contralateral or ipsilateral side or ipsilateral side of treatment meridian. For yin meridians used as the treatment ones to divert the obstructed flow, all of them must choose the opposite side to the diseased meridian, except for TxIII. On the other hand, for yang meridians used, all must choose the same side as the diseased meridian, except for TyI.

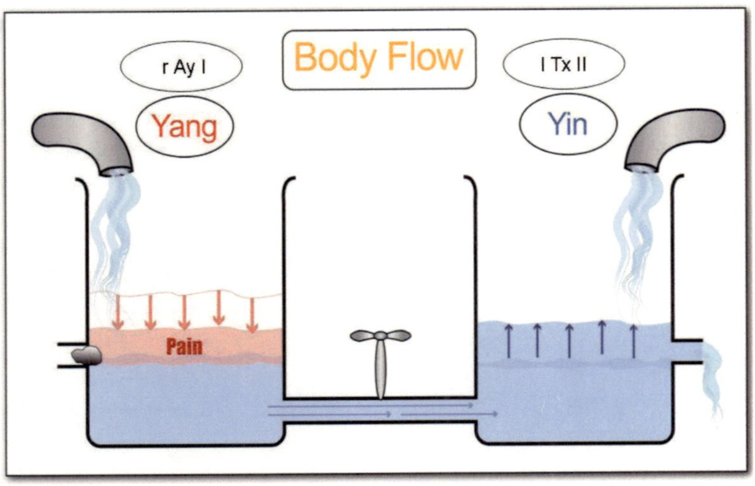

Fig. 6. Illustratin of the proposed mechanism of pain reduction.

2.5 Clinical reports for application in pain management

Case studies have shown the effectiveness of CMT on the treatment of intractable pain (Wong et al, 2006). Patients suffering from intricate chronic pain, such as post-herpetic neuralgia and complex regional pain syndrome, are responded dramatically to the CMT treatment (Wong et al, 2007). Moreover, CMT is also observed effectively on local musculoskeletal pain that resulted from such injuries as sprains or strains and demonstrated positive effect on shoulder pain relief after laparcoscopic surgery (Yeh et al, 2008). CMT is also an effect technique to reduce painful dysmenorrhea (Lin et al, 2010). Moreover, CMT is also highly effective in the treatment of post-neuraxial block backache in patients who were failed to treated by the conventional treatment (Yeh et al, 2009). Over the post few years, Dr. Ko and his team have repeatedly demonstrated positive results of this therapy through workshops, courses and pain clinics throughout Japan., Taiwan, Singapore and the United States (Hoka et al, 2008). A mini-symposium on CMT was also offered in the 13th World Society of Pain Clinicians Congress for the World Institute of Pain Meeting in 2008.

Meridian in CMT	Meridian in TCA	C-Point	Actual anatomical location
TxI	Lung	1	On the junction of the metaphysis and diaphysis over the distal radius. The pressure should be applied on the radial side of the flexor carbi radialis directly on the bone; pressure to the radial artery should be avoided (Fig. 7a).
TxII	Pericardia	2	Approximately three finger breadths proximal to the TxI/a (Fig. 7b).
TxIII	Heart	1	On the radial depression of the flexor carbi ulnaris at the junction of the metaphysis and diaphysis over the distal ulna (Fig. 7a).
AxI	Spleen	b	On the tangent line to the plantar-medial depression at the junction of the metaphysis and diaphysis over the proximal end of first metatarsal bone (Fig. 9a, b).
AxII	Liver	2	Approximately 1 cm posterior to the AxI/2 at the same horizontal level as AxI/2 (Fig. 9a).
AxIII	Kidney	a	On the tangent line to the posterior border of the medial malleolus (Fig. 9a).
TyI	Large Intestine	3	On the tangent line to the ulnar side of the radius at the musculotendinous junction (Fig. 8a).
TyII	Triple Energizer	2	Between the distal ulna and radius about one-sixth of the distance above TyII/a toward the olecranon (approximately three finger breadths proximal to TyII/a) (Fig. 8b).
TyIII	Small Intestine	3	On the tangent line to the radial border of the dorsal ulna at the musculotendinous junction (Fig. 8a).
AyI	Stomach	3	At the same horizontal level as AyIII/3, approximately one finger breadth posterior to the anterior crest of the tibia (Fig. 10a).
AyII	Gall Bladder	2	On the tangent line to the anterior border of the fibula at the same horizontal level as AyIII/3 (Fig. 10a).
AyIII	Bladder	3	First identify the Chinese traditional acupoint BL57 (Chengshan), which is in the depression below the belly of the gastrocnemius when the leg is stretched or the heel is lifted. After pressing BL57, find two lines running from it lateroinferiorly and medioinferiorly; AyIII/3 point is at the lateroinferior end on the tangent line to the posterior surface of the fibula (Fig. 10a, b).

CMT: Collateral Meridian Therapy; TCA: Traditional Chinese Acupuncture

Table 1. Anatomical location of C-points.

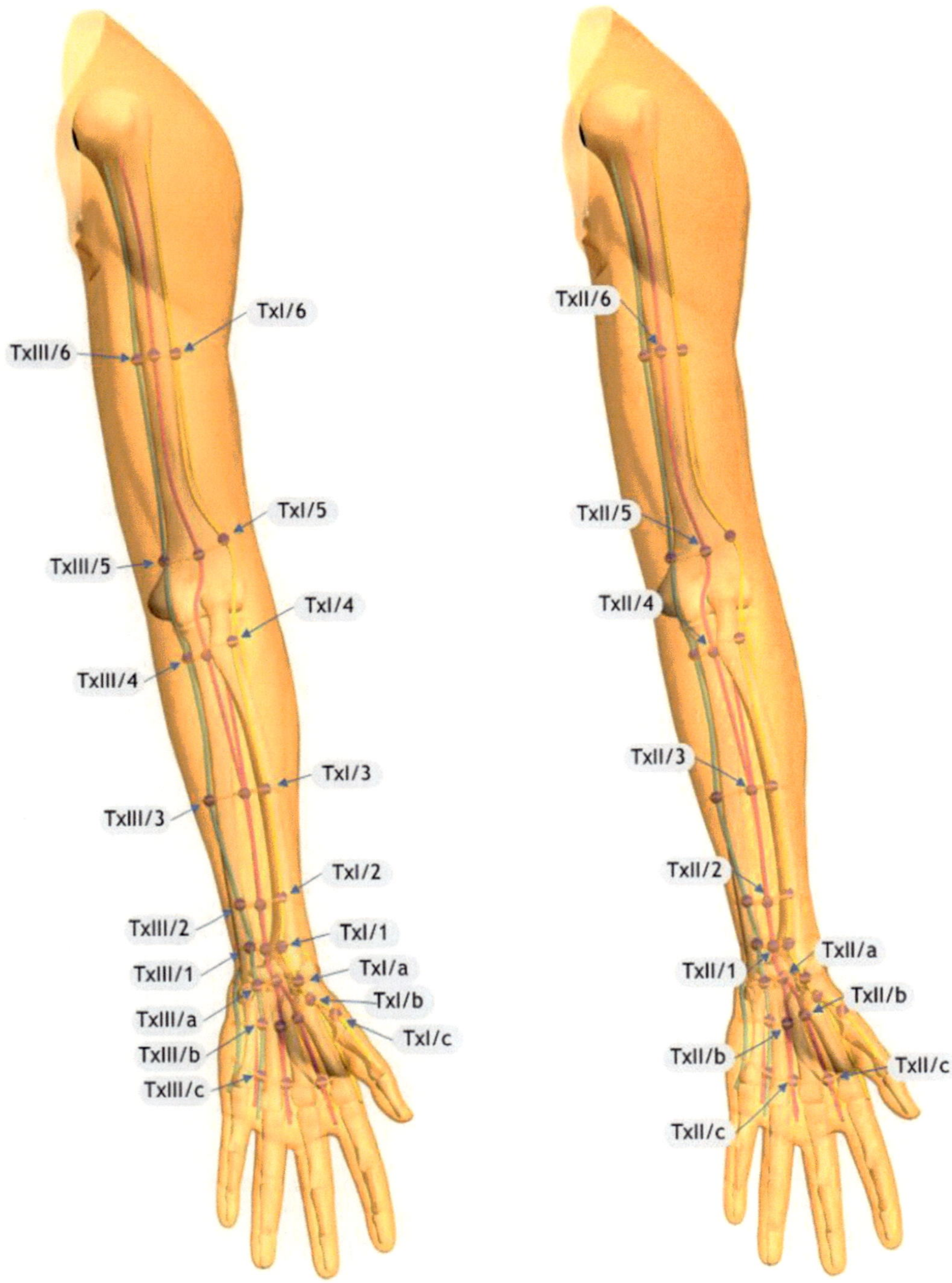

Fig. 7. (a) Volar view of upper extremity for localization of acupoints on TxI and TxIII. (b) Volar view of upper extremity for localization of acupoints on TxII.

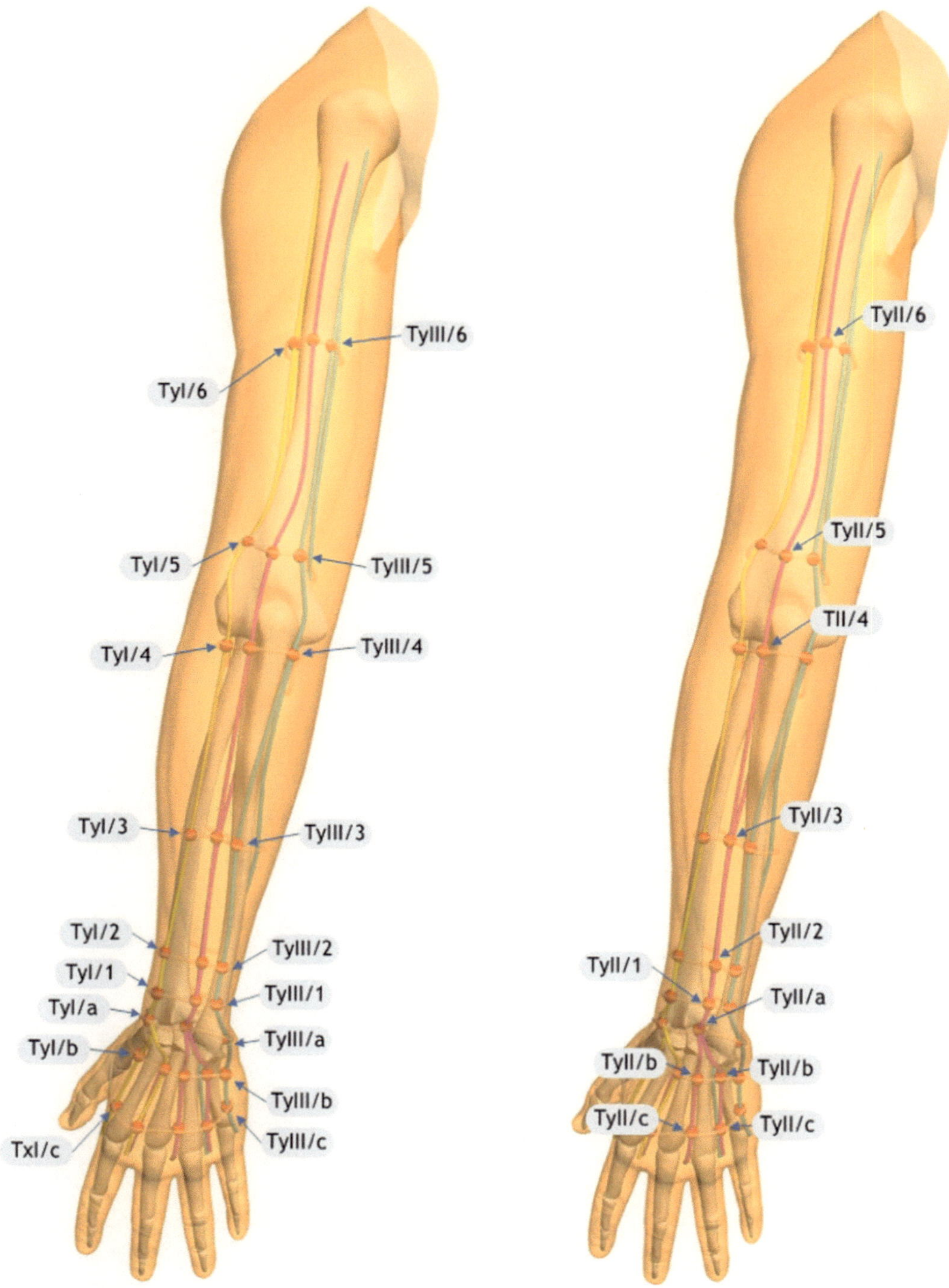

Fig. 8. (a) Dorsal view of upper extremity for localization of acupoints on TyI and TyIII. (b) Dorsal view of upper extremity for localization of acupoints on TyII.

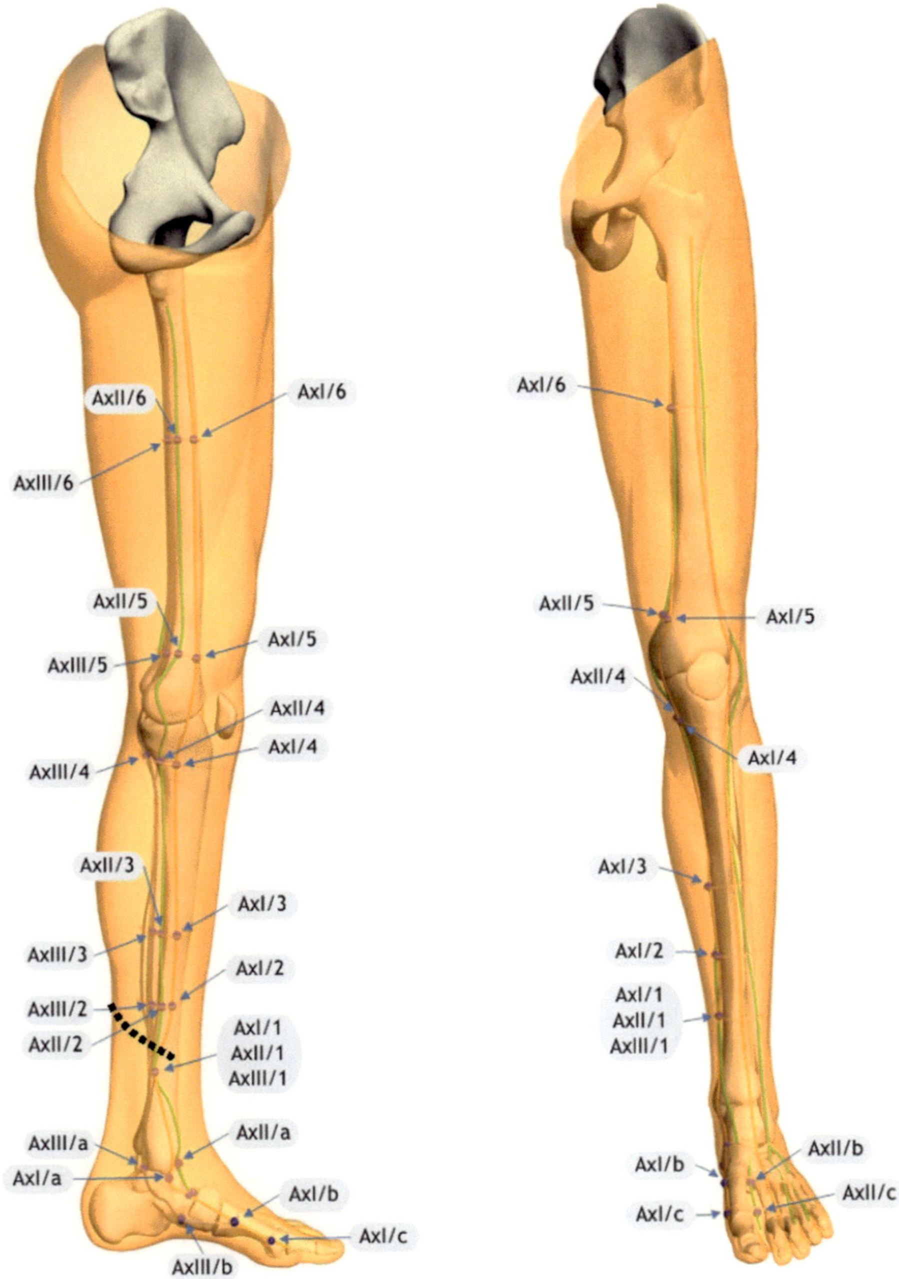

Fig. 9. (a) Medial view of lower extremity for localization of acupoints on AxI and most of AxII and AxIII (except for AxII/b AxII/c and AxIII/c). (b) Anterior view of lower extremity for localization of on AxI and AxII. The dotted line is extended along the curve of the lower border of the medial gastrocnemius belly.

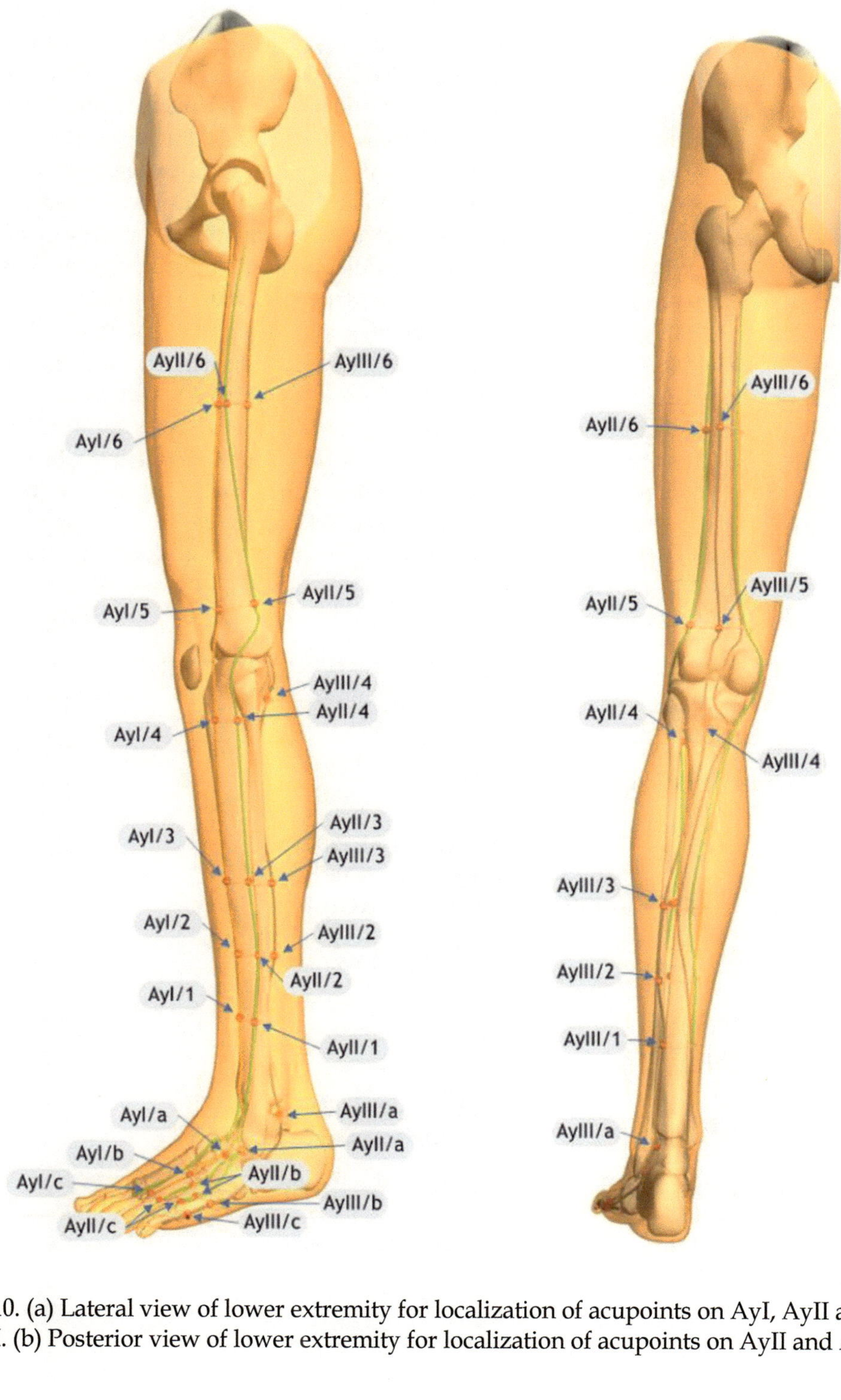

Fig. 10. (a) Lateral view of lower extremity for localization of acupoints on AyI, AyII and AyIII. (b) Posterior view of lower extremity for localization of acupoints on AyII and AyIII.

The National Institute of Health consensus, published in 1998, states that acupuncture shows effectiveness in the treatment of postoperative and chemotherapy induced nausea and vomiting and postoperative dental pain. The statement concludes that acupuncture may be useful in other conditions, including myofascial pain, osteoarthritis, low back pain, menstrual cramps and so on. In addition, we conducted a MEDLINE search and found that acupuncture therapy is also effective for low back pain (LBP) and myofascial pain. From prospective randomized controlled trials published in the peer-reviewed medical literature after 1998, we summarize the acupoints/meridians use for TCA and CMT in the management of LBP in table 2. According to the rules that we have introduced in this article, we can choose the corresponding healthy meridian and formats a set of acupoints for the treatment of LBP, whereas in TCA, one usually uses the diseased meridian, with different acupoints chosen in different reports (Ezzo et al, 2001; Leibing et al, 2002; Meng et al, 2004; Trinh et al, 2007; Wang et al, 2008; Yeh et al; 2009). Based on our literature review, patients with LBP received at lease short-term pain relief after TCA treatment; the CMT also provides significant pain relief via different approach with a standardized formulated protocol. Table 3 shows as summary of published CMT clinical reports for different types of pain (Wong et al, 2006; 2007; Hoka, 2008; Yeh et al, 2008; 2009, Lin et al, 2010). Furthermore to date, no clinical reports described the use of TCA to treat complex regional pain syndrome which patients may not tolerate the direct stimulation/acupuncture to the painful area. In contrast, CMT provides a promising technique for treating complex regional pain syndrome that can be used without touching the painful sites (Wong et al, 2007; Hoka, 2008).

Meridian	TCM [ref]	CMT [ref]
Governing vessel meridian	(+) Wang et al (2008) Leibing et al (2002)	
Urinary bladder meridian (AyIII)	(+) Wang et al (2008) Leibing et al (2002) Meng et al (2004) Ezzo et al (2001) Trinh et al (2007)	
Lung meridian (TxI)		(+) Yeh et al (2008)
Heart meridian (TxIII)		(+) Yeh et al (2008)
Spleen meridian (AxI)	(+) Wang et al (2008) Carlsson & Sjolund (2001)	
Large intestine meridian (TyI)	(+) Wang et al (2008)	

TCM: traditional Chinese medicine; CMT: collateral meridian therapy. (+): treatment meridian. Number: reference number.

Table 2. Acupunture points/meridians used for TCM and CMT in the management of low back pain and lumbar myofascial pain syndrome

First author (year) [Ref]	Condition treated	Post intervention	
		Pain reduction	Physical function recovery
Wong et al (2006)	Acute and chronic intractable pain	+	+
Lin et al (2010)	Primary dysmenorrhea	+	–
Wong et al (2007)	Complex regional pain syndrome	+	+
Hoka et al (2008)	Complex regional pain syndrome	+	+
Yeh et al (2008)	Shoulder-tip pain	+	+
Yeh et al (2009)	Post-regional anesthesia/analgesia backache	+	+

CMT, collateral meridian therapy. +, Yes; –, Not observed

Table 3. Clinical reports of CMT for pain management

3. Conclusion

CMT provides a different approach for managing intractable pain and various illnesses. It may play a role in the field of complementary and alternative medicine. The role of CMT in pain management looks promising for both acute and chronic pain, even including intractable pains, even though published randomized controlled trials are so far lacking. It is our hope that future research can focus on methodologically strong randomized controlled trials to validate the efficacy of CMT with high evidence level. The purpose of this article is to introduce the theory of CMT to interest physicians to achieve a greater awareness and understanding of this technique and theory.

4. Acknowledgment

The authors thank the Ko Medical System Inc. for providing the illustrations and figures for this chapter.

5. References

Carlsson C, Sjolund B. Acupuncture for chronic low back pain: a randomized placebo-controlled study with long-term follow-up. *Clin J Pain* 2001, 17:296-305.

Ezzo J, Hadhazy V, Birch S, Lao L, Kaplan G, Hochberg M, Berman B. Acupuncture for osteoarthritis of the knee: a systematic review. *Arthr Rheum* 2001, 44:819-25.

Hariharan J, Lamb GC, Neuner JM. Long-Term Opioid Contract Use for Chronic Pain Management in Primary Care Practice. A Five Year Experience. J of Gen Intern Med 2007, 22: 485-490.

Hoka S, Kanai A, Ko SC, Suzuki A. Collateral Meridian Therapy Alleviates Intractable Pain and Disablity in CRPS Patients. *ASA meeting* 2008: A904 .

Ko SC, Chao HR. Atlas of Ko medicine pressure points. (ISBN:978-986-83890-0-7, 2007)

Laxmaiah M, Mark VB, Vijay S, Ramsin M. B, Bert F, Salahadin A, Ricardo M B, Ann C, Sukdeb D, Richard D, Frank JE F, Stephanie E, Sudhir D, Salim M. H, Standiford H, Allan T. P, David M S, Howard S S, Lee R W, Joshua A H. Interventional techniques: evidence-based practice guidelines in the management of chronic spinal pain. *Pain Physician* 2009; 12: 699-802.

Leibing E, Leonhardt U, Koster G, Goerlitz A, Rosenfeldt J, Hilgers R, Ramadori G. Acupuncture treatment of chronic low-back pain- a randomized, blinded, placebo-controlled trial with 9-month follow up. *Pain* 2002, 96:189-196.

Lin JA, Wong CS, Lee MS, Ko SC, Chan SM, Chen JJY, Chen TL. Successful treatment of primary dysmenorrhea by collateral meridian acupressure therapy - a time series case report. *J Manipulative Physiol Ther* 2010, 33:70-5.

Meng C, Wang D, Ngeow J, Lao L, Peterson M, Paget S. Acupuncture for chronic low back pain through adjuvant electrical versus manual auricular acupuncture. *Anesth Analg* 2004, 98:1359-64.

Trinh K, Graham N, Gross A, Goldsmith C, Wang E, Careron I, Kay T. Acupuncture for neck pain disorder. *Spine* 2007, 32:236-43.

Wagner E, Ehrenhofer B, Lackerbauer E, Pawelak U, Siegmeth W. Rehabilitation of non-specific low back pain. Results of a multidisciplinary in-patient program. Schmerz 2007, 21: 228-33.

Wang SM, Kain ZN, White PF. Acupuncture Analgesia: II. Clinical Considerations. *Anesth Analg* 2008, 106:611-21.

Wong CS, Kuo CP, Ko SC. Can we do better, in addition to the pharmacological treatment, on pain: collateral meridian therapy. *Acta Anaesthesiol Taiwanica* 2006, 44:59-60.

Wong CS, Kuo CP, Fan YM, Ko SC. Collateral meridian therapy dramatically attenuates pain and improves functional activity of a patient with complex regional pain syndrome. *Anesth Analg* 2007, 104:452.

Yeh CC, Ko SC, Huh BK, Kuo CP, Wu CT, Cherng CH, Wong CS. Shoulder-tip pain following laparoscopic surgery analgesia by collateral meridian acupressure (shiatsu) therapy—report of two cases. *J Manipul Physiol Therap* 2008, 31:484-8.

Yeh CC, Wu CT, Huh BK, Lee SM, Wong CS. Collateral Meridian Acupressure Therapy Effectively Relieves Post-Regional Anesthesia/Analgesia Backache –The Report of Five Cases. *South Med J* 2009, 102:1179-1182.

Part 7

Nursing and Pain

25

When Theoretical Knowledge Is Not Enough: Introduction of an Explanatory Model on Nurse's Pain Management

Katrin Blondal[1] and Sigridur Halldorsdottir[2]
[1]*Landspitali -National University Hospital of Iceland, University of Iceland, School of Health Sciences, Faculty of Nursing, Reykjavik,*
[2]*School of Health Sciences, University of Akureyri, Akureyri, Iceland*

1. Introduction

Relieving the suffering of patients is a paramount responsibility for all health professionals. The fact that hospitalised patients still suffer from pain despite increasing technology and a wealth of research during recent decades, calls for an audit and new approaches in pain management. Nurses are professionally responsible for pain assessment and the administration of analgesia and are often considered the key persons in the management of pain. However, for many reasons nurses are unable to achieve the desired results of pain relief. Our study on nurses' experiences of caring for patients in pain indicates that previous studies in this field have often been limited to isolated aspects of pain management (Blondal & Halldorsdottir, 2009). Furthermore, they have been rather negative towards nurses. Our position is that many researchers have not appreciated the complexity of the nurse's multifaceted assignment of caring for patients in pain. We suggest that knowledge, in this respect, may often have been too narrowly defined. We challenge statements that propose that nurses do not believe that pain relief is a priority for nurses (Brockopp et al., 1998) or their responsibility (Twycross, 2002). Successful pain relief may provide satisfaction for the nurses involved (Blondal & Halldorsdottir, 2009), which is a rarely identified outcome by means of professional achievements. Various research results indicate that nurses' knowledge is less than adequate (Howell et al., 2000; Kuuppelomäki; 2002a; Van Niekerk & Martin, 2002). Therefore, the main methods that have previously been employed in order to improve nurses' performance and to achieve better pain control are formal education about pain assessment and the use of pain medication. Interestingly, programmes that aim at increasing this knowledge, however, often fail to help in diminishing patients' pain. Some programmes may demonstrate changes in practice (e.g. Carr, 2002) where other findings are contradictory regarding their effectiveness, indicating that the effect of nurses' re-education is not maintained over time (Howell et al., 2000) and that more theoretical knowledge does not necessarily correlate with patients reporting less pain (Watt-Watson et al., 2001). Furthermore, Wilson's (2007) survey on nurses' knowledge of pain also indicates that nurses may be incapable of managing pain, despite their knowledge of the existence of the patients' pain. It is, therefore, important to search for other explanations for inadequate pain management of nurses. Therefore, perhaps other patterns of knowledge are needed in addition to the often traditional emphasis on formal education about pain assessment and analgesics.

1.1 Aim of the theory

Theory is the acknowledged foundation to practise methodology, professional identity and the growth of formalized knowledge. Practice must not only be evidence based but also theory based. Hence, pain management must be theory based because theories serve as a broad framework for practice and may also articulate the goals of a profession and its core values. Our aim was to develop a theory, an explanatory model, which can explain nurses' complex task of pain management.

2. Methodology

In our evaluation of the various methods for this theory development we found *theory synthesis* as described by Walker and Avant (2004) a good method for constructing our explanatory model. They posit that more theory synthesis is needed to advance practice disciplines so we found a perfect fit. In the theory synthesis the theorists combine isolated pieces of information that may even be theoretically unconnected. Theory synthesis entails constructing a theory from study findings and scholarly writings, which may be numerous. It enables the theorist to organise and integrate a large number of findings into a single theory which can be presented as a model. The theory put forth in this chapter is based on 11 study findings, e.g. on our own phenomenological study on nurses' experience of taking care of patients in pain and ten other research findings from various researchers about: nursing advocacy; moral obligation; organisational barriers; patient based hindrances; and the nurse-doctor relationship (see Table 1). All these different studies helped us to clarify the manifold task of a nurse's pain management. This method can be compared with painting a picture where in step one the picture is drawn and step two (the literature in this case) is used to compare the "picture" drawn with other similar "pictures" for confirmation and clarification. In step three the picture is presented (Figure 1).

3. Findings

The theory provides a holistic view of the complicated task of relieving pain. The main tenets of this theory are: *the role of the nurses as the patient's advocates, multiple patterns of knowledge* and *the doctor-nurse relationship*. The theory is introduced in the form of an exploratory model which illustrates the main tenets, how they interact and how other aspects simultaneously mould nurses' actions and reactions while taking care of patients in pain (Figure 1).

3.1 The explanatory model

To understand and explain the nurses' central role of caring for patients in pain and their potential for providing adequate pain management, their position may be portrayed as that of *patients' advocates* (Mallik, 1997) within a goal-directed mission aimed at patients' pain relief. In figure 1, this journey is presented in an explanatory model where its main tenets have been arranged into a figure with a definite beginning and an end from top to bottom. As may be seen from the four central tenets of the model, acting as *patient's advocate, moral obligation, formal and tacit knowledge, knowing persons* and *the system,* initially dominate, followed by the concepts of *internal and external hindrances,* as well as *potential outcomes.*

Authors, published	Research	Participants, N	Data collection
Blondal & Halldorsdottir, 2009	The challenge of caring for patients in pain: from the nurse's perspective	Nurses caring for patients with pain in hospital wards, N= 10	20 in-depth interviews
De Schepper et. al, 1997	Feelings of powerlessness in relation to pain: ascribed causes and reported strategies	Community nurses caring for cancer patients with pain, N= 24	13 individual and 3 group interviews
Jenks, 1993	The pattern of personal knowing in nurse clinical decision making	Nurses working in various hospital settings, N= 23	Four focus groups/ participant observation
Kuuppelomäki, 2002	Pain management problems in patients' terminal phase as assessed by nurses in Finland	Nurses on inpatient wards of 32 municipal health centres, N= 328	Questionnaire and an open end question
Mallik, 1997	Advocacy in nursing – perceptions of practising nurses	Experienced nurses from various settings, N= 104	Focus group interviews
Malloy et al, 2009	Culture and organizational climate: nurses' insights into their relationship with physicians	Nurses from various settings in 4 countries, N= 42	Focus groups
Nagy, 1999	Strategies used by burns nurses to cope with the infliction of pain on patients	Nurses within paediatric and adult burn units, N= 32	84 unstructured interviews
Nash et al., 1999	Pain and the administration of analgesia: what nurses say	Registered nurses and BSc nursing students in acute and community settings, N= 19	Three focus group interviews
Oberle & Hughes, 2001	Doctors' and nurses' perceptions of ethical problems in end-of-life decisions	7 doctors and 14 nurses working in acute care adult medical-surgical areas, N= 21	Unstructured interviews
O'Connor & Kelly, 2005	Bridging the gap: a study of general nurses' perceptions of patient advocacy in Ireland	Practicing nurses in hospitals, N= 20	3 focus group interviews
Van Niekerk & Martin, 2002	The impact of the nurse-physician professional relationship on nurses' experience of ethical dilemmas in effective pain management	Nurses within public and private settings, N= 1,015	Questionnaire

Table 1. Key research used to develop the theory

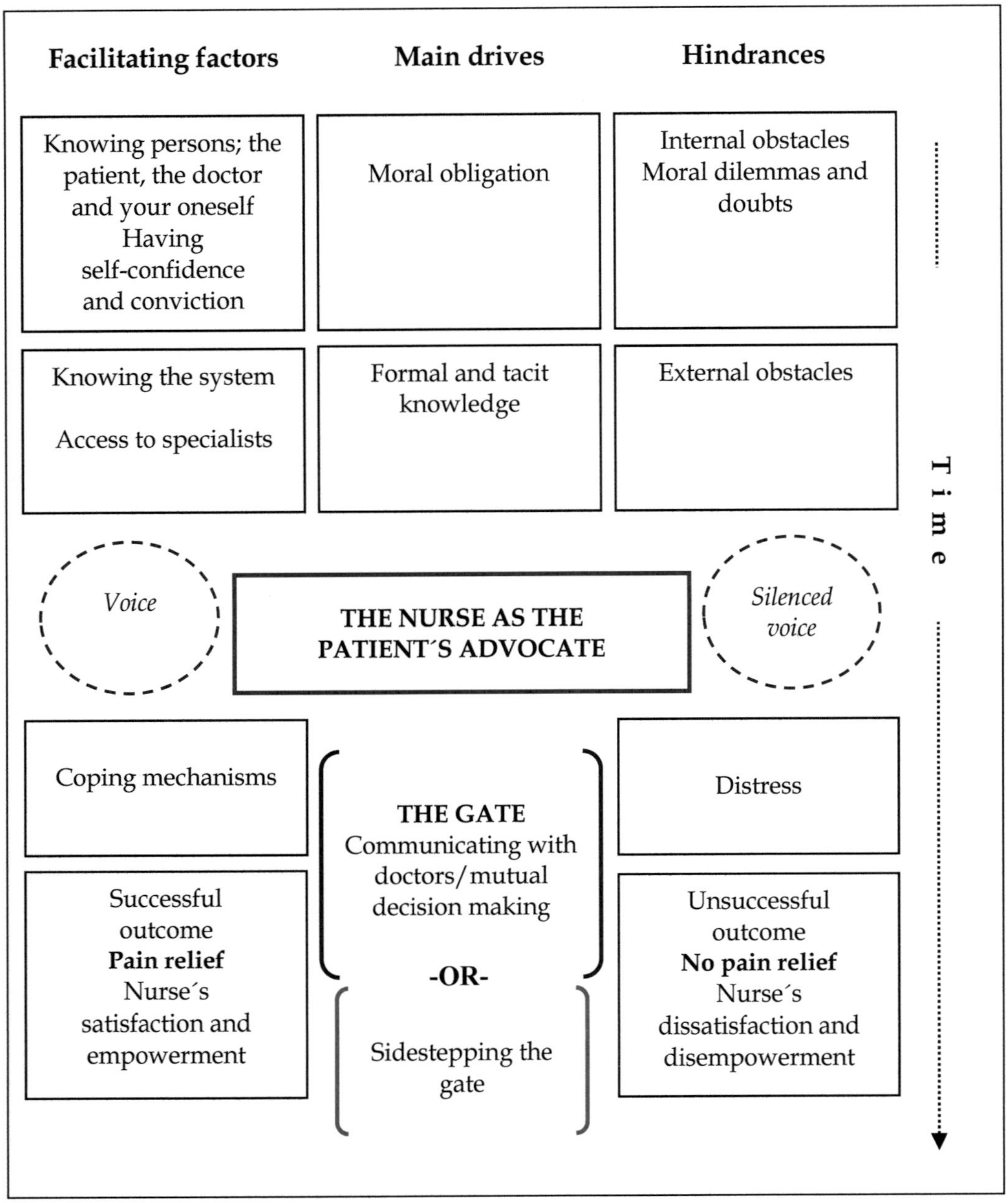

Fig. 1. An explanatory model of nurses´ pain management

3.2 Nurses' two main drives: Moral obligation and formal and tacit knowledge

The first two concepts we introduce in our explanatory model are *moral obligation* (Mallik, 1997; Oberle and Hughes, 2001) and *formal and tacit knowledge* (Blondal & Halldorsdottir, 2009; Mallik, 1997; Nash et al., 1999). We propose that on the nurses' journey to fulfil their mission of relieving patients' pain these two important drives prevail, as illustrated in figure 2 in the shadowed boxes.

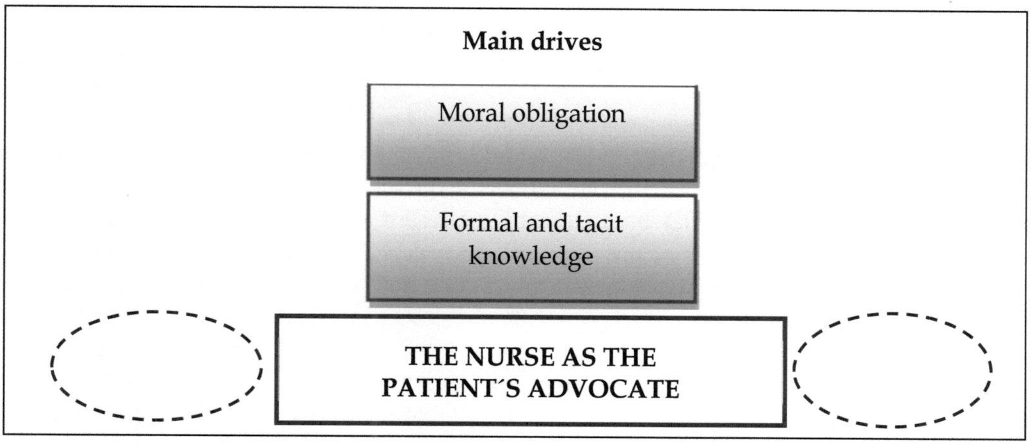

Fig. 2. Nurses' moral obligation and formal and tacit knowledge

The nurses' moral orientation is displayed in accounts like this one: "If the patients report pain, then they're in pain … and of course you must do something about it" (Blondal & Halldorsdottir, 2009, p. 4). Possessing *formal or theoretical knowledge* about pain assessment, pain management and medication is of importance but *tacit knowledge* is no less important, as experience and learning from other colleagues creates a sense of self confidence and increased empowerment in following their convictions to be the *patient's advocate* (Blondal & Halldorsdottir, 2009; Mallik, 1997; Nash et al., 1999). "I suppose I believe advocacy is utilizing our own clinical knowledge as well as our own knowledge of the patient and putting the two of them together and then doing what you feel is best for the patient." (O'Connor & Kelly, 2005, p. 460). This approach assists nurses to keep on advocating and relating with patients and doctors (Blondal & Halldorsdottir, 2009).

3.3 The nurse as the patient's advocate

As may be seen from our model, its central tenet portrays the position of the nurse as the *patient´s advocate* (Figure 3). Here, the mission's journey begins with the nurse's assessment of the patient's pain, which leads to further decisions and reactions and where the nurse will direct his or her responses; what she or he can solve alone and what problems must be referred to physicians (Blondal & Halldorsdottir, 2009).

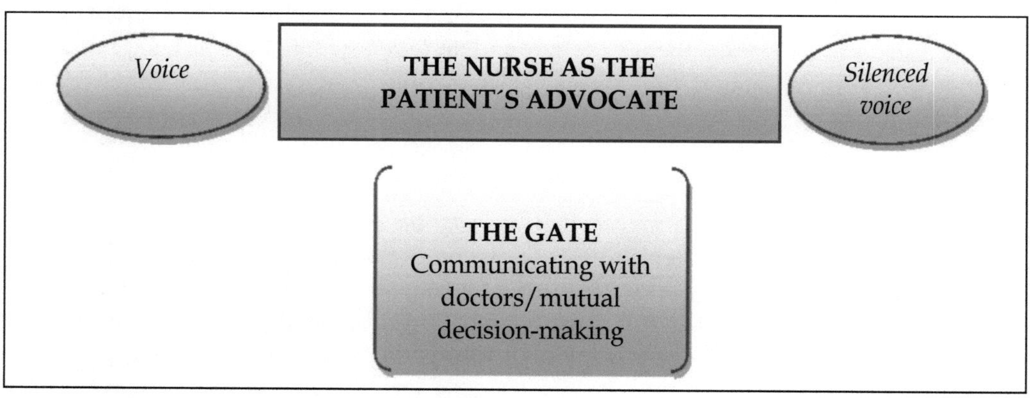

Fig. 3. Central position of the nurse as the patient's advocate

3.3.1 Communicating with doctors at the gate/mutual decision-making

Since medication is often the major pain treatment, and physicians are required to be responsible for all drug prescriptions, a crucial element in this process is the nurses' contribution to mutual *decision-making with the doctor,* where nurses assume the responsibility of advocates (Blondal & Halldorsdottir, 2009). At this point, which may be referred to as "*the gate*", *having a voice* is pivotal for nurses (Blondal & Halldorsdottir, 2009; Van Niekerk and Martin, 2002) because they represent the patient, and by using their influence they try to fulfil their mission (Blondal & Halldorsdottir, 2009; Jenks, 1993; O'Connor & Kelly, 2005). As two different nurses put it: "Well, unfortunately the decision-making is not ours. We are restricted to what's ordered… I mean, if the doctor's ordered it, you can't very well make a decision" (Nash et al., 1999, p. 186), and further: "I don't stand by and watch the patients and do nothing if I think they are wild with pain, I keep on pushing until something is done." (Blondal & Halldorsdottir, 2009, pp. 5-6). If the nurse and the doctor do not reach reciprocal decision or agreement the nurses may have to keep on insisting or else give up -- feeling *silenced* (Malloy, 2009; Blondal & Halldorsdottir, 2009). "We don't have any final authority - perhaps that's what's most difficult…and we have to put up with that, naturally, but it's very important, of course, that we feel we are listened to, that our voice is heard." (Blondal & Halldorsdottir, 2009, p. 2901). Furthermore, to maintain trust between all involved, the nurses sometimes take on the role of a mediator or intermediary (Blondal & Halldorsdottir, 2009; O'Connor & Kelly, 2005), but the importance of co-operation and holding a mutual vision crystallises in this description: "I just think it´s lot of give and take between doctors and nursing staff and patients; you´ve got to work together to actively relieve pain." (Nash et al., 1999, p. 185).

3.4 Facilitating factors for a successful outcome

The main drives, moral obligation and formal and tacit knowledge may not be enough for successful pain management. There are several facilitating factors which are necessary to make use of, together with the main drives, in order to achieve a positive outcome of pain management (See Figure 4).

3.4.1 Knowing the patient

One of the *facilitating factors* that are important motivating factors for advocacy (Mallik, 1997), requires that the nurse *knows the patient as a person,* that is, as an individual, which allows the nurse to interpret information and select individualised interventions (Jenks, 1993). "I think, knowing the patient's background and seeing more than just, say, a medical condition or a surgical wound, that makes you more able to advocate." (O'Connor & Kelly, 2005, p. 459).

3.4.2 Knowing the doctor

In the explanatory model we propose that *to know the gatekeeper,* i.e. the doctor, greatly influences the nurse's success (Jenks, 1993). "Sometimes I think the nurses are underheard if you go and you're telling the doctor, this patient is in pain. This patient is in pain, ah yeah, we'll change this. The patient is still in pain. Sometimes they don't actually listen to what you're saying. It depends on how you say it, or who you're actually saying it to." (Malloy et al., 2009, p. 726). Then on the other hand, "It's a good feeling when you know that someone respects your opinion and respects your assessment of the patient also." (Jenks, 1993, p. 403).

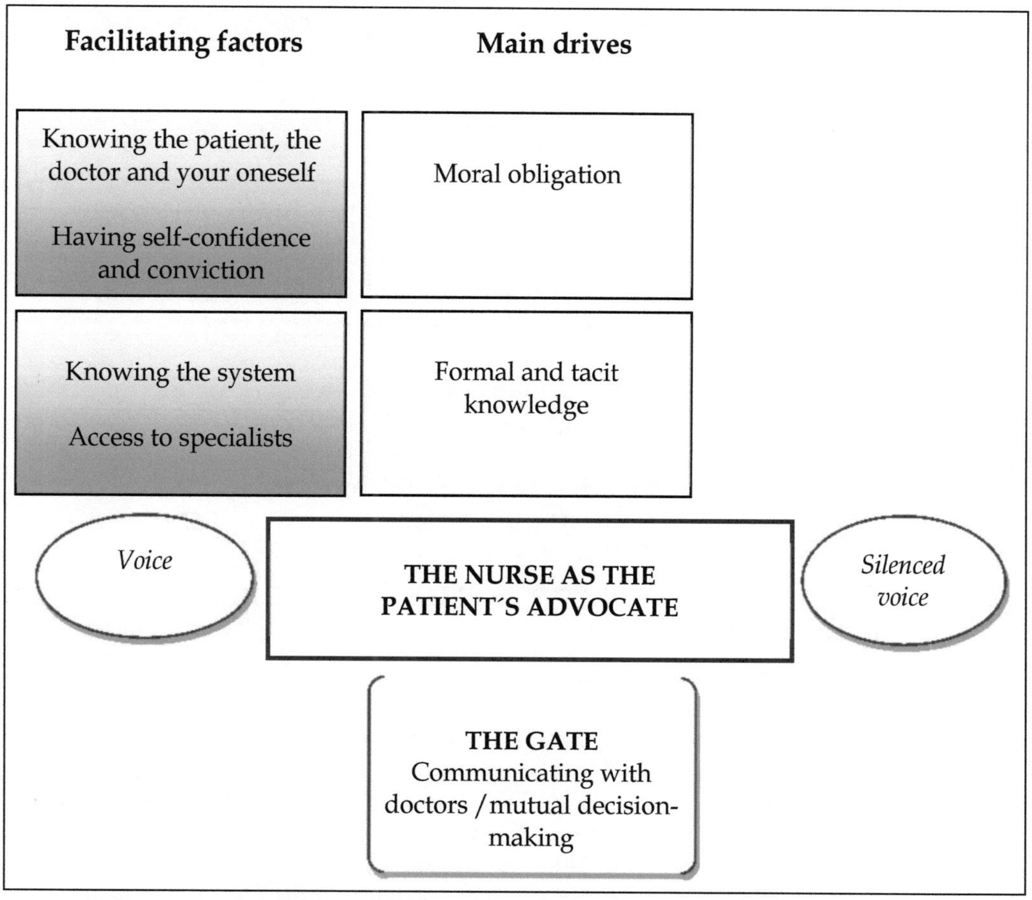

Fig. 4. Facilitating factors; Knowing persons and knowing the system

3.4.3 Knowing your own self, having self-confidence and conviction

It is no less important for nurses to know their own potential and believe in themselves, since experience creates a *sense of self-confidence* and increased empowerment in following their own *convictions*. Therefore, individual factors influence nurses' decisions on pain management; "I'm quite happy to make those decisions, because I'm happy to be answerable for them…so I do things that I am comfortable with and I feel that I am doing the best for the patient." (Nash et al., 1999, p. 185)

3.4.4 Knowing the system and access to specialists

Organizational knowledge, to *know how the system works*, together with knowledge of the wishes of patients, allows nurses to advocate in an effective way; therefore "[A]n advocate to me would be somebody who uses whatever knowledge they have in a situation to do the best for the patient." (O'Connor & Kelly, 2005, p. 460). Then *having access to a specialist in pain management* and pain teams within the organisation is of utmost importance as they serve as nurses' guides and help to turn distress into satisfaction (Blondal & Halldorsdottir, 2009).

3.5 Hindrances to successful pain management

This journey is complicated, however, by several obstacles that emerge either as *internal* or *external obstacles* (see figure 5).

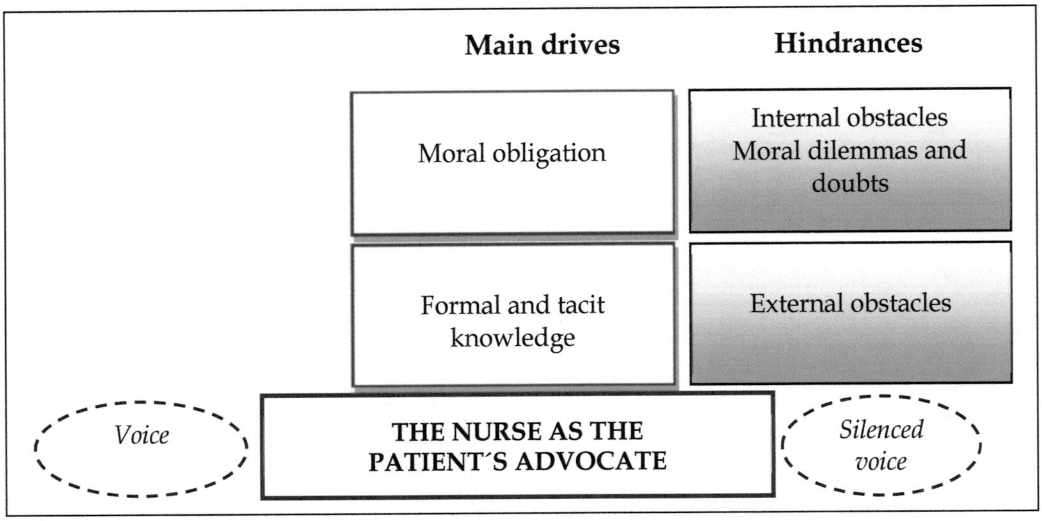

Fig. 5. Internal and external obstacles

3.5.1 Internal obstacles

Internal obstacles that can complicate this process are the nurses' inner struggle of *moral dilemma and doubt,* of doing right and trusting one's own judgement, that appear to be the result of tension between doubt and duty. Here a prevailing feature includes the fear of giving too much medication and caring for addicts (Blondal & Halldorsdottir, 2009; Nash et al., 1999). "I felt it [to give pain medication to an addict] was a strain, really, on human nature - are you doing something wrong? Or are you doing right? Or are you just cruel to refuse to give it to him? - really, what should you do?"(Blondal & Halldorsdottir, 2009, p. 5).

3.5.2 External obstacles

External obstacles are connected to organisational structures (Kuuppelomäki, 2002a) such as absence of or an inadequate prescription, lack of access to accountable physicians, and the lack of directions and clear rules. Moreover, decisions regarding palliative care are imperative for successful pain relief (Blondal & Halldorsdottir, 2009; Kuuppelomäki, 2002a); "Accepting death and the transition from acute care to terminal care are a problem." (Kuuppelomäki, 2002a, p. 706). External hindrances may also be patient related, such as their unwillingness to report pain and to accept analgesics (Blondal & Halldorsdottir, 2009; Kuuppelomäki, 2002a), which further complicates the assessment of pain and pain relief. "He was a difficult man and so withdrawn. You just couldn't get through [to] him and you don't know why not. Cases like that make me feel so uncertain, I start to doubt myself." (De Schepper et al., 1997, p. 424).

3.6 Coping mechanisms

Further action can involve the use of various *coping mechanisms* in order to share the burden, seek better solutions for the patient and/or control their feelings (Blondal & Halldorsdottir, 2009; Nagy, 1999). (See figure 6.)

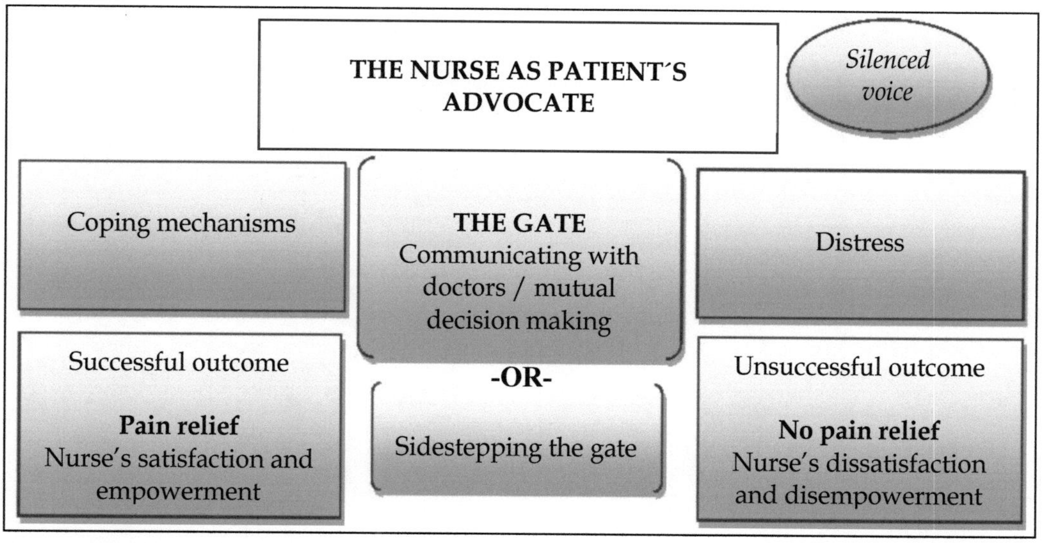

Fig. 6. Coping mechanisms

The most important factor is support provided by colleagues (De Schepper et al., 1997; Nagy, 1999) and specialists in pain management that serve as their guides (Blondal & Halldorsdottir, 2009). "The people that we work with. You can go up and say 'So-and-so, I can't cope with this any longer! Can you either give me a hand or do it for me?' And people where we are working at the moment will do that. So if we're getting too fed up someone else will either help you out or do it for you so you can go and have a rest. They understand what it's like!" (Nagy, 1999, p. 1433). Furthermore, "I get a lot of support from the team here. They give me [the] feedback I need and I can have a good moan." (De Schepper et al., 1997, p. 426). Assistance can, therefore, like other coping strategies, transform *distress* into *satisfaction* (Blondal & Halldorsdottir, 2009) which may keep them satisfied despite unfavourable outcomes. Some nurses do *sidestep the gate* by using independent nursing interventions, take control and thread the risky road of bypassing the gate by altering the medication on their own initiative or bend existing rules and directions (Blondal & Halldorsdottir, 2009). But this also may be the result of the distress mentioned above.

3.7 Potential outcomes

As suggested by this model, the nurse's journey has two potential outcomes, based on the degree to which nurses are able to fulfil their commitments (see figure 7).
Successful pain relief leads to nurses' *satisfaction* and *empowerment* and *patients' satisfaction* and possibly mutual trust (Blondal & Halldorsdottir, 2009). Conversely, pain management is burdensome when the patients' sufferings are not relieved (Nagy, 1999) or the nurses are *silenced*, with consequent *dissatisfaction and distress* (De Schepper et al., 1997; Oberle and Hughes, 2001), *disempowerment* and possibly mutual distrust. "I think, really, it's one of the more difficult things one experiences… I was so upset inside… so angry inside, not being able to help and not really knowing where to turn, because the doctors said just that [dose of medication], and it didn't work at all, so I was somehow defenceless about what to do." (Blondal & Halldorsdottir, 2009, p. 6). However, importantly, we want to point out that perceived discomfort or *dissatisfaction* with the outcome can serve as a drive for further action (Blondal & Halldorsdottir, 2009; Mallik, 1997).

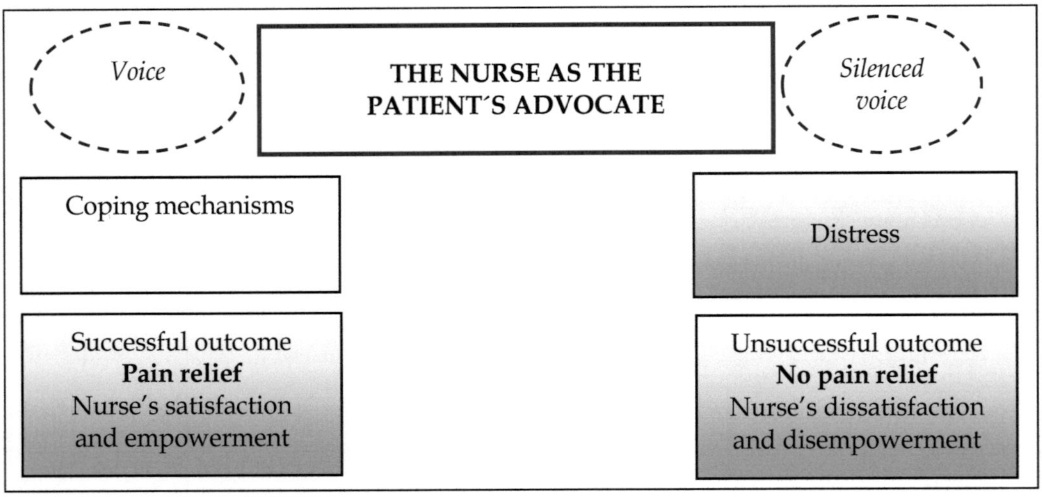

Fig. 7. Potential outcomes

From this overview we conclude that theoretical knowledge is only one aspect of nurses' pain management. They require knowledge from various other sources, ethical, personal, and aesthetic, as well as many skills, e.g. communication and negotiation skills, in order to fulfil their obligations and role. In our view, lack of recognition of these other kinds of knowledge may stem from the fact that many studies focus only on isolated aspects of pain management. All too commonly the studies provide only a somewhat fragmented analysis of isolated factors of pain management. In contrast, the explanatory model presented here provides a more holistic view of the nurses' complex situation when caring for patients in pain and may reveal that neglecting these other facets may have contributed to the permanent inadequacy in pain management of patients that is so widely described.

4. Discussion

This explanatory model clarifies how nurses require various coexisting patterns of knowledge, within a favourable organisational environment, to be able to perform in accord with their role as key persons in pain management and how their performance may predict a positive or negative outcome for the patient and the nurse. This model further explains the relationships of nurses with patients and physicians where nurses seek to act as patients' advocates and how having a voice is pivotal for nurses. Furthermore, we depict how internal and external barriers can hinder the performance of nurses and how an unsuccessful outcome that evokes profound distress may concurrently stimulate further actions and turn a negative outcome into a more favourable one. This explanatory model of a nurse's journey therefore denotes nurses' encounters with, and reactions to, the multiple demanding assignments they continually meet on their mission towards pain relief.

4.1 Nurses´ two main drives: Moral obligation and formal and tacit knowledge

4.1.1 Knowledge of ethical origins

According to our explanatory model *the role of ethical knowledge in pain management must be highlighted,* as it may be the fundamental component needed for nurses to act as advocates and to initiate the process of pain management. Our notion of nurses' obligation to relieve pain is supported by several studies (Oberle and Hughes, 2001; O'Connor & Kelly, 2005; Rejeh et al., 2009). However, it may have been underestimated up till now because even if nurses possess the relevant theoretical knowledge, they may not necessarily make use of it without the requisite motivation.

We want to emphasize that non-professional and professional *moral values* that motivate and direct individuals' choices can be inculcated through education or socialisation (Omery, 1989), and nurses recognise that a sense of responsibility in pain management needs to be learned (Rejeh et al., 2009). Taylor et al. (1993) also conclude that nurses' education about pain management must include professional ethical obligations and the suitability of their professional values. Importantly, moral values may also be generated by an organisation's philosophy statement or policy (Omery, 1989) and moral values should, therefore, be part of nursing education as well as organisational statements.

4.1.2 Formal and tacit knowledge

In accordance with our propositions, professional responsibility and moral obligation are considered key initiates for advocacy. Twycross (2002) posits that in order to advocate, a theoretical knowledge base is needed. Vaartio et al. (2006) and O'Connor & Kelly (2005) add to this by stating that theoretical as well as practical knowledge of pain management is a necessary antecedent of advocacy. Where sound empirical knowledge about pain assessment and various methods for management of pain are vital, it must be kept in mind that nurses learn no less through experience, where they learn to utilise their own potential and personal knowledge through their own practice and role modelling. This drive for taking action by using theoretical or formal knowledge along with experience and self-confidence is congruent with Mallik's (1997) statement that 'intervening conditions' facilitate advocacy. These factors have also been found important for nurses' decision-making (Nash et al., 1999). Where knowledge of theoretical origins may be the type of knowledge that is most easily recognised and is emphasised during formal education at school and in continuous education, we stress that the role of tacit knowledge gained through experience and role modelling has more rarely been pointed out, perhaps because it is rather of personal and aesthetic origins. Importantly, as we see it, this knowledge supplements formal knowledge, for instance in the early stages of the process where nurses assess the patient's pain.

4.2 The nurse as patient's advocate in pain management

Patients in pain have been recognised as a vulnerable group of patients that are in need of nurses to advocate on their behalf (Ware et al., 2011), and nurses see it as their role to safeguard their interests (Blondal & Halldorsdottir, 2009; Ware et al., 2011). As portrayed in our explanatory model nurses assume a central role in assessing and managing patients' pain. However, since doctors are responsible for prescribing analgesia, nurses' concerns about pain relief are often affected by their relationship with the doctors (Kuuppelomäki, 2002a; Taylor et al., 1993; Van Niekerk and Martin, 2002).

4.2.1 Communicating with doctors at "*the gate*" and mutual decision-making

On the nurses' journey *the gate*, where they enter these relations with *the gatekeeper*—the doctor, is an important turning point (Blondal & Halldorsdottir, 2009). Having a *voice* at the gate is pivotal, because there the nurses represent the patient, and by using their influence try to fulfil their mission. Subsequently, the doctor decides what medication the patient can or cannot receive; i.e. whether the nurses pass through the gate (Blondal & Halldorsdottir, 2009). Within the *gate* the nurses can also assume the role of 'conciliator' or 'intermediary'. Nurses' accounts of their advocating position have, therefore, also been described as 'bridging the gap' between the patients and the medical profession. This involves the translation of information between patients and doctors and in both directions (O'Connor & Kelly, 2005). As we envision it, yet another aspect of personal knowledge is revealed here where, inevitably, nurses must communicate with doctors to achieve the best outcome for patients.

Many nurses do not find it difficult to communicate with doctors or to confront them and are ready to push boundaries to acquire what the patient needs (Blondal & Halldorsdottir, 2009; Vaartio et al., 2008; Ware et al., 2011). For others, communicational problems are a matter of fact and they feel uncomfortable about trespassing on the doctors´ domain (De Schepper et al. 1997; Willson, 2000). Nurses in cancer-related home care, for instance, complain about physicians' lack of knowledge and collaboration, and problems with contacting them (Ferrell et al., 1993). Nurses then also describe physicians' fear of overmedicating patients with dementia or delirium in medical wards (Coker et al., 2010). Communicational problems cause feelings of powerlessness and distress (Blondal & Halldorsdottir, 2009; Malloy et al., 2009) and ethical dilemmas and they are sometimes punished for their advocating activities (Clabo, 2008; Mallik, 1997; Malloy et al., 2009). Mallik (1997) maintains that to achieve their goals, advocates often play the doctor-nurse game of recommending actions without appearing to do so (Stein et al., 1990) or assume the attitude of a 'stubborn rebel' with an over-determined and even hostile behaviour (Stein et al., 1990). In our study, however, the nurses emphasise assertiveness, rather than pushiness, for success (Blondal & Halldorsdottir, 2009). When nurses are straightforward in their requests, this could be explained by their perceptions of being respected and *having a voice*, and therefore in keeping with Van Niekerk and Martin (2002) that nurses who feel adequately consulted by physicians are more likely to initiate the consultation process. The use of assertiveness further matches the argument of Keenan et al. (1998) that conveying ideas in a forceful and confrontational manner increases the likelihood for successful collaboration. We claim that when nurses choose to bypass the *gate* by bending rules (Blondal & Halldorsdottir, 2009; Ware et al., 2011) despite the risk of jeopardising their career, this might indicate a lack of self-confidence, negotiating competence or communicational competence skills. For nurses, ethical problems may often be related to their hierarchical position, where their voices are not heard or they are being silenced in spite of their professional knowledge (Blondal & Halldorsdottir, 2009; Malloy et al., 2009; Oberle and Hughes, 2001). From this, it might be understood that the views of nurses and doctors are incompatible, for instance because of the different orientation of *care* versus *cure* (Malloy et al., 2009). However, doctors can also experience an inability to exercise moral agency and experience powerlessness, because of hierarchical structures, and they are faced with the same kinds of ethical dilemmas as nurses. Furthermore, the obligation to respond is the same for all and this difference could rather be explained by different roles and responsibilities and unawareness of each others' responses (Oberle and Hughes, 2001). This also may reflect the reality that nurses and doctors act independently, without mutually agreed principles or practices rather than as a team in managing pain (Kuuppelomäki, 2002a). Although this statement is made in regard to end-of-life situations, we conclude that this could also apply to other pain management decisions and call for more discussions about the ethical aspects of pain management across professions.

4.3 Facilitating factors for a successful outcome

As represented in our explanatory model, facilitating factors for successful advocacy and a favourable outcome require knowing persons and the system. Jenks' (1993) exploration of nurses' clinical decision-making, proposing that clinical decisions depend on the quality and dynamics of nurses' interpersonal relationships is in harmony with our interpretation of the process from pain assessment to reaction. However, we also want to add the dimension of knowing your own self and the organisation that also are essential facilitating factors. These important features that enhance nurses' possibilities for using their knowledge and moral motivation are opposed to the factors that hinder them in making use of their potential, and may, to some degree, be used to overcome their negative effects.

4.3.1 Knowing the patient

As repeatedly has been pointed out, insufficient pain assessment by nurses interferes with successful pain relief (Carr, 2002). According to McCaffery (Pasero et al., 1999, as cited in McCaffery, 1968) "[P]ain is whatever the experiencing person says it is, existing whenever he says it does" (p. 17). However, because individuals express pain very differently, this definition creates some problems for nurses. For instance, although the risk of addiction is minor (McCaffery et al., 1990), caring for a patient who is, or is suspected of being, an abuser can be very stressful (Blondal & Halldorsdottir, 2009; Nash et al., 1999). Moreover, McCaffery and Ferrell (1997) assert that nurses must appreciate that "the only scientific tool for measuring pain intensity is the patient's report using a pain rating scale" (p. 183). These scales may, however, be difficult to use with patients that are disoriented (Coker et al., 2010) or unconscious (Kuuppelomäki, 2002a) and many nurses are hesitant to use them (Schafheutle et al., 2001). Then many elderly patients suffer in silence with their pain and discomforts and do not seek help and more effort is required if those with pain are to be identified, supported and cared for as Gudmannsdottir & Halldorsdottir (2009) suggest. Whereas the use of various pain scales for pain assessment build on theoretical knowledge, conversely, *knowing the patient* as a person can greatly assist nurses to assess the patient's pain (Blondal and Halldorsdottir, 2009); this approach is more related to personal and aesthetic knowledge. Knowing the patient as a person strongly facilitates the assessment of patients' needs and clinical decision-making (Liaschenko, 1997), and allows nurses to interpret information and select individualised interventions (Takman and Severinsson, 1999). Furthermore, the nurse-patient relationship is a motivating factor for advocacy (Mallik, 1997; O'Connor & Kelly, 2005) and analysing the patient and the situation is a fundamental element of advocacy (Vaartio et al., 2008). Therefore, we suggest that more emphasis is given to this special aspect of pain management. Still, yet another pattern of knowledge may also be needed here; *unknowing the patient.* When nurses admit to themselves that they do not know the patient and his or her point of view, it allows them to hold their former biases and prejudices in abeyance (Munhall, 1993). We suggest that assuming this type of knowledge is of utmost importance as it may prevent nurses from making assumptions about patients´ pain intensity that is based on diagnosis and course of treatment (Clabo, 2008; Manias, 2003; Schafheutle et al., 2001) that is associated with underestimation of pain (Sjöström et al., 2000), and a barrier to effective pain relief (Schafheutle et al., 2001). Adopting this stance of unknowing could also avoid the stereotyping of patients, such as those who may be addicts, homeless or prisoners (Rejeh et al., 2009) or with a lifestyle that may affect nurses' pain management behaviours (Wilson, 2007). Therefore, we advise that strategies nurses use to connect to patients which may be based on personal knowledge (Carper, 1978) and unknowing (Munhall, 1993) are highlighted along with the current emphasis on using pain rating scales (e.g. Paice and Cohen, 1997).

According to our model, competent communication with patients may be a powerful way to overcome internal hindrances in addition to theoretical knowledge about pain assessment, addiction, respiratory depression and other possible side effects of pain medication that also may stem from the ethical orientation of preventing harm to the patients. When nurses' emphasise individualised pain management, knowing the patient as a person, recognising his/her special needs and responding to these needs on the basis of envisioned results, portrays the importance of aesthetic knowledge and comprehension of the particularity of the situation (Carper, 1978). Empathy is also an important component mode of the aesthetic pattern in nursing (Carper, 1978), and apparent in nurses' accounts of pain management (Blondal & Halldorsdottir, 2009; Rejeh et al., 2009) and should be not only acknowledged but utilised more often.

4.3.2 Knowing the doctor

Since nurses call for equality, mutual decision-making and respect for their judgement (Blondal & Halldorsdottir, 2009), knowing the doctor is a factor worth further exploration. In accordance with our explanatory model Jenks (1993) maintains that *knowing the doctor* creates mutual trust in each others' perceptions. Therefore, a good nurse-physician relationship, in accordance with our metaphor of nurses passing through the *gate*, knowing *the gatekeeper* may add to optimal pain relief and consequently affects nurses' and patients' wellbeing. It is, therefore, imperative that both doctors and nurses be aware of the need for good rapport and be knowledgeable about good communication techniques and that both groups of professionals make every effort to encourage collaboration and to find ways to get to know each other as persons. Again, we propose that personal knowledge and communicational skills that nurses must use in relations with patients and doctors is vital because, as before, possessing theoretical knowledge and the motivation to use it (moral orientation) may become of little use if not employed because of lack of communication or negotiating abilities or lack of self-confidence or if nurses cannot react because their voice is silenced. Therefore, nurses must be taught to act as the patients' advocates, represent themselves and act like the patients' representative.

4.3.3 Knowing oneself, having self-confidence and conviction

We further want to draw attention to how nurses' awareness of their feelings such as distress and empathy, recognition of their own capabilities, self-confidence and persistence may be important facilitating factors. As mentioned before, motivational factors such as experience and self-confidence are congruent with Mallik's (1997) 'intervening conditions' that facilitate advocacy and are important for nurses' decision-making (Nash et al., 1999). As further discussed later, emotional responses such as anger and frustration are also potent motivators for advocacy (Mallik, 1997). Such knowledge is of both personal and aesthetical origins and nurses must learn to identify and accept such feelings and be empowered to use them to be capable of following their convictions, both for their own sakes and for the good of the patient. According to our model, nurses that hold such knowledge and believe in themselves are more capable of entering into and coping positively with difficult relations with others —patients, families and doctors, and are more likely to gain what is needed for a positive outcome both for the patients and themselves.

4.3.4 Knowing the system

Yet another facet that is worth more consideration is nurses´ knowledge of the organisation. Knowing the system and the environment is part of nurses' advocacy, for instance when nurses must mediate between the patient and the system through interpretation of medical terminology or advocating for a group of patients (O´Connor et al., 2005). It also seems necessary to recognise what options or resources are available within the organisation, for instance whom to turn to for assistance. Here, the support of professionals — specialists in pain management within organisations, must be present at all times to assist them in dealing with difficult cases (Blondal and Halldorsdottir, 2009; Nash et al., 1999). Moreover, nurses must recognise the availability of specialists and when they should be contacted and involved.

4.4 Hindrances for successful pain management

As the model portrays, some inhibiting factors hinder nurses´ potentials for taking action and therefore interfere with their drives, moral obligation, and formal and tacit knowledge. It may also be seen that these factors are somewhat in opposition to the facilitating factors. The main obstacles are grouped as external — originating in the nurses´ environment, or internal — concerned with inner doubts or dilemmas. This gives an example of how these model elements are interconnected and should not be taken out of the immediate context.

4.4.1 Internal hindrances

As previously mentioned, nurses´ moral motivation is complicated by some dilemmas as the nurses encounter variable decisional and ethical conflicts (Taylor et al. 1993) that directly affect the pain management process and its outcome. The dilemma of inflicting pain to serve other goals of treatment (De Schepper, 1997; Willson, 2000), fear of giving too much pain medication because of respiratory depression (Ferrell et al., 1991; Howell et al., 2000; Wilson, 2007), sedation (Howell et al., 2000), fear of the addictive properties of narcotics (Brockopp et al., 1998), and doubt whether the pain is real (Nash, 1999; Rejeh et al., 2009) has repeatedly been described. So are the difficulties of distinguishing between physical pain and psychological distress (Kuuppellomäki, 2002a), patients' non-compliance in accepting analgesia (Kuuppellomäki, 2002a), patients' reticence (De Schepper et al 1997; Rejeh et al., 2009) and nurses' concerns about giving a dying person the last dose (Brockopp et al., 1998), as for some, hastening death through pain relief is morally unacceptable (O'Rourke, 1992). Ethical problems may also arise from a lack of permission to be honest with patients (Rejeh et al., 2009) or because of the attitudes of family members towards pain medication (Kuuppelomäki, 2002a). Nurses also frequently describe how difficult it is for them to care for patients that are known abusers or suspected of being addicts, and believing their words (Blondal & Halldorsdottir, 2009; Nash et al., 1999; Rejeh et al., 2009). Dilemmas may also be caused by preconceived notions about certain groups of patients that negatively interfere with nurses' decision-making (Brockopp et al., 2003). Interestingly, Van Niekerk and Martin (2002) point out that nurses with greater knowledge of pain assessment are less likely to experience ethical conflicts regarding overmedication, addiction or doubt about the existence of pain. Hence, more knowledge could prevent such ethical conflicts. Accounts like this further sustain our claims about how the separate parts introduced in our model are interconnected and cannot be separated from the complete picture.

4.4.2 External obstacles

Organisational barriers have formerly been extensively described, where lack of time, workload (Ware et al., 2011; Rejeh et al., 2009) financial restraints and staffing cutbacks (Oberle and Hughes, 2001; Rejeh et al., 2009), restraints of routine (Willson, 2000), insufficient prescribing of analgesics (Schafheutle et al., 2001; Kuuppelomäki, 2002a) based on habits instead of individualised needs (Boer et al, 1997), and unavailability of physicians (Kuuppelomäki, 2002a; Rejeh et al., 2009) interfere with pain relief. Other related hindrances that are part of the system have also been identified such as unavailable non-pharmacological pain relief measures and disorganised systems of care (Coker et al., 2010). Rejeh et al. (2009) also point out that defective equipment and interruptions can lead to ethical problems in pain management. The importance of a decision on palliative care for good pain relief is endorsed by Kuuppelomäki (2002b) who reports physicians' hesitancy about starting terminal care, and delayed decisions of using a strong analgesia (Kuuppelomäki, 2002a). The organisation must, therefore, provide an *optimal organisational environment* since organisational barriers such as unclear rules, lack of prescriptions or time and resources such as specialised pain services, may hinder nurses from acting according to their best knowledge, potential and goals. The presence of prescriptions, rules and directives are important to be able to give the patient what she or he needs. Inflexible protocols and strict policies or routines, on the other hand, impede good pain management (Rajeh et al., 2009; Willson, 2000) resulting in the nurses giving up and leaving them feeling silenced and disempowered (Blondal & Halldorsdottir, 2009; Malloy et al., 2009). Alternatively, nurses may feel compelled to choose to bypass the *gate*, by bending rules (Blondal & Halldorsdottir, 2009; Ware et al., 2011), to obtain favourable results for the patient, as is portrayed in our model. Our emphasis on organisational structures is supported by the results of Willson's (2000) participant observation study on factors affecting analgesia administration; Willson suggests that because of the interplay between multiple organisational and interpersonal features, more education of the nurses will not necessarily improve the administration of analgesics.

4.5 Coping mechanisms

How nurses *cope* with their challenges predicts to some extent how they perceive the outcome of pain relief and they seem to use various methods to cope and protect themselves. Applying methods such as concentrating on patients' positive attributes is a component of strategies that prevent burnout (Simoni and Paterson, 1997), and sharing feelings with colleagues (De Schepper et al., 1997; Nagy, 1999) and having the opportunity to stand back from situations (De Schepper et al., 1997; Rejeh et al., 2009) are consistent with strategies that reduce powerlessness (De Schepper et al., 1997). Seeking and receiving support from pain teams and specialists in pain management is vital, and such assistance can transform distress into satisfaction. Ironically, those who accept the responsibility as seeing to pain relief run the risk of experiencing ethical problems which may lead to a sense of loss of control and subsequently burnout, resulting in decreased quality of care (Schmitz et al., 2000). If nurses give up their advocating efforts and instead assume *coping methods* such as avoidance, which indicates unsuccessful coping (Simoni and Paterson, 1997), it may desensitise them to patients' needs (Nagy's, 1999), which means in turn that they may not be willing or able to attend to patients' suffering. Such strategies should, therefore, be detected, and those nurses helped to adopt more constructive coping strategies.

4.6 Potential outcomes of pain management and advocacy

Effective pain relief may provide *satisfaction*, both by means of professional achievements and benefits for the patient and the nurse (Blondal & Halldorsdottir, 2009; De Schepper et al. 1997; Vaartio et al., 2008). However, such positive outcomes are seldom mentioned. We believe that this aspect should receive more attention and nurses should be enabled to reap satisfaction from overcoming challenges and learning from them. As successful pain relief may enhance autonomy and a sense of *empowerment*, this is relevant to both quality of pain management and job satisfaction. Conversely, much more attention is given to the negative aspects: dissatisfaction, distress and frustration (e.g. Nagy, 1998; Söderhamn and Idvall, 2003) following insufficient or unsuccessful pain management that leads in turn to nurses' suffering and *disempowerment* (Blondal & Halldorsdottir, 2009; Oberle and Hughes, 2001).

4.6.1 Dissatisfaction and distress as motivators for a successful outcome

Since *dissatisfaction* and nurses´ *distress* may be the inevitable results of nurses' inability to ease the patients' pain, for instance because of silencing or lack of resources, it is important to note that nurses' distress can impel further actions. This is in agreement with Mallik's (1997) argument that emotional responses of anger and frustration can be potent motivators for advocacy. It, therefore, seems important that nurses accept and recognise such feelings, not least because those who acknowledge and try to deal with feelings of powerlessness are more capable of coping (De Schepper et al., 1997). All these responses require, once again, both personal and aesthetic knowledge where nurses as individuals must learn to know themselves and their reactions and be able to develop and maintain a view of what they want to achieve with their actions. Here we come back to earlier discussion about nurses' requirements of knowing their own "selves", their own feelings and capabilities.

5. Further development of this theory

Theory provides a more complete picture of practice than factual knowledge alone, and theories formulate, identify, and articulate the science and practice of every discipline (Butcher, 2006). Nursing scholars need to identify and articulate the processes and components of the art and science of pain management. This theory is an attempt to do so in an endeavour to continue the discipline's development by assisting in the understanding and practice of creating further theoretical discourse, processes and products for pain management, similar to what Kagan (2006) has described. All theories are reconstructed in the light of new data. The theory presented here is, therefore, seen as always being in the process of emerging, as is our world view. According to Walker and Avant (2004), the next steps in the phases of our theory development are: theory testing involving concept revision, statement revision, and theory revision, followed by further theory testing. We encourage our colleagues to critique the theory and use it to generate research questions and take part in testing the theory as well as in concept, statement and theory revision.

6. Implications for practice and future research

From our explanatory model many suggestions can be made about how to contribute to changes in the education of nurses, their work environment and future research.

6.1 Nurses' knowledge and formal education

Firstly, we propose that alterations should be made within nurses' basic education at school and continuous education at the institutional level. Nurses' formal education at school must include extensive knowledge about pain assessment and pain management and it is also necessary that courses are offered regularly within all health care settings on pain assessment, analgesia, adverse reactions, and respiratory depression. However, in addition to the traditional emphasis on the use of pain scales for the assessment of patients' pain, it is also important to emphasise *personal and aesthetic knowledge* that contains strategies that contribute to knowing and involving the patient, and nurses' availability. Then education about the pain management of dying patients, addiction and prejudices must also be increased, both at schools and within organisations. The *ethical aspects of pain management* should be included in all courses along with empirical knowledge and should contain discussions about moral responsibility, bioethical principles, nurses' professional code of conduct and the Patients' Rights Act together with religious discussions about pain management. Furthermore, despite differences in educational programmes and the cultures of nurses and doctors, these professions must reach a mutual understanding to achieve suitable and consistent care for their patients (Malloy et al., 2009). One method to bring together their views could, therefore, be to organise courses that these professionals attend together. That said, as nurses' socialisation occurs to a great extent during their nursing education (Stein et al., 1990), nursing students should be taught to make claims for mutual decision-making, to recognise their own potential, and be *empowered* to make claims for resources and improvements. As many nurses may lack the vocabulary for ethical decision-making, thus contributing to the silenced voices of nurses (Malloy et al., 2009), *advocating competence* should be taught at school. Moreover, they should be prepared for the need for *negotiation*, assertiveness, and effective *communication*. It is necessary that nurses are encouraged to reflect on their experience both as nurse students and as practicing nurses and also to establish positive working relationship with doctors. Moreover, since nurses seem to learn strategies such as self-confidence through role modelling we emphasize that during their nursing education and as novice nurses they should have access to role models for guidance that relate to their use of personal and aesthetic knowledge. During courses about pain management nurses' coping methods should be addressed, and they should be taught to recognise destructive methods and adopt more constructive ones. The method of *structured reflection* (Johns, 1995), for instance, could be used to assist nurses in learning about their own abilities and responses. However, not only should negative aspects of their practice or difficult cases be inspected, but also the positive ones.

6.2 Organisational environment

Firstly, it is imperative that pain relief is highlighted within all health care settings and organisational nursing policies or visions for nursing, which must reflect this important aspect of care. It should be stressed that pain management is a priority and recognised that time and adequate resources are important aspects of pain management. Protocols that exemplify the responsibility of each member of the health care team should exist, but all rules that are created should also be flexible; for instance nurses must be enabled to choose an analgesic from a range of individualised prescriptions. It also seems vital that clear directives exist for the pain relief of addicts and access to support from specialists in the management of this group of patients available at all times. Support from specialists in pain management and psychological support at all times are also fundamental. Moreover, the opportunity to discuss difficult cases with philosophers or leaders from different faiths and denominations should be provided in every health care setting. Subsequently, conversations about nurses' ethical responsibilities and dilemmas should be offered and should be open for both nurses and doctors. As pain assessment is partly dependent on positive nurse-patient relationships and knowing the patient as a person, nursing models and interventions that encourage such relations should be introduced and supported. Another aspect of organisational culture that may enhance successful pain management is good collaboration and maintenance of trust between nurses and in the nurse-physician relationships. All efforts that strengthen dialogue and a culture that enables nurses to seek support and advice from colleagues and encourages open discussions about feelings and coping may therefore have positive outcomes in this respect. Lastly, an atmosphere of persistence and seeking the best available solution should be supported.

6.3 Future research

The explanatory model can be a great source of ideas for future research. Firstly, a quantitative study could be conducted, to assess nurses' level of empirical, aesthetic and ethical knowledge along with personal knowledge regarding pain relief; including communication, collaboration and coping. Secondly, it would be interesting to explore the ethical component of the nursing and medical curricula and further to investigate to what extent nurses and doctors are guided by moral values in their pain relief at work. Thirdly, studies on how nurses' moral orientation is balanced with the effectiveness of the pain relief they provide could also be conducted. Fourthly, it seems necessary to conduct more studies where the communication of nurses and doctors connected with pain management is explored, for instance by using an ethnographic approach. Fifthly, it seems important to run more field studies within each organization to identify the main obstructions for effective pain management. It seems vital to begin with identifying what hindrances are most prominent before embarking on a campaign for better pain management within organisations. A part of these studies could be to inspect the effects of workload, lack of time and constraining directives on nurses' potentials for providing optimal pain relief.

7. Conclusion

Our explanatory model is at odds with statements proposing that pain relief is not the nurses' priority (Brockopp et al., 1998) or their responsibility (Twycross, 2002). We assert, however, that various reasons inhibit the nurses' potential for taking action. We conclude that nurses are the patients´ advocates in pain management and successful pain management is rewarded with a sense of satisfaction, empowerment and fulfilment of their duty. They are in a key position to assess and manage pain and their mediatory position within the hospital is unique. It is vital that nurses are adequately prepared for their role educationally by possessing multidimensional knowledge about pain management. We assert that good theoretical knowledge may be inadequate if the nurse does not have the right motivation, i.e. the *moral inclination* to use it in practice. Furthermore, *personal knowledge* that nurses must use in relations with patients and doctors is also necessary because theoretical knowledge alone may be of little use if it cannot be employed because of lack of communication or negotiation competence or because their voice is silenced. They also need personal knowledge for self-knowledge, and to reflect on their own strengths and weaknesses in order to make better use of their own abilities. Therefore, nurses must be taught to act as the patient's advocate and the patients' representative. This also requires nurses to use their *aesthetic knowledge* to appreciate the needs of every individual patient. Furthermore, nurses must acknowledge how little they know about some patients who could beforehand be labelled as "difficult". These patterns of knowledge in pain management are interrelated and should therefore be assessed as a whole if pain management is to be enhanced within an organisation or pain management skills in nurses' primary or continuing education. The organisation in turn must provide an *optimal environment*; a clear statement about pain management and clear but flexible rules on pain management, and provide ample time and resources such as specialised pain services, that otherwise may hinder nurses from acting according to their best knowledge, potentials, and nursing goals. Teamwork and good collaboration between health care professionals must also be supported. The structure and prevailing culture of organisations must therefore be scrutinised before organising improvements in pain management.

All the factors previously mentioned coexist and are interdependent and cannot be taken out of the immediate context, as may be seen from our model. Therefore, developments in pain management that focus only on one aspect of pain management may be ineffective, as many factors affect this process. We, therefore, propose that knowledge in this respect has often been too narrowly defined and we call for a more holistic approach in pain management by nurses and other health care personnel where multiple types of knowledge and skills as well as the organisational context are included and taken into consideration during educational efforts and reform of pain management within organisations.

8. References

Blondal, K. & Halldorsdottir, S. (2009). The challenge of caring for patients in pain: From the nurse's perspective. *Journal of Clinical Nursing*, Vol.18, No.20, pp. 2897–2906, ISSN 0962-1067

Boer, C., Treebus, A.N., Zuurmond, W.W.A. & de Lange, J.J. (1997). Compliance in administration of prescribed analgesics. *Anaesthesia*, Vol.52, No.11, pp. 1177- 1181, ISSN 1365-2044

Brockopp, D.Y., Ryan, P. & Warden, S. (2003). Nurses' willingness to manage the pain of specific groups of patients. *British Journal of Nursing*, Vol.12, No.7, pp. 409-415, ISSN 0966-0461

Brockopp, G., Warden, S., Wilson, J., Carpenter, J.S. & Vandeveer, B. (1998). Barriers to change: A pain management project. *International Journal of Nursing Studies*, Vol.35, No.4, pp. 226-232, ISSN 0020-7489

Butcher, H.K. (2006). Review of Walker and Avant's newest theory development text. *Nursing Science Quarterly*, Vol.19, No.2, pp.174-177, ISSN 0894-3184

Carper, B.A. (1978). Fundamental patterns of knowing in nursing. *Advances in Nursing Science*, Vol. 1, No. 1, pp. 13–23, ISSN 0161-9268

Carr, E.C.J. (2002). Refusing analgesics: Using continuous improvement to improve pain management on a surgical ward. *Journal of Clinical Nursing,* Vol.11, No.6, pp. 743-752, ISSN 0962-1067

Clabo, L.M.L. (2008). An ethnography of pain assessment and the role of social context on two postoperative units. *Journal of Advanced Nursing,* Vol.61, No.5, pp. 531–539, ISSN 0309-2402

Coker, E., Papaioannou, A, Kaasalainen, S., Dolovich, L., Turpie, I. & Taniguchi, A. (2010). Nurses' perceived barriers to optimal pain management in older adults on acute medical units. *Applied Nursing Research,* Vol.23, No.3, pp. 139-146, ISSN 0897-1897

De Schepper, A.M.E., Francke, A.L. & Abu-Saad, H.H. (1997). Feelings of powerlessness in relation to pain: ascribed causes and reported strategies: A qualitative study among Dutch community nurses caring for cancer patients with pain. *Cancer Nursing,* Vol.20, No.6, pp. 422-429, ISSN 0162-220X

Ferrell, B.R., Eberts, M.T., McCaffery, M. & Grant, M. (1991). Clinical decisionmaking and pain. *Cancer Nursing,* Vol.14, No.6, pp. 289-297, ISSN 0162-220X

Ferrell, B.R., Taylor, E.J., Grant, M., Fowler, M. & Corbisiero, R.M. (1993). Pain management at home: Struggle, comfort, and mission. *Cancer Nursing,* Vol.16, No.3, pp. 169-178, ISSN 0162-220X

Gudmannsdottir, G.D. & Halldorsdottir, S. (2009). Primacy of existential pain and suffering in residents in chronic pain in nursing homes: A phenomenological study. *Scandinavian Journal of Caring Sciences,* Vol.20, No.3, pp. 317-327, ISSN 0283-9318

Howell, D., Butler, L., Vincent, L., Watt-Watson, J. & Stearns, N. (2000). Influencing nurses' knowledge, attitudes, and practice in cancer pain management. *Cancer Nursing,* Vol.23, No.1, pp. 55-63, ISSN 0162-220X

Jenks, J.M. (1993). The pattern of personal knowing in nurse clinical decision making. *Journal of Nursing Education,* Vol.32, No.9, pp. 399–405, ISSN 1938-2421

Johns, C. (1995). Framing learning through reflection within Carper's fundamental ways of knowing in nursing. *Journal of Advanced Nursing,* Vol.22, No.2, pp. 226-234, ISSN 0309-2402

Kagan, P. (2006). Review of Walker and Avant's newest theory development text. *Nursing Science Quarterly,* Vol.19, No.2, pp. 177–179, ISSN 0894-3184

Keenan, G.M., Cooke, R. & Hillis, S.L. (1998). Norms and nurse management of conflicts: Keys to understanding nurse-physician collaboration. *Research in Nursing and Health,* Vol.21, No.1, pp. 59-72, ISSN 1098-240X

Kramer, M. & Schmalenberg, C. (1993). Learning from success: autonomy and empowerment. *Nursing Management,* Vol.24, No.5, pp. 58-64, ISSN 0744-6314

Kuuppelomäki, M. (2002a). Pain management problems in patients' terminal phase as assessed by nurses in Finland. *Journal of Advanced Nursing,* Vol.40, No.6, pp. 701-709, ISSN 0309-2402

Kuuppelomäki, M. (2002b). The decision-making process when starting terminal care as assessed by nursing staff. *Nursing Ethics,* Vol.9, No.1, pp. 20-35, ISSN 0969-7330

Liaschenko, J. (1997). Knowing the patient? In Thorne S.E. & Hayes, V.E. (Eds.), *Nursing Praxis: Knowledge and Action*, pp. 23–38, Sage, ISBN 0761900101, London

Mallik, M. (1997). Advocacy in nursing - perceptions of practising nurses. *Journal of Clinical Nursing*, Vol.6, No.4, pp. 303-313, ISSN 0962-1067

Malloy, D.C., Hadjistavropoulos, T., McCarthy, E.F., Evans, R.J., Zakus, D.H., Park, I., Lee, Y. & Williams, J. (2009). Culture and organizational climate: Nurses' insights into their relationship with physicians. *Nursing Ethics*, Vol.16, No.6, pp. 719-33, ISSN 0969-7330

Manias, E. (2003). Pain and anxiety management in the postoperative gastro-surgical setting. *Journal of Advanced Nursing*, Vol.41, No.6, pp. 585-594, ISSN 0309-2402

McCaffery, M. & Ferrell, B.R. (1997). Nurses' knowledge of pain assessment and management: How much progress have we made? *Journal of Pain and Symptom Management*, Vol.14, No.3, pp. 175-188, ISSN 0885-3924

McCaffery, M. & Pasero, C. (1999). Assessment: Underlying complexities, misconceptions, and practical tools. In McCaffery, M. & Pasero, C. (Eds.), *Pain: clinical manual* (2nd ed.), pp. 35-102, Mosby, ISBN 081515609X, St. Louis

McCaffery, M., Ferrell, B., O'Neil-Page, E., Lester, M. & Ferrell, B. (1990). Nurses' knowledge of opioid analgesic drugs and psychological dependence. *Cancer Nursing*, Vol.13, No.1, pp. 21-27, ISSN 0162-220X

Munhall, P.L. (1993) 'Unknowing': toward another pattern of knowing in nursing. *Nursing Outlook*, Vol.41, No.3, pp. 125-128, ISSN 0029-6554

Nagy, S. (1999). Strategies used by burns nurses to cope with the infliction of pain on patients. *Journal of Advanced Nursing*, Vol.29, No.6, pp. 1427-1433, ISSN 0309-2402

Nash, R., Yates, P., Edwards, H., Fentiman, B., Dewar, A., McDowell, J. & Clark, R. (1999). Pain and the administration of analgesia: What nurses say. *Journal of Clinical Nursing*, Vol.8, No.2, pp. 180-189, ISSN 0962-1067

O'Rourke, K. (1992). Pain relief: The perspective of catholic tradition. *Journal of Pain and Symptom Management*, Vol.7, No.8, pp. 485-491, ISSN 0885-3924

Oberle, K. & Hughes, D. (2001) Doctors' and nurses' perceptions of ethical problems in end-of-life decisions. *Journal of Advanced Nursing*, Vol.33, No.6, pp. 707-715, ISSN 0309-2402

O'Connor, T. & Kelly, B. (2005). Bridging the gap: A study of general nurses' perceptions of patient advocacy in Ireland. *Nursing Ethics*, Vol.12, No.5, pp. 453-67, ISSN 0969-7330

Omery, A. (1989). Values, moral reasoning, and ethics. *Nursing Clinics of North America*, Vol.24, No.2, pp. 499-508, ISSN 0029-6465

Paice, J.A. & Cohen, F. L. (1997) Validity of a verbally administered numeric rating scale to measure cancer pain intensity. *Cancer Nursing*, Vol.20, No.2, pp. 88-93, ISSN 0162-220X

Pasero, C., Paice, J.A. & McCaffery, M. (1999). Basic mechanisms underlying the causes and effects of pain. In McCaffery, M. & Pasero, C. (Eds.), *Pain: Clinical manual* (2nd ed.), pp. 15-34, Mosby, ISBN 081515609X, St. Louis

Rejeh, N., Ahmadi, F., Mohamadi, E., Anoosheh, M. & Kazemnejad, A. (2009). Ethical challenges in pain management post-surgery. *Nursing Ethics*, Vol.16, No.2, pp. 161-72, ISSN 0969-7330

Schafheutle, E.I., Cantrill, J.A. & Noyce, P.R. (2001). Why is pain management suboptimal on surgical wards? *Journal of Advanced Nursing*, Vol.33, No.6, pp. 728-737, ISSN 0309-2402

Schmitz, N., Neumann, W. & Oppermann, R. (2000). Stress, burnout and loss of control in German nurses. *International Journal of Nursing Studies*, Vol.37, No.2, pp. 95-99, ISSN 0020-7489

Simoni, P.S. & Paterson, J.J. (1997). Hardiness, coping, and burnout in the nursing workplace. *Journal of Professional Nursing*, Vol.13, No.3, pp. 178-185, ISSN 8755-7223

Sjöström, B., Dahlgren, L.O. & Haljamäe, H. (2000). Strategies used in post-operative pain assessment and their clinical accuracy. *Journal of Clinical Nursing*, Vol.9, No.1, pp. 111-118, ISSN 0962-1067

Söderhamn, O. & Idvall, E. (2003). Nurses' influence on quality of care in postoperative pain management: A phenomenological study. *International Journal of Nursing Practice*, No.9, Vol.1, pp. 26-32, ISSN 1322-7114

Stein, L.I., Watts, D.T. & Howell, T. (1990). The doctor-nurse game revisited. *New England Journal of Medicine*, Vol.322, No.8, pp. 546-549, ISSN 0028-4793

Takman, C. & Severinsson, E.I. (1999). A description of health care professionals' experiences of encounters with patients in clinical settings. *Journal of Advanced Nursing*, Vol.30, No.6, pp. 1368-1374, ISSN 0309-2402

Taylor, E.J., Ferrell, B.R., Grant, M. & Cheyney, L. (1993). Managing cancer pain at home: The decisions and ethical conflicts of patients, family caregivers, and homecare nurses. *Oncology Nursing Forum*, Vol.20, No.6, pp. 919-927, ISSN 0190-535X

Twycross, A. (2002). Educating nurses about pain management: The way forward. *Journal of Clinical Nursing*, Vol.11, No.6, pp. 705-14, ISSN 0962-1067

Vaartio, H., Leino-Kilpi, H., Salanterä, S. & Suominen, T. (2006). Nursing advocacy: How is it defined by patients and nurses, what does it involve and how is it experienced? *Scandnavian Journal of Caring Sciences*, Vol.20, No.3, pp. 282-92, ISSN 0283-9318

Van Niekerk, L.M. & Martin, F. (2002). The impact of the nurse-physician professional relationship on nurses' experience of ethical dilemmas in effective pain management. *Journal of Professional Nursing*, Vol.18, No.5, pp. 276-288, ISSN 8755-7223

Walker, L.O. & Avant, K.C. (2004). *Strategies for theory construction in nursing* (4th ed.). Prentice Hall, ISBN 0838586880, Englewood Cliffs, NJ

Ware, L.J., Bruckenthal, P., Davis, G.C. & O'Conner-Von, S.K. (2011). Factors that influence patient advocacy by pain management nurses: Results of the American society for pain management nursing survey. *Pain Management Nurs*ing, (Epub 2010 Jul 24), Vol.12, No.1, 25-32., ISSN 1524-9042

Watt-Watson, J., Stevens, B., Garfinkel, P., Streiner, D. & Gallop, R, (2001). Relationship between nurses' pain knowledge and pain management outcomes for their postoperative cardiac patients. *Journal of Advanced Nursing*, Vol.36, No.4, pp. 535-545, ISSN 0309-2402

Willson, H. (2000). Factors affecting the administration of analgesia to patients following repair of a fractured hip. *Journal of Advanced Nursing*, Vol.31, No.5, pp. 1145-1154, ISSN 0309-2402

Wilson, B. (2007). Nurses' knowledge of pain. *Journal of Clinical Nursing*, Vol.16, No.6, pp. 1012–1020, ISSN 0962-1067

Wilson, B. (2009). Can patient lifestyle influence the management of pain? *Journal of Clinical Nursing*, Vol.18, No.3, pp. 399–408, ISSN 0962-1067

Part 8

Complex Regional Pain Syndrome and Reflex Sympathetic Dystrophy

26

Complex Regional Pain Syndrome

Gabor B. Racz[1] and Carl E. Noe[2]
[1]*Department of Anesthesiology, Pain Center, Texas Tech University Health Sciences Center,*
[2]*Department of Anesthesiology and Pain Management, Eugene McDermott Center for Pain Mangement, Univerisity of Texas Southwestern Medical Center, USA*

1. Introduction

Complex regional pain syndromes (CRPS) are pain syndromes characterized by pain out of proportion to an inciting injury, swelling, discoloration, stiffness, hyperhidrosis (sudomotor), temperature (vasomotor) and trophic changes. Also commonly seen are fine tremor and less often spasms involving upper and lower extremities. Dr. Silas Wier Mitchell described CRPS II, or causalgia, during the American Civil War. CRPS I was described about the end of the 19th century by Sudek (Sudek's atrophy). Evans described reflex sympathetic dystrophy (RSD). Numerous other terms used to describe similar syndromes include algodystrophy and shoulder- hand syndrome. Bonica described 3 stages of RSD. Roberts described sympathetically maintained pain.

2. Diagnostic criteria

Specific inclusion criteria are needed for research studies but from a clinical perspective, many patients seem to have a constellation of signs and symptoms of CRPS without meeting strict criteria. The diagnosis is made by the process of exclusion. While avoiding over diagnosing and over treatment, the patients need to be treated.

3. Prognosis

The prognosis for CRPS is highly variable and to a large extent is influenced by the treatment. Functional restoration and involving the patient in ongoing range of motion and resistive exercises is helpful. Timely pain relief and interventional pain procedures, as well as psychological support, are important. Patients need to be followed closely and treatments adjusted accordingly. Timely and appropriate referral to experienced pain physicians that are able to offer multimodal therapies may prevent costly delays and complications.

4. Theories of mechanisms

Multiple possible mechanisms exist for CRPS including psychological, inflammatory, vascular, neurogenic and combinations of several mechanisms. Debate regarding definitions of neuropathic pain has led to the notion that CRPS may not be neuropathic pain. Psychogenic pain could be construed as being "pain arising as a direct consequence of a lesion or disease affecting the somatosensory system" but few would think of it as neuropathic pain which should be treated with anticonvulsants.
CRPS II is generally agreed to be caused by an injury to a peripheral nerve. CRPS 1 is caused by a lesion in or injury to a small nerve or multiple small nerves. It is difficult to accept that it is not neuropathic pain since it resembles CRPS II so closely. Denial of care based on psychological explanations is neither reasonable nor justifiable yet in rare instances pain can be of psychological origin. Commonly the onset of CRPS is 1- 3 months after the injury.

5. History

The diagnosis is made by process of exclusion following history of pain that is out of proportion to an injury or period of immobilization. Swelling, temperature asymmetry, stiffness, atrophy, hair, skin nail, bone changes. Tremor or spasms and asymmetry in sweat function are all potential signs. It is important to remember that many injuries are associated with pain, discoloration and swelling without being CRPS. Infection and other causes of inflammation are sometimes mistakenly thought to be CRPS. A number of patients have CRPS symptoms following stroke and classifying this as central pain or CRPS is problematic.

6. Physical exam

Observation of upper extremity guarding or antalgic gait for lower extremity is important. Range of motion of affected joints is particularly important as many patients develop permanent stiffness without analgesia for specific range of motion therapy. Discoloration or asymmetrical coloration, swelling, atrophy and allodynia are other physical findings. The allodynia may be tactile or cold induced.

7. Diagnostic tests

Bone scans, sweat tests and sympathetic blocks have been used but the diagnosis is a clinical one and can be made without confirmatory tests. Thermography has been used, but more commonly, the documentation of temperature differences is adequate. Early on in the evolution of the condition there may increased temperature and later reduction with the increased sympathetic activity. Three phase bone scan often show corresponding changes.
Comparing contra lateral x-ray images can show osteopenia in the involved area. EMG usually does not change from the CRPS but may show nerve injury.

8. Differential diagnosis

While it important to be vigilant in diagnosing CRPS, as is important to avoid misdiagnosis and over- diagnosis. Many patients have "pain out of proportion", swelling and

discoloration after injuries and will improve within a month with usual therapeutic interventions.
Infection is always a concern after surgery or other penetrating trauma. Other causes of acute inflammation, swelling and discoloration need to be considered such as malignancy, deep venous thrombosis as well as peripheral nerve entrapment, peripheral neuropathy and other neuropathic pains.

9. Stages

3 stages of RSD have been described however it is unclear that staging has much value regarding decision making.

10. Timing

Much has been made about early sympathetic blocks and failure to diagnose early. There is no data to support "emergent" sympathetic blocks and some patients have a favorable natural history.

11. Spreading

Pain from CRPS can spread, in rare instances, proximally and contra- laterally. (Shah, Racz) Lower extremity pain can spread to upper extremities and vice versa.

12. Bone loss

Osteopenia and fractures can occur in severe cases and aquatic therapy is useful to rehabilitate these patients.

13. Natural history

The natural history of CRPS 1 is variable but in an interesting report, approximately 25% of patients that had Colles' fractures developed signs of CRPS. (Atkins) Approximately 40% of these patients improved in 6 months. This suggests that mild cases may not require extensive treatment. Not treating the patients early can be problematic if the condition worsens. Appropriate examination and follow up is important where the disease can take a benign course. Patients obtain information on the Internet that is usually about catastrophic cases that needs to be dealt with by educating patients in an appropriate and caring manner where therapy is timely yet one can avoid catastrophizing based on inaccurate information.

14. Dogma

Much of "standard care" is not evidence based, but good outcome based. Additionally, it is based on physician experience and the outcome is superior in the hands of better-trained physicians. As new information becomes available, dogma can be weeded out and treatments based on randomized controlled trails can be incorporated into treatment guidelines.

15. Cases

One lady had not worn high-heeled shoes for a long time and then wore a pair for several hours at an event. She developed classic signs and symptoms of RSD. She experienced profound analgesia with sympathetic blockade and the condition resolved completely.

Another case was a woman who had a paper cut on her distal index finger on the job. She had classic signs and symptoms of CRPS, which resolved with a series of blocks. Both of these cases were challenged by insurance companies since the inciting injury was so minor but both patients were legitimate. The point is that physicians caring for these patients must be willing to serve as advocates for the patient even in an environment of cost containment. We have to be mindful of our "report cards" but not at the expense of a patient's outcome.

16. Overmedication pain syndrome (OPS)

Approximately 20 years ago, a movement began to improve the quality of pain care for cancer patients worldwide. The WHO analgesic ladder was promoted for cancer pain and then it was applied for other types of pain. Many patients are now taking large doses of opioid for chronic pain.

Overmedication pain syndrome is characterized by a chronic treatment program consisting of high doses of multiple analgesic medications without associated functional productivity and psychological coping ability.

Opioids are the most important class of drugs in pain management; however, it is clear that they are two edged swords and overmedication with opioids and other drugs classes have become a problem. Abuse may not be the largest problem. Lack of efficacy, unintended overdose, diversion, development of drug dependence, habituation and resistance to recovery and other unintended consequences may be more common.

Opioid induced hyperalgesia is a real clinical phenomenon and may be a subtle barrier to analgesia in many patients. Pain that is only incrementally responsive to opioid is also common.

Pseudo-addiction is defined in behavioral terms which are similar to addiction but related to pain and not addiction. The problem is that there are not good means to differentiate behaviors between the setting of pain and the setting of addiction.

Some have reported a lack of data to support doses of opioid over 200 mg/day of morphine equivalents. Also, there are no long term randomized controlled trials of opioid versus placebo. Additionally, fracture rates have been reported to be increased in patients on doses above 100 mg/day. (Sullivan) Overdose rates have been reported to increase above 50 mg/day. (Dunn) Drug interactions with other medications, reported and unreported to the treating physician, have been causes of fatalities.

Urine drug testing, opioid contracts and extensive documentation guidelines fail to help answer the clinical question: is the dose just too high?

Patients who are taking opioids chronically should be considered for an evaluation for a lack of meaningful efficacy, fall and fracture risk and overdose risk. An interdisciplinary evaluation may be a way to accomplish these objectives. Patients who are clearly doing well may be less likely to accept dose reductions. Patients who are working or similarly productive and are without signs of poor coping and physical disability may need to continue taking the effective dosages. On the other hand, patients, who have been on stable doses for a long time may need age related dose reductions.

Washington State has new guidelines limiting the dose of opioid to 120 mg/day of morphine equivalents. Patients, who require doses above this level, are guided to seek a pain management consultation. The purpose and intervention of a medical pain management consultation is unclear. The practitioner doing the evaluation needs to have additional training and qualification as well as be informed and knowledgeable in treatment options in addition to opioid management.

JCAHO, Press Gainey and other organizations have changed the environment with respect to patient rights regarding pain. In the past, if a patient wasn't happy with their opioid dose, their recourse was limited. Now, patient satisfaction is used as a factor to determine healthcare provider's compensation. The implication is that patients can pressure providers to prescribe more opioid, which is dangerous for patients and providers.

Regulators have become more active due to the increased rate of diversion and its consequences. However, the accidental overdose rate increase is even more concerning.

Most drugs have dose limits. For example, antibiotics and drugs for hypertension are increased to upper limits but there are limits. Perhaps it is time to limit doses of opioids regardless of pain severity for patients with non palliative care pain syndromes and find another way to treat the patient.

Other drugs classes that are problematic include benzodiazepines, muscle relaxers, sleeping pills and even anticonvulsants and antidepressants. Benzodiazepines are not prominent in the pain literature as analgesics. Baclofen and tizanidine are probably the first line muscle relaxers of choice. Hypnotic drugs are used too often for chronic sleep disturbances without sleep hygiene treatment or other medications which are better for long term use. Anticonvulsant use for chronic pain has exploded as opioids have. Antidepressants, even those not associated with analgesia, are prescribed for pain.

The costs of these drugs are significant and usually of incremental benefit. Most patients with chronic pain go without an interdisciplinary evaluation and many who receive an evaluation do not complete treatment with cognitive behavioral therapy, education and conditioning physical therapy. Treatment goals are frequently not established and some patients just go through the motions and are considered as a treatment failure. There is very little evidence for the multidisciplinary and physical therapy based treatments specifically for CRPS. Reimbursement has suffered for these kinds of therapies.

The cognitive effects and psychological effects of chronic opioid treatment are not well known.

Testosterone levels in males are known to decrease with chronic opioid administration.

It is proposed that patients with chronic pain have a short term trial of low dose opioid to access functional improvement before a treatment plan is finalized. Blinding patients to their drug and dose may be very helpful but has its critics on ethical and regulatory grounds.

Patients who are on doses above 50 mg/ day of morphine equivalents need to have access to interdisciplinary pain and addictionology evaluations and treatment if needed. Treatment goals should include dose reduction to below 200mg/day of morphine equivalents for those taking more than that. Intermediate term treatment goals for patients taking less than 200 mg/day should strive for less than 100 mg/day and patients taking less than 100 mg/day, 50 mg/day.

There is no data to support this approach but there was no data 20 years ago to support using the WHO analgesic ladder for headaches, fibromyalgia, back pain or any other condition. Data for limited doses of opioid for arthritis and neuropathic pain exists and prescribing for opioid responsive pain should not be overly scrutinized by regulators. Never the less, diversion, addiction, opioid induced hyperalgesia and other adverse events associated with opioids need to be avoided more effectively before the first prescription is written.

Many patients in drug treatment programs were initially treated with opioid for perfectly legitimate pain. The patient and the doctor may not be the biggest problems. The biggest problem may be the drug and the dosage.

17. Treatment guideline history

In 1994, the International Association for the Study of Pain (IASP) revised the terminology from RSD and causalgia to CRPS type I and II. 15 years ago we proposed an analgesic ladder for CRPS /RSD which included 3 steps. (Racz) Since then, well-respected groups have advanced other guidelines. (Van Eijs) (Stanton-Hicks)

Our initial proposal was:

Step 1. TENS, opioids, topicals, Tricyclic antidepressants, supportive psychotherapy, vocational rehabilitation, patient education, physical therapy and occupational therapy

Step 2. Regional or sympathetic block, evaluation and treatment of the emotional component of pain, IV regional block, peripheral block-infusion, carbamazepine, baclofen, clonidine, corticosteroid, NSAID, mexiletine, other drug trials

Step 3. Sympathectomy/sympatholysis, peripheral nerve decompression, lysis, continuous local anesthetic infusion epidural and or regional for five to seven days, Spinal Cord Stimulation (SCS), Peripheral Nerve Stimulation (PNS), intrathecal/epidural analgesia.

At that time, little data existed to guide treatment and the initial analgesic ladder was based on opinion. Since that time, additional data has been produced leading to modifications to the analgesic ladder. This is categorically not intended to estabish a standard of care since data to do such is inadequate. Rather, our intention is to share our beliefs in hopes of helping patients with this disorder.

18. New principles and information

Our current analgesic ladder promotes several concepts:

1. Interdisciplinary pain treatment is recommended rather than multidisciplinary care which tends to be fragmented. Interdisciplinary treatment specifically provides coordinated medical care, education, cognitive behavioral therapy for pain, physical therapy and outcome documentation by the interdisciplinary team. Patients who receive care at different clinics for each component of care by a group of providers who do not meet on a weekly basis nor document comprehensive outcomes are not receiving interdisciplinary pain management.

2. Interdisciplinary care is not isolated from medical pain management. Analgesic treatments are necessary to provide pain relief and allow functional restoration.
3. The course of an individual patient is highly variable and adjustments to the treatment plan should be made in a highly flexible manner.
4. Limiting opioid doses to below 200mg/day morphine equivalents
5. Numerous randomized controlled trials have been performed since our initial analgesic ladder was proposed and these findings are incorporated.
6. However if there is treatment failure and functional restoration failure the patient needs to be referred to centers or individuals with recognized experience to be specialists in the field.

Sympathetic blocks have been recommended early on in the management of the disorder but little data exists to support this practice. Only recently has any data from a randomized controlled trial been published to demonstrate efficacy of sympathetic blockade. (Meier)
Spinal cord stimulation has been shown to produce significant analgesia even after 5 years of treatment. (Klemer) Cortical stimulation has been shown to have some benefit. (Velasco)
Deep brain stimulation has been shown to be ineffective. Vitamin C has been studied by multiple investigators for the prevention of CRPS and has some effect. (Besse) Intravenous magnesium has been reported to be effective in an initial study. (Collins) Clodronate has been shown to be partially effective. (Varenna) Mirror therapy has been reported to have benefit in stroke patients with CRPS. (Cacchio) Multicenter comparison of spinal cord stimualtion and peripheral nerve stimulation showed that PNS is more effective than SCS but the best outcome was where both modalities were utilized. (Calvillo)
Intravenous regional anesthesia with the addtion of vasodilators such as phentolamine, reserpine and bretylium allow manipulation of hands without post procedure edema and speed up functional restoration without the pain associated with physical therapy. (Heavner, Calvillo, Racz)
An evidenced based review endorses bisphosphonates (alendronate, pamidronate, clodronate), corticosteroid, gabapentin, physiotherapy and psychotherapy/relaxation techniques as treatments. (Baron) Additionally intrathecal baclofen for associated dystonia and spinal cord stimulation for refractory caes are recommended. Topical DMSO and sympathetic blocks are not strongly recommended. Intravenous regional blocks with guanethidine are not recommended as specific treatment (Van Eijs)

19. Treatments to avoid

Amputation is less common nowadays because it was rarely effective and usually resulted in a phantom pain plus different pain of greater severity
IV regional with guanethidine has been shown to be ineffective in several studies as sole agent.
Deep brain stimulation has been shown to be ineffective.
High dose opioid should be avoided if possible due to possible opioid induced hyperalgesia, addiction, diversion risk and over-dosage.

20. Proposed treatment

Step 1.
Screening for substance abuse, affective disorders and disability
Education

Physical therapy
Occupational therapy
Vocational rehabilitation
Topical lidocaine for allodynia
Tricyclic antidepressants
Gabapentin
Tramadol
Opioid doses limited to less than 200mg morphine equivalents per day and below 50mg/day if possible
Corticosteroid

Step 2.

Interdisciplinary pain evaluation including psychological testing (MMPI-RF) and treatment (cognitive behavioral therapy, group psycho educational therapy and psychotropic medication management, addictionology, physical and occupational therapy, in a coordinated goal directed, outcome documenting rehabilitation program)
Sympathetic block
IV Regional block
Peripheral block
Other drug trials

Step 3.

Spinal cord stimulation
Sympathectomy/sympatholysis
Peripheral nerve stimulation
Peripheral nerve decompression/lysis
Intrathecal/epidural analgesia

21. Interdisciplinary care

Interdisciplinary pain management is a term that is poorly understood. It is best reserved to describe a team of healthcare professionals led by a physician and including a psychologist and physical therapist at a minimum. A care team of multiple physicians from different specialties is not an interdisciplinary team for pain management nor is a psychologically based treatment program in isolation from medical pain management. Cognitive behavioral therapy, education and functional rehabilitation must be provided in an interdisciplinary pain care model in addition to medical pain management therapies. Case management, psychiatry, outcome database management, nursing, vocational rehabilitation, occupational therapy, medical direction and program direction and administrative support are key disciplines to include in a mature pain program. Nutrition, chaplaincy and other medical specialties are needed for tertiary programs.

22. Conclusion

Complex regional pain syndrome is a challenging pain problem that frequently requires a comprehensive interdisciplinary assessment and treatment plan. Until a mechanism is discovered and a specific treatment for the syndrome is developed, an interdisciplinary approach, including pharmacologic and interventional pain management in a step wise fashion, will likely remain as the best route to follow.

23. References

Atkins, R.M., Duckworth, T., Kanis, J.A.: Algodystrophy following Colles' Fracture.Journal of Hand Surgery (British Volume, 1989) 14B: 161-164

Baron, R., Naleschinski, D., Hullemann, P., Mahn, F.: Complex Regional Pain Syndrome: A neuropathic disorder? Pain 2010- An updated Review: Refresher Course Syllabus. IASP Press p. 109-117. 2010

Besse, J., Gadeyene, S., Galand-Desme, S., et.al: Effect of vitamin C on prevention of complex regional pain syndrome in foot and ankle surgery. Foot and Ankle Surgery 15:179-182, 2009

Cacchio, A., De Blasis, E., De Blasis, V., at.al.:Mirror Therapy in Complex Regional Pain Syndrome Type 1 of the Upper Limb in Stroke Patients. Neurorehabilitation and Neural Repair 23: 792-799, 2009.

Calvillo O, Racz GBN, Diede J, Smith K: Neuroaugmentation in the treatment of complex regional pain syndrome of the upper extremity. Acta Orthopaedica Belgica, 64-1, 57-63, 1998.

Collins, S., Zuurmond, W.W.A., de Lange, J.J., et.al.: Intravenous Magnesium for Complex Regional Pain Syndrome Type 1 (CRPS 1) Patients: A Pilot Study. Pain Medicine 10:930-940, 2009.

Dunn KM, Saunders KW, Rutter CM, et al.: Opioid prescriptions for chronic pain and overdose: a cohort study. Annals of Internal Medicine 2010; 152:85-92

Heavner JE, Calvillo O, Racz GB: Thermal grill illusion and complex regional pain syndrome Type I Reflex Sympathetic Dystrophy. Regional Anesthesia 22(3): 257-259, 1997.

Klemer M.A., de Vet, H.C., Barendse, G.A.M., et.al.: Effect of spinal cord stimulation for chronic complex regional pain syndrome Type I: five-year follow-up of patients in a randomized controlled trial. Jounal of Neurosurgery 108:292-298, 2008.

Meier, P.M., Zurakowski, D., Berde, C. B., Sethna, M.B.: Lumbar sympathetic blockade in Children with Complex Regional Pain Syndromes. Anesthesiology 2009, 111: 372-80.

Racz, Gabor B., Heavner, James E., Noe, Carl E.: Definitions, classification and Taxonomy: an overview Sympathetic pain syndromes: reflex sympathetic dystrophy and causalgia. Physical Medicine and Rehabilitation: State of the Art Reviews Vol 10 No 2 June 1996 Hanley and Belfus, Philadelphia

Shah RV, Racz GB. Recurrence and spread of complex regional pain syndrome due to distant site surgery: a case report. Am J Orthop (Belle Mead NJ). 2006 Nov; 35(11): 523-6.

Stanton-Hicks, M., Baron, R., Boas, R., et.al: Complex regional pain syndromes: guidelines for therapy. Clinical Journal of Pain 14:155-166, 1998.

Sullivan, M.D.: Who gets high dose opioid therapy for chronic non-cancer pain? Pain 151:567-568, 2010.

Van Eijs, F., Stanton -Hicks, M., Van Zundert, J., et. al.: Complex Regional Pain Syndrome. Pain practice 11:70-87, 2010.

Varenna, M., Zucchi, F., Ghiringhelli, D., et.al.: Intravenous clodronate in the treatment of reflex symathetic dystrophy syndrome. Journal of Rheumatology 27:1477-83, 2000

Velasco, F., Carrillo-Ruiz, J.D., Castro, G., et.al.: Motor cortex stimulation applied to patients with complex regional pain syndrome. Pain 147:91-98, 2009.